Impacts of the Covid-19 Pandemic

International Laws, Policies, and Civil Liberties

Edited By

Nadav Morag
Department of Security Studies
Sam Houston State University
Texas, USA

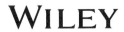

Registered Office
John Wiley & Sons, Inc., 111 River Street, Hoboken, NJ 07030, USA

Editorial Office
111 River Street, Hoboken, NJ 07030, USA

For details of our global editorial offices, customer services, and more information about Wiley products visit us at www.wiley.com.

Wiley also publishes its books in a variety of electronic formats and by print-on-demand. Some content that appears in standard print versions of this book may not be available in other formats.

Library of Congress Cataloging-in-Publication Data Applied for:
Hardback ISBN: 9781119812159

Cover image: © Yuichiro Chino/Getty Images
Cover design: Wiley

Set in 9.5/12.5pt STIXTwoText by Straive, Chennai, India

Contents

Notes on Contributors

Donald Abenheim is Professor Emeritus, Naval Postgraduate School.

Georges C. Benjamin is the Executive Director of the American Public Health Association.

Wendy E. Braund is the Covid-19 Response Director at the Pennsylvania Department of Health.

Iain Cameron is a Professor in public international law at Uppsala University. He is the author of numerous books and articles in the field of international and constitutional law.

Lisa Carayon is a Lecturer in law at the University of Paris, North. She is the Principal Investigator of "Localex" project on local and regional normative dynamics in France in the Covid-19 pandemic.

Andres de Castro is a Subject Coordinator at the National Distance Education University (UNED), Spain.

Jacinta I-Pei Chen is a Senior Manager at the Saw Swee Hock School of Public Health, National University of Singapore and National University Health System, Singapore.

Christelle Chidiac is a Research Collaborator at the School of Advanced Social Sciences and a PhD candidate in Public Law at the University of Paris Nanterre. She is a member of the "Localex" project on local and regional normative dynamics in France in the Covid-19 pandemic.

Ronan Cormacain is a Senior Research Fellow at the Bingham Centre for the Rule of Law, British Institute of International and Comparative Law, and an editor of Theory and Practice of Legislation. He is also a consultant legislative counsel and has drafted a number of pieces of coronavirus legislation.

Anna Jonsson Cornell is a Professor of comparative constitutional law and Vice Dean of the Faculty of Law at Uppsala University. She is also the Secretary General of the International Association of Constitutional Law.

François Delerue is an Assistant Professor of Law at IE University, Madrid, Spain. He is a member of the "Army" project on the role of the armies in the "war" against the coronavirus and its perception by the population.

Elena Demichelis is a lawyer practicing in Turin.

Duncan Fairgrieve is Senior Research Fellow in Comparative Law and Director of the Product Liability Forum at the British Institute of International and Comparative Law. He is also Professor of Comparative Law at Université de Paris Dauphine in France.

Alan Greene is a Reader in Constitutional Law and Human Rights and Deputy Head of Research at the Birmingham Law School, University of Birmingham.

Carolyn Halladay is a Senior Lecturer in the Department of National Security Affairs at the Naval Postgraduate School.

Jeremy Lim is an Associate Professor and Director of the Leadership Institute for Global Health Transformation (LIGHT) at the Saw Swee Hock School of Public Health, National University of Singapore and National University Health System, Singapore. He is also Vice-Chairman of Health-Serve, a Singapore-based migrant worker health charity.

Cheryl Lin is Co-director of the Policy and Organizational Management Program at Duke University.

Anna Malandrino is a Research Fellow in the Department of Political and Social Sciences at the University of Bologna and in the KPM Center for Public Management at the University of Bern.

Florina C. Matei is a Lecturer at the Center for Homeland Defense and Security, Naval Postgraduate School.

Jewel Mullen is Associate Professor in the Department of Population Health and Associate Dean for Health Equity at the Dell Medical School, University of Texas at Austin.

Nguyen Q. Duong is an official at the Vietnamese Ministry of Foreign Affairs.

Nguyen T. Trung is a Research Fellow at the Max Planck Institute Luxembourg for International, European and Regulatory Procedural Law.

Florian Opillard is a Researcher at the IRSEM (Institute for Strategic Research of the Military School), French Ministry of Defense. He is a scientific coordinator of the "Army" project on the role of the armies in the "war" against the coronavirus and its perception by the population.

Angelique Palle is a Researcher at the IRSEM (Institute for Strategic Research of the Military School), French Ministry of Defense. She is a scientific coordinator of the "Localex" project on local and regional normative dynamics in France in the Covid-19 pandemic and the "Army" project on the role of the armies in the "war" against the coronavirus and its perception by the population.

Margherita Paola Poto is an Associate Professor in Administrative Law at the University of Turin and Research Professor at the Faculty of Law, UiT The Arctic University of Norway.

Peak Sen Chua is an Independent Consultant based in Kuala Lumpur, Malaysia, and has worked with the US National Academy of Medicine, Collaborative Consulting, and the Saw Swee School of Public Health, National University of Singapore and National University Health System, Singapore.

Iffath U. Syed is an Assistant Professor in Health Policy and Administration at The Pennsylvania State University, Shenango.

Sharon H.X. Tan is a Research Fellow at the Saw Swee Hock School of Public Health, National University of Singapore and National University Health System, Singapore.

Yuichiro Tsuji is a Professor in the Department of Law at Meiji University.

Pikuei Tu is Director of the Policy and Organizational Management Program at Duke University.

Felix Uhlmann holds a Chair for Constitutional and Administrative Law as well as Legislative Studies at the University of Zurich. He is also Co-Director of the Centre for Legislative Studies.

Adriaan J. Wierenga is a senior researcher at the Centre for Public Order, Anti-social Behavior and Security from the Faculty of Law, University of Groningen.

Jorrit Westerhof is a Student Assistant at the University of Groningen.

Jason Chin-Huat Yap is an Associate Professor and Vice Dean (Practice) of the Saw Swee Hock School of Public Health, National University of Singapore and National University Health System, Singapore.

Foreword

Impacts of the Covid-19 Pandemic: International Laws, Policies, and Civil Liberties

Nadav Morag

Department of Security Studies, Sam Houston State University, Texas, USA

At the time of this writing, December 2021, the global pandemic caused by a novel coronavirus – the SARS-CoV-2 virus (commonly known as Covid-19) – first identified in Wuhan, China, in December 2019, has claimed an estimated 5.3 million lives. This is an official estimate, though the exact number is unknowable and almost certainly significantly larger. For example, one estimate of the overall global death toll puts the number of lives lost at 21.2 million.[1] No one knows how much the death toll will increase as this will depend on a wide variety of factors including the nature of new variants of the virus, the number of persons receiving vaccinations, the efficacy (over time) of these vaccinations, and a host of other variables.

The desire to reduce transmission of the virus and otherwise protect their respective populations has led countries across the globe to devise a wide range of laws and policies in response to the current pandemic. As with other forms of security, achieving higher levels of health security requires considering trade-offs between maximizing security and minimizing the negative impact that higher levels of security mean for the exercise of civil liberties and personal freedoms. In the context of pandemic response, there are two features that stand out in particular in terms of presenting a challenge to national, regional, and local governments in trying to maintain a balance between the provision of health security on the one hand and the maintenance of civil liberties on the other: contact tracing and quarantine. Contact tracing, particularly in the earlier phases of the current pandemic, was used to slow the spread of the virus through trying to determine who may have been exposed to individuals who tested positive for the virus, regardless of whether they were exhibiting symptoms of Covid-19. Given what was eventually found to be a high transmissibility rate of this coronavirus (roughly equivalent to that of the SARS virus and the 1918 Influenza virus), contact tracing, if properly implemented, was deemed to help slow the spread of the disease and thus buy time for the development of vaccines and better treatments, as well as to avoid overwhelming healthcare facilities. Over time, as community spread has dramatically increased in many Western countries, contact tracing has arguably become less critical and has been replaced with, in some Western countries, vaccination requirements, particularly as vaccines have become much more readily available and proven to be efficacious in reducing transmissibility and in reducing severe manifestations of disease. However, in many countries in east Asia, where minimizing community spread and "zero Covid" policies are in place, contract tracing is still a high priority despite increasing vaccination rates. Not surprisingly, when governments can trace who an individual has come in contact with, when, and where they have been, this raises a host of questions

---

1 "The Pandemic's True Death Toll," *The Economist*, December 15, 2021, available at: https://www.economist.com/graphic-detail/coronavirus-excess-deaths-estimates (accessed, December 15, 2021).

about implications for privacy rights. Quarantines represent another potential violation of civil liberties – in this case, freedom of movement. Quarantines are a long-standing public health measure stretching back centuries and can be efficacious in reducing spread, though they can also result in a range of psychological and economic challenges. At the same time, all democracies require some sort of legal due process before impinging on individuals' right to freedom of movement and forced quarantine on a large scale does not involve such a process. As with privacy rights, the right to freedom of movement during a pandemic will necessarily be balanced against health security.

The attempt to achieve maximal levels of public safety while, at the same time, avoiding negative impacts on economic activity and individual freedoms should be familiar to students of Homeland Security (or as it is often termed in Europe, Civil Security). This is one of the core dilemmas in legislating and policymaking in this area as, in many cases, this is a zero sum game. Maximum security, whether it pertains to limiting the threat of terrorism, large-scale criminal activity, public health threats, or even the regulation of activity in the immediate wake of a natural disaster, necessarily means less freedom of movement, privacy, and/or other basic rights. On the other hand, maximum levels of individual freedom and civil liberties protections can be taken advantage of by negative actors (terrorists, criminal enterprises, hostile nation-states, etc.) as well as by viruses and bacteria, to generate threats to public safety. No one can say definitively where the balance must lie between public safety and individual freedoms as this is largely a subjective matter (both for the individual and for the society and state) and will necessarily vary in time as a function of both the perception of the nature of the threat facing a given population during a given time period and the culture and history of the society in question. Some societies are more willing to subordinate specific civil liberties in favor of enhancing security than are others. In some cases, this parallels cultural and social tendencies toward collectivism as opposed to individualism (with the latter often less willing to subordinate civil liberties to public safety needs). The willingness to accept restrictions on individual freedoms in the name of public safety also often correlates with the level of trust in government. Those countries whose citizens generally exhibit a higher trust in government are often more willing to accept restrictions, even voluntary ones, than those countries where the population is more distrustful of government.

This volume will focus on a broad swath of countries in the context of laws, policies, and institutions that play a role in coping with the challenge posed by Covid-19, as well as the significance these laws and policies have with respect to the maintenance of individual civil liberties. Every country surveyed in this book has taken a slightly different approach, and in some cases a radically different approach, to trying to minimize the impact of Covid on society, the economy, and the health of their respective population. They have all done so through their own attempts to balance civil liberties with health security and each thus provides a distinct model for legislation, governance, and public health measures for the Covid-19 era and beyond.

This book represents the collaborative efforts of a number of international scholars specializing in areas including: law, governance, and public health, and surveys the laws, policies, and governance frameworks in 16 countries: Sweden, the United Kingdom, Germany, Italy, Switzerland, Canada, Singapore, Romania, Vietnam, Taiwan, the Netherlands, Ireland, Japan, France, Spain, and Austria. In order to facilitate an assessment of the various national approaches and frameworks, these countries have been grouped into four categories based on a range of commonalities in policies, governance structures, and/or laws within each group (though, in general, the differences between countries in each group are greater than their similarities). The initial chapters of the book will focus on a group of country analyses that focus on the *rule of law and the provision of civil liberties* in the context of: The Netherlands, Ireland, Switzerland, Germany, and the United Kingdom. The next set of chapters will focus on countries that *have made extensive use of emergency laws and have generally followed a securitized approach* (through the use of security agencies) to dealing with the Covid pandemic: Italy, Spain, Romania, and France. The third group of countries can be characterized by *focusing heavily on gathering information about their respective population and on controlling their movements*: Taiwan, Vietnam, and Singapore. Finally, the fourth group of countries can be characterized by taking an approach based on *fostering popular trust in government, emphasizing social welfare, and limiting sanctions and restrictions*: Sweden, Japan, Germany, Canada, and Austria.

In Chapter 1, Adriaan Wierenga and Jorrit Westerhof examine the pandemic response in the Netherlands through the lens of laws promulgated to maintain the constitutional balance and fundamental rights and reduce reliance on problematic emergency laws. In Chapter 2, Alan Greene assesses the constitutional checks and balances that, in some cases, facilitated the government's pandemic response measures and, in other cases, hindered them – with a view toward evaluating the rule of law implications of these measures. In Chapter 3, Felix Uhlmann looks at Switzerland's policies, particularly the restrictions imposed on the population, in the context of the country's laws as well as the balance between its federal institutions. In Chapter 4, Carolyn Halladay examines Germany's constitutional order and the country's decision to respond to the pandemic via the existing constitutional order without recourse to emergency powers. In Chapter 5, Ronan Cormacain and Duncan Fairgrieve explore the United Kingdom's coronavirus response and the fact that, despite a rapid and constantly changing response, the approaches taken have been based firmly within the existing legal order. In Chapter 6, Anna Malandrino, Margherita Poto, and Elena Demichelis address Italy's efforts to address the pandemic in the context of the use of emergency legislation and its implications for constitutional rule and civil liberties. In Chapter 7, Carolyn Halladay, Andres de Castro, and Florina Cristiana Matei focus on Spain's use of emergency legislation (state-of-alarm declarations) that involved, among other things, a sharp move toward centralization in what is normally a decentralized country with significant local autonomy. In Chapter 8, Florina Cristiana Matei looks at Covid-19 measures in Romania and, in particular, the implications of the use of emergency declarations such as the "State of Siege" and "State of Emergency" and what this has meant for fundamental rights. In Chapter 9, Angelique Palle, Lisa Carayon, Florian Opillard, François Delerue, and Christelle Chidiac analyze the use of securitized approaches in France including, in particular, the use of the armed forces. In Chapter 10, Cheryl Lin, Pikeui Tu, Wendy Braund, Jewel Mullen, and Georges Benjamin consider Taiwan's extensive use of contact tracing, quarantine, and other restrictions in the country's efforts to control its rate of infection. In Chapter 11, Than Nguyen and Quynh Nguyen describe Vietnam's success in dealing with the pandemic via strong contract tracing, quarantine, and social distancing measures. In Chapter 12, Jacinta Chen, Sharon Tan, Peak Chua, Jeremy Lim, and Jason Yap explore Singapore's efforts to control infections through social distancing and public shaming of those involved in noncompliance as well as the use of technology to enhance contact tracing efforts and enforce quarantines. In Chapter 13, Ian Cameron and Anna Cornell assess Sweden's unique approach to dealing with the pandemic, which relied on the use of ordinary laws and the fostering of trust. In Chapter 14, Yuichiro Tsuji addresses Japan's model for coping with the pandemic, which, absent legislation with strong sanctions, relied to a great extent on public trust and cooperation. In Chapter 15, Iffath Syed examines Canada's approach to the pandemic, which has been focused on maintaining a balance between federal and provincial governments and a significant focus on social welfare, including addressing the economic effects on individuals of measures designed to reduce transmission. In Chapter 16, Donald Abenheim and Carolyn Halladay explore the Austrian Covid response, which was characterized by a focus on the social dimensions of governance (specifically that the state and society act to advance social welfare) while also trying to cope with the nexus between vaccine hesitancy and extreme right-wing politics.

It should be noted that this book does not deal with the United States and its approach (or, rather, the varying approaches of its 50 states, as it is they who have authority over the lion's share of public health measures), as one of the objectives of this volume is to demonstrate to an American audience the wide range of options for improving pandemic measures in the United States based on examples from other countries. At the same time, the book should be useful to audiences outside the United States for similar reasons.

Preface

One of my main areas of research focuses on international homeland security law, institutions, and policy. If one can conclude anything about efforts around the world to improve homeland security – which I define as the ability to prevent, prepare for, respond to, and recover from events that can potentially significantly undermine the ability of government, the economy, and society to function – it is that each country is trying to find its own path, in some cases learning from the successes and failures of other countries. Each country's path will be unique because each country's history, laws, institutions, culture, threat environment, etc., is unique. Despite improvements, no country has found the "answer" – assuming there is one – to achieving optimal homeland (or as it is referred to in some countries "civil") security. At the same time, new and often unforeseen challenges (or, what is rather more common, challenges that were foreseen by some, but not taken seriously enough by those in charge of policy and budgets) demonstrate yet again that whatever progress may have been achieved in some areas of homeland security law and policy, there is still much to do.

Nothing illustrates this point better than the global scramble to cope with the Covid-19 pandemic. In putting together this edited volume, I was motivated by the desire to catalog and understand some of the ways in which various national governments attempted to cope with the pandemic and how they modified their laws and policies over time in response to it. I was also particularly interested in understanding how the various national approaches impacted their citizens in a wide range of areas, not least the impact of contact tracing on privacy rights and the impact of quarantine and isolation on the right to freedom of movement. Hopefully, this book will provide the reader with useful insight into laws, policies, and institutions that proved effective, and those that did not, and expand the reader's understanding of the wide range of approaches that were taken to cope with this very grave homeland security challenge – one that has resulted in major loss of life globally and significant disruption to economies and societies worldwide.

I would like to thank the distinguished international scholars who produced the 16 topical chapters that comprise this book. Their expertise and insight lie at the core of this book and are what will, hopefully, make it a useful source of information and analysis for readers.

Section 1

Countries with a Focus on the Rule of Law and Legal Protections of Civil Liberties

1

The Netherlands: Dutch COVID-19 Policy Viewed from a Fundamental Rights Perspective

Adriaan J. Wierenga and Jorrit Westerhof[#]

Centre for Public Order and Safety, University of Groningen, The Netherlands

1.1   Introduction

In the early months of the COVID-19 outbreak in China late 2019, many Dutch people thought of it as something that was only happening somewhere far away. This sentiment changed after a large number of cases of infection were observed in Italy and Spain. A growing fear arose that the Netherlands would be hit by COVID-19 as well. That fear materialized on 27 February 2020. While appearing on a talk show, the Minister of *Medische Zorg en Sport* (Medical Care and Sport) received a note informing them that the first COVID-19 case had been observed in the Netherlands (Keulemans 2020).[1] Although the national government initially reacted by providing urgent hygiene advice, the first legally enforceable COVID-19 measures were announced on 13 March 2020, a month after the first COVID-19 infection was observed.

The Dutch government has tried to control the pandemic through various legal routes. In the first period of the crisis – March to December 2020 – only limited use was made of existing infectious disease control legislation because it proved to be insufficient to combat the pandemic. Therefore, it was subsequently significantly bolstered by municipal emergency law.[2]

The prolonged nationwide use of municipal emergency powers in addition to existing national legislation led to several constitutional bottlenecks. That is why in December 2020, the *Tijdelijke wet maatregelen COVID-19* (Interim COVID-19 Measures Act, Twm COVID-19) 2020 was implemented in order to provide for a constitutionally sound legal basis for COVID-19 measures that were over time increasingly unlawfully imposed through municipal emergency decrees in the absence of sufficient powers based in national laws. Later, additional measures were deemed necessary. Some of

---

[#] Adriaan Wierenga is a researcher at the University of Groningen's Centre for Public Order and Safety. He is one of the Netherlands's most renowned experts in crisis, emergency and disaster law. Wierenga consults, among others, the Police Academy of the Netherlands, the Dutch Safety Board, the House of Representatives of the Netherlands, the Council of State, the Ministry of Justice and Security and the Dutch Association of Mayors. Earlier, he published an overview article on the topic of this chapter in the Dutch legal journal Ars Aequi (Wierenga 2021). Jorrit Westerhof is his research assistant.

[1] During the first period of the COVID-19 crisis, the Minister of Medical Care and Sport, a minister falling under the Ministry of *Volksgezondheid, Welzijn en Sport* (Health, Welfare, and Sport, HWS), carried out the Minister of HWS's tasks on infectious disease control. Later, these tasks were performed by the Minister of HWS. Therefore, we will only refer to the Minister of HWS for the remainder of this chapter.

[2] In the Netherlands, government power is divided in three levels, consisting of the national government on a central level, provinces (12) – or in the case of disaster management: security regions (25) – on a regional level, and municipalities (352). National legislation overrules provincial legislation, while provincial legislation overrules municipal legislation.

Impacts of the Covid-19 Pandemic: International Laws, Policies, and Civil Liberties, First Edition. Edited by Nadav Morag.
© 2023 John Wiley & Sons, Inc. Published 2023 by John Wiley & Sons, Inc.

these measures, however, could find no basis in the Twm COVID-19. Therefore, long-term dormant national emergency legislation was used, in particular to impose a curfew.

In this chapter, we will focus on the various legal instruments the Dutch government used to combat COVID-19 and the administrative bodies that were involved. We will consider the constitutional obstacles the government encountered, paying special attention to the limitation of fundamental rights protected by the *Grondwet voor het Koninkrijk der Nederlanden* (Dutch Constitution) – which originated in 1815, the European Convention for the Protection of Human Rights and Fundamental Freedoms (ECHR) 1950, and the International Covenant on Civil and Political Rights (ICCPR) 1966.[3] We will start the next section with an introduction to the Dutch legislative framework for disaster management.

1.2   Disaster Management in the Netherlands

Article 1 of the *Wet veiligheidsregio's* (Security Regions Act, Wvr)[4] – a national Act part of the legal framework on regional and municipal emergency law – 2010 defines a disaster as "a major accident or other event that seriously damages or threatens the life and health of many people, the environment or major material interests and that requires the coordinated deployment of services or organizations from different disciplines to remove the threat or limit the adverse effects thereof." Needless to say, the massive spread of COVID-19 – the COVID-19 crisis – falls within the scope of this definition. Because of this, combating COVID-19 is covered by regional and municipal emergency law.[5]

1.2.1   Functional and General Chain of Command

Dutch emergency law is adopted in either a "functional chain of command" or the "general chain of command," depending on the type of disaster. These chains of command are enshrined in legislation that determines which administrative body is responsible for the preparedness, prevention, and recovery of a specific type of disaster, and who has the authority over the emergency services and the other organizations and institutions involved in the response to a disaster. The legislation also assigns emergency powers to these authorities in order for them to take response measures during a disaster.

A functional chain of command exists when there is legislation, specifically made for the response to the specific type of disaster at hand. In many such cases, the responsibility for disaster management lies with a specialized administrative body at the central/national level, such as a specialized minister. Examples thereof include the legislation on major maritime accidents, whereby the Minister of *Infrastructuur en Waterstaat* (Infrastructure and Water Management) is

---

3 In addition to the Dutch Constitution and the ECHR, several other fundamental rights sources are relevant for the Netherlands. For instance, by virtue of its membership of the European Union (EU), the Netherlands is bound to the Charter of Fundamental Rights of the European Union 2000. However, the fundamental rights in this charter only apply to the member states of the EU to the extent that they apply EU law. Since infectious disease control falls within the responsibility of the EU member states themselves, we will not discuss the charter in this chapter.

The Netherlands is also a member state to the European Social Charter (ESC) 2006 and the International Covenant on Economic, Social, and Cultural Rights (ICESCR) 1966. However, both charters have no direct effect on the Dutch legal order and therefore will not be considered in this chapter.

4 Also translated as Safety Regions Act.

5 Occasionally, the term "COVID-19 crisis" is used. A disaster falls under the scope of the term "crisis." The term "crisis," however, has a wider scope than the term "disaster." In relation to COVID-19, the term "COVID-19 disaster" could be used instead of "COVID-19 crisis." However, in this chapter, we will use the more commonly used umbrella term "COVID-19 crisis."

assigned the responsibility for disaster response (Article 7 ff *Wet bestrijding maritieme ongevallen,* Maritime Accidents Act, 2015), and the legislation on nuclear and other radiation disasters, whereby the Minister of *Justitie en Veiligheid* (Justice and Security, J&S) is assigned the responsibility for the disaster response (Article 40 *Kernenergiewet,* Nuclear Energy Act, 1963). In the legislation of these examples, the minister is granted special powers that should enable them to effectively respond to the disaster at hand. The rules on infectious disease control are also enshrined in a functional chain of command, which is laid down in the *Wet publieke gezondheid* (Public Health Act, Wpg) 2008. We will discuss this in further detail in Section 1.3.

If there is no specific legislation for the specific type of disaster at hand, the general rules for disaster management of the general chain of command are applicable. This is, among others, the case in the event of a major fire or a severe multiple-vehicle collision. In principle, the responsibility for disaster management within the general chain of command lies with the local authorities, which, for instance, means that, in response to a disaster, a municipality's mayor has the power to impose emergency decrees (Article 5 Wvr).

Another important actor in the general chain of command is the chair of the security region. A security region is a cooperative network of several municipalities that jointly carry out various tasks connected to disaster management. For instance, the security region has the duty to identify the risks of fires, disasters, and crises, and is responsible for setting up and maintaining a fire brigade (Articles 1 and 10(a) and (e) Wvr). All 352 Dutch municipalities are allocated among 25 security regions, which are managed by the mayors of the participating municipalities (Articles 8 and 11 Wvr). The mayor of the largest municipality is usually the chair of the security region.

If a regional disaster or supra-local disaster – a disaster with effects crossing municipal borders (Wierenga 2017) – occurs in a security region, the chair of the security region has an important role in the response to a disaster. The chair is the sole executive body to manage that regional disaster, excluding all other mayors involved in the security region (Article 39 Wvr).

1.2.2 The COVID-19 Crisis

From March to December 2020, disaster response relating to the COVID-19 crisis was based on both the functional chain of command for infectious disease control (the Wpg) and the general chain of command. The fact that powers from the general chain of command were primarily used as the basis for COVID-19 measures, while there is a functional chain of command for infectious disease control, can be explained by the fact that the functional chain lacked the provisions that provided the necessary powers to battle the COVID-19 crisis.[6]

1.3 The Public Health Act 2008 (Functional Chain of Command)

The Netherlands has had special legislation for combating infectious diseases since the nineteenth century.[7] Today, the legal framework for infectious disease control is set out in the *Wet publieke gezondheid* (Public Health Act, Wpg), which came into force in 2008.[8] That Act implements the

---

6 This is not unusual. The functional and general chain do not exclude each other, in many situations they (partly) coincide.

7 The first infectious disease control acts were the *Wet op de uitoefening der geneeskunst* (Medicine Practice Act) 1885 and the *Wet ter wering en beteugeling van besmettelijke ziekten* (Prevention and Control of Infectious Diseases Act) 1872.

8 The Wpg replaced three acts: The *Infectieziektenwet* (Infectious Diseases Act) 1998, the *Wet collectieve preventie volksgezondheid* (Public Health Preventive Orders Act) 1990, and the *Quarantainewet* (Quarantine Act) 1960.

2005 International Health Regulations, a treaty regarding international health protection established under the auspices of the World Health Organization.[9]

The Wpg distinguishes four classes of infectious diseases: A, B1, B2, and C. This classification is based on contagiousness, seriousness, and the likely impact on public health.[10] Class A is the most severe category (Timen et al. 2009, pp. 156–158). The Minister of *Volksgezondheid, Welzijn en Sport* (Health, Welfare, and Sport, HWS) is authorized to add infectious diseases to these classes or to recategorize them (Article 20 Wpg).

According to the Wpg, an infectious disease epidemic exists when the number of new patients suffering from the infectious disease of one of the aforementioned classes steeply increases in a short period of time (Article 1(i) Wpg). The disease control measures that may be imposed depend on the class to which the infectious disease belongs. The most severe measures may be applied during an epidemic of a Class A infectious disease. The classification also determines who is in charge of combating the epidemic and which bodies are authorized to take disease control measures.

On 28 January 2020, the Minister of HWS designated COVID-19 as a Class A infectious disease (*Ministeriële regeling 2019-nCoV 28-01-2020,* Ministerial Regulation 2019-nCoV 28 January 2020). In the case of a Class A infectious disease epidemic or the threat thereof, the chair of the security region takes care of its control, as stated in Article 6(4) Wpg. According to Article 7(1) Wpg, the Minister of HWS is in charge of disease control operation. Thereby, they can instruct the chair of the security region on how to manage the response to the epidemic. This includes the power to give the chair of the security region an instruction regarding the deployment of specific disease control measures.

1.3.1 National Crisis Structure

As follows from the foregoing, the Minister of HWS is in charge of disease control operation during the COVID-19 crisis. Thereby, the minister is assisted and advised by the *Centrum infectieziektebestrijding* (Centre for Infectious Disease Control, CIb), which is part of the *Rijksinstituut voor Volksgezondheid en Milieu* (National Institute for Public Health and the Environment, RIVM), a government agency under the Ministry of HWS.[11] Following the outbreak of COVID-19, the CIb convened an Outbreak Management Team (OMT). This team consists of (medical) experts in the area of infectious disease control. The OMT played an important role during the COVID-19 crisis by providing the Minister of HWS advice regarding the necessary policy decisions.

Before the minister proceeds to implement the OMT's advice, it is discussed in the *Bestuurlijk afstemmingsoverleg infectieziekten* (Administrative Consultative Committee on Infectious Diseases, BAO) to test its administrative feasibility and desirability (Article 7(4) Wpg and Article 2(1) *Instellingsbesluit bestuurlijk afstemmingsoverleg infectieziektebestrijding*, Instituting Decree Administrative Consultative Committee Infectious Disease Control, 2004). The BAO consists of officials from the ministries involved and representatives of the organizations involved, such as the *Vereniging Nederlandse gemeenten* (Association of Dutch Municipalities, VNG) (Article 3 *Instellingsbesluit bestuurlijk afstemmingsoverleg infectieziektebestrijding*, Instituting Decree Administrative Consultative Committee Infectious Disease Control, 2004). The BAO exists to ensure the separation of science from political decision-making (Dute 2021).

---

9 The IHR binds 196 member states, including 194 WHO member states, and is based on the 1946 Constitution of the World Health Organization.

10 Class A contains, for instance, diseases such as polio and hemorrhagic fever. Class B1 includes diseases such as diphtheria, the plague, and rabies. Class B2 contains illnesses such as hepatitis A, B, and C and measles. Class C contains, for instance, anthrax, malaria, and tetanus.

11 See also: *Wet op het RIVM* (RIVM Act) 1966.

Following the discussion of OMT advice in the BAO, the minister will coordinate the intended disease control measures with their fellow ministers. Initially, this coordination took place within the *Ministeriële Commissie Crisisbeheersing* (Ministerial Committee for Crisis Management, MCCb), but during the COVID-19 crisis, a special ministerial committee was established: the *Ministeriële Commissie COVID-19* (Ministerial Committee COVID-19, MCC-19). Within the MCC-19, all ministers involved jointly decide on the infectious disease control policy and on an integrated approach to the consequences of the COVID-19 crisis (*Kamerbrief,* Letter to Parliament, 1760471-212563-PDC19).

1.3.2 Measures

In line with the advice of the OMT, at the start of the COVID-19 crisis, the national government gave urgent hygiene advice and imposed some relatively light measures instead of imposing stricter legally enforceable measures. The prime minister provided the public in a number of press statements with urgent advice on regular hand-washing, sneezing into the elbow, refraining from shaking hands, maintaining a social distance of 1.5 meters, working from home as much as possible, and avoiding busy places.

Instead of imposing drastic legally enforceable measures, such as those imposed in southern European states (which involved a measure amounting to home detention), the Dutch government referred to their policy as an "intelligent lockdown" with less drastic measures (Hendriks and Toebes 2021). Although a "soft approach" is preferable from a human rights perspective, over time the government deemed this approach insufficient to counter the wide and rapid spread of COVID-19. The national government considered it necessary to impose legally enforceable measures that also affected the healthy part of the population. For instance, events and gatherings in groups were forbidden, and the hospitality sector, shops, and schools were closed.

The Wpg, which is specifically meant for infectious disease control, offered insufficient powers for such general measures. The Wpg mainly enables the imposition of measures on individuals who are suffering from an infectious disease, individuals who could justifiably be regarded as being infected, and on buildings, goods, and transport means that are presumed or actually contaminated with an infectious disease. Examples of these measures are admission to a hospital in isolation, accompanied by compulsory medical examination, quarantine at home or elsewhere, and the partial or complete closure of buildings (Articles 6(4), 34(1) and (3), 35, and 47(3)(a) Wpg).

To deal with the insufficiency of the Wpg and still be able to introduce general measures, the Minister of Health, Welfare, and Sport invoked their power to issue instructions, as defined in Article 7(1) Wpg. This power enables the minister to instruct the chair of a security region to deploy disease control measures in the case of a Class A infectious disease epidemic. As earlier mentioned in this section, the chair has an executive role in infectious disease control in the case of a Class A epidemic in their security region, supervised by the Minister of HWS (Roozendaal and Van Sande 2020).

Interestingly, the power to issue instructions was not used to instruct the deployment of measures under the Wpg (the functional chain of command), but rather to take measures based on the power to issue emergency orders given to the chair of the security region within the general chain of command (see Section 1.4). Whether the Minister of HWS, in their capacity within the functional chain of command, was authorized to instruct the deployment of powers in the general chain of command is not undisputed. Cammelbeeck (2021), for instance, argues that the power to issue instructions does not have and may not have such a broad scope. Dute (2021) is slightly more cautious and merely considers that the Minister of HWS interpreted Article 7 Wpg quite liberally. We believe that on methodological and teleological grounds, the argument that the legislator intended this scope, or at least did not wish to exclude it, can be justified. This would particularly be the case if it were done for a short period of time in an unexpected, very grave situation such as the COVID-19 crisis (Brainich and Helsloot 2020; Wierenga 2021).

1.4   Municipal Emergency Powers (General Chain of Command)

The core of the municipal emergency powers consists of the power to issue emergency orders and emergency decrees as laid down in Articles 175 and 176 of the *Gemeentewet* (Municipalities Act, Gemw) 1992, respectively. The power to issue emergency decrees (Article 176 Gemw) gives the mayor – or the chair of the security region in case of a regional disaster or crisis – the authority to issue generally binding regulations needed to maintain public order or contain danger in cases of major disorder or disaster, or of serious fear of their occurrence. The power to issue emergency decrees thus provides for the possibility of promulgating some sort of temporary emergency laws. These may, for instance, include an area ban or a mandatory evacuation in case of imminent flooding or chemical fire (De Jong 2015; Wierenga et al. 2016). An emergency decree may derogate from existing legislation and regulations but may not derogate from the Dutch Constitution, as is explicitly stated in Article 176(1) Gemw. Therefore, emergency decrees do not form a legal basis for long-term mandatory quarantine or isolations measures, since they result in a far-reaching limitation of the right to privacy, as protected by Article 10 of the Constitution.

As previously stated, the power to issue emergency decrees was used to administer national infectious disease control measures during the COVID-19 crisis. Since the COVID-19 crisis is a disaster on an international scale and affects the entire country, it also constitutes a regional disaster in all 25 security regions in the Netherlands. Therefore, the powers within the general chain of command were employed by the chairs of the security regions.

On 13 March 2020, the chairs of the security regions rolled out a patchwork of 25 emergency decrees across the Netherlands. The Security Council – the consultative body of the 25 security regions – played an essential role in this process.[12] It compiled emergency decree models that included the instructions of the Minister of Health, Welfare, and Sport. The respective chairs of the various security regions then based their emergency decrees on these models. Despite the existence of these models, regional differentiation existed across the security regions.[13] Between 13 March and 30 November 2020, the 25 security regions issued at least 15 consecutive emergency decrees (De Jong 2021). Never before had the municipal power to issue emergency decrees been applied so intensively and for such a prolonged period of time to regulate society so drastically.

1.4.1   Areas of Tension

As stated, the deployment of emergency decrees during the COVID-19 crisis is an exceptional legal phenomenon. In particular, because the legislator intended Article 176 Gemw to be used to impose short-term measures to control local and regional emergencies, not national emergencies. The power to issue emergency decrees has always been used in this way since its introduction in 1851. The exceptional application in the COVID-19 crisis led to several constitutional tensions. Not only is the power to issue an emergency decree a power of the mayor for local disasters, the issued emergency decrees were in effect for a relatively long time.

---

12 The Security Council is intended for strategic and the integral security coordination between the security regions. The Wvr, however, does not grant a specific role to the Security Council during the "hot phase" of a crisis.
13 The security regions of Rotterdam-Rijnmond and Amsterdam-Amstelland, for instance, introduced an obligation to wear a face mask in public places on 5 August 2020, while all other security regions did not. Also, security regions differentiated in their regulations on street markets.

1.4.2 Debatable Limitations of Fundamental Rights

In addition to the discrepancy between the use and the nature of the power to issue emergency decrees, it is, in principle, unlawful to derogate from the Dutch Constitution in an emergency decree.[14] Such limitations of fundamental constitutional rights did, however, take place on a large scale as a result of COVID-19 emergency decrees. For example, restrictive measures, such as the general ban on visits to certain care institutions, or the maximum number of allowed visitors at home-situations represent both far-reaching limitations of the right to respect for privacy, as protected by Article 10 Dutch Constitution, and the right of inviolability of the home, as protected by Article 12 Dutch Constitution (De Jong 2020). Furthermore, for a long time, the number of persons permitted to attend religious meetings was capped. In principle, such a measure cannot be adopted in an emergency decree either, because this results in a limitation of the freedom of religion, as laid down in Article 6 Dutch Constitution.

However, the aforementioned tensions notwithstanding, this does not automatically mean that the emergency decrees were unlawful. An important exemption from the principle that emergency decrees may not derogate from the Dutch Constitution exists in cases of real and immediate danger to life. This exemption relates to the positive obligations of governments to protect the life of their nationals, which follows from the right to life, as protected by Article 2 ECHR.[15] The ECHR is a European fundamental rights treaty signed by 47 European member states, including the Netherlands, documenting legally enforceable fundamental rights. It is possible that an obligation under the national constitution conflicts with an obligation under a fundamental rights treaty, such as the ECHR. This amounts to a so-called conflict of fundamental rights. In cases of such a conflict, the government must weigh the conflicting interests of the fundamental rights in question. The COVID-19 crisis resulted in a severe threat of real and immediate danger to the lives of Dutch citizens. Therefore, the national government's decision to grant a greater weight to the positive obligation under Article 2 ECHR than, for example, the right to privacy is justifiable (Wierenga et al. 2016; Brouwer and Schilder 2020; Wierenga et al. 2020).[16]

The courts have upheld emergency decrees that restrict fundamental constitutional rights on more than one occasion.[17] Nevertheless, in light of the aforementioned, the legality of the emergency decree approach in the COVID-19 crisis became increasingly controversial as time went on, as is also noted by the Council of State's Advisory Division, a High Council of State that operates as the Dutch legislature's most important advisor on legislative issues (*Voorlichting Raad van State*, Advise by the Council of State, 2020). Over time, it may be expected from the government to adopt COVID-19 measures by means not conflicting with the rules on the lawful limitation of constitutional rights. The national government's argument that the far-reaching limitation of fundamental constitutional rights is legitimized by the conflict of those rights with the ECHR's right to life becomes increasingly fragile over time. This is especially the case, since several months had passed wherein the national government could have lawfully limited fundamental constitutional rights through national legislation, as the Dutch Constitution requires for lawful limitation of fundamental constitutional rights.

---

14 See also the advice of the Council of State on the subject: *Kamerstukken II* (Parliamentary Papers House of Representatives), 2020/21, 25295, no. 742.
15 See for instance: ECtHR 30 November 2004 (Öneryildiz/Turkey), ECLI:CE:ECHR:2004:1130JUD004893999, par. 71; Council of State Administrative Court Division 9 December 2020, ECLI:NL:RVS:2020:2839, with annotation of J.G. Brouwer and A.E. Schilder.
16 See also: Council of State Administrative Court Division 9 December 2020, ECLI:NL:RVS:2020:2839, with annotation of J.G. Brouwer and A.E. Schilder (*AB* 2020/183).
17 See for example: The Hague Court 19 June 2020, ECLI:NL:RBDHA:2020:5865; The Hague Court 27 June 2020, ECLI:NL:RBDHA:2020:5865; Amsterdam Court 19 August 2020, ECLI:NL:RBAMS:2020:4057.

Aside from the limitations of constitutionally protected fundamental rights, the COVID-19 emergency decrees frequently constitute limitations of fundamental rights protected under the ECHR and the ICCPR.[18] However, these limitations do not result in legal problems because both the ECHR and the ICCPR have relatively lenient rules on lawful limitation of fundamental rights.[19] Both the ECHR and the ICCPR require that a limitation is provided for by law. "Law" in this sense is interpreted materially, which means that it may be any type of regulation. An emergency decree in the sense of Article 176 Gemw therefore falls under this definition.[20]

Additionally, the ECHR and the ICCPR require the limitation to be necessary in view of a prescribed interest. Concerning the right to respect for private and family life, for instance, the ECHR states that a limitation may only be imposed if it is "necessary in the interests of national security, public safety or the economic well-being of the country, for the prevention of disorder or crime, for the protection of health or morals, or for the protection of the rights and freedoms of others." The COVID-19 measures serve more than one of these aims.

The ECHR contains an additional requirement not included in the ICCPR: limitations of fundamental rights must be necessary in a democratic society. This requirement first of all stipulates that limitations to fundamental rights must be proportional to the objective pursued through the establishment of the specific limitation. Secondly, the measure can only be legitimate if the same objective cannot be achieved through measures that are less restrictive. In other words, the default must always be to use less restrictive measures if these can accomplish the objective. Many of the COVID-19 measures can clearly be seen to satisfy all of the ECHR and ICCPR requirements for lawful limitation of fundamental rights (*Voorlichting Raad van State*, Advise by the Council of State, 2020).

1.4.3 Democratic Control and Administrative Supervision

The lawfulness of the COVID-19 measures based on emergency decrees came under increased pressure because of the lack of democratic control and administrative supervision. When a mayor issues an emergency decree during a local disaster, the Gemw provides for a system of democratic control and administrative supervision.

With respect to democratic control, the Gemw not only provides for a system of political accountability of the mayor to the municipal council – the democratically elected body that has the legislative powers in the municipality under normal circumstances, but also requires the mayor to inform the municipal council immediately after promulgating an emergency decree. At its next meeting, the municipal council is expected to vote on the ratification of that decree (Article 180 and 176(2) and (3) Gemw). Even though non-ratification has only happened once in the history of the Netherlands, this procedure is an essential element of the democratic control over generally binding rules imposed by government-appointed bodies.[21]

With respect to administrative supervision, the Gemw gives the King's Commissioner (the Netherlands is a constitutional monarchy) – the presiding member of the provincial executive – the power to suspend the effect of emergency decrees (Article 176(2) and (6) Gemw).

18 The Dutch Constitution, the ECHR, and the ICCPR overlap considerably in the sphere of the protection of human rights. For instance, both the Dutch Constitution and the ECHR contain the right to respect for privacy (Article 10 Dutch Constitution and Article 8 ECHR, respectively), and all sources contain the right of freedom of religion (Article 6 Dutch Constitution, Article 9 ECHR, and Article 18 ICCPR).
19 Although Article 176 Gemw does not explicitly prohibit limitations on fundamental rights as protected in treaties, emergency decrees may not limit these rights. This rule derives from Article 94 Dutch Constitution.
20 ECtHR 18 June 1971 (De Wilde, Ooms and Versyp/Belgium), ECLI:NCE:ECHR:1971:0618JUD000283266, par. 96.
21 In the Netherlands, a mayor is appointed by the Minister of *Binnenlandse Zaken en Koninkrijksrelaties* (Interior and Kingdom Relations, IKR) after nomination by the municipal council (Article 61 Gemw).

The national government has a similar power. It may suspend the effect of decisions of the municipality executive, such as the promulgation of an emergency decree, when this decision is contrary to the common interest (Article 132(4) Dutch Constitution; Article 268 Gemw).

The mechanisms of democratic control and administrative supervision, however, do not work when the chair of the security region takes over the power to issue emergency decrees during a regional disaster. Firstly, because the (appointed, not democratically elected) chair of the security region is merely obligated to send written reports on the use of their powers to the municipal councils of the municipalities involved, after the crisis (Article 40 Wvr). This can result in a significant democratic deficit with respect to the emergency decrees issued, especially if these decrees are deployed by the chair of the security region for a long period of time. Secondly, because the only way in which the King's Commissioner can exercise administrative supervision is through giving instructions regarding the use of emergency powers to the chair of the security region (Article 42 Wvr). During the COVID-19 crisis, however, the Minister of Health, Welfare, and Sport already used their power to give instructions to the chairs of the security regions. In such a situation, it is unlikely the King's Commissioner will also give instructions. Finally, the national government is unlikely to use its earlier mentioned power to suspend the effect of an emergency decree during the COVID-19 crisis, since it played a prominent role in determining the contents thereof.

In conclusion, the use of emergency decrees to address a long-term crisis such as the COVID-19 crisis brought with it several constitutional objections. The Council of State's Advisory Division also criticized this controversial approach (*Kamerstukken II,* Parliamentary Papers House of Representatives, 2020 25295, no. 742). On 13 July 2020, the legislative proposal for the Twm COVID-19 (also referred to as the COVID-19 Act) was submitted to the *Tweede Kamer der Staten-Generaal*, the Dutch House of Representatives. The Act was intended to bring this controversial emergency decree approach to an end (*Kamerstukken II*, Parliamentary Papers House of Representatives, 2020 35526, nos. 1-3). After lengthy debate and radical amendment of the legislative proposal, the *Eerste Kamer der Staten-Generaal* – the Dutch Senate – adopted the Act.[22] The Twm COVID-19 went into force on 1 December 2020. Given the abovementioned objections to the use of municipal emergency powers (emergency decrees), the Act came far too late.

1.5 Interim COVID-19 Measures Act (Addition to the Functional Chain of Command)

With the Twm COVID-19, the legislator added a temporary chapter – Chapter Va – to the Wpg, titled: "Temporary provisions for combating the COVID-19 epidemic." The chapter was initially intended to be in force for three months, after which it would terminate automatically. However, the extension procedure of Article VIII Twm COVID-19 has since been used twice. This procedure permits the national government to extend the application of the Twm COVID-19 by three months. The Council of State must be consulted for each extension (Article 58t Wpg). Currently, the expiration date of Chapter Va is 1 September 2021 (*Besluit van 17 mei 2021, (…),* Decree of 17 May 2021, Providing for the Second Extension of the Duration of the Interim Covid-19 Measures Act). Because of a recent amendment to the Twm COVID-19, the House of Representatives as well as the Senate may terminate the effect of this chapter at any time (Article 1 *Wet van 14 juli 2021 (…),* Act of 14 July 2021 Amending the Interim COVID-19 Measures Act in Relation to the Required Approval by Act of Parliament of a Royal Decree of Extension).

---

22 The realization of an act needs the approval of the national government, the House of Representatives, and the Senate. See: Article 81 Dutch Constitution.

Chapter Va provides for powers to take the same measures that were previously being adopted through emergency decrees. These powers reside with the Minister of HWS, who can deploy them through "ministerial regulations" (legislation enacted by a minister). Thus, the minister remains in charge of combating the COVID-19 crisis after the Twm COVID-19 entered into force. Hereby, the Minister of HWS must still seek consensus with the other ministers involved, as well as the opinion of the national government (Article 58c(1) Wpg). A newly created clause requires that the minister be obliged to report on a monthly basis to both houses of the Dutch parliament about the implementation or extension of measures and the grounds therefore (Article 58s(1) Wpg).

1.5.1 Improvements and Shortcomings

The Twm COVID-19 is a solution to many of the problems of the emergency decree approach. Firstly, because the Twm COVID-19 is an Act of Parliament. An Act of Parliament is legislation, made by the national government, the House of Representatives, and the Senate (Parliament) jointly. The fundamental rights as protected in the Dutch constitution may only be restricted when they are based on such an Act of Parliament.[23]

1.5.2 Legitimate Limitation of Fundamental Rights

With the coming of the Twm COVID-19, the legislator provided for a legally sound basis for COVID-19 measures that constitute a limitation of fundamental rights, protected by the Dutch Constitution.[24] For example, after 1 December 2020, the Dutch government decided to impose the highly controversial obligation to wear a face mask in public places. This measure infringes the right to respect for privacy (Article 10 Dutch Constitution) and could therefore not lawfully be imposed through an emergency decree (Article 58j(1)(a) Wpg).

Although some new measures were made possible,[25] several orders that had been adopted through emergency decree were explicitly prohibited under the Twm COVID-19. Article 58o Wpg, for instance, determined that the total ban on visits to care institutions, in force for a long time under emergency decrees, was no longer permitted. Likewise, restrictions on the number of people allowed at home visits or religious gatherings were no longer allowed (Article 58g(1) and (2)(c) Wpg).

The Twm COVID-19 not only provides for constitutionally legitimate grounds for the limitation of fundamental rights, it also puts a greater emphasis on the requirements for restricting fundamental rights as protected additionally by the ECHR and the ICCPR. In this regard, Article 58b(2) Wpg states that the powers given by the Wpg may only be applied to the extent that it is necessary in view of the severity of the threat to public health, a lawful aim for restricting rights protected under the ECHR and the ICCPR. Furthermore, the application of powers from the Wpg must be consistent with the principles of a democracy based on the rule of law and should limit fundamental rights as little as possible and be proportionate to the envisaged objective, all these being conditions for the lawful limitation of fundamental rights as provided for by the ECHR.

---

23 In this respect, the rules on the lawful limitation of fundamental constitutional rights are stricter than the rules to lawful limitation of fundamental rights protected by the ECHR or the ICCPR. The latter two allow limitations based on any type of law.

24 For instance, the 1.5 m measure (Article 58f Wpg), the maximization of groups (Article 58g Wpg), the closure or conditional opening of public places (Article 58h Wpg), and the regulation or prohibiting of events (Article 58i Wpg).

25 Examples of such disease control measures are measures concerning care institutions (Article 58o Wpg), passenger transport (Article 58p Wpg), educational activities (Article 58g Wpg), and childcare services (Article 58r Wpg); all measures that previously had not been included in the Wpg.

1.5.3 Stricter Democratic Control

With the introduction of the Twm COVID-19, the democratic control of policy regarding the implementation of COVID-19 measures was significantly improved. Firstly, because both the House of Representatives and the Senate were involved in the creation of the Twm COVID-19, and the House of Representatives assumed a prominent role in the legislative process by drastically amending the legislative proposal.[26] Secondly, mayors were given a more prominent role in the execution of measures and were required to account for their enforcement policies before municipal councils. Finally, attempts were made to strengthen the democratic control by the House of Representatives. It demanded the insertion of a veto right in the Twm COVID-19 regarding all COVID-19 measures (*Kamerstukken II,* Parliamentary Papers House of Representatives, 2020 35526 B). This veto implies that every proposed measure must be sent to the House of Representatives for approval before coming into effect (Article 58c(2) Wpg). The provision may be deviated from in very urgent circumstances, but even then, the House of Representatives plays an important part: it votes on the continuation of the measure after it has come into effect (Article 58c(3) Wpg).

Although the veto power of the House of Representatives in theory strengthens the democratic legitimacy of the COVID-19 measures, in practice the veto largely remained unused because of the urgency in which many of the measures needed to be introduced. The veto can be regarded as a very unfortunate and unusual construction in emergency law. Leading constitutional law scholar Bovend'Eert (2021) even described it as a constitutional monstrosity. He rightly points out that in times of crisis, it is essential that the national government has sufficient leeway to take measures independently. The "co-manager" role that the House of Representatives has acquired through its veto impedes decisive decision-making, and decisiveness is essential during emergency situations. Emergency situations are often characterized by time pressures and rapid, successive, and evolving developments. The short duration under which the House of Representatives must perform its controlling role could make sound democratic control illusory (Wierenga 2021). There are also proponents of the House of Representatives' veto right. Brouwer and Schilder (2020) consider that it is a correct response to the constitutional disorder created by the system of emergency decrees. According to them, the democratic control mechanism fits well with a prolonged crisis situation such as the COVID-19 crisis.

In early December 2020, the national government used the Twm COVID-19 to impose a second lockdown. The Twm COVID-19 provided a purer legal basis and better democratic legitimacy for many of the measures deemed necessary during this lockdown in contrast with the measures employed during the first lockdown. However, situations wherein the Twm COVID-19 offered no solution still emerged. For instance, the national government decided that persons travelling to the Netherlands must be obligated to show a negative PCR test result (Regeling van de ministers van VWS, J&V en BZK 1806234-216586-WJZ, Regulation issued by the Minister of Health, Welfare and Sport, the Minister of Justice and Security, and the Minister of the Interior and Kingdom Relations of 24 December 2020, reference number 1806234-216586-WJZ, to amend the Interim COVID-19 Measures Act regarding the requirement of a negative test result for international public transport). This measure infringes the right to inviolability of the body, as laid down in Article 11 Dutch Constitution. As mentioned in Section 1.5.1, a limitation of a fundamental constitutional right requires sufficient specific basis in an Act of Parliament (Nieuwenhuis et al. 2017, pp. 131–133). The court that reviewed the measure decided that the Wpg did not yet provide the necessary specific basis.[27]

---

26 In the legislative process, only the House of Representatives is allowed to propose amendments. The Senate only votes on the (amended) legislative proposal. See Article 84(2) Dutch Constitution.

27 The Hague Court (preliminary relief judge) 31 December 2020, ECLI:NL:RBDHA:2020:13643, par. 10. Article 7 Wet buitengewone bevoegdheden burgerlijk gezag (Civil Authority Special Powers Act, Wbbbg) 1996 provides a similar option.

This is why the legislature decided to create a more specific basis for that measure in the Wpg (*Wet van 8 januari 2021 (…)*, Act of 8 January 2021 to amend the Public Health Act regarding clarification of the interim legal basis for issuing rules concerning admission to and use of passenger transport services). A similar situation occurred when the national government decided to introduce a curfew in January 2021, when the British mutation of COVID-19 started its rise in the Netherlands. Even after the addition of Chapter Va, the Wpg did not provide for the possibility to introduce a curfew. The national government could have chosen to try and add this possibility to the Wpg, but in view of the urgency of the situation, this route was not taken. The government instead sought refuge in national emergency law.

1.6   National Emergency Law

National emergency law is the legal framework regarding exceptional circumstances wherein the central government cannot carry out its tasks within the ordinary (constitutional) framework. It is an additional legal framework to that on infectious disease control (Wpg, supplemented by the Twm COVID-19), as already discussed in previous sections, and that on municipal emergency powers (emergency decrees based on the Gemw), which were used as the basis for the COVID-19 measures up to the introduction of the curfew.

Since the nineteenth century, the Dutch Constitution includes a system of national emergency law wherein the national government has the power to impose emergency measures during a so-called "state of exception." At the center of national emergency law lies Article 103 Dutch Constitution. This Article states that an Act of Parliament must provide for the conditions under which a state of exception may be declared for the protection of the internal or external security of the state.

The 1968 *Coördinatiewet uitzonderingstoestanden* (Exceptional Situations Coordination Act, CWU) implements Article 103 Dutch Constitution and provides for the power to declare two types of states of exception: the general state of emergency and the limited state of emergency. Both states of exception are declared by Royal Decree, a decree originating from the national government (Article 2 CWU). After making such a decision, both the House of Representatives and the Senate must be informed immediately. In united assembly, these bodies may then decide to end the state of exception if they are of the opinion that it must no longer continue (Article 3(a) CWU). The national government also has the power to end the state of exception. It must do so as soon as the circumstances permit.

Article 103(2) Dutch Constitution determines that during a state of exception, deviations may be made from five constitutionally protected rights, including the freedom of religion of Article 6 and the freedom of assembly and demonstration of Article 9.

Also the ECHR and the ICCPR recognize the power to declare a state of emergency. When a member state uses this power, some of the fundamental rights laid down in the ECHR/ICCPR may lawfully be limited. Thereby, both the ECHR and the ICCPR require a notification of the announced state of emergency. Furthermore, the member state must notify which rights are being restricted during that state of emergency (Article 15(1) and (3) ECHR; Article 4(1) and (3) ICCPR). It should be noted that certain fundamental rights cannot lawfully be restricted, even during a state of emergency. The ECHR and the ICCPR qualify the right to life and the prohibition of torture as so-called *notstandfeste* rights; rights that may not be deviated from even during a state of emergency (Article 15(2) ECHR; Article 4(2) ICCPR).

In the Netherlands, the type of state of emergency declared determines which powers the national government may use to respond to the emergency situation. During a "limited state of emergency," the national government may use the emergency provisions of the CWU's List A, while during a "general state of emergency," the government may use those of List B. List B contains all the provisions of List A, supplemented by provisions that may result in further-reaching limitations of fundamental rights. The provisions of lists A and B contain emergency powers that remain "inactive" in normal times. The national government can activate them if a state of emergency calls for it. Examples of emergency powers listed in lists A and B include the power of the Minister of *Economische Zaken en Klimaat* (Economic Affairs and Climate Policy) to take measures to discourage the hoarding of goods (Article 3 Hamsterwet, Hoarding Act, 1962) and the power of the Ministers of *Binnenlandse Zaken en Koninkrijksrelaties* (Interior and Kingdom Relations, IKR) and the Minister of *Defensie* (Defence) to order a mandatory evacuation of the population (Article 2a Wet verplaatsing bevolking, Population Evacuation Act, 1952).

Declaring a state of emergency also permits the activation of Article 54 of the Wvr. This article enshrines the Minister of Justice and Security's power to wholly or partially assume the powers of mayors, or other decentral executive bodies. Between March and November 2020, the minister could have used these powers autonomously to exercise mayoral authority to issue emergency decrees to impose national COVID-19 measures.[28] This could have saved a lot of the time that had been lost in, for instance, the Security Council's drafting of model emergency decrees and the implementation thereof throughout the 25 individual security regions.[29] It would also have given the parliament a better position to perform its democratic control tasks over the national government's COVID-19 policy. Instead, the enforcement of these measures was in the hands of the – as previously discussed – limited democratically controlled security regions. The national government, however, did not take this course of action. Furthermore, national emergency law legislation was outdated and at various points no longer relevant (Vink 2020). This, however, would not have been an obstacle for the use of this provision during the COVID-19 crisis.

1.6.1 Separate Implementation

Throughout history, the Dutch government has been reluctant to declare a state of emergency, since such a declaration is regarded as a far-reaching action that can have an escalating effect. Therefore, the declaration of a state of emergency should be avoided for as long as possible (*Kamerstukken II,* Parliamentary Papers House of Representatives, 1994 23790 no. 3). Also during the COVID-19 crisis, the national government refrained from declaring a state of exception.[30] During a debate in the Senate, the Minister of J&S even remarked that declaring the state of emergency does not fit the Dutch mentality (*Handelingen I,* Proceedings Senate, 2021 12 no. 26).

Even without declaring a state of emergency, it is possible to activate certain emergency powers provided for by national emergency law. This is referred to as "separate activation." Separate activation may take place when a situation occurs in which the activation of a specific power of national emergency law is necessary, whereas the declaration of a state of emergency is not. An example of the use of separate activation is the activation of a provision from the *Distributiewet* (Rationing Act)

---

28 Article 7 Wet buitengewone bevoegdheden burgerlijk gezag (Civil Authority Special Powers Act, Wbbbg) 1996 provides a similar option.

29 The measures announced on 23 March 2020, for instance, were only enshrined in emergency decrees on 26 or 27 March.

30 W. Boonstra, '*Noodtoestand afkondigen "niet aan de orde"'* (Declaring the State of Emergency 'Out of order'), www.binnenlandsbestuur.nl 10 June 2020. Moreover, the Netherlands has not used Article 15 ECHR and Article 4 ICCPR to lawfully set restrict the rights under these treaties during a state of emergency. With respect to the ECHR, the Netherlands follows the example of certain European states such as Sweden and Spain. Other European states did make use of Article 15 ECHR. These states include Armenia, Georgia, Romania, and Serbia. See "Notifications" coe.int.

1939 during the 1973 Dutch oil crisis in order to ration petrol. The separate activation of that provision and the use of the power laid down therein achieved the desired effect without declaring a national emergency.

The Dutch government also used separate activation of national emergency law powers during the COVID-19 crisis. On 22 January 2021, the national government decided to separately activate Article 8 of the *Wet buitengewone bevoegdheden burgerlijk gezag* (Civil Authority Special Powers Act, Wbbbg) 1996 (Article 1 Besluit van 22 januari 2021 (…), Decree of 22 January 2021, Providing for the Entry Into Force and Activation of Article 8(1) and (3) Civil Authority Special Powers Act). This section provides the Minister of J&S the power to restrict movement of persons outdoors. The procedure for separate activation of this power is laid down in the CWU in conjunction with Article 1(1) Wbbbg and allows the national government to activate several powers from the Wbbbg – including the powers from Article 8 Wbbbg – independently of a state of emergency when exceptional circumstances require it.

Determining whether an emergency situation amounts to such an exceptional circumstance is a task of the national government. One major factor that must be considered thereby is whether the circumstances are such that ordinary legal powers are insufficient to respond effectively to the emergency situation. After an emergency power based on Article 1(1) Wbbbg has been activated separately, the national government must immediately send the House of Representatives a legislative proposal concerning the continuation of the activation of that power. If that legislative proposal is not adopted, the national government must deactivate the power immediately (Article 1(1) and (2) Wbbbg).

Article 8 Wbbbg distinguishes two procedures to use the power to restrict movement of persons outdoors (for instance, by imposing a curfew). Under Article 8(2), an order restricting the movement of persons outdoors may be laid down in a governmental decree. In urgent situations, such a measure may be laid down in a ministerial regulation, Article 8(3) provides.[31] In the latter case, no rules for publication of the order apply; the order enters into force immediately after its announcement. During the COVID-19 crisis, the Minister of J&S used the "urgency option" of Article 8(3) Wbbbg to impose a curfew. This curfew prohibited remaining out of doors between 9.00 p.m. and 4.30 a.m. (*Article 1 Besluit van 22 januari 2021, (…)*, Decree of 22 January 2021, Providing for the Entry Into Force and Activation of Article 8(1) and (3) Civil Authority Special Powers Act; Article 1 *Tijdelijke regeling landelijke avondklok covid-19*, Interim Regulation National Curfew COVID-19, 2021).

1.6.2 Criticism

Given the urgency of the situation as asserted by the national government, the "urgency option" of Article 8(3) Wbbbg provided a sound legal basis for the introduction of the curfew. However, the national government decided to ensure a majority in the House of Representatives in favor of the measure through a debate before the curfew was implemented. This led to a delay of about three days. Although consulting the House of Representatives strengthened the democratic legitimacy of the curfew, it raised legal questions on at least two issues. Firstly, consultation of the House of Representatives before implementing an emergency measure is not in line with the system of national emergency law, which is based on the idea of an independently operating administration that needs to respond to emergency situations quickly and decisively. In this system, democratic control is carried out swiftly, but only after the measure has been imposed. Since national emergency law thus

---

31 A governmental decree is legislation made by the national government as a whole, consisting of all ministers and the King. A ministerial regulation is legislation made by a single minister.

provides for ex post facto democratic control, the House of Representatives had to provide its opinion on the curfew for a second time in the extension procedure under national emergency law. Such a duplication of procedures in times of crisis is contrary to all logic (Cammelbeeck 2021; Wierenga 2021).

Secondly, consulting the House of Representatives in advance is not in line with the asserted urgency of the situation that justifies the use of the urgency procedure of Article 8(3) Wbbbg. The Council of State also pointed out the discrepancy between the use of the urgency procedure and the debate in the House of Representatives (*Kamerstukken II,* Parliamentary Papers House of Representatives, 2021 35722 no. 4). An interest group opposing the COVID-19 measures requested the national government to suspend the curfew as it allegedly had not been based on proper legal grounds. When the national government dismissed that request, the group decided to start legal proceedings against the state.[32] These proceedings were followed with great interest by the Dutch society.

1.6.3 The Curfew Case

On 16 February 2021, the preliminary relief judge of the The Hague court ruled in the "curfew case" that the curfew was based on incorrect legal grounds. The effects of the court's ruling were, however, very far-reaching: the national government was ordered to suspend the curfew immediately.[33] In a special procedure on the same day, the Court of Appeal decided to suspend the effects of the preliminary relief judge's decision.[34]

Nevertheless, the national government decided to be on the safe side and provide for a second legal basis for a curfew. On 22 February 2021 – four days after submitting the legislative proposal – an Act was adopted that added a power to impose a curfew to the temporary Chapter Va of the Wpg (*Tijdelijke wet beperking vertoeven in de openlucht covid-19*, Interim Restriction on Staying Outdoors COVID-19 Act, 2021; Article 58j(1)(f) Wpg).[35] In the appeal procedure, the Court of Appeal judged that the Wbbbg does offer a proper legal ground for the introduction of the curfew. That was a correct judgment. However, the Court of Appeal relatively quickly disregarded the explicit requirement of urgency, which follows from the incorrectly chosen Article 8(3) Wbbbg procedure.[36]

In the preliminary relief case, the court also considered the proportionality and subsidiarity of the curfew in addition to the requirement for urgency. According to the court, the curfew resulted in a limitation of the freedom of movement under Article 2 ECHR and of the right of protection of privacy of Article 8 ECHR.[37] As mentioned in Section 1.4.2, the ECHR requires that such limitation must be necessary in a democratic society (Nieuwenhuis et al. 2017, p. 111). This requirement implies that the limitation must be proportional and comply with the principle of subsidiarity, which, as noted earlier in the chapter, means that the severity of the restriction must be proportionate to the intended objective and that less severe means to achieve the same goal are not available.

---

32 The Hague Court (preliminary relief judge) 16 February 2021, ECLI:NL:RBDHA:2021:1100, paras. 2.6. and 3.2.
33 The Hague Court (preliminary relief judge) 16 February 2021, ECLI:NL:RBDHA:2021:1100, par. 5.1.
34 Court of Appeal of The Hague 16 February 2021, ECLI:NL:GHDHA:2021:252.
35 Article 8 Wbbbg was deactivated after the Interim Restriction on Staying Outdoors COVID-19 Act entered into force. See: Besluit van 22 februari 2021, houdende buitenwerkingstelling van artikel 8, eerste en derde lid, van de Wet buitengewone bevoegdheden burgerlijk gezag (Decree of 22 February 2021, Providing for Deactivation of Article 8(1) and (3) Wbbbg).
36 Court of Appeal of The Hague 26 February 2021, ECLI:NL:GHDHA:2021:285, paras. 6.4.-6.11.
37 The court was also of the opinion that the curfew order indirectly restricted the freedom of religion (Article 9 ECHR) and the freedom of assembly and demonstration (Article 11 ECHR). See The Hague Court (preliminary relief judge) 16 February 2021, ECLI:NL:RBDHA:2021:1100, par. 4.1.

The court ruled that the government had not shown sufficient evidence that the curfew would have an impact on the number of infections, nor that the aim could have been achieved in a less severe manner.[38]

This superfluous reasoning in the Court's decision certainly does not demonstrate the required judicial restraint. As follows from ECtHR case law, ECHR member states have wide margin of appreciation in assessing whether a limitation is necessary in a democratic society. Because of this margin of appreciation, a court – especially in cases of emergency and urgency – should exercise restraint when judging a case.[39] It was therefore not unexpected that the Court of Appeal judged that there were no reasons to assume that the requirements of proportionality and subsidiarity had not been fulfilled.[40]

1.7 Conclusion

During the COVID-19 crisis, the Netherlands had to cope with a disaster of unprecedented scope and duration. Initially, the government tried to contain the crisis with a "soft approach," mainly consisting of hygiene advice, but soon the national government took a stricter approach which included legally enforceable measures.

The Dutch legal framework concerning infectious disease control soon proved to be utterly insufficient for taking the required measures in response to the COVID-19 crisis. With evolving insight and under pressure of time, the national government had to find the necessary legal grounds for far-reaching measures to combat COVID-19. This explains why the national government in the first phase of the crisis did not always follow a legally pure path, resulting in constitutional objections.

The power to issue emergency decrees, used by the Minister of Health, Welfare, and Sport in collaboration with the chairs of the 25 security regions, for instance, provided no lawful means for restricting constitutionally protected rights for a prolonged period of time. Furthermore, the measures only had a limited democratic legitimization and were only limitedly subject to democratic control.

It may reasonably be stated that the use of emergency decrees in the fight against COVID-19 went on too long. Only in December 2020, when the Twm COVID-19 added temporary Chapter Va to the Wpg, did this controversial approach come to an end. It not only ended the poor legal basis for the limitation of constitutionally protected fundamental rights, it also strengthened the democratic control and administrative supervision of the COVID-19 policy to a level that is acceptable within the Dutch understanding of the rule of law.

The amended legislation concerning infectious disease control also had to be reviewed and supplemented several times. For instance, to provide for a power to impose a curfew after this measure was contested, as it had allegedly been wrongly based on national emergency law.

The COVID-19 crisis revealed that Dutch infectious disease control legislation, as laid down in the Public Health Act (Wpg), is in need of substantial review. Infectious diseases have been present throughout the ages, and the COVID-19 crisis will not be the last the Netherlands has to cope with. We recommend that not only the Wpg but also the municipal emergency powers and the outdated national emergency law be overhauled once this crisis is over. We also note that the use of these legal instruments during the COVID-19 crisis revealed several constitutional

---

38 The Hague Court (preliminary relief judge) 16 February 2021, ECLI:NL:RBDHA:2021:1100, paras. 4.11.–4.14.

39 See for example: ECtHR 7 December 1976 (*Handyside/United Kingdom*), ECLI:CE:ECHR:1976: 1207JUD000549372.

40 Court of Appeal of The Hague 16 February 2021, ECLI:NL:GHDHA:2021:252, par. 6.15.

flaws in those legal instruments. Consequently, it is important to secure meaningful democratic control and administrative supervision of the use of far-reaching emergency powers such as those employed during the Covid-19 crisis. This proved essential during a long-lasting crisis like the COVID-19 crisis. In order to enable the authorities to act decisively and to limit the risk that sound democratic control should become illusory, the democratic control function of elected bodies must not be allowed to reach a point in which it virtually shares its emergency powers with the executive.

Finally, due consideration must be given to the acceptability of limitations on fundamental rights during emergency situations. Thought should be given to which limitations should be deemed justified and under what circumstances. Reflection on that question and further grounding it in legislation will provide a better assessment framework for future crises.

References

Books

Brainich, E.T., and Helsloot, I. (2020). Commentaar op artikel 39 Wet Veiligheidsregio's (Comments on Article 39 Safety Regions Act). In: *Tekst & Commentaar Openbare Orde en Veiligheid (Text & Comments on Public Order and Safety Law)* (ed. E.R. Muller, E.T. Brainich, J.G. Brouwer et al.), 805–809. Kluwer: Deventer.

De Jong, M.A.D.W. (2015). Noodbevel en noodverordening (Emergency Order and Emergency Decree). In *Openbare orde (Public order)* (ed. E. Backx, A. van den Berg and J. van der Grinten et al.). Nijmegen: Ars Aequi Libri.

Dute, J.C.J. (2021). De Wet publieke gezondheid als instrument voor de bestrijding van de COVID-19-epidemie. Gewogen en te licht bevonden? (The Public Health Act as an Instrument to Combat the COVID-19 Epidemic. Tried and Found Wanting?). In: *Gezondheidsrecht in tijden van crisis: de COVID-19-pandemie (Health Legislation in Times of Crisis: the COVID-19 Pandemic)* (J.G. Sijmons, N.V. Alexandrov, J.A.R. Koot, et al.), 67–86. The Hague: Sdu.

Hendriks, A.C., and Toebes, B.C.A. (2021). Gezondheidsrecht in tijden van crisis: de COVID-19-pandemie (Health Legislation in Times of Crisis: the COVID-19 Pandemic). In: *Gezondheidsrecht in tijden van crisis: de COVID-19-pandemie (Health Legislation in Times of Crisis: the COVID-19 Pandemic)* (J.G. Sijmons, N.V. Alexandrov, J.A.R. Koot, et al.), 43–66. The Hague: Sdu.

Nieuwenhuis, J., Den Heijer, M., Hins, A.W. (2017). *Hoofdstukken grondrechten (Chapters on Fundamental Rights)*. Nijmegen: Ars Aequi Libri.

Timen, A., Van Wijngaarden, J.K., and Van Steenbergen, J.E. (2009). De (on)zichtbare scheiding tussen een uitbraak en een crisis (The (In)visible distinction between an outbreak and a crisis). In: *Crisis: Studies over crisis en crisisbeheersing (Crisis: Studies on Crisis and Crisis Control)* (ed. Dat moet zijn Muller, E., Rosenthal, U., Helsloot, I.), 156–158. Deventer: Kluwer.

Wierenga, A.J., Post, C., and Koornstra, J. (2016). *Naar handhaafbare noodbevelen en noodverordeningen. Een analyse van het gemeentelijke noodrecht (To Enforceable Emergency Orders and Emergency Decrees. An Analysis of Municipal Emergency Law), Politiekunde 84 (Politie & Wetenschap) (Police Studies 84, Police & Science)*. Amsterdam: Reed Business.

Wierenga, A.J (2017). Noodbevelen en noodverordeningen in tijden van bijzondere noodsituaties: Over de aantasting van de noodrechtelijke autonomie van de burgemeester (Emergency Orders and Emergency Decrees in Times of special Emergencies: On the Impairment of the Mayor's Autonomy in Emergency Law). In: *In dienst van het recht, Brouwer bundel (In Service of the Law, Brouwer Essays)* (ed. P.A.J. Van den Berg and G. Molier), 41–54. The Hague: Boom juridisch.

Journal articles

Bovend'Eert, P.P.T. (2021). Parlementaire betrokkenheid in de tijdelijke Coronawet. Niet voor herhaling vatbaar (Parliamentary involvement in the interim COVID-19 Act. Not to be repeated). *Nederlands Juristenblad* 2641 (39): 2990–2994.

Brouwer, J.G., and Schilder, A.E. (2020). Parlementair vetorecht bij ministeriële coronamaatregelen – Juiste reactie op staatsrechtelijke wanorde (Parliamentary veto regarding ministerial COVID-19 measures – the right reaction to a consitutional disorder). *Nederlands Juristenblad* 3053 (44): 3391–3393.

Cammelbeeck, T.D. (2021). Van noodsprong naar bijzondere noodwet, het failliet van het staatsnoodrecht? (From Desperate Move to Special Emergency Legislation, the Bankruptcy of National Emergency Law). *RegelMaat* 37(3): 25–42.

De Jong, M.A.D.W. (2020). Onder druk wordt alles vloeibaar. Over noodverordeningen en het wetsvoorstel Tijdelijke wet maatregelen covid-19 in relatie tot de persoonlijke levenssfeer (Everything becomes liquid under pressure: about emergency decrees and the interim COVID-19 measures act in relation to privacy). *Tijdschrift voor Constitutioneel Recht* 11 (4): 364–381.

De Jong, M.A.D.W. (2021). Tijd voor een Wet maatregelen virusuitbraak? (Time for a disease outbreak measures act?). *RegelMaat* 37 (3): 7–24.

Roozendaal, B. and Van Sande, S. (2020). COVID-19 in het publiekrecht – een overzicht (COVID-19 in public law – an overview). *Nederlands Juristenblad* 879 (14): 938–947.

Vink, J. (2020). Het Nederlandse staatsnoodrecht. Wat te doen met de EHBO-trommel die niet op orde is? (The Dutch emergency powers legislation. How to work with a failing first-aid kit?). *Nederlands juristenblad* 1134 (18): 1308–1316.

Wierenga, A.J., Schilder, A.E., and Brouwer, J.G. (2020). Aanpak coronacrisis niet houdbaar (COVID-19 crisis approach not tenable). *Nederlands Juristenblad* 1135 (18): 1317.

Wierenga, A.J. (2021). De ongekende opleving van het noodrecht in de coronacrisis (The unprecedented recrudescence of emergency law during the COVID-19 crisis). *Ars Aequi* 7 (8): 660–670.

Legislation

Besluit van 22 januari 2021, houdende inwerkingtreding en inwerkingstelling van artikel 8, eerste en derde lid van de Wet buitengewone bevoegdheden burgerlijk gezag (Decree of 22 January 2021, Providing for the Entry Into Force and Activation of Article 8(1) and (3) Civil Authority Special Powers Act), Article 1.

Besluit van 22 februari 2021, houdende buitenwerkingstelling van artikel 8, eerste en derde lid, van de Wet buitengewone bevoegdheden burgerlijk gezag (Decree of 22 February 2021, Providing for Deactivation of Article 8(1) and (3) Wbbbg).

Besluit van 17 mei 2021, houdende de tweede verlenging van de geldigheidsduur van de Tijdelijke wet maatregelen covid-19 (Decree of 17 May 2021, Providing for the Second Extension of the Duration of the Interim Covid-19 Measures Act).

Charter of Fundamental Rights of the European Union 2000.

Constitution Of The World Health Organization 1946.

Coördinatiewet uitzonderingstoestanden (Exceptional Situations Coordination Act) 1968, Articles 2, 3(a).

European Convention for the Protection of Human Rights and Fundamental Freedoms 1950, Articles 2, 8-11, 15.

European Social Charter 2006.

Gemeentewet (Municipalities Act) 1992, Articles 61, 175, 176, 180, 268.

Grondwet voor het Koninkrijk der Nederlanden (Dutch Constitution) 1815, Articles 6, 8-10, 12, 81, 84(2), 94, 103, 132(4).

Hamsterwet (Hoarding Act) 1962, Article 3.

Infectieziektenwet (Infectious Diseases Act) 1998.

Instellingsbesluit bestuurlijk afstemmingsoverleg infectieziektebestrijding (Instituting Decree Administrative Consultative Committee on Infectious Disease Control) 2004, Articles 2(1) and 3.

International Covenant on Civil and Political Rights 1966, Articles 4, 18.

International Covenant on Economic, Social and Cultural Rights 1966.

International Health Regulations 2005.

Kernenergiewet (Nuclear Energy Act) 1963, Article 40.

Ministeriële regeling 2019-nCoV 28-01-2020 (Ministerial Regulation 2019-nCoV 28 January 2020) 2020.

Quarantainewet (Quarantine Act) 1960.

Regeling van de Ministers van Volksgezondheid, Welzijn en Sport, van Justitie en Veiligheid en van Binnenlandse Zaken en Koninkrijksrelaties van 24 december 2020, kenmerk 1806234-216586-WJZ, tot wijziging van de Tijdelijke regeling maatregelen covid-19 in verband met het vereisen van een negatieve testuitslag voor internationaal openbaar Vervoer, Regulation issued by the Minister of Health (Welfare and Sport, the Minister of Justice and Security, and the Minister of the Interior and Kingdom Relations of 24 December 2020, reference number 1806234-216586-WJZ, to amend the Interim COVID-19 Measures Act, Twm COVID-19 regarding the requirement of a negative test result for international public transport).

Tijdelijke regeling landelijke avondklok covid-19 (Interim Regulation National Curfew COVID-19) 2021, Article 1.

Tijdelijke wet beperking vertoeven in de openlucht covid-19 (Interim Restriction on Staying Outdoors COVID-19 Act) 2021.

Tijdelijke wet maatregelen covid-19 (Interim COVID-19 Measures Act, Twm COVID-19) 2020.

Wet bestrijding maritieme ongevallen (Maritime Accidents Act) 2015, Article 7ff.

Wet buitengewone bevoegdheden burgerlijk gezag (Civil Authority Special Powers Act, Wbbbg) 1996, Articles 1, 7, 8.

Wet collectieve preventie volksgezondheid (Public Health Preventive Orders Act) 1990.

Wet op de uitoefening der geneeskunst (Medicine Practice Act) 1885.

Wet op het RIVM (RIVM Act) 1996.

Wet publieke gezondheid (Public Health Act) 2008, Articles 1(i), 6(4), 7(1) and (4), 20, 34(1) and (3), 35, 47(3)(a), 58b(2), 58c, 58f-58j(1)(a) and (f), 58o, 58p, 58r-58t.

Wet publieke gezondheid BES (BES Public Health Act) 2010.

Wet ter wering en beteugeling van besmettelijke ziekten (Prevention and Control of Infectious Diseases Act) 1872.

Wet van 8 januari 2021 tot wijziging van de Wet publieke gezondheid in verband met een verduidelijking van de tijdelijke grondslag voor het stellen van regels over de toegang tot en het gebruik van voorzieningen voor personenvervoer (Act of 8 January 2021 to amend the Public Health Act regarding clarification of the interim legal basis for issuing rules concerning admission to and use of passenger transport services).

Wet van 14 juli 2021 tot wijziging van de Tijdelijke wet maatregelen covid-19 in verband met regeling van het vereiste van goedkeuring bij wet van een koninklijk besluit tot verlenging als bedoeld in artikel VIII, derde lid, van de Tijdelijke wet maatregelen covid-19 (Act of 14 July 2021 Amending the Interim COVID-19 Measures Act in Relation to the Required Approval by Act of Parliament of a Royal Decree of Extension in the Sense of Article VIII(3) Interim COVID-19 Measures Act), Article 1.

Wet veiligheidsregio's (Safety Regions Act) 2010, Articles 1, 5, 8(appendix), 10(a) and (e), 11, 39, 40, 42.

Wet verplaatsing bevolking (Population Evacuation Act) 1952, Article 2a.

Case law

ECtHR 18 June 1971 (De Wilde, Ooms and Versyp/Belgium),
ECLI:NCE:ECHR:1971:0618JUD000283266, par. 96.

ECtHR 7 December 1976 (*Handyside/United Kingdom*), ECLI:CE:ECHR:1976:1207JUD000549372.

ECtHR 30 November 2004 (Öneryildiz/Turkey), ECLI:CE:ECHR:2004:1130JUD004893999, par. 71.

The Hague Court 19 June 2020, ECLI:NL:RBDHA:2020:5865.

The Hague Court 27 June 2020, ECLI:NL:RBDHA:2020:5865.

Amsterdam Court 19 August 2020, ECLI:NL:RBAMS:2020:4057.

Council of State Administrative Court Division 9 December 2020, ECLI:NL:RVS:2020:2839, with
annotation of J.G. Brouwer an A.E. Schilder (*AB* 2021/183).

The Hague Court (preliminary relief judge) 31 December 2020, ECLI:NL:RBDHA:2020:13643, par. 10.

The Hague Court (spreliminary relief judge) 8 January 2021, ECLI:NL:RBDHA:2021:63, par. 4.4.

The Hague Court (preliminary relief judge) 8 January 2021, ECLI:NL:RBDHA:2021:282, par. 1.6.

The Hague Court (preliminary relief judge) 28 January 2021, ECLI:NL:RBDHA:2021:600.

The Hague Court (preliminary relief judge) 16 February 2021, ECLI:NL:RBDHA:2021:1100, paras. 2.6.,
3.2., 4.1., 4.11.-4.14., and 5.1.

Court of Appeal of The Hague 16 February 2021, ECLI:NL:GHDHA:2021:252, paras. 6.4.-6.11, and 6.15.

Parliamentary documents

Handelingen I (Proceedings Senate) 2020/21, no. 26, 12.

Kamerbrief (Letter to Parliament) 'Antwoorden op de vragen van het Kamerlid Asscher (PvdA) over de
besluitvorming in de coronapandemie' (Answer to MP Asscher's Questions About Decision-making
During the COVID-19 pandemic) of the Minister of Health, Welfare, and Sport, reference
1760471-212563-PDC19.

Kamerstukken II (Parliamentary Papers House of Representatives) 1993/94, 23790, no. 3, p. 7.

Kamerstukken II (Parliamentary Papers House of Representatives), 2020/21, 25295, no. 742.

Kamerstukken II (Parliamentary Papers House of Representatives) 2020/21, 35526, no. 30

Kamerstukken I (Parliamentary Papers Senate) 2020/21, 35526, B, amended legislative proposal.

Kamerstukken II (Parliamentary Papers House of Representatives) 2020/21, 35695, no. 3.

Newspaper articles

Keulemans, M. (2020). Eerste coronapatiënten in Nederland, wat betekent dit? (First COVID-19
Patients in the Netherlands, What Does it Mean?). *De Volkskrant* (27 February 2020).

2

Emergencies, Executive Power, and Ireland's Response to the Covid-19 Pandemic

Alan Greene

Reader in Constitutional Law and Human Rights, Birmingham Law School, Birmingham, United Kingdom

2.1 Introduction

On 12 March 2020, the Taoiseach (Irish Prime Minister) Leo Varadkar announced in an address to the nation that schools, colleges, and childcare facilities would close until 29 March 2020 due to COVID-19.[1] The Taoiseach made his remarks in Washington where he was attending annual St. Patrick's Day events. Exactly one year later on 12 March 2021, Varadkar who was now Tánaiste (Deputy Prime Minister) admitted that he believed the first lockdown would only last six weeks; instead, Ireland experienced substantial coronavirus restrictions for well over a year. At the time of writing (July 2021), many of these restrictions are still in effect.[2]

Ireland has taken a relatively robust response to the pandemic as evidenced by this lengthy lockdown. That stated, Ireland, often touted as an "open economy" heavily dependent upon foreign direct investment, has also been considerably reluctant to restrict international travel. Moreover, the two jurisdictions on the island made it politically difficult, if not impossible to restrict travel between Ireland and the United Kingdom (UK). The Irish Government has frequently stressed that its decisions are backed by science and that they are following the recommendations of the expert National Public Health Emergency Team (NPHET).[3] However, the Government has also deviated from NPHET advice at certain pivotal moments, most notably in the lead up to Christmas 2020 in pursuit of the Government's stated objective of allowing people a "meaningful Christmas."[4] Ireland's pandemic response thus illustrates the complex tapestry of scientific, normative, economic, domestic political, and international political factors that influence the state's emergency response.

This complex political tapestry will form the background to this chapter's analysis of the key restrictions Ireland enacted in response to the COVID-19 pandemic. A comprehensive analysis of Ireland's entire pandemic response measures would not be possible in this brief chapter. Therefore,

1 'Taoiseach's full statement: "I need to speak to you about coronavirus"' *RTÉ News* (12 March 2020) https://www.rte.ie/news/coronavirus/2020/0312/1121849-taoiseach-full-statement-coronavirus-ireland/ accessed 13 July 2021.
2 'Varadkar admits he expected Ireland's first lockdown to last only six weeks' *The Irish Times* (12 March 2021) https://www.irishtimes.com/news/politics/varadkar-admits-he-expected-ireland-s-first-lockdown-to-last-only-six-weeks-1.4508474 accessed 13 July 2021.
3 'National Public Health Emergency Team (NPHET) for COVID-19: Governance structures' *Department of Health* (28 April 2020, last updated 24 September 2020) https://www.gov.ie/en/publication/de1c30-national-public-health-emergency-team-nphet-for-covid-19-governance-/ accessed 24 July 2021.
4 Simon Carswell, 'How did Ireland jump from low Covid base to world's highest infection rate?' *The Irish Times* (16 January 2021) https://www.irishtimes.com/news/health/how-did-ireland-jump-from-low-covid-base-to-world-s-highest-infection-rate-1.4459429 accessed 24 July 2021.

Impacts of the Covid-19 Pandemic: International Laws, Policies, and Civil Liberties, First Edition. Edited by Nadav Morag.
© 2023 John Wiley & Sons, Inc. Published 2023 by John Wiley & Sons, Inc.

focus will be on particular measures that most people in Ireland have experienced directly; namely, measures restricting a person's liberty and movements, and what businesses, events, and associations were permitted to operate. Focus shall also be on how these measures were enacted and the degree to which constitutional checks and balances facilitated or curtailed the state's response. In addition, this article shall evaluate the rule of law implications of these measures. Ultimately, this article argues that Ireland's response to the COVID-19 pandemic and the impact this response has had on key constitutional values, such as human rights, the separation of powers, and the rule of law, bears all the hallmarks of an emergency response albeit without a formal declaration of a state of emergency. While there are strong public health and human rights justifications underpinning the state's robust response to the pandemic, not least the necessity to prevent catastrophic loss of life; it is nevertheless the case that this "de facto state of emergency" may have long-term damaging consequences for these constitutionalist values in Ireland beyond the pandemic. Moreover, the political tapestry of factors that affect government decision-making, beyond simply scientific advice underlies the importance of legal and political accountability mechanisms for pandemic decision-making.

2.2   Ireland's Constitutional Emergency Framework

Like many states, Ireland enacted an emergency response to the COVID-19 pandemic. An emergency response is understood here as:

> A crisis identified and labelled by a state to be of such magnitude that it is deemed to cross a threat severity threshold, necessitating urgent, exceptional, and, consequently, temporary actions by the state not permissible when normal conditions exist.[5]

Ireland enacted numerous exceptional measures in response to this threat of substantial magnitude that, at the time of writing, had caused the deaths of over 5,000 people in the Republic of Ireland and over 7,000 deaths on the island as a whole.[6] In order to understand the exceptionality of these measures, it is first necessary to set out the constitutional and other legal standards against which such a response can be appraised. Formerly a constituent part of the UK, 26 of the 32 counties of Ireland gained dominion status from the UK in 1921 resulting in the creation of the Irish Free State. The resultant Irish Free State Constitution was subsequently replaced by the Constitution enacted in 1937 and which continues in effect to this date. Preserving its common law tradition, the 1937 Constitution established a parliamentary democracy with a muscular judiciary empowered to invalidate legislation if incompatible with constitutional norms.[7] These constitutional norms entail various enumerated and unenumerated human rights,[8] as well as key provisions pertaining to the separation of powers such as the nondelegation of legislative functions to authorities other than the Oireachtas – Ireland's bicameral legislature consisting of Dáil Éireann (lower house) and the Seanad (upper house).[9]

---

5 Alan Greene, *Permanent States of Emergency and the Rule of Law: Constitutions in an Age of Crisis* (Hart Publishing, 2018), 30.
6 'Ireland: coronavirus cases' *Worldometer* (last updated 26 July 2021) https://www.worldometers.info/coronavirus/country/ireland/ accessed 26 July 2021; 'Coronavirus (COVID-19) statistics' *Northern Ireland Statistics and Research Agency* (last updated 26 July 2021) https://www.nisra.gov.uk/statistics/ni-summary-statistics/coronavirus-covid-19-statistics accessed 26 July 2021.
7 Article 34.3.2°, Constitution of Ireland.
8 Article 40, Constitution of Ireland. The concept of unenumerated constitutional rights was first identified in *Ryan v Attorney General* [1965] IR 294.
9 Article 15.2.1°, Constitution of Ireland.

The Irish Constitution does make express provision for a state of emergency to be declared by the Oireachtas. Subject to three amendments to date, Article 28.3.3° of the Irish Constitution currently reads as follows:

> Nothing in this Constitution other than Article 15.5.2° shall be invoked to invalidate any law enacted by the Oireachtas which is expressed to be for the purpose of securing the public safety and the preservation of the State in time of war or armed rebellion, or to nullify any act done or purporting to be done in time of war or armed rebellion in pursuance of any such law. In this subsection "time of war" includes a time when there is taking place an armed conflict in which the State is not a participant but in respect of which each of the Houses of the Oireachtas shall have resolved that, arising out of such armed conflict, a national emergency exists affecting the vital interests of the State and "time of war or armed rebellion" includes such time after the termination of any war, or of any such armed conflict as aforesaid, or of an armed rebellion, as may elapse until each of the Houses of the Oireachtas shall have resolved that the national emergency occasioned by such war, armed conflict, or armed rebellion has ceased to exist.[10]

The breadth of the powers afforded to the state under Article 28.3.3° is striking. Essentially, no provision of the Constitution, other than Article 15.5.2°, can be used to invalidate and Act of Parliament which derives its validity from Article 28.3.3°.[11] Article 15.5.2° that prohibits the introduction of the death penalty was introduced to the Constitution in 2001 meaning that from 1939 to 1995, when a declaration of emergency under Article 28.3.3° was in effect, the Oireachtas essentially had carte blanche to respond to the emergencies as it saw fit.[12] Article 28.3.3° could not, however, be used in response to the COVID-19 pandemic as it only permits an emergency "in time of war or armed rebellion." The meaning of "time of war" in Article 28.3.3° has been amended twice to allow for the declaration of an emergency in response to a war in which the state is not a belligerent, and to cover the period after the cessation of the conflict but during which emergency powers may still be necessary.[13] Despite this expansion of the meaning "time of war," a pandemic clearly falls outside of this definition and so any legislation enacted in response to the pandemic had to be compatible with the ordinary parameters of the Constitution.[14] As a result, Ireland did not enter into a de jure state of emergency during the COVID-19 pandemic. Nevertheless, as we shall see, the idea of necessary, exceptional, temporary powers that would not previously have been contemplated accurately describes Ireland's response to the COVID-19 pandemic. To this end, Ireland experienced a "de-facto emergency," where officially, a state of normalcy was in existence but the state, nevertheless, enacted exceptional powers in response to a crisis represented as an extreme aberration from the status quo.[15]

This official state of normalcy did not necessarily mean that Ireland's response to the pandemic would be unduly restrained by the Constitution; in contrast, the Irish courts have frequently demonstrated a considerable willingness to stretch the meaning of constitutional provisions to accommodate exceptional powers without the need to declare a state of emergency. A recent

---

10 Article 28.3.3°, Constitution of Ireland.
11 See Alan Greene, 'The historical evolution of Article 28.3.3° of the Irish constitution' (2012) 47(1) *Irish Jurist* 117.
12 ibid 140–141; James Casey, *Constitutional Law in Ireland,* (3rd ed Roundhall, 2000) 181.
13 First Amendment of the Constitution Act 1939, Second Amendment of the Constitution Act 1941; Greene (n 9) 130–135.
14 It should be noted, however, that the Supreme Court has expressly refused to say whether or not the decision to declare a state of emergency is amenable to judicial review. See *Re Emergency Powers Bill 1976* [1977] IR 159.
15 On the term "de facto emergency," see 'Study of the Implications for Human Rights of Recent Developments Concerning Situations Known as States of Siege or Emergency,' UNESC E/CN4/Sub2/1982/15 (27 July 1982) 26.

example of this can be seen from the Supreme Court case taken by Joan Collins TD challenging the vast powers conferred on the Minister for Finance by the Credit Institutions (Financial Support) Act 2008 in response to the 2008 financial crisis. There, the Supreme Court upheld the constitutionality of these powers as they were "a permissible constitutional response to an exceptional situation."[16] This was so, despite the fact that no emergency was (or even could have been) declared using Article 28.3.3°. A similar deferential approach can be seen through the Court's jurisprudence on the existence of special courts established under Article 38.3.1°. While such courts may only be established when "the ordinary courts are inadequate to secure the effective administration of justice, and the preservation of public peace and order," the current inception of the nonjury Special Criminal Court has been in operation since 1972 and is now "hard-wired" into the state's criminal justice system.[17] This is largely due to the fact that the courts have substantially deferred to the executive's assessment of the question as to whether "the ordinary courts are inadequate to secure the effective administration of justice, and the preservation of public peace and order" to such an extent that it is almost nonjusticiable.[18] It is only if mala fides on the part of the executive can be shown will such a declaration be unlawful; however, the courts have also found that the executive has no duty to give reasons to justify this, making it almost impossible to demonstrate mala fides.[19] Irish courts have therefore demonstrated the willingness to defer to the elected branches of government in times of crisis, interpreting constitutional norms to facilitate rather than constrain exceptional state power.[20] While, at the time of writing, jurisprudence pertaining to the pandemic is sparse, it is likely a similarly deferential approach may be taken by the course in response to COVID-19. The consequences of such deference may, in turn, have implications long after the pandemic recedes.

2.2.1 International Human Rights Law

In addition to constitutional norms, Ireland is also a signatory to several international human rights treaties relevant to the state's response to the pandemic. For instance, Ireland is a signatory to the International Covenant on Civil and Political Rights (ICCPR) and was one of the founding members of the Council of Europe and signatory to the European Convention on Human Rights (ECHR). The ECHR was incorporated into domestic law through the European Convention on Human Rights Act 2003 (ECHRA 2003). The ECHRA 2003 requires "every organ of the state" to "perform its functions in a manner compatible with the State's obligations under the Convention provisions."[21] The Act also places a duty on courts to interpret legislation compatibly with the Convention "so far as is possible to do so,"[22] and also empowers courts to declare legislation incompatible with the ECHR when this is not possible. Unlike a finding of unconstitutionality a declaration of incompatibility with the ECHR does not, however, affect the validity of the legislation in question.[23] Relatedly, while Article 15 ECHR does permit derogations from most Convention rights "In time of war or

---

16 *Collins v Minister for Finance* [2016] IESC 73.
17 See Fionnuala Ní Aoláin, 'The special criminal court: a conveyor belt of exceptionality' in Mark Coen (ed), *The Offences Against the State Act 1939 at 80: A Model Counter-Terrorism Act?* (Hart Publishing, 2021) 59, 70–71.
18 *Kavanagh v Ireland* [1996] I IR 321.
19 *Re MacCurtain,* [1941] IR 83.
20 This is a common feature of what Oren Gross terms the 'business as usual approach' to emergency responses. See Oren Gross, 'Chaos and rules: should responses to violent crises always be constitutional' (2003) 112 *Yale Law Journal* 1011, 1043–1058.
21 Section 3(1) ECHRA 2003.
22 Section 2 ECHRA 2003.
23 Section 5 ECHRA 2003.

other public emergency threatening the life of the nation," Ireland chose not to derogate in response to the COVID-19 pandemic.[24]

Ireland is also a signatory to several human rights treaties pertaining to specific groups such as the Convention on the Rights of Persons with Disabilities, the UN Convention on the Elimination of all Forms of Discrimination against Women (CEDAW), and the UN Convention on the Rights of the Child. Many of these treaties contained provisions acutely affected by the pandemic as its impact, and the impact of pandemic responses enacted were not dispersed evenly throughout society. Finally, Ireland has ratified several treaties pertaining to socioeconomic rights; rights which come to the fore in a pandemic where the state response is to shut down vast sectors of the economy, and require people who may be infected to stay at home and not go to work. Consequently, Ireland's pandemic response had to conform with various constitutional and international human rights standards.

2.3 Ireland's Pandemic Response and Constitutional Constraints

As noted, for the entire duration of the pandemic, Ireland has remained in a de jure state of normalcy, despite the exceptional nature of both the threat posed by COVID-19 and the state's response contained in the legislation enacted and the powers conferred on the executive. Nevertheless, the Oireachtas and the Government has deployed the language of "emergency" to frame the state's response to the pandemic and to politically demarcate it from the status quo prior to the outbreak of the pandemic in March 2020. This de facto state of emergency was further underlined through the use of sunset clauses in pandemic-related legislation to signal the temporary nature of the measures, and the expedited manner in which the Oireachtas enacted the emergency legislation in question conveying its urgency and necessity.[25]

Following the Irish general election result of February 2020, a hung parliament was returned with the three largest parties all within three seats of each other. With the prospect of extended coalition negotiations looming, it fell on the outgoing government – some of whom had lost their seats in the February election – to steer Ireland's emergency response in the early days of the pandemic. To confront the pandemic, Ireland enacted at least 14 pieces of primary legislation.[26] Ireland's initial legislative response to the pandemic was contained in the Health (Preservation and Protection and other Emergency Measures in the Public Interest) Act 2020 (hereinafter the Health Act), and the Emergency Measures in the Public Interest (Covid-19) Act 2020 (hereinafter the Emergency Act). Both acts passed the Oireachtas without a formal vote with all parties in agreement as to the necessity of the measures enacted. In so doing, the Oireachtas demonstrated a key feature of state emergency responses: convergence among the political spectrum as to the necessity of the measures enacted and the conferral of vast, discretionary power on the executive branch of government as a result.[27]

---

24 Article 15 ECHR.
25 John Ferejohn and Pasquale Pasquino, 'The law of the exception: a typology of emergency powers' (2004) 2 *International Journal of Constitutional Law* 210, 217–221; John Ip, 'Sunset clauses and counterterrorism legislation' (2013) *Public Law* 74.
26 Eoin Carolan and Ailbhe O'Neill, 'Ireland: legal response to Covid-19' in Jeff King and Octavio Ferraz (eds), *The Oxford Compendium of National Legal Responses to COVID-19* (Oxford University Press, 2021) https://oxcon.ouplaw .com/view/10.1093/law-occ19/law-occ19-e19 accessed 24 July 2021, 4–5.
27 Alan Greene, *Permanent States of Emergency and the Rule of Law: Constitutions in an Age of Crisis* (Hart Publishing, 2018) 24–25.

2.3.1 Pandemic Rent Controls and Constitutional Constraints

While the Health Act 2020 contained the majority of exceptional powers enacted to confront the pandemic, the Emergency Act 2020 centered more on the state's initial economic response to the crisis, as well as relaxing regulations pertaining to employing health professionals and armed forces personnel who recently retired or left the profession. Due to its financial focus, the Emergency Act 2020 was initially subject to a three-month sunset clause whereby it was believed that a new government would be formed following coalition negotiations. This new government would then have the requisite legitimacy to enact further financial measures to confront the pandemic. Consequently, many of the subsequent statutes pertaining to the pandemic were to give effect to various financial measures enacted by the new government which took office in June 2020.[28] This government consisted of the two centre-right parties of Fianna Fáil and Fine Gael, and the Green Party.

The most exceptional aspect of the Emergency Act 2020 was the prohibition of rent increases during the emergency pandemic period. The subject of rent freezes was a high-profile issue during Ireland's general election campaign at the start of 2020.[29] Parties of the left argued that a rent freeze was a necessary response to what they termed Ireland's "housing emergency" caused by a substantial housing shortage which had its origins in the 2008 financial crash.[30] In contrast, centre-right parties opposed rent freezes, with Fianna Fáil arguing that rent freezes would be unconstitutional due to their impact on the right to private property protected by Article 43 of the Constitution.[31] This was based on a tenuous reading of a narrow Supreme Court judgment where rent controls on certain arbitrarily selected dwellings were found to be unconstitutional.[32] Concerns as to the constitutionality of a rent freeze to deal with the pandemic, however, were conspicuous by their absence during the debate on the Emergency Act 2020, notwithstanding the lack of a de jure state of emergency under the Constitution. In July 2021, however, Fianna Fáil Taoiseach Micheál Martin ruled out further rent freezes or linking rent increases to inflation, resurrecting the argument that they were unconstitutional.[33] The debate surrounding the constitutionality of rent restrictions in Ireland demonstrates how the language of emergency can be used to both justify *and* delegitimize certain measures. Despite the lack of a de jure emergency, the exceptionality of the pandemic was used to justify the temporary freezing of rents with this temporal limit factored into the proportionality of the restriction on property rights. A permanent rent freeze or permanent, stricter rent controls are then ruled out precisely because they lack this time limit. This is so, notwithstanding the fact that the proportionality question should be based on a holistic assessment of the regime as a whole, not simply on the basis of the presence or absence of one specific safeguard.[34] The Government's contention that linking rents to inflation would be unconstitutional has been subject to substantial

---

28 Marie O'Halloran, Fiach Kelly and Pat Leahy, 'Micheál Martin elected Taoiseach as head of coalition' *The Irish Times* (27 June 2020) https://www.irishtimes.com/news/politics/miche%C3%A1l-martin-elected-taoiseach-as-head-of-coalition-1.4290529 accessed 19 July 2021.

29 Jennifer Bray, 'Election 2020: FF decides against rent freeze on "legal advice"' *The Irish Times* (21 January 2020) https://www.irishtimes.com/news/politics/election-2020-ff-decides-against-rent-freeze-on-legal-advice-1.4146755 accessed 24 July 2021.

30 Hayley Halpin, 'Q+A: Here's where Ireland's political parties stand on housing and homelessness ahead of the election' *The Journal.ie* (4 February 2020) https://www.thejournal.ie/housing-homelessness-general-election-4985853-Feb2020/ accessed 25 July 2021.

31 Hugh O'Connell, '"It's unconstitutional" – Martin says FF won't back rent freeze despite admitting staff committed to measure' *Irish Independent* (31 January 2020) https://www.independent.ie/irish-news/election-2020/its-unconstitutional-martin-says-ff-wont-back-rent-freeze-despite-admitting-staff-committed-to-measure-38915674.html accessed 19 July 2021.

32 *Blake v Attorney General* [1981] ILRM 34.

33 Aoife Moore, 'Taoiseach rules out another rent freeze as "unconstitutional"' *Irish Examiner* (14 July 2021) https://www.irishexaminer.com/news/politics/arid-40336928.html accessed 19 July 2021.

34 *Heaney v Ireland* [1994] 3 IR 593.

academic critique as corroborating the contention that Irish governments often use constitutional constraints and legal advice as scapegoats to mask what are, in reality, ideological objections to the policy proposals in question.[35]

2.3.2 Executive Supremacy and the COVID-19 Pandemic

While one may have expected a statute entitled the "Emergency Act" to contain the state's principal response to the pandemic; in reality, it was the Health Act 2020 which contained the most striking emergency provisions. The Health Act 2020 amended the Health Act 1947 which was itself enacted in response to outbreaks of tuberculosis and was described as providing "a complete code of the law relating to the prevention of the spread of infectious disease." The key aspect of the Health Act 2020 was Part III which conferred on the Minister for Health powers to make regulations for the broadly defined purpose of "preventing, limiting, minimising or slowing the spread of Covid-19." Section 10 of the Health Act 2020 empowered the Minister for Health to pass regulations that could include the power to restrict travel to or from the state, require persons to stay in their homes, and prohibit the holding of events. Section 10(i) further expanded upon these already broad powers to allow the minister to enact "any other measures the Minister considers necessary in order to prevent, limit, minimise or slow the spread of Covid-19." It was through these powers that Ireland's lockdown was implemented and amended over the course of the pandemic.

The scope of measures enacted under Part III of the Health Act 2020 was substantial. Businesses and schools were closed, often for long periods of time, with some businesses staying closed from March 2020 to July 2021.[36] Large gatherings were prohibited and the right to protest substantially curtailed; sporting and live music events were cancelled, and strict attendance limits on funerals and other religious services were introduced. On 13 July 2020, a requirement to wear face coverings on public transport was introduced by the Minister under the powers conferred upon him by the Health Act 1947. This measure was originally due to expire on 5 October 2020 but was extended until 9 June 2021. It was then further extended to November 2021 with a possible further extension to February 2022. A similar obligation to wear face-masks in certain businesses and premises such as shops was introduced in August 2020 and was also extended to June 2021 and again until November 2021 with a possible further extension to February 2022.[37]

The breadth of executive power conferred by the Health Act 2020 raises a number of questions from a constitutionalist perspective. Article 15.2.1° vests the sole and exclusive law-making power for the state in the Oireachtas and unfettered delegation of law-making powers to an authority other than the Oireachtas will be unconstitutional. However, the courts have often adopted a hands-off approach to this question only striking down legislation if "that which is challenged is more than the mere giving effect to principles and policies which are contained in the statute itself."[38] The parent act must also contain sufficient principles and policies to guide the exercise of the delegated power in question.[39] Consequently, it is unlikely that a court would find Section 10 of the Health Act unconstitutional, notwithstanding the breadth of discretion afforded to the executive. This is

---

35 See David Kenny and Conor Casey, 'A one person Supreme Court? The Attorney General, constitutional advice to government, and the case for transparency' (2019) 42 *Dublin University Law Journal* 89.

36 Jade Wilson, '"Day of relief" as indoor hospitality reopens after some venues have been closed almost 500 days' *The Irish Times* (26 July 2021) https://www.irishtimes.com/news/ireland/irish-news/day-of-relief-as-indoor-hospitality-reopens-after-some-venues-have-been-closed-almost-500-days-1.4630233 accessed 26 July 2021.

37 Jennifer Bray, 'Cabinet to extend sweeping pandemic powers until November' *The Irish Times* (18 May 2021) https://www.irishtimes.com/news/politics/cabinet-to-extend-sweeping-pandemic-powers-until-november-1 .4568608 accessed 21 July 2021.

38 *Cityview Press v AnCo* [1980] IR 381, 399.

39 See *Bederev v Ireland* [2016] IESC 34.

particularly so given the propensity of Irish courts to defer to the political branches in times of crisis.[40]

That stated, Henry VIII clauses – powers conferred on the executive to amend primary legislation – are not permitted under the Irish Constitution as such would be a violation of the Oireachtas' power to legislate.[41] Moreover, section 5 of the Health Act 1947 states that regulations made under the Act must be laid before each House of the Oireachtas as soon as possible after being made. Either House may then annul the regulation by resolution within 21 days. Casey et al., however, note that in reality, such powers are almost never used, not least owing to the fact that the government has a built-in majority in the Dáil, with additional mechanisms in place to also ensure executive dominance of the Seanad.[42] Indeed, to even get a debate on a resolution regarding the annulment of a regulation is difficult with Casey et al. noting that in the week of 11 May 2020, some 14 sets of COVID-related regulations were laid before each House but only on one occasion did a deputy manage to move a motion to annul a set of regulations.[43]

Throughout the pandemic, legislative oversight has also been severely impacted by the difficulty in convening both houses due to social distancing requirements. While many states implemented measures for remote hearings,[44] the Ceann Comhairle (Speaker of the Dáil) received legal advice that remote hearings would be unconstitutional owing to the requirement that Article 15.1.3° of the Constitution states that "The Houses of the Oireachtas shall sit in or near the City of Dublin or in such other place as they may from time to time determine." This, it was contented, stipulated a *physical* sitting. This hyper-literal interpretation of the Constitution was critiqued by several commentators, arguing that a purposive approach to Article 15.1.3° reveals that the provision was designed to ensure the integrity of the voting record.[45] There were therefore no good constitutional or practical reasons why remote hearings could not take place so long as systems were developed to ensure the integrity of the voting record. Instead, the Oireachtas moved to the Convention Centre in Dublin and sat in a diminished capacity. Moreover, no ordinary committees of the Oireachtas sat between January and October 2020.[46]

Part III of the Health Act was initially subject to a sunset clause and was due to expire on 9 November 2020. In October 2020, the measures were renewed until 9 June 2021; however, there was considerable controversy over the fact that only 45 minutes of Oireachtas time would be set aside to debate the motion. When this was extended to an extent, some TDs nevertheless still protested.[47] On 2 June 2021, the measures were again extended until 9 November 2021. In the Seanad, the Health Minister Stephen Donnelly stated that the powers would only be extended, if necessary, for another three months after that date up to February 2022. If further similar powers were necessary, he proposed that a new bill would be introduced.[48] Legislative oversight of the powers conferred

---

40 Alan Greene, 'A less exceptional state of exception: the offences against the state act as an emergency response' in Mark Coen (ed), *The Offences Against the State Act 1939 at 80* (n 15) 221, 234-237.

41 Carolan and O'Neill (n 23) [7].

42 For instance, Article 18.3 of the Constitution empowers the Taoiseach to nominate 11 of the 60 Senators that constitute the Seanad.

43 Conor Casey, Oran Doyle, David Kenny and Donna Lyons, *Ireland's Emergency Powers During the Covid-19 Pandemic* (Irish Human Rights and Equality Commission, February 2021) https://www.ihrec.ie/documents/irelands-emergency-powers-during-the-covid-19-pandemic/ accessed 3 July 2021, 49–50.

44 Alan Greene, *Emergency Powers in a Time of Pandemic* (Bristol University Press, 2020) 101–108.

45 ibid 106–107.

46 Casey et al. (n 38) 49.

47 ibid 26.

48 Marie O'Halloran and Harry McGee, 'Emergency Covid-19 powers will end in February 2022, Minister for health Stephen Donnelly says' *Irish Times* (25 May 2021) https://www.irishtimes.com/news/politics/oireachtas/emergency-covid-19-powers-will-end-in-february-2022-minister-for-health-stephen-donnelly-says-1.4575006 accessed 23 July 2021.

on the executive therefore has been light-touch at best; at worst, the impact of the pandemic has stymied even the ordinary legislative functions of the Oireachtas, weakening the ability of TDs and Senators to scrutinize legislation and hold the Government to account.

Overall, Ireland's pandemic response has resulted in the legislature conferring vast discretionary power on to the executive. As noted, this is a common feature of emergency responses generally. However, in contrast to national security emergencies where the executive can claim to have access to sensitive information that the legislature or judiciary does not or cannot have access to, the same cannot necessarily be said in the case of a public health emergency or pandemic. Thus, while the executive may be able to claim superior expertise in a national security emergency that the other branches of government should defer to, this argument is considerably less persuasive in a public health emergency.[49] It is distinctly disappointing therefore that the Oireachtas has been stymied in its effectiveness and important constitutional role in holding the government to account in an emergency where the arguments in favor of executive supremacy are considerably weaker.

2.4   Ireland's Pandemic Response and Human Rights

As noted, Ireland's pandemic response had to comply with various constitutional and international human rights protections and many of the measures the state enacted had significant and, at times, severe impacts on these rights. For instance, Article 40.6.1°ii, for example, protects the right of citizens "to assemble peaceably and without arms." Social distancing measures clearly impact upon the right to publicly protest and to organize and hold meetings of political organizations and trade unions.[50] This right is fundamental in a democratic society. However, like similar provisions in international treaties such as Article 11 ECHR, this right can be interfered with if meetings "are determined in accordance with law to be calculated to cause a breach of the peace or to be a danger or nuisance to the general public." Proportionality will be key and this will vary as the pandemic progresses.[51]

2.4.1   The Pandemic and the Right to Liberty

Like many states, the right to liberty and freedom of movement of persons were interfered with in a variety of ways. The Health Act 1947 originally introduced a detention regime for infected individuals or individuals who may be infected. These detention provisions in the 1947 Act were themselves designed to replace similar powers under the Emergency Powers (No. 46) Order 1940. This latter regime was enacted under the Emergency Powers Act 1939, which derived its validity from a declaration of emergency under Article 28.3.3° of the Constitution in force as a result of the outbreak of World War II. It was therefore not subject to constitutional constraints. That stated, the constitutionality of the detention powers in the 1947 Act were upheld in 2009 with the High Court finding that they supported an important public interest objective. Moreover, a detained person could have recourse to a habeas corpus petition at any time to challenge their detention.[52] Despite these existing powers, however, in response to the COVID-19 pandemic, section 11 of the Health

---

49 Greene (n 44) 117.
50 Despite this, some high-profile anti-lockdown protests did take place. See Conor Lally, Ronan McGreevy and Conor Pope, 'Large Garda presence sustained in Dublin for anti-lockdown protests' *The Irish Times* (17 March 2021) https://www.irishtimes.com/news/crime-and-law/large-garda-presence-sustained-in-dublin-for-anti-lockdown-protests-1.4512885 accessed 26 July 2021.
51 *Heaney* (n 34).
52 Carolan and O'Neill *S v HSE and Others* [2009] IEHC 106 (High court).

Act 2020 introduced new powers of "detention and isolation of persons in certain circumstances." A person could be detained under these provisions by a "medical officer of health" acting "in good faith." A detained person must be examined as soon as possible "and in any event no later than 14 days from the time the person has been detained. There was, however, no express time-limit on the duration which a person can be detained for under these provisions. A detained person can request that their detention be reviewed by a medical officer of health other than the officer who made the initial order on the grounds that they are not a potential source of infection." However, the appeal process to the Minister for Health under the 1947 Act is not applicable to somebody detained under the Health Act 2020. Nevertheless, as an Article 28.3.3° emergency is not in effect, the constitutional safeguards pertaining to *habeas corpus* set out in Article 40.4 still applied. Like many other provisions of the Health Act 2020, section 11 was originally due to sunset in November 2020; however, it was renewed on several occasions and, at the time of writing, is now scheduled to sunset in November 2021. As the powers under Schedule 11 do not appear to have been utilized during the pandemic, this raises substantial questions as to their stated necessity and, in turn, the efficacy of Oireachtas oversight of the Government's pandemic powers.

The Health Act 2020 also introduced substantial changes to the ordinary provisions pertaining to the detention of persons on mental health grounds, weakening key procedural safeguards regarding the right to a fair hearing. The justification for such changes were that it was alleged that such procedural safeguards would be too cumbersome and resource intensive during a pandemic; however, this argument has been vociferously critiqued as many state institutions have shown their capacity to still operate during the pandemic. Relatedly, Casey et al. state that whatever legitimacy this argument attracted at the outset of the pandemic, this was certainly not the case when the measures were renewed in October 2020 when the immediate urgency and uncertainty surrounding the pandemic has abated to an extent.[53]

2.4.1.1 Mandatory Hotel Quarantine

Despite the breadth of the powers conferred on the minister by the Health Act 2020, it was not the vehicle through which Ireland introduced mandatory hotel quarantine for those entering the state from "designated states" in March 2021. Instead, it was introduced through new legislation in the form of the Health (Amendment) Act 2021. The 2021 Act amended Section 2 of the 1947 Act, empowering the Minister to declare a state a "designated state" "where there is known to be sustained human transmission of Covid-19 or any variant of concern or from which there is a high risk of importation of infection or contamination with Covid-19 or any variant of concern by travel from that state."[54] Mandatory hotel quarantine had been suggested by NPHET as early as June 2020; however, the Government was reluctant to proceed with it for a variety of political and legal reasons. In February 2020, in response to a question from opposition leader Mary Lou McDonald, the Taoiseach heavily implied that mandatory hotel quarantine would be unconstitutional:

> There are compelling legal reasons [why] it is not possible to do what Deputy McDonald is suggesting. We have our Constitution, which has a clear framework concerning personal liberties and freedoms. Balancing is required, therefore, in respect of getting something in place which can be robust in resisting legal challenge.[55]

This prompted several responses from Irish constitutional academics in public fora with Conor O'Mahony arguing that while Article 40.4 of the Constitution proved that "No citizen shall be

---

53 Casey et al. (n 43) xii.
54 Section 38E(1).
55 Dáil Deb 3 Feb 2021 vol. 1003 No.7 (Mary Lou McDonald).

deprived of his personal liberty save in accordance with law" and that 14-day quarantine would certainly amount to a deprivation of liberty; nevertheless, the issue as to such a regime's constitutionality would come down to the question of proportionality.[56] This proportionality would be assessed by means of the test as laid down in *Heaney v Ireland* and that such a measure: first, pursues an objective of sufficient importance; second, is rationally connected to that objective and is not arbitrary or unfair; and finally, that it impairs the right as little as possible.[57] When making such a designation, the legislation set out several mandatory considerations the Minister must take into account when exercising their discretion to designate a state as necessitating mandatory hotel quarantine for arrivals. One important consideration was the requirement to consult the Minister for Foreign Affairs, demonstrating the complex geopolitical factors that were taken into consideration when placing a country on the designated list. Consequently, the decision was not solely based on scientific advice or wholly objective criteria such as virus circulation levels or "variants of concern" in specific states. As a result, several high-profile controversies arose over certain countries being labeled as designated states and others not. For instance, there was reportedly substantial opposition from the Minister for Foreign Affairs over the adding of EU countries and the United States as designated states.[58] The list of designated states was dominated by South American, sub-Saharan African, and Middle Eastern states, implying that geopolitical considerations other than the circulation of "variants of concern" were key factors in drawing up this list.[59] However, such factors do potentially undermine both the efficacy of the policy in mitigating the effects of the pandemic and preventing new variants emerging in Ireland, and the necessity of the deprivation of liberty of those in the hotel quarantine system due to arbitrariness. The ICCL, for example, argued that Israel's inclusion on the list on 5 April 2021 when its 14-day incidence rate per 100,000 was 58 was arbitrary as at the same time, the equivalent incidence rate in Ireland was 157.1.[60] Moreover, the Expert Advisory group suggested that France and the United States be categorized as designated states in March but they were not included until 15 April 2021.[61] Such arbitrariness has the potential to undermine the necessity of the detention of those who are subject to hotel quarantine.

Some limited exemptions to mandatory hotel quarantine were included in the scheme, the most notable being passengers who are fully vaccinated with documentation to prove this.[62]The period of mandatory hotel quarantine for arrivals from a designated state was 14 days; however, this period could end early on receipt of a negative PCR test taken pm day 10 of quarantine. The Act contained several grounds of appeal which could form the basis of a challenge against detention including if an individual needed urgent medical attention or if the detainee provided necessary care to a

56 Conor O'Mahony, 'The constitutionality of mandatory hotel quarantine' *Constitution Project @UCC* (4 February 2021) http://constitutionproject.ie/?p=792 accessed 6 July 2021. Similar arguments were also made by David Kenny in The Irish Times. See David Kenny, 'Mandatory quarantine allowable under the constitution' *The Irish Times* (4 February 2021) https://www.irishtimes.com/opinion/mandatory-quarantine-allowable-under-the-constitution-1 .4476110 accessed 6 July 2021.

57 *Heaney v Ireland* (n 31) 607.

58 Jack Horgan-Jones, Jennifer Bray and Paul Cullen, 'State facing pressure from EU countries after expanding quarantine list' *Irish Times* (12 April 2021) https://www.irishtimes.com/news/ireland/irish-news/state-facing-pressure-from-eu-countries-after-expanding-quarantine-list-1.4536562 accessed 26 July 2021.

59 Rónán Duffy, '20 countries to be on Ireland's mandatory hotel quarantine list' *TheJournal.ie* (11 February2021) https://www.thejournal.ie/mandatory-hotel-quarantine-list-5351005-Feb2021/ accessed 26 July 2021.

60 Irish Council for Civil Liberties, *Human Rights in a Pandemic: A Human Rights Analysis of the Irish Government's Response to COVID*-19 (May 2021) https://www.iccl.ie/wp-content/uploads/2021/06/Human-Rights-in-a-Pandemic .pdf accessed 26 July 2021, 56.

61 ibid 56.

62 'Mandatory hotel quarantine: your questions answered' *Department of Health* (23 March 2021, last updated 29 June 2021) https://www.gov.ie/en/publication/3b8e1-mandatory-hotel-quarantine-your-questions-answered/# exemptions-from-mandatory-hotel-quarantine accessed 24 July 2021.

vulnerable person.[63] Several high-profile legal challenges were taken against the requirement to quarantine, including one from a fully vaccinated person required to travel to Israel for work. He returned to Ireland upon hearing the news that his father was dying and, despite having a series of negative COVID-19 test results was still required to remain in hotel quarantine. He was then released after the High Court directed an inquiry into his detention.[64] In July 2021, the Mandatory Hotel Quarantine Scheme was extended to 31 October 2021.[65]

2.4.2 Quarantine and Detention at Home

In light of the fact that the detention regime under Section 11 of the Health Act 2020 was never used, mandatory hotel quarantine was the only exceptional form of institutional detention actually utilized. Instead, throughout various stages of the pandemic, substantial restrictions on people's movements and obligations to "stay at home" were in effect. In March 2020, Ireland moved quickly from a containment to mitigation stage of pandemic management and essentially remained in this mitigation stage for the duration of the pandemic to date. The World Health Organisation (WHO) divides pandemic responses into two stages: containment and mitigation. In the containment stage, states attempt to prevent the establishment of in-community transmission of the disease in the first place. Such measures are often targeted at specific areas or persons; for instance, people arriving into the state from a country where a disease is known to be circulating, or individuals in a certain area within a state where a disease has been detected. Quarantine regimes are often a key feature in containment stages of the pandemic. If and when containment fails and in-community transmission of the disease is detected, pandemic management moves to the mitigation stage. Unlike the containment stage where the goal is to fully suppress and eliminate the virus or, at least, prevent it from establishing in-community transmission, the goal of the mitigation stage is to reduce the rate of reproduction (R Number) of the virus to temper the numbers of people infected at any one time. In this way, states seek to "flatten the curve" of the epidemic, preventing health services from being over-whelmed. It is in the mitigation stage of pandemic management that steps such as lockdowns tend to be introduced. Lockdowns do not necessarily seek to separate infected or possibly infected persons from others. Certainly, there may be more draconian restrictions on such individuals but these will not be the only steps taken; rather, lockdowns seek to reduce the spread of a virus through a reduction in social interactions. Such measures may include the closure of schools, workplaces, businesses, places of worship, restrictions on the size of groups of people, and restrictions on people's movements. Lockdowns therefore:

> … are more porous than quarantines; they do not necessarily require confining people behind physical barriers. Lockdowns thus look different to classic or "paradigmatic" models for depriving individuals of their liberty. Under this human rights lens, lockdown measures may appear less draconian than quarantines for the people subjected to them; however, in another way, they are stricter, applying to all persons rather than just specific persons.[66]

Lockdowns can also be introduced in the containment stage, as has been the approach taken by New Zealand and Australia; however, these lockdowns tend to be at the extreme end of the scale regarding restrictions on individuals to the extent that they are closer in nature to quarantines.

---

63 Health (Amendment) Act 2021, s38B(16).
64 'Son of dying man released from hotel quarantine' *RTÉ News* (11 April 2021) https://www.rte.ie/news/coronavirus/2021/0411/1209125-court-quarantine/ accessed 24 July 2021.
65 Dáil Deb 14 July 2021 Vol.1010 No. 5.
66 Greene (39) 63–64.

In Ireland, as case numbers began to fall, and, in particular, the numbers of patients suffering COVID-19 in hospitals reduced, lockdown measures were eased. At no point was what has been termed a "Zero Covid" approach taken. Again, due to Ireland's proximity to Europe and the fact that it shared a land border with a constituent part of the UK, it was felt that such an approach was not feasible. Consequently, a level of in-community transmission was always foreseeable; from the state's perspective, the goal was to keep this in-community transmission level as low as possible. However, the lifting of restrictions can, in turn, result in an increase in the R-Number and Ireland has experienced several "waves" of infection with the severity of COVID restrictions in effect oscillating accordingly. As a result, Ireland has enacted one of the longest periods of lockdown in the world, although such lockdowns were not as extensive as those seen in, for example, Australia or New Zealand; nevertheless, people's human rights such as freedom of movement and association, and liberty were substantially curtailed.

Throughout the most severe levels of restrictions, people were not allowed to leave their homes without a "reasonable excuse." Such "reasonable excuses" included travel to and from work, shopping for essential items, and exercise. However, the list of what constituted a reasonable excuse was non-exhaustive, raising questions as to the clarity of the provisions.[67] Strict geographical limitations to the distance which a person could travel for exercise were introduced. At one stage early in the pandemic, this was limited to 2 km only from a person's home.[68] In September 2020, the Irish Government launched its Resilience and Recovery 2020–2021: Plan for Living with COVID-19, which was described as guiding "Ireland's response to saving lives and managing the pandemic over the next seven months."[69] The key aspect of this plan was to introduce a series of "Levels" of various restrictions with Level 1 being the least restrictive and Level 5 being the most restrictive.[70] Levels 3–5 included geographical restrictions on people's movements with Level 3 and 4 requiring individuals to stay within their counties except for essential work, education, and other essential purposes; while Level 5 reduced this geographical zone to 5 km from a person's home. In the early stages of the pandemic in April 2020, this zone was only 2 km.[71] For Level 5 level of restrictions introduced in the National Framework for living with COVID-19 in September 2020, this geographical limit was 5 km. In Level 4, this was extended to permit travel within one's county.

All of Ireland entered Level 5 restrictions on 19 October 2020 for six weeks, with the Government seeking to suppress virus levels to the extent that it would facilitate greater socializing opportunities and what it termed a "meaningful Christmas."[72] However, following an escalation of virus levels as a result of this increased socialization and the circulation of the "Alpha variant" of COVID-19, the Government announced that from 24 December, the entire state would enter Level 5, albeit with a requirement to stay in your country rather than 5 km from home. On 30 December, "full Level 5"

---

67 ICCL (n 60) 30.

68 Marie O'Halloran, 'Coronavirus: 2 km limit is restriction most want lifted, survey finds' *Irish Times* (27 April 2020) https://www.irishtimes.com/news/ireland/irish-news/coronavirus-2km-limit-is-restriction-most-want-lifted-survey-finds-1.4238792 accessed 25 July 2021.

69 'Government sets out plan for Covid-19 resilience and National Recovery' *Department of the Taoiseach* (15 September 2020) https://www.gov.ie/en/press-release/5ff8c-government-sets-out-plan-for-covid-19-resilience-and-national-recovery/ accessed, 26 July 2020.

70 'National framework for living with Covid-19' *Government of Ireland* (15 September 2020) https://assets.gov.ie/87604/405b1065-055a-4ca8-9513-390ce5298b10.pdf accessed 26 July 2021.

71 Rónán Duffy, 'Explainer: What exactly ARE the current Covid-19 restrictions and when can we expect them to change?' *TheJournal.ie* (22 April 2020) https://www.thejournal.ie/explainer-restrictions-ireland-5080859-Apr2020/ accessed 24 July 2021.

72 Pat Leahy, Jack Horgan-Jones, Jennifer Bray and Shauna Bowers, 'Covid-19: state moves to Level 5 for six weeks with hopes of "meaningful" Christmas celebrations' *The Irish Times* (19 October 2020) https://www.irishtimes.com/news/ireland/irish-news/covid-19-state-moves-to-level-5-for-six-weeks-with-hopes-of-meaningful-christmas-celebrations-1.4384986 accessed 16 July 2021.

was introduced with the 5 km restriction in effect.[73] This would remain until 12 April where it was replaced with a countywide or 20 km – whichever was larger – restriction. As of July 2021, there were no restrictions on domestic travel within Ireland in effect.

2.5 Data Protection, Surveillance, and Discrimination Issues

In July 2020, the Irish Health Service Executive (HSE) launched the CovidTracker App, which was designed to assist with track and trace efforts.[74] The compatibility of such a contact tracing app with the right to privacy enshrined in the Irish Constitution and international human rights treaties such as Article 8 ECHR will depend upon the proportionality of the interference with this right and the degree to which it is directed toward a legitimate aim – here, the suppression of the virus and, in turn, the protection of the health and lives of others. In this regard, Ireland's CovidTracker app took a "decentralized" approach to data management meaning that the vast majority of data were stored locally on a person's device, with the minimal necessary data being shared with the central authority.[75] Such a "decentralized" model can be contrasted with "centralized" models in which the vast bulk of people's data are shared with a central server and accessible and managed by a central authority which can mine these data for relevant and ancillary information. Centralized models thus raise much more profound human rights concerns, particularly regarding the right to privacy, than decentralized models owing to the amount of data shared with the center and the personal information that can be extrapolated from these data.[76] Nevertheless, some concerns do remain with a decentralized model such as Ireland's CovidTracker App. Notably, concerns centered on the requirement of Android users to have Google Play switched on which would result in highly sensitive personal data being sent to Google. Human rights concerns are not simply abated by the fact that such data are being collected by private organizations rather than the state; instead, such data collection raises issues pertaining to the rise of surveillance capitalism and the possibility of private corporations manipulating people's behavior.[77] The ICCL also raised concerns app's effectiveness, which, in turn, affects whether the interferences with rights caused by the app are necessary. The CovidTracker App was complemented by a manual system of contact tracing involving individuals disclosing places they have been and people they have been in touch with to a phone operator who would then contact the relevant people in question. Businesses also had to keep a record of persons on their premises for up to 28 days in order to facilitate contact tracing.[78] Again, no formal emergency was in effect from which such powers could derive their validity from. It remains to be seen therefore whether bulk information gathering technology and regulation could pave the way for similar technology to be deployed outside of a pandemic in response to a "less objective" crisis, such as in response to a national security threat.[79]

---

[73] 'Statement by the Taoiseach, Micheál Martin, on the reintroduction of Level 5 restriction of the Plan for Living with Covid-19' *Department of the Taoiseach* (20 December 2020) https://www.gov.ie/en/speech/8753b-statement-by-an-taoiseach-micheal-martin-on-the-reintroduction-of-level-5-restrictions-of-the-plan-for-living-with-covid/ accessed 26 July 2021.

[74] 'HSE launch the COVID Tracker App' *HSE* (7 July 2020) https://www.hse.ie/eng/services/news/media/pressrel/hse-hpsc-launch-the-covid-tracker-app.html accessed 26 July 2021.

[75] Joint Committee on Human Rights, *Human Rights and the Government's Response to COVID-19: Digital Contact Tracing,* Third Report of the JCHR Session 2019-2021 (6 May 2020) https://publications.parliament.uk/pa/jt5801/jtselect/jtrights/343/343.pdf accessed 26 July 2021.

[76] ibid.

[77] See Shoshana Zuboff, *The Age of Surveillance Capitalism* (Profile Books, 2019); Greene (n 44) 133.

[78] ICCL (n 60) 60–61.

[79] Greene (n 44) 132–135.

2.5.1 Vaccination and Vaccine Passports

In 2021, Ireland began its vaccination programme against COVID-19. This raised the possibility of developing bespoke vaccination regimes for vaccinated and unvaccinated persons and, in turn, raising the possibility of discriminatory treatment of persons. To facilitate international travel, Ireland signed up to the EU Digital COVID Certificate (EUDCC). The EUDCC was designed to allow EU citizens and residents to travel between the 27 EU member states and some additional third-party states that also signed up to the scheme. The EUDCC entailed a QR code that when scanned showed whether a person had been vaccinated against COVID-19, received a negative test result, or that the person had recovered from COVID-19. An EU wide approach to the question of what have been termed "COVID Passports" were adopted on the basis that such documents needed to be "interoperable" in order to protect and vindicate individuals' rights to free movement throughout the EU.[80] Furthermore, unilateral steps by states were considered to "have the potential to cause significant disruption to the exercise of the right to free movement and to hinder the proper functioning of the internal market."[81] That stated, unilateral moves by states to restrict freedom of movement are, nevertheless, a permitted response during the pandemic as evidenced by Ireland's hotel quarantine requirement for certain EU member states; however, as noted, Ireland was criticized by some EU states for taking this approach.[82] Like contact tracing apps, vaccine passports raise the problem of highly sensitive personal data being shared with organizations and individuals other than the patient and their health-care professional.

Vaccine passports also raise the possibility of discriminatory treatment between the vaccinated and unvaccinated. This discriminatory potential is not limited to the ability to travel beyond states. At the time of writing in July 2021, the Irish Government was in the process of introducing new legislation to facilitate the reopening of the hospitality sector. This legislation would entail allowing only fully vaccinated persons or persons who had recovered from COVID-19 to access indoor dining. The pace at which the legislation was enacted was criticized by Irish human rights organizations and opposition politicians. The Health (Amendment No.2) Bill 2021 was introduced to the Dáil on 12 July 2021 and passed all stages of the Oireachtas by 16 July. During the second stage, David Cullinane TD remarked that:

> It [the Health (Amendment No.2 Bill)] is rushed through the Dáil. The health committee has been told there would be no pre-legislative scrutiny even though there was a vote on it. That was rammed through by the Government. There was very little time for any amendments. I suspect that not a single amendment posed by the Opposition will be accepted by the Government because it has decided it is just going to push this through. There will certainly be no engagement of any substance with the Opposition at all.[83]

Well over a year into the pandemic and members of the Oireachtas were accusing the Government of sidelining proper legislative oversight. While such responses may be understandable at the outset of an emergency when it initially erupts and time is of the essence, the same cannot be said 16 months later. The Government defended its position, arguing that similar approaches were taken by Denmark and Germany.[84] Throughout the debate, opposition concerns centered on

---

80 Article 8, Regulation (EU) 2021/953 on a framework for the issuance, verification, and acceptance of interoperable COVID-19 vaccination, test, and recovery certificates to facilitate free movement during the COVID-19 pandemic.

81 Article 9 Regulation (EU) 2021/953.

82 Horgan-Jones et al. (n 58).

83 Dáil Deb 14 July 2021 vol. 1010 No. 5 (David Cullinane).

84 Marie O'Halloran, 'Indoor dining law passed in Dáil, Donnelly rejects discrimination claims' *The Irish Times* (14 July 2021) https://www.irishtimes.com/news/politics/oireachtas/indoor-dining-law-passed-in-d%C3%A1il-donnelly-rejects-discrimination-claims-1.4620639 accessed 15 July 2021.

the discriminatory potential of the Bill and the different treatment vaccinated and unvaccinated persons would be subjected to. Many people have medical conditions and disabilities that prevent them from taking a vaccine and vaccination passports could open the door for indirect discrimination. Fears were also raised that introducing such a requirement before everybody in Ireland had been offered a vaccine could also run the risk of breaking down social cohesion and people's willingness to conform with the state's pandemic response more generally.[85]

2.6   COVID-19 and the Rule of Law in Ireland

Like many states, Ireland's response to the pandemic has varied, with the powers and regulations in effect changing from time to time, often rapidly and sometimes with no advance warning. To document every regulation in effect at every specific time would be a Herculean task and to expect individuals to keep track of these changes raises profound concerns as to the clarity and certainty of the laws in effect and the degree to which Ireland's pandemic response conformed with even the thinnest formalist conceptions of the rule of law.[86] The conferral of vast discretionary power on decision makers can, for instance, give rise to the arbitrary application of these rules. In September 2020, the Garda Síochána (Irish police force) were given powers to issue "fixed penalty notices" to individuals who were found leaving their homes without a reasonable excuse. The recourse to the criminal law to enforce regulations raises further concerns regarding the clarity of the phrase "reasonable excuse." In its July 2021 report on the operation of COVID-19 police powers by An Garda Síochána, the Policing Authority noted that 52% of all Covid-related Fixed Charge Notices (FCNs) were issued to 18–25-year olds and 74% were issued to males.[87] No data, however, are contained in the report regarding the race or ethnicity of those subjected to FCNs; however, Casey et al. note that it is worrying that a recent internal Garda Survey suggested that substantial numbers of frontline Gardaí had negative attitudes toward Traveller and Roma, Arab, Black African, and Indian and Pakistani communities.[88]

This rule of law problem is further amplified by the propensity of Ireland's pandemic response to blur the lines between legally enforceable restrictions, and mere government advice or "guidelines." Often government guidelines would be announced prior to any legally enforceable change being in effect.[89] While the reliance on guidance over enforceable law or "nudging" may be considered to be less intrusive on individual freedom and thus more compliant with human rights obligations, several difficulties emerge.[90] For instance, the initial closure of Irish businesses announced by the Taoiseach in March 2020 led to some insurance companies to refuse to pay out compensation to businesses on the basis that the decision to close was entirely voluntary.[91]

Confusion can also result in both individuals and state actors not knowing how to conduct their own behavior. A high-profile example of this confusion can be seen from the issue surrounding the closure of places of worship during the second lockdown under Level 5 of the state's regulations. Although the Minister for Health had informed the Dáil that holding religious services in person

---

85 Dáil Deb 14 July 2021 vol. 1010 No. 5 (Alan Kelly).

86 Joseph Raz, *The Authority of Law* (2nd ed Oxford University Press, 2009) 226.

87 Policing Authority, 'Report on policing performance by the Garda Síochána during the COVID-19 health crisis' (19 July 2021) https://www.policingauthority.ie/assets/uploads/documents/Report_on_Policing_Performance_by_the_Garda_S%C3%ADoch%C3%A1na_during_COVID-19_Health_Crisis_-_19_July_2021.pdf, 3.

88 Casey et al. (n 38) 89; Pavee Point, 'Submission to the Department of Justice and equality: towards the development of a strategy for the criminal justice system' (August 2020).

89 Casey et al. (n 43) 13–14; ICCL (n 60) 18–19; Carolan and O'Neill (n 26) [34].

90 On the idea that guidance is more compatible with human rights law than legally enforceable obligations, see *Reverend Dr William JU Philip and others for Judicial Review of the closure of places of worship in Scotland* [2021] CSOH 32.

91 Carolan and O'Neill (n 26) [46].

was not a criminal offence, but that services were "required to move online."[92] Several reports did emerge of An Garda Síochána threatening prosecution of those seeking to attend services. In May 2021, the Irish High Court refused to hear a challenge to the regulations on religious worship as these regulations had lapsed and so were moot. This was so, notwithstanding the fact that both parties had agreed not to raise the issue of mootness during the proceedings.[93] This approach stands in sharp contrast to that of the Scottish Court of Session which found the closure of places of worship during the pandemic to be an unjustified infringement of their right to manifest their religious beliefs under Article 9 ECHR and to associate with others under Article 11 ECHR. The Scottish court rejected the idea that the fact that the restrictions were to be lifted rendered the question moot.[94] However, the Scottish Court also substantially downplayed the strong human rights arguments that can be used to justify pandemic responses; for instance, to protect the right to life.[95]

The result of the Irish approach is that there is an acute lack of clarity regarding the scope of the state's COVID-19 powers. Reliance on soft law approaches such as guidance may be understood as more beneficial from a human rights perspective as state coercion and force is avoided in favor of less intrusive modes of behavior modification, it is also the case that confusion over the scope of rules can also impact upon behavior and, in turn, raise serious rule of law concerns. A fundamental aspect of even the thinnest, formalist conceptions of the rule of law is that rules are clear and ex-ante prescribed. Reliance upon guidance rather than clear legal rules impacts upon this certainty. It affects not just individuals whose behavior the government is seeking to alter – religious worshipers wishing to attend a congregation – but also state actors – the Gardaí – in terms of how they exercise their powers.

2.7 Conclusions

At the time of writing (July 2021), much of the legal apparatus of the pandemic response remains in effect. Ireland has been noticeably more reluctant than its closest neighbor the UK to ease COVID restrictions. While emergency powers pertaining to national security threats such as terrorism often have a propensity of becoming permanent due to their oft-perceived democratic popularity among the electorate, the UK government has instead pursued a strategy of what can be described as a "rush to normalcy."[96] This phenomenon is not unique to the UK but is seen in many countries across the globe. It is also seen in states where governments have been reluctant to implement any steps to contain or mitigate the pandemic in the first place. The rush to normalcy implies that the risk of pandemic emergency powers becoming permanent is low. Given the negative impact that these measures have on the economy, coupled with the substantial impact they place on people's lives, it is reasonable to assume that these pressures incentivize democratic governments to restore normalcy as soon as possible or sometimes even too soon.[97] That stated, this is not to assume that there are no negative or permanent consequences to pandemic responses from a constitutional and human rights perspective. The introduction of such measures without a formal declaration of emergency, runs the risk of creating a precedent for the introduction of different powers but with

---

92 Oran Doyle, 'Religious services and the rule of law: authority and coercion' *COVID-19 Law and Human Rights Observatory* (9 March 2021) https://tcdlaw.blogspot.com/2021/03/religious-services-and-rule-of-law.html accessed 26 July 2021.
93 Mary Carolan, 'Declan Ganley's case of Covid-19 restrictions on Mass now moot, judge says' *The Irish Times* (18 May 2021) https://www.irishtimes.com/news/crime-and-law/courts/high-court/declan-ganley-s-case-over-covid-19-restrictions-on-mass-now-moot-judge-says-1.4568591 accessed 26 July 2021.
94 *Philip and Others* (n 90).
95 See Alan Greene, 'Closing places of Worship and COVID-19: towards a culture of justification?' (2021) *Edinburgh Law Review* (forthcoming).
96 Greene (n 44) 120–126.
97 ibid.

a similar effect outside of the discrete conditions of a pandemic. Relatedly, existing constitutional safeguards may be reinterpreted and stretched to accommodate novel and exceptional pandemic emergency powers. This juristic accommodation can then be used to justify future emergency powers for "less objective" de facto emergencies.[98]

In principle, emergencies justify exceptional and unpalatable but ultimately necessary measures. It is this idea of necessity that explains why states make such "unpalatable choices." Necessity implies a constraint in choice. It suggests that the decision maker has either no choice at all or that they must choose between the lesser of two evils. In the context of emergencies, necessity implies that the decision maker had no choice but to take the steps it did to respond to the threat. If the state did not respond in the way it had, the threat would have come to fruition and the consequences that would flow from this would be catastrophic.[99] Pandemic responses thus fall within this classic emergency paradigm. Unpalatable constraints on individual freedoms, delegated powers to the executive with minimal oversight, and broad, ill-defined rules are all enacted to confront the virus.

At the time of writing, the pandemic has taken the lives of over 7,000 people on the island of Ireland. In terms of lives lost, the magnitude of the threat posed by COVID-19 far exceeds that posed by even paramilitary violence at the height of the conflict known as the Troubles that raged from the 1970s to the 1990s. The high death toll experienced by states, even those such as in Ireland where robust pandemic responses were implemented, can certainly justify emergency responses on the grounds of necessity. That stated, Ireland's experience of the pandemic also shows that an array of factors are often taken into account when an emergency response is enacted. Certainly, the introduction and relaxation of measures were often done in line with scientific advice, to such an extent that the government was accused of outsourcing its decision-making to NPHET, or that Ireland was now run by technocrats rather than elected officials.[100] The emphasis that governments place on following scientific advice to legitimate pandemic responses can give such advisory bodies powerful soft power, granting them the ability to frame public understandings of the pandemic and set the agenda for what responses should be enacted. Ultimately, decision-making resides in the Government and, consequently, so too does accountability for these decisions.

Ultimately, claims to necessity cannot be wholly justified as objective due to these complex variables that must be taken into account by a decision maker. It follows that, Ireland's experience of the pandemic demonstrates the importance of accountability mechanisms in a democratic constitutional order. At the time of writing, groups in Ireland are calling for public inquiries into the handling of aspects of the pandemic, most notably the high levels of deaths in Irish nursing homes.[101]

Claims that "nothing was done other than that which inexorable necessity demanded" must and should be challenged and decision makers must be held to account through democratic and legal methods.[102] All constitutions both facilitate and limit power; what matters is how such power is controlled and how individuals are held to account when such power is abused. Despite the lack of a formal state of emergency, Ireland's constitutional provisions have demonstrated an elastic capacity to accommodate the exceptional response required. Yet, despite the necessity of many of the measures enacted, the legacy of this elastic accommodation may prove problematic. Weak legislative oversight of the Executive's response, coupled with an overly deferential judiciary can result in justifiable pandemic responses leaving a problematic legacy. It remains to be seen whether such is the fate of Ireland.

---

98 Gross (n 20) 1131–1134.
99 Greene (n 5) 26–27.
100 'Letters: NPHET and the Government' *The Irish Times* (6 October 2020) https://www.irishtimes.com/opinion/letters/nphet-and-the-government-1.4372770 accessed 24 July 2021.
101 Neil Michael, 'Group backs call for "wide-ranging inquiry" into Covid deaths' in nursing homes' *Irish Examiner* (15 June 2021) https://www.irishexaminer.com/news/arid-40313798.html accessed 23 July 2021.
102 Frederick C Hicks, *Human Jettison* (St Paul, 1937) 109.

3

COVID-19: Legal Lessons Learned in Switzerland

*Felix Uhlmann**

Constitutional and Administrative Law as well as Legislative Studies, University of Zurich, Zurich, Switzerland

3.1 Introduction

The COVID-19 pandemic hit many countries hard, and Switzerland is no exception.[1] This chapter deals with how Switzerland reacted to the crisis. In particular, it will discuss the restrictions to the daily life that were in place and will assess these restrictions from a legal standpoint. Contact tracing apps and vaccinations will also be discussed.

3.2 Legal Framework

3.2.1 Legal Framework before COVID-19 (Swiss Epidemics Act)

3.2.1.1 Scope and Goals

The Epidemics Act[2] (EpidA) has been in force since 1 January 2016. In contrast to other federal acts, there exists no (unofficial) English translation but only the (official) versions in German, French, and Italian.[3] The act contains 88 articles and is regularly compiled, meaning that later amendments have been fully included in the legal text. This makes the act – as all legislation in Switzerland – comparably easy to read, not the least because the legislative process in Switzerland is comparably slow but usually technically sound and because legislation is drafted with regard to the ideal that ordinary citizens should be able to understand it.[4]

The Epidemics Act defines its scope as follows: "This law regulates the protection of people from communicable diseases and provides the necessary measures" (Article 1 EpidA). The main purpose "is to prevent and control the outbreak and spread of communicable diseases" (Article 2 paragraph 1 EpidA), more specifically to "monitor communicable diseases and provide basic knowledge of

---

* Prof. Dr. Felix Uhlmann, LL.M., holds a Chair for Constitutional and Administrative Law as well as Legislative Studies at the University of Zurich (Switzerland). The author thanks Martin Wilhelm, MLaw, for his help with the editing of this chapter.

1 Until 22 July 2021, Switzerland registered 712,633 cases of COVID-19 and 10,389 COVID-19-related deaths. On 4 November 2020, the seven-day average infection rate peaked at 90.2 cases per 100,000 persons, cf. Federal Office of Public Health (2021).
2 Federal Act on the Control of Communicable Human Diseases (Epidemics Act, EpidA) of 3 December 2010 (SR [Classified Compilation of federal law] 818.101).
3 Which are accessible through Fedlex, the publication platform for federal law, https://www.fedlex.admin.ch/eli/cc/2015/297/de (accessed 26 July 2021).
4 For the so-called requirement of comprehensibility ("Verständlichkeitsgebot") cf. Höfler (2018), p. 67 ff.

Impacts of the Covid-19 Pandemic: International Laws, Policies, and Civil Liberties, First Edition. Edited by Nadav Morag.
© 2023 John Wiley & Sons, Inc. Published 2023 by John Wiley & Sons, Inc.

their spread and evolution" (Article 2 paragraph 1 lit. a EpidA), to "detect, assess and avoid the dangers of the outbreak and spread of communicable diseases" (Article 2 paragraph 1 lit. b EpidA), to "induce individuals, certain groups of people and institutions to contribute to the prevention and control of communicable diseases" (Article 2 paragraph 1 lit. c EpidA), to "create the organizational, technical and financial prerequisites for the detection, monitoring, prevention and control of communicable diseases" (Article 2 paragraph 1 lit. d EpidA), to "ensure access to facilities and resources for protection against transmissions" of communicable diseases (Article 2 paragraph 1 lit. e EpidA), and to "reduce the impact of communicable diseases on society and those affected" (Article 2 paragraph 1 lit. f EpidA).

The Epidemics Act defines some crucial legal terms, e.g. "communicable disease" as a "disease that can be transmitted to humans through pathogens or their toxic products" (Article 3 lit. a EpidA). The introductory part of the law further contains goals and strategies of the Confederation (Article 4 EpidA) and national programs (Article 5 EpidA) with regard to the detection, monitoring, prevention, and control of communicable diseases.

3.2.1.2 Normal, Particular, and Extraordinary Situations

The Epidemics Act introduces a three-part model applicable to normal, particular, and extraordinary situations, respectively; terms that were of high importance during the current pandemic.[5] In a *normal situation*, most competencies to fight an epidemic lie within the cantonal (state) authorities which is in line with the federalist system of Switzerland. The cantons have quite a strong position as the Swiss Constitution of 1848 has copied many ideas from the United States (bicameral Parliament, enumerated federal powers, etc.).[6] In a *particular (special) situation*, the competencies shift toward the Confederation. After hearing the cantons, the Federal Council (executive branch) may order measures against individual persons, measures against the population, require doctors and other health professionals to participate in the fight against communicable diseases, and make vaccinations compulsory for vulnerable population groups, for particularly exposed people and for people who carry out certain activities such as medical staff (Article 6 paragraph 2 EpidA). I will come back to these measures.

A *particular situation* has to be assumed if the enforcement agencies are unable to prevent and control the outbreak and spread of communicable diseases and if there is an increased risk of infection and spread, a particular threat to public health or a serious impact on the economy or other areas of life (Article 6 paragraph 1 lit. a EpidA). A particular situation exists also if the World Health Organization (WHO) has established that there is an international health emergency which threatens public health in Switzerland (Article 6 paragraph 1 lit. a EpidA).

From a particular situation, the level may further increase to the highest level of urgency, to an *extraordinary situation*. It is noteworthy that the Epidemics Act is rather taciturn in this situation. The relevant provision (Article 7 EpidA) stipulates only:

> *If an extraordinary situation so requires, the Federal Council can order the necessary measures for the whole country or for individual parts of the country.*

When Parliament enacted the Epidemics Act, there was little discussion on this article – too little, one may state with hindsight. It is safe to assume that no one expected this provision to become relevant. This assumption was not so wrong in the light of the fact that the particular situation already attributes important competencies to the Confederation. In other words, an "ordinary" epidemic

---

5 The three-part model has first been established in the context of security policy, cf. Rechsteiner (2016), p. 3; Trümpler (2012), p. 42 f.
6 Cf. Kley (2020b), p. 252 f.

such as the 2002–2004 SARS (severe acute respiratory syndrome) outbreak, still undoubtedly very dangerous, would have been qualified as a particular situation,[7] giving the Confederation ample means to fight the epidemic.

It is interesting that the Federal Council was relatively quick to declare an extraordinary situation at the wake of the COVID-19 pandemic.[8] From a purely legal standpoint, if one analyzes the measures taken by the Federal Council, many of them would have had a sound footing in the competencies of the Federal Council in case of a particular situation. The main legal "advantage" for the Federal Council in an extraordinary situation is that it must not take into account the views of the cantons before taking measures.[9] The views of the cantons are not binding but it would be highly unusual – and politically unwise – if the Federal Council would enact measures against considerable opposition of the cantons, not the least as the cantons are in charge of implementing federal measures. On 13 March 2020, the declaration of an extraordinary situation had mainly a symbolic function, i.e. to underline the urgency of the situation to the citizens.[10]

This is not to say that Article 7 EpidA did not play a role in this crisis and will not in the future. Indeed, the provision is vague to the extreme and as far-reaching as a legal norm can possibly be:[11] If an extraordinary situation so requires, the Federal Council can order the "necessary measures" or whatever it takes.

However, Article 7 EpidA is not a *carte blanche* to the executive branch. It must be seen in the light of further legal provisions, namely the Constitution.[12] Indeed, the dispatch[13] of the Federal Council to the Epidemics Act considered the article as a mere repetition of the emergency clause of the Federal Council that lies in Article 185 paragraph 3 Constitution, reading as follows:

> *[The Federal Council] may in direct application of this Article issue ordinances and rulings in order to counter existing or imminent threats of serious disruption to public order or internal or external security. Such ordinances must be limited in duration.*

Indeed, many scholars doubt that Article 7 EpidA has a legal existence of its own besides the Constitution,[14] an opinion that is in line with the (sparse) legal materials in connection with the

---

7 Cf. Rüefli et al. (2018), p. 12.

8 The Federal Council declared an extraordinary situation on 13 March 2020, cf. Federal Council (2020a).

9 Wyss (2020), Para. 4.

10 Cf. Bernard (2020), p. 21. Later, the Federal Council enacted several emergency ordinances outside of the scope of the Epidemics Act which were based on Article 185 paragraph 3 Constitution. Even for these, the declaration of an extraordinary situation was not necessary, as the existence of an extraordinary situation is not a legal requirement of the Federal Council's authority to enact emergency measures under Article 185 paragraph 3 Constitution, cf. Trümpler (2012), p. 43. However, the Federal Council's authority under Article 185 paragraph 3 Constitution is seen as a means to handle extraordinary situations, cf. Saxer (2014), para. 9.

11 Cf. Trümpler and Uhlmann (2020), p. 575; Waldmann (2021), p. 13.

12 Federal Constitution of the Swiss Confederation of 18 April 1999 (SR 101).

13 The Federal Council submits its bills to the Federal Assembly together with a dispatch that provides justification for the bill and comments on the individual provisions. In addition, it analyzes specific points in particular such as the legal background, the consequences for constitutional rights, compatibility with superior law and the relationship with European law, the delegation of powers provided for in a draft act, the points of view debated in the preliminary stages of the legislative process and their alternatives, the planned implementation of the enactment, the planned evaluation of its implementation and the assessment of the planned implementation that took place in the preliminary stages of the legislative process, the consequences for staffing and finances of the bill and its implementation for the federal government, cantons, and communes, the methods for meeting the costs and the cost–benefit ratio, etc., see Art. 141 Federal Act on the Federal Assembly of 13 December 2002 (Parliament Act, ParlA; SR 171.10).

14 Brunner et al. (2020); Trümpler and Uhlmann (2020), p. 574 f.; Rechsteiner (2020), p. 122; Flückiger (2020), p. 144; Bernard (2021), p. 143; cf. also Stöckli (2020), p. 22. Waldmann (2021), p. 14, highlights that while Article 7 EpidA refers to Article 185 paragraph 3 Constitution, the Federal Council is, during an extraordinary situation, still

adoption of this article.[15] The question is not only of scholarly interest but has legal consequences. It is already clear from the constitutional language in Article 185 paragraph 3 that emergency legislation of the Federal Council must be limited in time, a condition not stipulated in Article 7 EpidA. Furthermore, Article 185 paragraph Constitution is embedded in a constitutional system that requires the Federal Council to involve Parliament in order to replace emergency legislation, again a condition lacking in Article 7 EpidA.[16] Last but not least, the competencies of the Courts vary according to the legal basis of federal ordinances. The Federal Supreme Court must apply federal laws even if it considers these laws unconstitutional (Article 190 Constitution),[17] meaning that it must accept the wide leeway of Article 7 EpidA in principle and may only intervene if the Federal Council oversteps its competencies under the Act or enacts an ordinance that is unconstitutional for other reasons.[18] In contrast, there is, in principle, full judicial scrutiny for ordinances based on Article 185 paragraph 3 Constitution.[19] This is a subtle difference (and a court may find ways to intervene also against ordinances based on Article 7 EpidA) but not one without importance if the Courts apply the correct doctrine when reviewing federal ordinances.

There have not been any court decisions on this question. In my view, Article 7 EpidA merely reiterates the Constitution. Apart from the legal materials supporting this view, it is questionable as to whether Parliament wanted to stretch the powers of the Federal Council over its constitutional limits, taking into account that these competencies are already quite extensive.

Speaking of Parliament, one should note that the Swiss Epidemics Act does not provide a role for Parliament. A particular or extraordinary situation needs not be declared, triggering the extended competencies of the Federal Council. It is the Federal Council that must assess whether the situation warrants particular or extraordinary measures.

3.2.1.3 Measures

Chapter 5 of the Epidemics Act is dedicated to fight an epidemic. It distinguishes measures to be taken against individuals (Articles 30–39 EpidA), measures to be taken against the population and certain groups of people (Article 40 EpidA), measures in international passenger traffic (Articles 41–43 EpidA) and special measures (Articles 44–49 EpidA), the latter including measures such as the safeguard of the supply chain with therapeutic products (Article 44 EpidA).

It is noteworthy that in connection with the measures to be taken against individuals, the Epidemics Act starts out with a principle: A measure may only be ordered if less drastic measures to prevent the spread of a communicable disease are insufficient and if the measure serves to avert a serious risk to the health of third parties (Article 30 paragraph 1 EpidA). The measure must

---

authorized to enact the measures the Epidemics Act allows for during a normal and during a special situation. In contrast to those maintaining that Article 7 EpidA refers to Article 185 paragraph 3 Constitution, Kley (2020a), p. 272 ff., Biaggini (2020), p. 258 ff., and Märkli (2020), p. 60 ff., argue that the scope of Article 185 paragraph 3 Constitution is not broad enough to cover measures aimed at providing economical and social stability while Article 7 EpidA does or at least should allow for such measures.

15 Federal Council (2010), p. 334, 337, and 365 f.

16 Brunner, Wilhelm and Uhlmann (2020), p. 689 ff.; cf. also Biaggini (2020), p. 243.

17 The Swiss Constitution bears resemblance to the US Constitution as the Swiss Constitution of 1848 has been strongly influenced by the United States, see Kley (2020b), p. 252 f. Still, Switzerland has not opted for a strong Supreme Court that may fully review federal laws. This system has come under pressure as this restriction does not prevent interventions of the European Court of Human Rights. Hence, the Federal Supreme Court has started to review federal law under the European Convention of Human Rights – but not the Swiss Constitution. Several attempts to extend the powers of the Federal Supreme Court have failed. See Griffel (2021), p. 436 ff.; Biaggini (2017), p. 1451 ff.

18 Brunner, Wilhelm and Uhlmann (2020), p. 694 and 697; Gerber (2020), p. 262; cf. also Federal Supreme Court, BGE 131 II 162, 166.

19 Cf. Stöckli (2021b), p. 17 f.; Trümpler and Uhlmann (2020), p. 585; Trümpler (2012), p. 164.

be necessary and reasonable (Article 30 paragraph 2 EpidA) which is arguably a reminder to the authorities to act proportionately, a principle that is laid down in Article 5 paragraph 2 Constitution. It is doubtful that the Epidemics Act stipulates a stricter reading of the proportionality as the constitution.

Measures against individuals encompass identification and notification of affected persons (Article 33 EpidA), medical surveillance of affected persons (Article 34 EpidA), quarantine and segregation (Article 35 EpidA), compulsory examination of affected persons (Article 36 EpidA), and compulsory medical treatment of affected persons (Article 37 EpidA). Affected persons may also be restricted in their professional activities (Article 38 EpidA).

A key provision of the Epidemics Act is Article 40, dealing with measures to be taken against the population and certain groups of people. Slightly simplified, it reads as follows:

1 *The competent cantonal authorities order measures to prevent the spread of communicable diseases in the population or in certain groups of people.*
2 *In particular, they can take the following measures:*
   a. *Prohibit or restrict events;*
   b. *Close schools, other public institutions and private companies or impose operating regulations;*
   c. *Prohibit or restrict entering and leaving certain buildings and areas as well as certain activities in defined locations.*
3 *The measures may only last as long as is necessary to prevent the spread of a communicable disease.*

Note that Article 40 EpidA speaks of the cantons (states) but as explained earlier, the Confederation may assume these powers in case of a particular or extraordinary situation.

3.2.2 Legal Framework Under COVID-19

3.2.2.1 First and Second Wave

The Epidemics Act remained in force during the outbreak of the COVID-19 pandemic and served as an important legal basis for many of the measures taken by the Confederation and the cantons (states). Still, it has been superseded by an impressive number of emergency ordinances of the Federal Council, partly based directly on the Constitution (Article 185 paragraph 3) and partly based on the competencies under the Epidemics Act. The choice was not always fully coherent.

In the wake of the crisis, the Federal Council has enacted several ordinances on the Corona virus. It started by prohibiting events with more than 1,000 participants (Article 2 paragraph 1 COVID-19 Ordinance[20]). It soon was evident that these measures were insufficient, and further interventions followed. One key ordinance, the so-called COVID-19 Ordinance 2[21] prescribed further measures. Those were still less strict than in most of Switzerland's neighbors. There was no curfew *per se* but the population and especially vulnerable persons (Article 10b paragraph 1 COVID-19 Ordinance 2) were urged to stay at home. Universities, schools, museums, restaurants, and most businesses with customers were closed (Article 5 paragraph 1 and Article 6 paragraph 2

---

20 Ordinance on Measures to Combat the Coronavirus (COVID-19) of 28 February (COVID-19 Ordinance; SR 818.101.24).
21 Ordinance 2 on Measures to Combat the Coronavirus (COVID-19) of 13 March 2020 (COVID-19 Ordinance 2; SR 818.101.24).

COVID-19 Ordinance 2) but not industry, supermarkets, and hotels (Article 6 paragraph 3 COVID-19 Ordinance 2). Indeed, it was still possible to spend holidays in Switzerland if you were able to enter Switzerland. The public was only urgently requested to stay at home over the Easter holidays in 2020. Leaving and entering Switzerland became complicated because of the many restrictions of cross-border traffic, especially targeting "unnecessary" leisure trips, including shopping, but allowing employees to cross the border (Article 3 ff. COVID-19 Ordinance 2). The latter was obviously vital for Switzerland, given its central position in Europe and heavily dependent on the large cross-border commuter workforce which amounts to 6.2% of the total workforce nationally and in some cantons (states) to as much as 28.8% (Ticino) or 24% (Geneva).[22] Generally, the measures were accompanied by a substantial information campaign. Switzerland was late issuing a mask mandate for public transport (Article 3a COVID-19 Special Situation Ordinance,[23] in force from 6 July 2020) and for publicly accessible indoor areas of businesses and establishments (Article 3b COVID-19 Special Situation Ordinance; in force from 19 October 2020), supposedly because of uncertain benefits, more truly because Switzerland lacked the necessary quantities of masks.[24] This raised some doubts about the truthfulness of the government's actions which were, in general, well received and accepted by the public.[25]

As in many countries, the situation eased over the summer 2020. As travelling in Switzerland was not restricted and many European countries relaxed their cross-border travel restrictions, many Swiss were able to spend their summer holidays either in Switzerland or in neighboring countries. Disregarding the omnipresence of masks, one could have assumed that life was "normal" again. It was a kind of "drôle de pandémie" (a term of the author but others had the same association of the French and British passive reaction after declaring war to Hitler Germany).

Still, the situation was anything but normal even from a legal point of view. Although the Federal Council had declared the end of the extraordinary situation per 19 June 2020 and rescinded the COVID-Ordinance 2, many restrictions stayed in place as the Federal Council transferred them to the new COVID-19 Ordinance Special Situation. Events with over 1,000 people were prohibited (Article 6 paragraph 1 COVID-19 Ordinance Special Situation), and publicly accessible establishments and businesses had to enforce either distancing or other protective measures or, if neither was possible, to record contact details of persons present (Article 4 paragraph 2 COVID-19 Ordinance Special Situation). The Federal Council also enacted additional measures during summer. Notably, it issued the aforementioned mask mandate for public transport per 6 July 2020 (Article 3a paragraph 1 COVID-19 Ordinance Special Situation).

From a factual standpoint, the situation in summer 2020 was not normal as experts expected and warned that in autumn, the number of infections would rise again.[26] Indeed, the second wave (some called it a "wall") hit Switzerland quite hard. Although the Federal Council did not declare an extraordinary situation again, many of the measures from spring 2020 had to be reintroduced.

---

22 Federal Statistical Office (2021a), p. 4.

23 Ordinance on Measures during the Special Situation to combat the COVID-19 Epidemic of 19 June 2020 (COVID-19 Special Situation Ordinance; SR 818.101.26).

24 During a press conference of the Federal Council on 16 March 2020, Daniel Koch, head of the section of infectious diseases of the Federal Office of Public Health, said that the use of masks worn by the general population was small. He also stressed that masks were, at this moment, a scarce good worldwide. See Schweizer Radio und Fernsehen (2020).

25 According to opinion surveys, a majority of the population supported the restrictions imposed by the Federal Councils beginning in March 2020 and all through March 2021. However, support for the restrictions was declining over time. See Bühler et al. (2021), p. 17 f.

26 Already on 3 July 2020, the National COVID-19 Science Task Force warned that the number of cases was growing exponentially and would reach, without any interventions, a level associated with massive consequences for public health and the economy, see National COVID-19 Science Task Force (2020), p. 1 f.

Public gatherings in public spaces were restricted to 15 persons (Article 3c paragraph 1 COVID-19 Ordinance Special Situation), most events were prohibited (Article 6 paragraph 1 COVID-19 Ordinance Special Situation), and universities had to switch to online lectures (Article 6d paragraph 1 COVID-19 Ordinance Special Situation). The Federal Council also enacted additional measures. In particular, it extended the mask mandate to publicly accessible areas indoor and outdoor areas of businesses and establishments (Article 3b paragraph 1 COVID-19 Ordinance Special Situation) and later to busy pedestrian zones (Article 3c paragraph 2 lit. a COVID-19 Ordinance Special Situation).

Again, as in many countries, the (latest) turning point appeared in spring 2021. Cases went down, not only because of the measures in place since autumn 2020 but also because of the better weather conditions and the positive effects of vaccinations. Restaurants, discotheques, cultural institutions, and sports facilities were allowed to reopen, and events were permitted again subject do different constraints including the requirement of a COVID-19 vaccination, recovery or test certificate to gain access to discotheques or take part in events with over 1,000 persons. The Federal Council enacted the corresponding rules in the revised COVID-19 Ordinance Special Situation[27] (Articles 6 and 10–24).

In the summer of 2021, many eyes were turned to the United Kingdom. The United Kingdom was more advanced in vaccinations than Switzerland but was nevertheless hit hard by the Delta variant.[28] Switzerland was catching, both in vaccinations and in cases caused by the Delta variant.[29] It remained in a relatively good position as it used mostly mRNA vaccinations providing reasonably good protection against the Delta variant.[30] Still, it remained an open debate whether one should accept numbers as high as in the United Kingdom. Hospital cases were under control, at least at the end of July 2021, but the effects of long COVID were still unexplored and it was unclear whether it posed a significant threat to children that were rarely vaccinated or not at all.

3.2.2.2 Financial Aid

The measures to fight the COVID-19 pandemic were flanked by a myriad of other ordinances of the Federal Council, many of them concerning financial aid, either in the form of money lent by private banks but fully guaranteed by the Confederation or lump sum payments. Because the Swiss economy was not shut down strictly speaking, the financial aid was mainly directed to businesses that were temporarily closed for customers, i.e. restaurants, cultural institutions, sports facilities, and entertainment venues. Still, in 2020 alone, the Swiss Confederation spent 15.0 billion Swiss Francs in connection with the COVID-19 pandemic and guaranteed loans totaling 17.5 billion Swiss Francs. In 2021, the Swiss Confederation was expected to spend further 24.4 billion Swiss Francs.[31] Not included herein are expenses of the cantons (states) and tax revenue losses. As the Epidemics Act did not provide any redress for most measures aimed at combating the COVID-19 pandemic, the Federal Council enacted the necessary provisions in spring 2020 as emergency ordinances

---

27 Ordinance on Measures during the Special Situation to combat the COVID-19 Epidemic of 23 June 2021 (COVID-19 Ordinance Special situation; SR 818.101.26).

28 On 19 July 2021, the 7-day average infection rate in United Kingdom reached a new peak at 71.7 cases per 100,000 persons. To this date, 68.5% of people aged 18 or older had been fully vaccinated. See Public Health England (2021).

29 From 30 June 2021 to 19 June 2021, the 7-day average infection rate in Switzerland rose from 1.2 cases per 100,000 persons to 6.2 cases per 100,000 persons. On 27 July 2021, 57.4% of people aged 18 or older had been fully vaccinated. See Federal Office of Public Health 2021.

30 Cf. Lopez Bernal et al. (2021); Sheik et al. (2021); Nasreen et al. (2022).

31 Federal Finance Administration (2021).

(e.g. Joint and Several Guarantee Ordinance[32]). Later, provisions that had to remain in force were incorporated in emergency acts adopted by Parliament (e.g. Joint and Several Guarantee Act[33]).

3.2.2.3 The Federal Council and Other Actors

At the beginning of a pandemic, the Epidemics Act as well as the Constitution transfer a lot of power to the Federal Council.[34] The Federal Council is the highest executive authority in Switzerland. It is composed of seven members that share equal rights (Articles 175–177 Constitution). This system of collective leadership is quite unique.[35] One may speculate whether the broader responsibility had an effect on the acceptance of the measures in the crises, compared e.g. to France and the United States where public attention was often focused on one person.

In any case, the Swiss system becomes less democratic and less federalistic in a pandemic, the latter far from obvious as in normal times, Swiss federalism is considered strong,[36] comparable to the United States, certainly stronger than in Germany[37] where the Länder (states) kept more competencies during the crisis,[38] to the surprise of many Swiss. It proved also quite difficult to transfer back competencies to the cantons (states) and the interplay between the Confederation and the cantons was rather complicated.

Likewise, in earlier emergencies, Parliament hardly played an active role as the emergency clause in Article 185 paragraph 3 Constitution was typically invoked for single cases or unique situations.[39] During the pandemic, Parliament struggled to find a proper role, having a false start at the very beginning by aborting the ongoing spring session 2020, which was not only legally doubtful but also politically badly received.[40] Also, the COVID-19 Act[41] – which mainly incorporated pandemic-related measures first enacted as emergency ordinances by the Federal Council in an emergency act adopted by Parliament – passed later on had arguably some legal flaws.[42]

3.3 Contact Tracing App

It has been pointed out that Swiss Parliament's reaction to the crisis was rather late and modest.[43] The contact tracing app (or, officially, proximity tracing (PT) system) is the exception that confirms this rule. Citing concerns about significant fundamental rights violations (i.e. of the right to privacy, Article 13 Constitution), Parliament insisted on being involved,[44] and indeed, inserted a new article (60a) in the Epidemics Act on 19 June 2020. Why Parliament was not as insistent on being involved with other issues remains unclear.

---

32 Joint and Several Guarantee Ordinance of 25 March 2020 (SR 951.261).
33 Joint and Several Guarantee Act of 18 December 2020 (SR 951.26).
34 See Section 3.2.1; cf. also Trümpler and Uhlmann (2020), p. 586.
35 Cf. Biaggini 2017; Brühl-Moser (2007), p. 480; Schweizer (1999).
36 Cf. Tiefenthal (2021), p. 6. See also below Section 3.2.1.1.
37 Braun (2003) characterizes Swiss federalism as "decentralized" and German federalism as "unitarian."
38 Cf. Münch (2020), p. 211 ff.
39 For an overview of relevant cases, see Saxer (2014), para. 107 ff.
40 Cf. Wilhelm and Uhlmann (2020), p. 9 ff.; Glaser and Gfeller (2020), p. 16 f.; Trümpler and Uhlmann (2020), p. 581; Caroni and Graf (2021), p. 6.
41 Federal Act on the Statutory Principles for Federal Council Ordinances on Combating the COVID-19 Epidemic of 25 September 2020 (SR 818.102).
42 Cf. Uhlmann and Wilhelm (2021), p. 50 ff. Nevertheless, the COVID-19 act was approved twice in a popular referendum, see below section 3.5.
43 Cf. Glaser and Gfeller (2020), p. 16 ff. Less skeptical Stöckli (2021b), p. 16.
44 Political Institutions Committee of the National Council (2020); Political Institutions Committee of the Council of States (2020).

As in many countries, the Swiss contact tracing app (available as "SwissCovid" app) recorded signals of nearby cell phones belonging to people who participated in the system and notified the users of the app when they had been potentially exposed to the coronavirus (Article 60a paragraph 1 EpidA).[45] A person who had been notified by the contact tracing app that she or he had been potentially exposed to the coronavirus could have tests carried out for infection with the coronavirus and for antibodies against the coronavirus free of charge if the notification was provided (Article 60a paragraph 4 EpidA).

Swiss public opinion and politicians were quite concerned about abuses, so the law clearly states that "the data may not be used for other purposes, in particular not to order and enforce measures according to Articles 33–38 by cantonal authorities or for police, criminal or intelligence purposes" (Article 60a paragraph 2 EpidA). The data protection legislation is fully applicable (Article 60a paragraph 6 EpidA) and the contact tracing must follow strict rules on data safety, decentralized data storage, data destruction, etc. (Article 60a paragraph 5 EpidA).

The skepticism is echoed in Article 60a paragraph 3 EpidA, which reads as follows:

> *Participation in the PT system is open to all volunteers. Authorities, companies and single persons may not favor or disadvantage any person because of their participation or non-participation in the PT system; deviating agreements are ineffective.*

This rule imposes a strict voluntariness on the use of the contact tracing app. Even between private parties, no advantage or disadvantage of any kind may be connected with the use of the app, which also means that companies and public institutions are not allowed to restrict the offer of their services or products to persons that are using the contact tracing app.[46] This regime has been criticized. It is indeed a contradiction in valuation that private enterprises may require vaccination under certain circumstances,[47] obviously a much more far-reaching condition than the simple use of an app on the mobile phone.[48] It is questionable that Parliament would still take the same decision, not the least in comparison to all the other burdens that were put on the population since June 2020.

By the same token, it is disputed as to how effective the contact tracing app has been. Until 11 July 2020, the SwissCovid app had been downloaded approximately 3.2 billion times, but only 1.7 billion apps were active on the same day.[49] Compared to 6.4 billion people aged 16–74 living in Switzerland[50] and 84% of those using the internet via mobile phone,[51] this is far from satisfactory.

The modest use of the contact tracing app had also the consequence that most of the contact tracing had to be done manually by civil servants, a system which was overwhelmed during the second wave of the pandemic in autumn 2020. The so-called contact tracers had to rely on extensive but largely unregulated private collections of contact data (e.g. contact data recorded by restaurants) as well as data provided by persons with positive test results. The Canton of Berne, as the only canton, authorized its Office for Health, Social Services, and Integration to run a database where all contact data registered at restaurants, bars, and clubs were centrally stored.[52]

---

45 As the pandemic subsided, the Federal Council suspended the use of the COVID-19 app per 31 March 2022. Article 60a EpidA remains in force until 31 December 2022.
46 Federal Council (2020b), p. 4473 f.
47 See Section 3.4.2.
48 Cf. Uhlmann and Wilhelm (2021), p. 56; Uhlmann (2021), p. 114 f.
49 Federal Statistical Office (2021b).
50 Federal Statistical Office (2020a).
51 Federal Statistical Office (2020b).
52 Article 3a Verordnung über Massnahmen zur Bekämpfung der Covid-19-Epidemie of 4 November 2020 (Covid-19 V; BSG 815.123). The provision was reviewed but upheld in court, cf. Federal Supreme Court, 2C_525/2021 of 27 October 2021.

3.4 Fundamental Rights (Civil Liberties)

3.4.1 Restrictions on Daily Life

There is no doubt that the COVID-19 pandemic brought not only a heavy toll on death and serious illness but also on side effects such as depression[53] and domestic violence associated with isolation,[54] knowledge gaps for schoolchildren,[55] and economic loss.[56]

It goes without saying that the measures meant a heavy hand limiting the enjoyment of fundamental rights. The restrictions on meeting friends and family affected the right to privacy (Article 13 Constitution) and the right to have a family (Article 14 Constitution). The prohibition of gatherings not only restricted the freedom of assembly (Article 22 Constitution) and the freedom of expression (Article 14 Constitution) but also religious freedom (Article 15 Constitution), artistic freedom (Article 21 Constitution), and political rights (Article 34 Constitution). Closed schools – the exception in Switzerland – touched upon the right to the basic education of children (Article 19 Constitution). Many restrictions directly targeted economic activities, hence affecting economic freedom (Article 27 Constitution). In short, it is plausible that more fundamental rights were restricted in this crisis than remained unaffected.

The Swiss Constitution sets out the frame of reference for restrictions of fundamental rights in Article 36. Restrictions must have a legal basis (Article 36 paragraph 1 Constitution), must be justified in the public interest or for the protection of the fundamental rights of others (Article 36 paragraph 2 Constitution), and must be proportionate (Article 36 paragraph 3 Constitution). Less relevant is Article 36 paragraph 4 Constitution in the current crisis: The essence of fundamental rights is sacrosanct.

It is obvious that much of a legal assessment depends on the *weighting of the public interest* to fight the pandemic, balanced against the interests protected by fundamental rights. The principle of proportionality not only requires that a state measure is suitable to achieving a certain public interest (suitability, effectiveness) and that the measure is the least intrusive (necessity) but also when balanced against the private interest, the importance of the public interest must prevail (reasonableness/balancing). The suitability of a state measure is a technical question in the sense that it mainly requires scientific knowledge to answer that question.[57] This is true also when comparing the effectiveness of different measures, yet the necessity test of the proportionality principle already includes a certain normative aspect in the sense that one must decide which measure is more or less intrusive.[58] The proportionality test becomes fully normative when balancing public and private interests.[59] It is obvious that such balancing also includes political elements and personal views, hence the legal result may depend substantially on a person's political and social preferences. Consequently, the legal result also reflects the standpoint of the author.

I would argue that most of the governmental measures were legally justified during the COVID-19 pandemic. The prevention of death and serious illness is a key public interest, if not the most basic function of a modern state. Indeed, there are no Court decisions or legal opinions

---

53 Cf. de Quervain et al. (2020).

54 According to police crime statistics, domestic violence did not rise significantly in Switzerland during 2020. However, according to the task force on domestic violence and corona, there is evidence that less severe domestic violence rose temporarily during the pandemic, cf. Federal Office for Gender Equality (2021).

55 There have not been any studies verifying this effect yet. According to Helm et al. (2021), section 6.1.2, surveys show that a significant part of students, parents, and teachers are expecting a negative impact of remote learning settings on results.

56 In 2020, the Swiss GDP fell by 2.9%, cf. State Secretariat for Economic Affairs (2021). For the public expenses related to the COVID-19 pandemic, see Section 3.2.2.2.

57 Uhlmann and Wilhelm (2021), p. 54 f.

58 Uhlmann and Wilhelm (2021), p. 55 f.

59 Uhlmann and Wilhelm (2021), p. 56.

that considered the general path taken by Swiss authorities as unconstitutional on the grounds of exaggerated restrictions on fundamental rights. In several decisions, the Federal Supreme Court as well as cantonal (state) courts upheld measures such as mask mandates, the prohibition of events, and the registration of customers' contact details as constitutional and lawful.[60] This may be partly explained by the tendency of Swiss legal scholars (and courts) to look upon state activities in a lenient manner – at least insofar as this has been claimed by critics. More importantly, it seems to me that Swiss authorities never took measures as drastic as those taken by many other countries, especially shying away from enforcing curfews and locking down the economy; the term "lockdown" was, whenever possible, carefully avoided. Regardless of any criticism, there was a feeling that Switzerland never lost a sense of proportion. The Swiss way through the pandemic might be called pragmatic but it also showed its limits when Switzerland was rather unprepared when hit by the second wave of the pandemic.

This positive overall assessment of the Swiss handling of the pandemic does not to mean that governmental authorities were without fault. Indeed, courts and legal scholars were critical in the following typical situations:

Incompetence: Typically, lower administrative authorities have no lawmaking power.[61] Ordinances must be enacted by the Federal Council and on the cantonal level by the cantonal government. Some measures were "disguised" as measures against defined objects (e.g. all Salsa clubs must be closed) but were abstract in nature and hence only the government was competent.[62]

Legality: Usually, the legal basis of measures was not critical as the Federal Council and the cantonal governments rightfully assumed the powers of the legislator in an emergency situation such as the pandemic. Still, it is debatable whether emergency powers included stiffer sanctions than just fines.[63]

Imbalance: Sometimes, the measures chosen were justifiable by themselves but not in comparison. There was a time during the pandemic when one could still visit soccer games but demonstrations on public grounds were strictly prohibited. Here, it was obvious that freedom of expression should be preferred over allowing sports games, the latter arguably not even covered by any fundamental right.

Lacking flexibility: Governments favored "simple" rules, which is perfectly understandable in times of a crisis. Still, sometimes the solutions were just too simple. The administrative court of Zurich intervened against a rule that no more than 15 people were allowed to gather in public places, without any exceptions for political rallies or other important purposes. Here, the rule lacked the necessary flexibility to balance the different interests and allowing more differentiated answers under the proportionality principle.[64]

Unrelated to the pandemic: Some rules were only loosely connected to the pandemic. The Federal Supreme Court found unconstitutional a restriction of access to courts in case of a dispute on cultural subsidies.[65] Again, such a rule may be considered comfortable from an authorities' perspective but obviously had no justification in the pandemic.[66] One may also doubt that a prohibition of open fires in the mountains[67] could be justified by the pandemic; the official reason was that firefighters might be needed for other duties during a pandemic – which is certainly a stretch to say the least.

---

60 Federal Supreme Court, BGE 147 I 450; 147 I 478; 147 I 393; Administrative Court of the Canton of Zurich, AN.2020.00018 of 21 January 2021.
61 Cf. Häfelin et al. (2020), p. 19; Wilhelm and Uhlmann (2021), p. 60.
62 Cf. Wilhelm and Uhlmann (2021), p. 62 ff.
63 Cf. Trümpler and Uhlmann (2020), p. 576 ff.; Uhlmann and Wilhelm (2021), p. 68 f.; Ege and Eschle (2020). Until summer 2021, lower courts had decided on the legality of criminal sanctions imposed based on emergency law provisions in a few cases which were still subject to review by higher courts, see Felber (2021).
64 Cf. Administrative Court of the Canton of Zurich, AN.2021.00003 of 29 April 2021.
65 Federal Supreme Court, BGE 147 I 333.
66 Cf. Brunner et al. (2020), p. 696.
67 As imposed by the government of the canton of Graubünden, AGS 2020-012 (Generelles Feuerverbot im Freien).

3.4.2 Vaccinations

There has been quite a discussion to what extent vaccinations could have been made compulsory. The Epidemics Act, drafted before the COVID-19 pandemic, is quite extensive. Article 22 EpidA reads as follows:

> *Compulsory vaccinations*
>
> *The cantons can make vaccinations compulsory for vulnerable population groups, particularly exposed persons and persons who carry out certain activities if there is a significant risk.*

Note that in a particular situation, the Federal Council can assume this power of the cantons (Article 6 paragraph 2 lit. d EpidA).

The language of Article 22 and Article 6 paragraph 2 lit. d EpidA suggests that a pandemic like COVID-19 was not anticipated by the legislator as compulsory vaccinations were envisaged only for certain groups ("… vulnerable population groups, particularly exposed persons and persons who carry out certain activities …") but not for the entire population which arguably could be envisaged under COVID-19. Still, one may contend that Article 22 and Article 6 paragraph 2 lit. d EpidA only cover the case of a *normal* and of a *particular situation* but not of an *extraordinary situation* in which are no explicit limits to the powers of the Federal Council as explained. The language of the provisions as well as the legal materials[68] suggest that a compulsory vaccination for everyone was not intended by Parliament, so it must be assumed that compulsory vaccinations are possible only for the groups explicitly mentioned in Article 22 and Article 6 paragraph 2 lit. d EpidA.

The reach of Article 22 and Article 6 paragraph 2 lit. d EpidA has not been tested before the courts as the Federal Council as well as the cantons clearly favored voluntary vaccinations. The question could have been relevant as vaccination data suggested that nursing staff in retirement homes were disproportionately skeptical about vaccinations. Compulsory vaccinations for this group would have fallen undoubtedly under Article 22 and Article 6 paragraph 2 lit. d EpidA and an older cantonal court decision as well as decisions by the European Court of Human Rights and the German Federal Constitutional Court suggest that courts might have upheld an obligation.[69]

There was an intensive debate to what extent unvaccinated persons could be excluded from certain state or private services. It was easy, in such situations, to claim discrimination. The legal questions surrounding possible discrimination are far from trivial as there are more groups than simply those willing to be vaccinated and those unwilling to be vaccinated.[70] It is yet unclear as to how many people must avoid vaccination for medical reasons. There is also the case of young children that do not have access to vaccinations (yet). Additionally, it is far from obvious in which situations alternatives such as tests, masks, etc., should be considered (legally) equal to vaccinations.

As a tendency, legal scholars assumed that vaccinations may be required for free time activities, typically private, but less so for vital services, typically public.[71] The denial of vital services would amount to a hidden compulsion which – arguably – is not covered by the law of the land. Also, the exclusion of groups that cannot be vaccinated is considered problematic as the Constitution explicitly forbids discrimination on the grounds of disabilities (Article 8 paragraph 2 Constitution).

Difficult cases can also be expected to emerge dealing with whether (public or private) employers may require vaccinations from their employees. Again, this is relatively easy to justify in case

---

68 Federal Council (2010), p. 380.
69 Verwaltungsgericht des Kantons St. Gallen, Judgment of 19 October 2006 = GVP 2006 Nr. 1; European Court of Human Rights, 47621/13 of 8 April 2021 (Vavřička and others v. The Czech Republic); Bundesverfassungsgericht, 1 BvR 2649/21 of 27 April 2022.
70 Cf. Langer (2021); Vokinger (2020).
71 Cf. Stöckli (2021a). Scholars disagree on whether employers are allowed to require employees other than healthcare workers to get vaccinated, see Vögeli Galli (2021), p. 112 f.; Vionnet (2021), p. 14.

of critical activities (hospitals, etc.) but less so in all other situations. Employers might prefer vaccinated persons for the sake of customers' and coworkers' safety, which undoubtedly would have to be considered as a legitimate interest – but would it be strong enough to put such a heavy incentive on employees skeptical to vaccinations? Court answers a difficult to predict.

3.5   Assessment

Are there legal lessons to be learned from the pandemic in Switzerland? It may be too early for a definitive answer but one may consider the following.

The lockdown in Switzerland was less severe than in other countries which bolstered acceptance of the governmental measures. This not to say that no mistakes were made. Conflicts of competence, sanctions in tension with the legality principle, imbalanced measures in comparison, inflexible rules, and provisions bearing no relation to the pandemic were all to be found. Still, given the omnipresence of daily life restrictions, one should not be too critical.

The Epidemics Act had its baptism of fire. True, for the extraordinary situation, the regulation was meager if not inadequate and Parliament as well as the cantons struggled to find their role. Further, the compensation rules were clearly missing for the case of a pandemic. Still, many measures were correctly pictured and regulated in this act, so again, the verdict should not be too strict.

The long-term effects of the pandemic on the Swiss political system are still hard to predict. To this date, no radical changes are in sight. This holds true both for the interaction of the Federal Council, Parliament, and the courts, as well as between the Federation and the Cantons. As usual, Switzerland fine-tunes its rather reliable but sometimes cumbersome system with foundations dating back to the nineteenth century. Parliaments debate and will enact rules on emergency meetings and one may expect that the role of Parliament will be better understood in future crises. The interaction of federal and cantonal governments may be optimized, not the least as far as communication is concerned – agencies have been rightly been ridiculed for relying on fax machines.[72] Preparation for future crises must be improved as far as stocking for medicines, etc., are concerned and responsibilities must be clear and properly controlled. These are necessary but not spectacular improvements, expected to be completed in reliable Swiss fashion.

This optimistic prediction may be proven wrong. The debate on vaccinations has been unusually fierce in Switzerland. At the time of writing, Switzerland has a disappointingly low rate of vaccination. A first popular referendum against the COVID-19 Act has been defeated by a 60 : 40% margin on 13 June 2021[73] – comfortably but not too comfortably, one may say. A second referendum which included the COVID-19 certificate[74] has been defeated on 28 November 2021 by a 62 : 38% margin.[75] The alleged "discrimination" of the unvaccinated and the possible intrusion to privacy

---

72 Hehli and Gafafer (2021).
73 Federal Council (2021).
74 COVID-19 certificates are issued for persons who have received a COVID-19 vaccination or have recovered from COVID-19 or have recently been tested negative for COVID-19. Article 6a COVID-19 Act authorizes the Federal Council to provide the cantons and third parties with a system for issuing certificates and to stipulate the necessary rules. As Article 6a COVID-19 Act is an amendment to the COVID-19 Act, it had to be approved in a separate popular referendum. The Federal Council issued the necessary rules on the COVID-19 certificate in the Ordinance on certificates to prove COVID-19 vaccination, COVID-19 recovery, or a COVID-19 test result of 4 June 2021 (COVID-19 Certificates Ordinance; SR 818.102.2). Neither the COVID-19 Act nor the COVID-19 Certificates Ordinance specify in which situations companies or public institutions are obligated or allowed to require a valid COVID-19 certificate. The Federal Council stipulated these rules in the COVID-19 Special Situation Ordinance. In summer 2021, a valid COVID-19 certificate was a requirement for participating in events with more than 1,000 persons (Article 17 paragraph 1 COVID-19 Special Situation Ordinance) as well as for entering clubs and discotheques (Article 13 paragraph 1 COVID-19 Special Situation Ordinance). Restaurants, bars, and other businesses and establishments in the culture, entertainment, leisure, and sports sectors were authorized to require a valid COVID-19 certificate on a voluntary basis (cf. Article 10 paragraph 2 COVID-19 Special Situation Ordinance).
75 Federal Council (2022).

rights, not only by way of economic and social pressure to be vaccinated but also that unvaccinated may wear masks, hence "shaming" them in public, cynically compared to the Jewish star in WWII, were key topics in the referendum campaign. The complex Swiss political system, balanced in many directions, requires a high willingness to compromise. It cannot be excluded that the pandemic will substantially damage this virtue. If the United States foreshadows Europe, as often, some fears are appropriate.

References

Bernard, F. (2020). La loi sur les épidémies à l'épreuve du nouveau coronavirus. *Jusletter* (30 March).

Bernard, F. (2021). Les pouvoirs extraordinaires du Conseil fédéral dans la lutte contre les épidémies. *Schweizerisches Zentralblatt für Staats- und Verwaltungsrecht* 122 (3): 131–152.

Biaggini, G. (2017). *BV Kommentar*. 2. Zürich: Orell Füssli.

Biaggini, G. (2020). «Notrecht» in Zeiten des Coronavirus – Eine Kritik der jüngsten Praxis des Bundesrats zu Art. 185 Abs. 3 BV. *Schweizerisches Zentralblatt für Staats- und Verwaltungsrecht* 121 (5): 268–276.

Braun, D. (2003). Dezentraler und unitarischer Föderalismus. Die Schweiz und Deutschland im Vergleich. *Swiss Political Science Review* 9 (1): 57–89.

Brühl-Moser, D. (2007). *Die schweizerische Staatsleitung*. Bern: Stämpfli.

Brunner, F., Wilhelm, M., and Uhlmann, F. (2020). Das Coronavirus und die Grenzen des Notrechts. *Allgemeine Juristische Praxis* 29 (6): 685–701.

Bühler, G., Craviolini, J., Hermann, M., et al. (2021). 7. SRG Corona-Monitor, Studienbericht. https://sotomo.ch/site/wp-content/uploads/2021/03/7.-SRG-Corona-Monitor.pdf (accessed 27 July 2021).

Caroni, A. and Graf, M. (2021). Wahrung der Sessionsteilnahmegarantie in einer Pandemie? *Jusletter* (15 February).

Ege, G. and Eschle, D. (2020). Das Strafrecht in der Krise. *sui generis* 2020: 279–295. https://doi.org/10.21257/sg.137 (accessed 28 July 2021).

Federal Council (2010). Botschaft zur Revision des Bundesgesetzes über die Bekämpfung übertragbarer Krankheiten des Menschen (Epidemiengesetz, EpG). *Bundesblatt* (BBl) 2011: 311–456.

Federal Council (2020a). Coronavirus: Federal Council declares "extraordinary situation" and introduces more stringent measures. Press release (16 March). https://www.admin.ch/gov/en/start/documentation/media-releases.msg-id-78454.html (accessed 26 July 2021).

Federal Council (2020b). Botschaft zu einer dringlichen Änderung des Epidemiengesetzes im Zusammenhang mit dem Corona-Virus (Proximity-Tracing-System). *Bundesblatt* (BBl) 2020: 4461–4480.

Federal Council (2021). Bundesratsbeschluss über das Ergebnis der Volksabstimmung vom 13. Juni 2021. *Bundesblatt* (BBl) 2021: 2135.

Federal Council (2022). Bundesratsbeschluss über das Ergebnis der Volksabstimmung vom 28. November 2021. *Bundesblatt* (BBl) 2022: 894.

Federal Finance Adminstration (2021). Covid-19: Impact on federal finances. https://www.efv.admin.ch/efv/en/home/aktuell/brennpunkt/covid19.html (accessed 15 July 2021).

Federal Office for Gender Equality (2021). Häusliche Gewalt während Corona-Pandemie – Wachsamkeit weiter nötig. Press release (22 March). https://www.ebg.admin.ch/ebg/de/home/das-ebg/nsb-news_list.msg-id-82772.html (accessed 28 July 2021).

Federal Office of Public Health (2021). Covid-19 Switzerland, Information on the current situation. https://www.covid19.admin.ch/en/ (accessed 26 July 2021).

Federal Statistical Office (2020a). Annual Population Statistics. https://www.bfs.admin.ch/bfs/en/home/statistics/population/effectif-change/age-marital-status-nationality.assetdetail.14087718.html (accessed 15 July 2021).

Federal Statistical Office (2020b). Omnibus 2019: Erhebung zur Internetnutzung, Mobile Internetnutzung. https://www.bfs.admin.ch/bfs/de/home/statistiken/kultur-medien-informationsgesellschaft-sport/informationsgesellschaft/gesamtindikatoren/haushalte-bevoelkerung/mobile-internetnutzung.assetdetail.12307308.html (accessed 15 July 2021).

Federal Statistical Office (2021a). Grenzgängerinnen und Grenzgänger in der Schweiz 1996–2020. https://www.bfs.admin.ch/bfsstatic/dam/assets/17205597/master (accessed 14 July 2021).

Federal Statistical Office (2021b). SwissCovid App Monitoring. https://www.experimental.bfs.admin.ch/expstat/en/home/innovative-methods/swisscovid-app-monitoring.html (accessed 15 July 2021).gener

Felber, T. (2021). Gericht uneins im Umgang mit Maskengegnern. *Neue Zürcher Zeitung* (23 July): 11.

Flückiger, A. (2020). Le droit experimental. *Sicherheit & Recht* 13 (3): 142–158.

Gerber, K. (2020). Rechtsschutz bei Massnahmen des Bundesrats zur Bekämpfung der Covid-19-Pandemie. *sui generis* 2020: 249–264.

Glaser, A. and Gfeller, K. (2020). Das Ringen des Parlaments um mehr Macht. *Jusletter* (5 October).

Griffel, A. (2021). Rechtsschutz, insbesondere Verfassungsgerichtsbarkeit. In: *Staatsrecht* (ed. G. Biaggini, T. Gächter, and R. Kiener), 413–444. 3. Zürich and St. Gallen: Dike.

Häfelin, U., Müller, G., and Uhlmann, F. (2020). *Allgemeines Verwaltungsrecht*. 8. Zürich and St. Gallen: Dike.

Hehli, S. and Gafafer, T. (2021). Die Schweiz hat die Digitalisierung des Gesundheitswesens verpasst – das rächt sich jetzt. *Neue Zürcher Zeitung* (2 February): 7.

Helm, C., Huber, S., and Loisinger, T. (2021). Was wissen wir über schulische Lehr-Lern-Prozesse im Distanzunterricht während der Corona-Pandemie? – Evidenz aus Deutschland, Österreich und der Schweiz. *Zeitschrift für Erziehungswissenschaften* 24: 237–311.

Höfler, S. (2018). Gute Gesetzessprache aus dem Blickwinkel der Verwaltung: Die Redaktionskommission der schweizerischen Bundesverwaltung. In: *Gute Gesetzessprache als Herausforderung für die Rechtsetzung* (ed. F. Uhlmann and S. Höfler), 65–100. Zürich and St. Gallen: Dike.

Kley, A. (2020a). «Ausserordentliche Situationen verlangen nach ausserordentlichen Lösungen.» – Ein staatsrechtliches Lehrstück zu Art. 7 EpG und Art. 185 Abs. 3 BV. *Schweizerisches Zentralblatt für Staats- und Verwaltungsrecht* 121 (5): 268–276.

Kley, A. (2020b). *Verfassungsgeschichte der Neuzeit*. 4. Bern: Stämpfli.

Langer, L. (2021). Immunitätsnachweis, Impfpass und Impfobligatorium. *Jusletter* (1 February).

Lopez Bernal, J., Andrews, N., Gower, C., et al. (2021). Effectiveness of Covid-19 Vaccines against the B.1.617.2 (Delta) Variant. *The New England Journal of Medicine*. https://doi.org/10.1056/NEJMoa2108891 (accessed 28 July 2021).

Märkli, B. (2020). Notrecht in der Anwendungsprobe – Grundlegendes am Beispiel der COVID-19-Verordnungen. *Sicherheit & Recht* 13 (2): 59–67.

Münch, U. (2020). Wenn dem Bundesstaat die Stunde der Exekutive schlägt: der deutsche (Exekutiv-)Föderalismus in Zeiten der Coronakrise. In: Jahrbuch Föderalismus 2020 (ed. Europäisches Zentrum für Föderalismus-Forschung Tübingen. Baden-Baden: Nomos. https://doi.org/10.5771/9783748910817-1 (accessed 28 July 2021).

Nasreen, S., Chung, H., He, S., et al. (2022). Effectiveness of COVID-19 vaccines against symptomatic SARS-CoV 2 infection and severe outcomes with variants of concern in Ontario. *Nature Microbiology* 7: 379–385. https://doi.org/10.1038/s41564-021-01053-0 (accessed 22 May 2022).

National COVID-19 Science Task Force (2020). National Covid-19 Science Task Force alarmiert über den rapiden Anstieg der Zahl der SARS-CoV-2-Infektionen in der Schweiz. https://sciencetaskforce .ch/wp-content/uploads/2020/10/National-COVID-19-Science-Task-Force-alarmiert-uber-Anstieg-der-SARS-CoV-2-Infektionen-03-July-20-GE.pdf (accessed 27 July 2021).

Political Institutions Committee of the Council of States (2020). Gesetzliche Grundlagen zur Einführung der Corona-Warn-App (Corona-Proximity-Tracing-App). Motion 20.3168 of 30 April 2020. https://www.parlament.ch/de/ratsbetrieb/suche-curia-vista/geschaeft?AffairId=20203168 (accessed 9 August 2021).

Political Institutions Committee of the National Council (2020). Gesetzliche Grundlagen zur Einführung der Corona-Warn-App (Corona-Proximity-Tracing-App). Motion 20.3144 of 22 April 2020. https://www.parlament.ch/de/ratsbetrieb/suche-curia-vista/geschaeft?AffairId=20203144 (accessed 9 August 2021).

Public Health England (2021). Coronavirus (COVID-19) in the UK. https://coronavirus.data.gov.uk/ (accessed 28 July 2021).

de Quervain, D., Aerni, A., Amin, E., et al. (2020). The Swiss Corona Stress Study: second pandemic wave, November 2020. Preprint. https://doi.org/10.31219/osf.io/6cseh (accessed 28 July 2021).

Rechsteiner, D. (2016). *Recht in besonderen und ausserordentlichen Lagen*. Zürich and St. Gallen: Dike.

Rechsteiner, D. (2020). Die Auswirkungen der Corona-Pandemie auf das Notrecht. *Sicherheit & Recht* 13 (3): 118–129.

Rüefli, Ch., Zenger, Chr, and Elser, D. (2018). Analyse besondere Lage gemäss EpG: Aufgaben, Zuständigkeiten und Kompetenzen des Bundes. Schlussbericht im Auftrag des Bundesamts für Gesundheit. https://www.bag.admin.ch/dam/bag/de/dokumente/mt/k-und-i/ ausbruchsuntersuchungen/BAS_180831_Schlussbericht%20Besondere%20Lage%20180831.pdf .download.pdf/BAS_180831_Schlussbericht%20Besondere%20Lage%20180831.pdf (accessed 13 July 2021).

Saxer, U. (2014). Artikel 185. In: *Die schweizerische Bundesverfassung, St. Galler Kommentar* (ed. B. Ehrenzeller, B. Schindler, R. J. Schweizer, et al.), 2956–2986. 3. Zürich and St. Gallen: Dike.

Schweizer, R.J. (1999). Die Ausgestaltung der Regierung des Bundes in der Schweizerischen Bundesverfassung von 1848. In: Executive and Legislative Powers in the Constitutions of 1848–1849 (ed. H. Dippel), 187–203. Berlin: Duncker & Humblot.

Schweizer Radio und Fernsehen (2020). Daniel Koch zum Tragen von Schutzmasken. *Video clip* (16 March). https://www.srf.ch/play/tv/news-clip/video/daniel-koch-zum-tragen-von-schutzmasken?urn=urn:srf:video:7af2dbfe-077b-48db-8553-8952df0e75be&startTime=30 (accessed 27 July 2021).

Sheik, A., McMenamin, J., Taylor, B., et al. (2021). SARS-CoV-2 Delta VOC in Scotland: demographics, risk of hospital admission, and vaccine effectiveness. *The Lancet* 397 2461–2462. https://doi.org/10 .1016/S0140-6736(21)01358-1 (accessed 28 July 2021).

State Secretariat for Economic Affairs (2021). Gross domestic product in the 4th quarter of 2020: a slowdown in recovery. Press release (26 February). https://www.seco.admin.ch/seco/en/home/seco/ nsb-news/medienmitteilungen-2021.msg-id-82489.html (accessed 28 July 2021).

Stöckli, A. (2020). Regierung und Parlament in Pandemiezeiten. *Zeitschrift für Schweizerisches Recht* special issue Pandemie und Recht: 9–54.

Stöckli, A. (2021a). Corona – mögliche Privilegien für Geimpfte. *Neue Zürcher Zeitung* (20 January): 19.

Stöckli, A. (2021b). Gewaltenteilung in ausserordentlichen Lagen – quo vadis? *Jusletter* (15 February).

Tiefenthal, J.M. (2021), *«Vielfalt in der Einheit» am Ende? Aktuelle Herausforderungen des schweizerischen Föderalismus*. Zürich: EIZ Publishing. https://doi.org/10.36862/eiz-402 (accessed 28 July 2021).

Trümpler, R. (2012). *Notrecht*. Zürich: Schulthess.

Trümpler, R., and Uhlmann, F. (2020). Problemstellungen und Lehren aus der Corona-Krise aus staats- und verwaltungsrechtlicher Sicht. In: *Covid 19 – Ein Panorama der Rechtsfragen zur Corona-Krise* (ed. Helbing Lichtenhahn Verlag). Basel: Helbing Lichtenhahn.

Uhlmann, F. (2021). Die Rolle des Rechts in der Pandemie. *Recht* 2021 (2): 113–116.

Uhlmann, F., and Wilhelm, M. (2021). Verwaltungsrechtliche Herausforderungen. In: *Notrecht in der Corona-Krise* (ed. F. Uhlmann and S. Höfler), 49–80. Zürich and St. Gallen: Dike.

Vionnet, R. (2021). Der Umgang mit Arbeitnehmern während der Corona-Krise. *ex ante* 2020 (1): 12–24.

Vögeli Galli, N. (2021). Covid-19-Impfung und Selbstbestimmungsrecht im Arbeitsverhältnis. *sui generis* 2020: 107–116. https://doi.org/10.21257/sg.174 (accessed 10 August 2021).

Vokinger, K.N. (2020). Impfobligatorium und Impfzwang – eine staatsrechtliche Würdigung. *Recht* 2020 (4): 257–274.

Waldmann, B. (2021). Staatsrechtliche Herausforderungen. In: *Notrecht in der Corona-Krise* (ed. F. Uhlmann and S. Höfler), 3–48. Zürich and St. Gallen: Dike.

Wilhelm, M., and Uhlmann, F. (2020). Herausforderungen für Parlamente in der Corona-Krise – Versuch eines Überblicks. *Parlament* 23 (2): 4–13.

Wilhelm, M., and Uhlmann, F. (2021). Handlungsformen in der Covid-19-Pandemie. *Sicherheit & Recht* 14 (2): 56–65.

Wyss, D. (2020). Sicherheit und Notrecht. *Jusletter* (25 May).

4

Not Dead Yet: Protest, Process, and Germany's Constitutional Democracy Amid the Coronavirus Response

*Carolyn Halladay**

National Security Affairs Department, Naval Postgraduate School, Monterey, CA, USA

Germany's democracy did *not* die of COVID-19 – or of the Federal Republic's response to the pandemic. In fact, the SARS-CoV-2 virus did not even seriously afflict the constitutional order, which remains alive and well, healthy and hale. The reader who has been exposed even casually to the fevered arguments in the old and new media in 2020 and 2021 might be forgiven for thinking otherwise, however; a great many scholars and experts – as well as a fair few cranks – have dedicated countless keystrokes to the question of whether/how Angela Merkel's grand-coalition government and its scientific enablers seized on the crisis to establish some kind of proto-dictatorship.

Such constitutional alarm marks an old fear in new personal protective equipment (PPE), as this chapter shows – and, more urgently, this specter of a creeping coup led by media-star virologists simply fails on the facts. The COVID-19 response in the Federal Republic of Germany (FRG) did not entail a declaration of a state of emergency. No provisions or procedures of the German constitution were suspended at any point. To be sure, the FRG's COVID response – including lockdowns, travel bans, hygiene rules, mask guidelines, distancing, testing, tracing, immunization plans, etc. – represents something other than business as usual. But this situation is hardly a state of emergency or even an "exceptional" situation, constitutionally speaking, as this term has operated since the Weimar Constitution or in the Third Reich. Rather, the Basic Law – the *Grundgesetz*, as the Federal Republic calls its constitution – has remained in full effect for the duration of the pandemic, as have all of the civil-liberties protections that the German state owes its citizens. Indeed, the legal/judicial process has resulted in substantive amendments to the German COVID response as the situation and knowledge about it evolved – change in favor of civil liberties, prosperity, and German democracy.

In contrast, both the Nazi jurist *cum* critic of the Federal Republic, Carl Schmitt, and the Weimar Republic's constitution (including the infamous Article 48, the emergency powers provision that allowed for the suspension of civil liberties amid ill-defined crisis and that ultimately and directly heralded the Nazified legal and social order in Germany in the 1930s and 1940s) are both dead – well and truly dead. Schmitt and his well-cited if camouflaged skepticism of liberal/parliamentary governance have enjoyed a startling reanimation amid the pandemic, at least as "ghosts" of lockdowns past and future.[1] One contemporary commentator characterized the politicized panic about

---

* The ideas and views expressed in this chapter are the author's alone, and they do not represent the official view or policies of the U.S. government, the U.S. Department of Defense, or the U.S. Navy. The author would like to thank Prof. Dr. Donald Abenheim for his invaluable assistance with the drafting and redrafting of this chapter, as well as LCDR. Cameron Jennison (USN), and Major Alicia Jobe (USMC) for their thoughtful reviews.

1 See, for example, Joseph Owen's analysis of an early statement by philosophy professor Giorgio Agamben: "Yet as our political and administrative leaders invoke the language of emergency and of enemy, the apparition of Carl

Germany's COVID response as culminating in the "fascistoid-hysterical rule of hygiene."[2] And observers within and without the Federal Republic have invoked the notorious Weimar-era emergency provisions, as if the FRG were hostage to the same laws and their poisonous effects on democracy.

The thing is, with apologies to Fritz René Allemann and his insights into the FRG of the 1950s: Berlin is not Weimar.[3] Even when, in late August 2020, a crowd of protestors – mostly Corona-skeptics, right-wing extremists, and QAnon conspiracy theorists, many of whom had been gathering repeatedly, usually without masks or much space between them, for demonstrations against ongoing COVID-related restrictions – attempted to penetrate the Reichstag while parliament was meeting, the FRG did not declare a state of emergency, suspend the constitution, or otherwise defer, derange, or disrupt Germany's democracy in the name of public-health expediency.[4]

In the event, Germany's COVID response embodies long-standing and long-considered legal frameworks that – whether or not they bespeak momentary political exigencies – serve the people and, thus, the democracy of the Federal Republic, especially in this pandemic. This chapter examines these frameworks and institutions, the popular and political responses in the FRG, and the historical context of the concern, or maybe *Angst*, that these measures have aroused, initially amid successful and then subsequently less successful measures to combat the pandemic in Germany.

4.1   The First Wave: So Far, So Good

According to the Federal Ministry of Health, Germany's first official case of COVID-19 occurred in a man in the southern state of Bavaria on 27 January 2020.[5] Federal Health Minister Jens Spahn appeared before reporters the next day and admonished the public to exercise "vigilant calm" (*wachsame Gelassenheit*) about the virus, amid other seasonal afflictions like the flu.[6]

No legal or administrative measures were immediately forthcoming, while health authorities awaited further guidance from the Robert Koch-Institut (RKI), the FRG's public center for infectious disease control within the broad purview of the Federal Ministry of Health. The RKI conducts research into infectious disease and response measures, and it advises the German government in this capacity.[7] It has no executive authority – or capability – but the federal *Infektionsschutzgesetz*

Schmitt, Agamben's great influence, ghosts into view." Owen, "States of Emergency, Metaphors of Virus, and COVID-19," 31 March 2020, https://www.versobooks.com/blogs/4636-states-of-emergency-metaphors-of-virus-and-covid-19.

2 Hans Michael Heinig, "Gottesdienstverbot auf Grundlage des Infektionsschutzgesetzes: Verfassungsrechtliche Rechtfertigung und Grenzen," in *Verfassungsblog, on Matters Constitutional*, 17 March 2020, https://verfassungsblog.de/gottesdienstverbot-auf-grundlage-des-infektionsschutzgesetzes/. Heinig's pithy turn of phrase is often reproduced without the key context. Writing of the early response measure to ban even religious gatherings of people, Heinig goes on to note: *Es handelt sich ja nicht um ein dauerhaftes Verbot, sondern um temporäre Maßnahmen, die einem gesundheitspolitisch nachvollziehbarem Plan folgen, um möglichst viele Menschenleben zu retten*—"It's not a matter of a long-term ban, rather of temporary measures that follow a justifiable health policy plan to save as many human lives as possible."

3 Fritz René Allemann, *Bonn ist nicht Weimar* (Cologne and Berlin: Kiepenheuer & Witsch, 1956).

4 "German Leaders Slam Extremists who Rushed Reichstag Steps," https://www.dw.com/en/german-leaders-slam-extremists-who-rushed-reichstag-steps/a-54758246.

5 Bundesministerium für Gesundheit, "Coronavirus-Pandemie (SARS-CoV-2): Chronik bisheriger Maßnahmen und Ereignisse," https://www.bundesgesundheitsministerium.de/coronavirus/chronik-coronavirus.html.

6 Bundesministerium für Gesundheit, "Coronavirus: Aktueller Stand 28.1," https://youtu.be/OGm0b9mn0kA. In this interview, Spahn speaks already of four cases – and admonishes Germans to sneeze into their elbows "rather than [sneezing] in others' faces." Spahn's primary concern in this interview is Germans who have been to China.

7 Robert Koch-Institut, "Das Robert Koch-Institut," https://www.rki.de/DE/Content/Institut/institut_node.html; jsessionid=803E5E82F679042D4893AC2DBAD37CB6.internet052.

(Infection Protection Law or IfSG) establishes the RKI's assessments as the baseline for various governmental policy actions and posits the RKI as the first and best resource for the 16 federal states (*Länder* – for example, Bavaria or Saxony).[8] As Germany is a federal republic, the 16 *Länder* are the principal executors of policy, including public health measures. More exactly, the main responsibility for implementation of COVID-response measures falls to the *Kommune*, the smallest subdivisions of each state, which led to some variation of policy and practice during the pandemic, particularly in the beginning. This arrangement is a matter of "concurrent jurisdiction," according to Art. 74 of the German constitution – that is, an area in which both the federal government and the several states retain some primacy.[9]

The RKI also communicates and coordinates with such international disease-control entities as the European Center for Disease Control (ECDC) and the World Health Organization (WHO).[10] The RKI's initial assessments were fairly restrained, limited by the preliminary nature of the COVID-related science. The RKI approached SARS-CoV-2 with the same three-part model as it would take to any other epidemic: containment, protection, and mitigation.[11] Its first recommendations – and, thus, Germany's initial pandemic policies – focused on containment, largely because the virus and the disease it causes appeared to be an external matter at this point.

By 2 February, 102 Germans who had been in or near Wuhan, China, arrived in the Federal Republic by special air evacuation, thence to spend two weeks in quarantine in an air force dormitory in the Palatinate.[12] The press was shown clean, bright suites with bunk beds; complete if perhaps not luxurious bathrooms; and burly Bundeswehr guards in the hallways, presumably to keep the returnees and the general public (to include even worried family members) apart for the 14-day duration of the quarantine.[13] Two of the returnees tested positive for COVID-19 by 2 February, further confirming the efficacy of the central quarantine policy, according to Health Minister Spahn.[14] The youthful minister toured the facility on 5 February.[15] On 7 February, a short public-service announcement outlined the then-prevailing basics of infection prevention: hand-washing and sneezing into an elbow as far away from others as possible.[16] By 12 February, there were 16 COVID cases in Germany.[17] As yet, Germans seemed willing to go along with such measures as long as it kept the "alien" virus out.

For much of February, with an eye toward the political significance of Germany's nationalists, Spahn remarked conspicuously and often on the connection between SARS-CoV-2 and China, and the ministry emphasized entry restrictions as the first line of defense – more of the initial

8 Andrea Kießling, *IfSG: Infektionsschutzgesetz: Kommentar* (Munich: C.H. Beck, 2020), p. 28.
9 Chancellor's Office, Bundesregierung, https://www.bundesregierung.de/breg-en/chancellor/basic-law-470510.
10 Gesetz zur Verhütung und Bekämpfung von Infektionskrankheiten beim Menschen (Infektionsschutzgesetz – IfSG), § 4 Aufgaben des Robert Koch-Institutes, http://www.gesetze-im-internet.de/ifsg/__4.html.
11 Robert Koch-Institut, Abteilung für Infektionsepidemiologie, "Ergänzung zum Nationalen Pandemieplan – COVID-19 – neuartige Coronaviruserkrankung," April 2020, https://www.rki.de/DE/Content/InfAZ/N/Neuartiges_Coronavirus/Ergaenzung_Pandemieplan_Covid.pdf?__blob=publicationFile, pp. 7–8.
12 SARS-CoV-2 was first identified in Wuhan, China, which informed the initial impulse among health experts and politicians to try to contain COVID-19 there. See, for example, https://www.cdc.gov/coronavirus/2019-ncov/cdcresponse/about-COVID-19.html.
13 Rheinische Post Online, "Coronavirus – So sieht die Quarantäne-Unterkunft in Germersheim aus," https://rp-online.de/leben/gesundheit/news/coronavirus-so-sieht-die-quarantaene-unterkunft-in-germersheim-aus_bid-48697409.
14 Bundesministerium für Gesundheit, "Coronavirus: Aktueller Stand 2.2," https://youtu.be/4878r4DXlLI.
15 Bundesministerium für Gesundheit, "Coronavirus-Pandemie (SARS-CoV-2): Chronik bisheriger Maßnahmen und Ereignisse," https://www.bundesgesundheitsministerium.de/coronavirus/chronik-coronavirus.html.
16 Bundesministerium für Gesundheit, "Fakten zum Coronavirus," https://youtu.be/qBoe_cbewcY.
17 Bundesministerium für Gesundheit, "Coronavirus-Pandemie (SARS-CoV-2): Chronik bisheriger Maßnahmen und Ereignisse," https://www.bundesgesundheitsministerium.de/coronavirus/chronik-coronavirus.html.

emphasis on containment.[18] By 24 February, however, the media focus had shifted to Italy, which had reported its first COVID-19 fatality three days earlier and which was about to post the world's highest COVID death rates until the United States outstripped it in mid-April 2020. The difficulty of imposing travel restrictions within the European Union (EU) became manifest, and the Europe-level response loomed larger in the Health Ministry's communications, although little more than mutual consultation happened in these early days.[19]

On 26 February 2020, Germany reported the first COVID cases, respectively, in the states of Baden-Württemberg and, more alarmingly, Germany's most populous *Land*, North Rhine-Westphalia. Both states established "crisis staffs," basically joint task forces, in accordance with their pandemic plans, supported by the federal government and the RKI. On 27 February, the federal government implemented its own *Krisenstab*, with the goals of "protecting the population and curbing the pandemic as much as possible"[20] – a discursive shift to the "protection" phase of response, in the RKI's three-phase model.[21] The principal method at this point remained entry controls and restrictions of nonessential travel into the country, as well as reporting requirements.

On 3 March 2020, the federal crisis staff, led by the Ministry of Health, urged an export ban on medical protective gear that proved to be in short supply, and the government effected the necessary measures, including covering certain breach-of-contract penalties for companies that faced such measures.[22] On 4 March, the RKI released its update to Germany's National Pandemic Plan (NPP), which document had guided (and been guided by) the FRG's response to earlier influenza epidemics since 2005.[23] On 9 March, Germany reported its first COVID deaths.[24] The WHO declared a global pandemic on 11 March. On 16 March, the FRG closed its land borders to all noncommercial surface traffic amid a rapidly worsening pandemic scenario in Europe.[25]

Within days, six *Länder* imposed various restrictions in an effort to slow the spread of the virus – mainly in the interests of keeping intensive-care beds available for the sickest of patients. On 17 March, amid an unprecedented official declaration of statewide disaster (but *not* of emergency), Bavaria became the first federal state to ban public gatherings, close schools, and shutter "nonessential" business, like restaurants – initially for two weeks.[26] In fact, the disaster declaration remained in effect for 92 days, ending in mid-June. The most obvious effect of the declaration of a *Katastrophenfall* was to activate a kind of whole-of-government Bavarian crisis staff – officially

---

18 Robert Koch-Institut, "VORBEREITUNGEN AUF MAßNAHMEN IN DEUTSCHLAND VERSION 1.0 (STAND 04.03.2020): Ergänzung zum Nationalen Pandemieplan – COVID-19 – neuartige Coronaviruserkrankung," https://www.rki.de/DE/Content/InfAZ/N/Neuartiges_Coronavirus/Ergaenzung_Pandemieplan_Covid.pdf?__blob=publicationFile, p. 7.

19 Bundesministerium für Gesundheit, "Coronavirus: Aktueller Stand 24.2," https://youtu.be/Z5vUNVlARQg.

20 Bundesministerium für Gesundheit, "Coronavirus-Pandemie (SARS-CoV-2): Chronik bisheriger Maßnahmen und Ereignisse," https://www.bundesgesundheitsministerium.de/coronavirus/chronik-coronavirus.html.

21 Robert Koch-Institut, Abteilung für Infektionsepidemiologie, "Ergänzung zum Nationalen Pandemieplan – COVID-19 – neuartige Coronaviruserkrankung," April 2020, https://www.rki.de/DE/Content/InfAZ/N/Neuartiges_Coronavirus/Ergaenzung_Pandemieplan_Covid.pdf?__blob=publicationFile, p. 7.

22 Bundesministerium für Gesundheit, Pressemitteilungen, "Gemeinsamer Krisenstab BMI/BMG fällt weitere Beschlüsse," 4 March 2020, https://www.bundesgesundheitsministerium.de/weiterere-beschluesse-krisenstab-bmi-bmg.html.

23 Robert Koch-Institut, Abteilung für Infektionsepidemiologie, "Ergänzung zum Nationalen Pandemieplan – COVID-19 – neuartige Coronaviruserkrankung," April 2020, https://www.rki.de/DE/Content/InfAZ/N/Neuartiges_Coronavirus/Ergaenzung_Pandemieplan_Covid.pdf?__blob=publicationFile.

24 Caroline Kantis, Samantha Kiernan, and Jason Socrates Bardi, "UPDATED: Timeline of the Coronavirus," Think Global Health, updated 26 March 2021, https://www.thinkglobalhealth.org/article/updated-timeline-coronavirus.

25 BBC, "Coronavirus: Germany latest country to close border," 16 March, 2020, https://www.bbc.com/news/world-europe-51905129.

26 Bayrisches Staatsministerium des Innern, für Sport und Integration, "Informationen zum Coronavirus," https://www.bayern.de/bericht-aus-der-kabinettssitzung-vom-17-maerz-2020/; https://www.corona-katastrophenschutz.bayern.de/lage/index.php (see the entries for 16 and 17 March, in particular).

called the *Führungsgruppe Katastrophenschutz* (Command Group for the Disaster Response) and given the unfortunate acronym FüGK – to coordinate for the entire state of Bavaria COVID-related first-response efforts, communications and information both among participating agencies and outward to the media and the public, and the acquisition and distribution of such necessities as PPE. The FüGK was also tasked with documenting its actions and decisions, including at least one self-congratulatory brochure available through the Bavarian Ministry of the Interior.[27]

Similarly, by 19 March, in the eastern state of Thuringia, a comprehensive list of restrictions went into effect for a month, banning all gatherings, shuttering all touristic and leisure venues (except for take-out service in restaurants), closing the playgrounds, and sites and modalities of prostitution.[28] In Nordrhein-Westfalen, closures and postponements proceeded voluntarily (and, therefore, haphazardly) until the state government issued a set of generally applicable orders on 22 March 2020.[29] Significant fines and even incarceration were included as the penalties for noncompliance. The same day, the state of Saxony issued its own policies, initially somewhat less restrictive or perhaps more focused than the measures that western *Länder* had undertaken – for example, closing nursing homes to visitors and limiting the number of people who could congregate in a weekend cottage or garden plot (*Kleingarten*).[30] The federal authorities continued to urge more uniformity among the several *Länder*.

With the Easter holidays looming in mid-April 2020, two significant COVID-related laws passed in the upper house of parliament, the Bundesrat (25 March), and then the lower house, the Bundestag (27 March), to take effect by or before 1 April. One was the COVID-19 Hospital Relief Bill (*COVID19-Krankenhausentlastungsgesetz*), which sought to remunerate/incentivize health-care facilities for modifications and acquisitions they made to accommodate COVID-19 patients – the kind of supply-chain intervention that the IfSG expressly anticipates.[31] By this time, the extent to which the disease demanded extensive and expensive medical intervention, at least for the acute cases, had become clear. The second law amended the *Infektionsschutzgesetz* in light of, as the title of the law momentously put it, "an Epidemic Situation of National Significance" – *Gesetz zum*

---

27 Bayrisches Staatsministerium des Innern, für Sport und Integration, "92 Tage Katastrophenfall: Corona-Pandemie in Bayern," August 2020, https://www.bestellen.bayern.de/application/eshop_app000002? SID=579476209&ACTIONxSETVAL(artdtl.htm,AARTxNR:03100094,USERxARTIKEL:index_portal.htm, AKATxID:283770,USERxPORTAL:FALSE)=Z.

28 The 19 March 2020 *Erlass* has become difficult to find. Its basic tenets, including the provisions specific to prostitution, appear more formally in Freistaat Thüringen, Ministerium für Arbeit, Soziales, Gesundheit, Frauen und Familie, "Thüringer Verordnungüber erforderliche Maßnahmen zur Eindämmung der Ausbreitung desCoronavirus SARS CoV 2," 26 March 2020, https://www.tmasgff.de/fileadmin/user_upload/Gesundheit/ COVID-19/Verordnung/20200326_ThuerSARS-CoV-2_EindmassnV0.pdf.

29 Landesregierung Nordrhein-Westfalen, "Landesregierung beschließt weitreichendes Kontaktverbot und weitere Maßnahmen zur Eindämmung der Corona-Virus-Pandemie," 22 March 2020, https://www.land.nrw/de/ pressemitteilung/landesregierung-beschliesst-weitreichendes-kontaktverbot-und-weitere-massnahmen-zur.

30 Sächsisches Staatsministerium für Soziales und Gesellschaftlichen Zusammenhalt, "Allgemeinverfügung/Vollzug des Infektionsschutzgesetzes Maßnahmen anlässlich der Corona-Pandemie/Ausgangsbeschränkungen/Bekanntmachung des Sächsischen Staatsministeriums für Soziales und Gesellschaftlichen Zusammenhalt," 22 March 2020, https://www.coronavirus.sachsen.de/download/AllgV-Corona-Ausgangsbeschraenkungen_22032020.pdf.

31 "Gesetz zum Ausgleich COVID-19 bedingter finanzieller Belastungen der Krankenhäuser und weiterer Gesundheitseinrichtungen (COVID-19-Krankenhausentlastungsgesetz)," 27 March 2020, https://www.bgbl.de/ xaver/bgbl/start.xav?startbk=Bundesanzeiger_BGBl&jumpTo=bgbl120s0580.pdf#__bgbl__%2F%2F*%5B%40attr_id %3D%27bgbl120s0580.pdf%27%5D__1614640622410. A directive from 30 March 2020 – *die Verordnung zur Abweichung von der Approbationsordnung für Ärzte bei einer epidemischen Lage von nationaler Tragweite* – provided a mechanism by which current medical students in Germany could aid the efforts against COVID-19 without prejudice to their studies. The second round of state board examinations, originally scheduled for April 2020, had been deferred amid concerns about mass gatherings, anyway.

Schutz der Bevölkerung bei einer epidemischen Lage von nationaler Tragweite.[32] (In all, three such supplemental laws had been passed in Germany by the end of November 2020.)

This turn of phrase – "an epidemic situation of national significance" – created both the threshold and the limit, however vaguely defined at first, of the federal German response. Pointedly, then, German lawmakers did not intend ever to activate all or even part of the coercive powers of the state to intervene in, for example, an outbreak of salmonella related to a local or regional egg producer. In contrast, an "epidemic situation of national significance" seemed to demand more of the federal government – though not necessarily a more federal response.

There followed a flurry of highly technical laws, rules, and directives on the federal level to fine-tune and further facilitate the first-wave response, including:

- *Arzneimittelversorgungsverordnung* (8 April 2020) – a directive that provided for home delivery of COVID medications, as well as various mechanisms to allow pharmacies to substitute drugs and to share supplies among themselves amid much streamlined medical oversight.[33]
- *Verordnung zur Beschaffung von Medizinprodukten und persönlicher Schutzausrüstung bei der durch das Coronavirus SARS-CoV-2 verursachten Epidemie* (9 April 2020) – a directive that allowed the federal government to cover any costs or damages that German firms might incur internationally as they shifted their production and delivery of pandemic necessities to the FRG first.
- *Verordnung zum Ausgleich COVID-19 bedingter finanzieller Belastungen der Zahnärztinnen und Zahnärzte, der Heilmittelerbringer und der Einrichtungen des Müttergenesungswerks oder gleichartigen Einrichtungen sowie zur Pflegehilfsmittelversorgung* (30 April 2020) – a directive that provided a one-time subsidy for health-care professionals whose regular business had been adversely affected by anti-COVID measures.

Similar measures continued to issue for the duration of the pandemic, all aimed at easing the economic effects of Coronavirus and/or honing the commercial sector for the response. Many measures and/or their effects proved to be controversial and attracted significant media scrutiny, especially of Spahn.[34]

By mid-April 2020, as the COVID crisis spread in Europe and North America, but undaunted by the high-profile delay of a tracking app amid concerns about digital surveillance, federal Health Minister Spahn declared that Germany had weathered the first wave of the Coronavirus.[35] The public, as well as the global media, seemed broadly to agree in this assessment, particularly as Germany began to reopen, albeit tentatively. On the one hand, shops with sufficient space as well as certain cultural institutions were allowed to reopen, depending on *Land*-level laws. On the other hand, major public sporting and cultural events were still off until at least the end of August; on 21 April,

---

32 "Gesetzzum Schutz der Bevölkerungbei einer epidemischen Lage von nationaler Tragweite," 27 March 2020, https://www.bgbl.de/xaver/bgbl/start.xav?startbk=Bundesanzeiger_BGBl&start=//*%5B@attr_id=%27bgbl120s0587.pdf%27%5D#__bgbl__%2F%2F*%5B%40attr_id%3D%27bgbl120s0587.pdf%27%5D__1614639649364.

33 Bundesministerium für Gesundheit, "SARS-CoV-2-Arzneimittelversorgungsverordnung," https://www.bundesgesundheitsministerium.de/service/gesetze-und-verordnungen/guv-19-lp/sars-cov-2-arzneimittelversorgungs-vo.html.

34 See, for example, Deutsche Welle, "Germany's health minister under scrutiny over mask purchases," 21 March 2021, https://www.dw.com/en/germanys-health-minister-under-scrutiny-over-mask-purchases/a-56946274.

35 Bundesministerium für Gesundheit, "Coronavirus-Pandemie (SARS-CoV-2): Chronik bisheriger Maßnahmen und Ereigniss," see especially the entry for 17 April 2020 for the quote. The link to the original Channel 1 morning show interview – https://www.daserste.de/information/politik-weltgeschehen/morgenmagazin/videos/Jens_Spahn-102.html – has gone dead in the meantime, but this author viewed the interview when it was still available. The digested account of the interview that still appears on the MOMA website refers only to Spahn's comments about elective surgeries and the pending return to a semblance of normalcy in the German health-care system.

the Premier Minister of Bavaria announced that, out of an abundance of caution, Oktoberfest 2020 was cancelled, an ill omen, whatever temporary success had been attained in public health.[36]

4.2 Proportionality and its Discontents

By this time, as part of the spirit of ferment in German domestic politics that has blossomed since the refugee crisis of 2015, German citizens had begun to circulate petitions on social media and such platforms as change.org, demanding more transparency in the Coronavirus decision-making, if not an end to the pandemic-related restrictions.[37] And sundry German legal experts and personalities chimed in with their own challenges. For example, in April 2020, a Berlin attorney launched a call for "reliable" Coronavirus data on which to base – or by which to revoke – lockdown policies and other COVID rules.[38] In her petition to Chancellor Angela Merkel, which closed out with nearly 85,000 signatures, Viviane Fischer disputes how the RKI attributes all deaths among people with COVID-19 to the disease (rather than, say, to the heart attack or pulmonary crisis that carried them away), and she asserts that a recount will show that "there is absolutely no excess mortality."[39] Dismissing the crisis as "likely nonexistent," Fischer notes portentously: "I truly fear for our democracy."[40]

In much the same vein, Uwe Volkmann, a law professor and legal philosopher at the Goethe University in Frankfurt, lamented in April 2020 that the imprecise models of "the virologists" whose prognostications were meant to guide German policy in the COVID response. In a widely cited commentary in the right-leaning *Frankfurter Allgemeine,* Volkmann points out archly that the Federal Republic sees between 3,000 and 4,000 traffic deaths a year; a particularly severe flu season might claim 25,000 lives – and even then, both society and its leaders satisfy themselves "by and large with mostly unheeded recommendations for immunization."[41] With the Coronavirus, however, he argues, the government seems obsessed with preserving human life at any cost – rather than emphasizing life with dignity, the principle with which the *Grundgesetz* begins in its very first clause.[42] Moreover, he writes, the lockdowns, quarantines, travel restrictions, and other response measures impinge on the fundamental right to the free development of personality enshrined in Art. 2 of the *Grundgesetz,* "which includes relations with other people."[43] Where Chancellor Merkel had, a month earlier, invoked her own experience in the "dictatorship of the proletariat" in East Germany – "Let me assure you: for someone like myself, for whom freedom of travel and

---

36 "Oktoberfest 2020 has been Cancelled: The Wiesn 2020 Cannot Take Place Because of Covid-19," 21 April 2020, https://www.oktoberfest.de/en/magazine/oktoberfest-news/2020/oktoberfest-2020-will-be-cancelled.
37 Danielle Celermajer and Dalia Nassar, "COVID and the Era of Emergencies: What Type of Freedom is at Stake?" *Democratic Theory*, Vol. 7, No. 2 (Winter 2020), pp. 12–24. The authors refer to several such petitions on pp. 15–17.
38 Viviane Fischer, "Conduct a base line study – we finally need reliable Corona data!" petition on OpenPetition.de, launched April 2020, https://www.openpetition.de/petition/online/conduct-a-base-line-study-we-finally-need-reliable-corona-data.
39 Viviane Fischer, "Conduct a base line study – we finally need reliable Corona data!" petition on OpenPetition.de, launched April 2020, https://www.openpetition.de/petition/online/conduct-a-base-line-study-we-finally-need-reliable-corona-data.
40 Viviane Fischer, "Conduct a base line study – we finally need reliable Corona data!" petition on OpenPetition.de, launched April 2020, https://www.openpetition.de/petition/online/conduct-a-base-line-study-we-finally-need-reliable-corona-data.
41 Uwe Volkmann, "Das höchste Gut," *Frankfurter Allgemeine Zeitung*, 1 April 2020, https://www.faz.net/aktuell/feuilleton/debatten/staatsrecht-und-die-wuerde-des-menschen-16705618.html?premium.
42 Uwe Volkmann, "Das höchste Gut," *Frankfurter Allgemeine Zeitung*, 1 April 2020, https://www.faz.net/aktuell/feuilleton/debatten/staatsrecht-und-die-wuerde-des-menschen-16705618.html?premium.
43 Uwe Volkmann, "Das höchste Gut," *Frankfurter Allgemeine Zeitung*, 1 April 2020, https://www.faz.net/aktuell/feuilleton/debatten/staatsrecht-und-die-wuerde-des-menschen-16705618.html?premium.

movement were hard-won rights, such restrictions can only be justified when they are absolutely necessary"[44] – Volkmann sees the Merkel government's pandemic response as the next-worst thing: "If you want to know what it would be like to wake up one morning in North Korea—complete with shelves empty of cleaning supplies—now is the chance to begin to form some impressions."[45]

North Korea? Really? Even Volkmann has to admit that, despite the purported overreach by a constitution-crushing government, he still has the freedom to disagree with the response without fear of repression or reprisal. He notes that "all measures are communicated transparently and can be overseen by independent courts."[46] Actually, he may be slightly optimistic in this aside – consider Fischer's petition – but this tossed-off comment is kind of the whole point of such expansive legalistic rhetoric. Volkmann grudgingly concedes that, yes, the federal and state legislatures are still meeting, despite the broader restrictions, and they are giving due consideration to the measures at issue. The courts are, too. That is to say that Germany's legal, political, and procedural democracy remains in full swing. One doubts that Pyongyang can say the same.

Volkmann's histrionics, even more than his formidable legal–professorial prose, obscure one false equivalency (because the state sends its citizens to fight and die in wars – and thereby effectively withdraws the citizen-soldier's right to life – the state cannot curtail one citizen's personality development in the name of saving another's life) AND one dubious chicken-and-egg proposition, where he insists that the government's restrictions would only be constitutional if, in fact, Germany faced a shortage of emergency-room beds or ventilators … as if the various measures enacted in March had not somehow contributed to the happy slack in the FRG's emergency medical system in spring 2020.

But he also raises a valid legal point in and about the German system of law and governance – as did Fischer, albeit obliquely, and as did, more seriously, Jessica Hamed, a lawyer from Mainz, who sued several *Länder* over COVID response measures. Ultimately at issue is the principle of proportionality (*Grundsatz der Verhältnismäßigkeit*), a cornerstone of German legal calculus, particularly as regards the protection and preservation of basic rights.[47] Proportionality entails three parts – and any law in the FRG that seeks to infringe fundamental liberties must meet all three requirements:

- Suitability (*Geeignetheit*): The measure must effectively achieve its aim.
- Necessity (*Erforderlichkeit*): The measure is needed to achieve its aim.
- Appropriateness (*Angemessenheit*): The measure must not impinge unduly on civil liberties, a calculation that involves an exact and exacting balancing (*Abwägung*) of individual and societal interests.

Suitability may be the easiest hurdle to clear.[48] One can imagine any number of measures (think: quarantine requirements in their variety) that would effectively inhibit the transmission of COVID-19. To be sure, questions about the underlying science – how long does the virus really live on surfaces? – might speak to this aspect of proportionality if, for example, a given restriction would have no real impact on the Coronavirus. But "effectiveness" does not really speak to the heart of proportionality. Critics who, for example, look to flu outbreaks as a point of comparison often touch on the matter of necessity; Volkmann's recitation of traffic-fatality

44 Deutsche Welle, "Merkel: Coronavirus is Germany's greatest challenge since World War II," 18 March 2020, https://www.dw.com/en/merkel-coronavirus-is-germanys-greatest-challenge-since-world-war-ii/a-52830797.
45 Uwe Volkmann, "Das höchste Gut," *Frankfurter Allgemeine Zeitung*, 1 April 2020, https://www.faz.net/aktuell/feuilleton/debatten/staatsrecht-und-die-wuerde-des-menschen-16705618.html?premium.
46 Uwe Volkmann, "Das höchste Gut," *Frankfurter Allgemeine Zeitung*, 1 April 2020, https://www.faz.net/aktuell/feuilleton/debatten/staatsrecht-und-die-wuerde-des-menschen-16705618.html?premium.
47 Nigel Foster and Satish Sule, *German Legal System and Laws*, 4th ed. (Oxford: OUP, 2010), p. 185.
48 See Foster and Sule on the "falconry case," Nigel Foster and Satish Sule, *German Legal System and Laws*, 4th ed. (Oxford: OUP, 2010), p. 186.

statistics – arguably, German society is content to lose a few thousand souls every year to ultimate driving machines, rather than implementing more restrictive rules of the road so as to preserve more human lives – pokes at the necessity, or not, of all of this pandemic legislation.

The real battleground is appropriateness, as Celermajer and Nassar write.[49] Is it appropriate to shut down all the schools, granted the detriment to the students that this measure entails? Is it appropriate to require that all Germans returning from visits to "hot spot" states strictly quarantine for two weeks, whether they can afford it or not? Is it appropriate for the government to require German manufacturers of PPE to supply the FRG first, regardless of contract or market provisions? In the event, many of the legal challenges to COVID-response measures in Germany failed – and therefore faced significant amendment, limitation, or repeal – on the grounds of appropriateness for these and other reasons.

It merits mention here, particularly if Volkmann wants to dismiss it as self-evident and somehow insignificant, that for the duration of the pandemic and the response, Germany's courts were available to hear and decide on these challenges, and the legislatures at all levels were able to revise the laws appropriately. That is, even if, as the record suggests, the FRG's initial measures to contain and protect – and eventually mitigate – SARS-Cov-2 were more than the German constitutional dedication to human dignity could abide, then Germans can take comfort in the fact that the law and their liberties ultimately prevailed. The process persisted.

In all, Germany's response to the first wave of Coronavirus infection managed to balance several constitutional obligations: the *individual* citizen's right to life and physical integrity (Art. 2 of the *Grundgesetz*,[50] which also forms the basis of all public health law in Germany, including the IfSG[51]); the FRG's fundamental orientation as a "social state" (Art. 20 and Art. 28 of the *Grundgesetz*; the more natural English phrasing might be "social welfare state"), which principle is mostly about socioeconomic equity, but which also encompasses deeply rooted popular expectations of basic services that the government should provide[52]; and the now-ingrained tenets of federalism (Arts. 70–74 of the *Grundgesetz*). The same legal structure facilitated a nimble political and practical response to the first wave of the pandemic in Germany. Thus, a relatively healthy and democratically intact FRG headed into the summer – with vacation on its collective mind.

4.3 Summer in the City

Germany's success with the first wave may have wrongly inflected overly buoyant expectations about successive waves – at all levels of politics and society – for better and worse. Either way, things were about to get weird in the FRG, although at first, the summer seemed to be shaping up rather nicely as SARS-CoV-2 restrictions eased. Some acute, if largely localized, COVID outbreaks in meat-packing plants around the FRG made headlines in the late spring and early summer of 2020.[53] Still, the response became increasingly differentiated and focused as lawsuits and cooler heads prevailed. Thus, for the most part, Germany and Germans were ready for a quasi-normal summer, even as other parts of the world stumbled into ever greater mass illness and death; most leaders at most levels continued to press for caution.

---

49 Danielle Celermajer and Dalia Nassar, "COVID and the Era of Emergencies: What Type of Freedom is at Stake?" *Democratic Theory*, Vol. 7, No. 2 (Winter 2020), pp. 12–24.
50 The Basic Law, https://www.bundesregierung.de/breg-en/chancellor/basic-law-470510.
51 Andrea Kießling, *IfSG: Infektionsschutzgesetz: Kommentar* (Munich: C.H. Beck, 2020), pp. 2–3.
52 Nigel Foster and Satish Sule, *German Legal System and Laws*, 4th ed. (Oxford: OUP, 2010), p. 187.
53 See, for example, Deutsche Welle, "Germany's meat industry under fire after COVID-19 outbreaks," 19 May 2020, https://www.dw.com/en/germanys-meat-industry-under-fire-after-covid-19-outbreaks/a-53502751.

The Federal Ministry of Health boiled this message down to a three-letter slogan: AHA – *Abstand, Hygiene, Alltagsmaske* (roughly: Distancing, Handwashing, and Masking).[54] Spahn urged Germans to maintain these practices and their vigilance even while they enjoyed their summer travels amid tentatively relaxed restrictions within Germany and Europe. Germany reopened its borders to most of its EU neighbors, with reciprocity, in mid-June. Spain had extended its state of emergency until 21 June, so travel restrictions lasted for a few days longer. Nonetheless, starting on 15 June, Germans were allowed to travel to the Balearics, facilitating a semblance of the ritual seasonal migration toward the sun. Returning vacationers were required to have a COVID test within three days of arrival back in Germany and to quarantine at home for two weeks. Eventually, this rule required people arriving from high-risk countries to be tested immediately in the arrival airport or train station or to provide evidence of a negative test result from just before their journey began. The concern remained keeping the virus outside German territory.

On 16 June 2020, the ministry launched its delayed Corona-Warn-App, an anonymous contact-tracing program for smart phones.[55] Presently, the Health Ministry's guidance became AHA+A (app) or AHA+C (Corona-Warn-App).[56]

At the same time, the German health leadership became expansive in its attention to European and global disease control efforts. The EU was not particularly prominent in the earliest phases of SARS-Cov-2 in Europe, even after the WHO proclaimed Europe to be the epicenter of the pandemic in March. But the first paragraph of Art. 168 of the Treaty on the Functioning of the European Union specifies that all Union action as regards public health should "complement" the national policies of the several member states.[57] In other words, the responsibility for public health policy and its execution remains wholly with the national governments. (The ECDC, thus, functions at the Union level, principally as a source of training, information, and broad guidance.[58])

Still, Para. 2 of Art. 168 directs the EU to "encourage cooperation" among the member states in the public-health realm,[59] which worked well enough as regards the easing of internal and external travel restrictions in the summer of 2020 (even if the initial unilateral travel bans and border closures among members surely bruised the Schengen promise of free movement within the Union). When the matter turned to money, however, the shadow side of German government in the Merkel era, namely the fetish of no-deficit spending, emerged with what has proven to be disastrous consequences. The acrimonious disagreements among member states, which the euro-crisis of 2008–2009 had sparked, threatened to reignite amid the run-up to negotiations for what became a €750 billion stimulus package in July. While the Germans had vociferously opposed an early plan for "Corona-bonds" – which would have made the EU's larger and/or more frugal states into guarantors – in the event, Merkel opted for European solidarity and voted in favor of the stimulus,

54 The rough translation speaks to the images on the posters, rather than the awkward literal translation. https://commons.wikimedia.org/wiki/File:Bundesgesundheitsministerium_%22AHA%22_COVID-19-Plakat.jpg
55 Bundesministerium für Gesundheit, "So funktioniert die #CoronaWarnApp," 16 June 2020, https://youtu.be/shoM2G-yecA; see also the ministry's Corona app web page: https://www.zusammengegencorona.de/informieren/die-corona-warn-app/.
56 By the autumn of 2020, amid evolving insights into COVID-19 and its transmission, the Federal Ministry of Health also recommended AHA+L (*Lüften*/ventilation).
57 "Consolidated versions of the Treaty on European Union and the Treaty on the Functioning of the European Union," https://eur-lex.europa.eu/legal-content/EN/TXT/HTML/?uri=CELEX:12012E/TXT&from=EN.
58 https://www.ecdc.europa.eu/en. To the extent that the ECDC relies on data from the member states, the overall picture of public health in the EU may not be as easily or clearly assembled as one might hope, however. In this connection, see the helpful volume on apples-to-apples statistics by Linda Hantrais and Marie-Thérèse Letablier, *Comparing and Contrasting the Impact of the COVID-19 Pandemic in the European Union* (London and New York: Routledge, 2021).
59 The ECDC's English-language website appears at: https://eur-lex.europa.eu/legal-content/EN/TXT/HTML/?uri=CELEX:12012E/TXT&from=EN.

which included significant grants (but not credits) to states hardest hit by the virus. Nonetheless, as Hantrais and Letablier note, this big-ticket compromise left "several countries less than satisfied with the outcome."[60]

A certain discontent was growing within Germany, as well. After years of a globalized boom in which the storied German export economy flourished, lockdowns and business closures augured an economic slowdown in the FRG and probably a Europe-wide recession. In short order, the EU's Covid-era stimulus agreement raised the specter of bailouts and other shades of the sovereign debt malaise 2008, the likes of which then had given rise, among other things, to the far-right, anti-EU, and anti-Merkel Alternative for Germany party (*Alternative für Deutschland* or AfD). The persistence of Coronavirus restrictions, despite the cheery blue and red of the AHA posters and the allure of Spanish beaches, exacerbated popular disgruntlement – even as the COVID infection rate started to rise again amid summer-vacation travel. Amid this darkening public mood, after first demanding that Germany close its borders and blaming migrants for the spread of SARS-CoV-2 in the FRG, the AfD, after some party-internal turmoil, ultimately threw its lot in with the noisiest of the Corona-skeptics, who had started gathering regularly in Germany's major cities to protest.[61]

"Corona-skeptic" is a broad notion in German – connotatively a term of opprobrium in pretty much all cases – that includes, depending on just who is deploying it, people who: object to business and/or school closures; reject masking and social distancing requirements; argue that the Coronavirus is less infectious/less lethal than influenza and, therefore, should not be such a concern; insist that the pandemic is a matter of media or scientific hype; claim that the "lying press" (*Lügenpresse*, a term that Josef Goebbels originated) has purposefully throttled discussion to abet the shadowy powers that gain from various COVID fictions; assert that vaccines are a form of social control; suggest that Microsoft founder Bill Gates has masterminded the pandemic; and/or believe in a global conspiracy in which many of the world's political and cultural leaders are engaged in a vast child sex-trafficking network that may or may not reveal the plotting and scheming of half-human, half-lizard aliens bent on world domination. Proponents of such theories in their number have illustrated their various points with slogans and imagery that evoke the anti-Semitic chestnut of the so-called blood libel plainly enough to have attracted the investigative attention of the Federal Office for the Protection of the Constitution (*Bundesverfassungsschutz* or BfV).

Without question, the protests drew a considerable cross section of participants, ranging from glittering stragglers from Berlin's now much subdued rave scene, through variously engaged citizens and more than a few gawkers, to extremists from both sides of the political spectrum who may have had ideologies to grind with the pandemic response or who may have simply come for the crowd. Conspiracy theorists provided much of the text – and the headlines. The "hygiene demos" gave German authorities a jolting look at the reach and grasp of QAnon, which had even claimed the minds and Twitter feeds of such celebrities as influencer and singer Xavier Naidoo and the Turko-German TV chef Attila Hildmann.[62]

They also saw the rise of homegrown entities like Querdenken 711. The name translates connotatively as "lateral thinking" in the sense of dissent, though "disruptive thinking," with its tech-sector overtones, might be more apt; 711 is the locality prefix for telephone numbers in tony Stuttgart, where the group's founder, Michael Ballweg, has his home and software business. In the initial

60 Linda Hantrais and Marie-Thérèse Letablier, *Comparing and Contrasting the Impact of the COVID-19 Pandemic in the European Union* (London and New York: Routledge, 2021), p. 94. See also Jens Kersten and Stephan Rixen, *Der Verfassungsstaat in der Corona-Krise* (Munich: C.H. Beck, 2020), pp. 138–140.
61 Deutsche Welle, "German far-right AfD in crisis," 18 May 2020 https://www.dw.com/en/german-far-right-afd-in-crisis/a-53487633.
62 Deutsche Welle, "Why the QAnon conspiracy theory is gaining popularity," 27 September 2020, https://www.dw.com/en/why-the-qanon-conspiracy-theory-is-gaining-popularity/a-55066593.

days of the pandemic, the middle-40s tech entrepreneur Ballweg had made something of a project of suing to repeal or at least roll back COVID-related restrictions along the lines of Jessica Hamed's work, although he was not the earliest adopter of this tactic, despite his claims in the spring of 2020.[63] Eventually, though, both Ballweg and his group oriented themselves more firmly toward QAnon-type conspiracy theories, with a bit of doomsday prepping thrown in for dramatic effect.[64] Ever fewer masks appeared among the protestors, but, while the authorities denied some demonstration permits to groups that refused to agree to the basic AHA guidelines and at least once broke up a protest of regulation-flouting opponents of the restrictions, the summer's agitations continued as a kind of seasonal happening.

For the most part, as Celermajer and Nassar point out, these protests represent a very healthy, very democratic response to the response – "democratic" in the sense of citizens taking their grievances directly to their government.[65] In this spirit, the demonstrations represent the antidote to Hannah Arendt's "hollowing out" of democracy in favor of totalitarianism and the "mass transfer of power from the people to a centralized state."[66]

Ultimately, however, many of the *Querdenker* and other groupings that appeared amid the hygiene demos coalesced around – or into – far-right extremism that is generally ascendant in worrisome parts of the European body politic more or less since 2013–2015. And then the protests acquired a very different character. The populists and other opponents of Germany's multicultural liberal democracy became prominent; for example, the *Reichsbürger*, as the FRG's native and nativist sovereign citizens call themselves – with their dogma that the Bonn and Berlin Republics are illegitimate usurpers of some eternal German Reich – were well represented among the carriers of black-white-red imperial banners[67] (a coded reference to Germany's nationalist past, albeit one that still passes muster with the BfV as far as public display goes in a way that, say, Nazi emblems do not).

On the last Saturday in August 2020, as the FRG closed in on 250,000 COVID-19 cases and 10,000 deaths,[68] several thousand demonstrators assembled in Berlin and, among other things, heard prominent anti-vaxxer Robert Kennedy, Jr., who was speaking at the Victory Column, proclaim that Bill Gates and the director of the U.S. National Institute of Allergy and Infectious Diseases, Anthony Fauci, had been cooking up this "crisis of convenience" for decades, in part to use the quarantine to impose 5G and virtual currency on the formerly free world.[69] Perversely invoking the famous words of his uncle, the late President John F. Kennedy – "Ich bin ein Berliner" – the younger Kennedy disputed the expected media characterization of the audience as a bunch of Nazis. Instead, he said of his assembly of alternate Berliners, "We are the frontline against totalitarianism."[70] Later, some hundreds of protestors – despite Kennedy's prediction, largely with extremist right-wing agendas,

---

63 Claudia Henzler, "Profil: Michael Ballweg," *Süddeutsche Zeitung*, 27 August 2020, https://www.sueddeutsche.de/politik/profil-michael-ballweg-1.5012098.

64 Claudia Henzler, "Profil: Michael Ballweg," *Süddeutsche Zeitung*, 27 August 2020, https://www.sueddeutsche.de/politik/profil-michael-ballweg-1.5012098.

65 Danielle Celermajer and Dalia Nassar, "COVID and the Era of Emergencies: What Type of Freedom is at Stake?" *Democratic Theory*, Vol. 7, No. 2 (Winter 2020), p. 13.

66 Danielle Celermajer and Dalia Nassar, "COVID and the Era of Emergencies: What Type of Freedom is at Stake?" *Democratic Theory*, Vol. 7, No. 2 (Winter 2020), p. 13.

67 Bundesamt für Verfassungsschutz, "Reichsbürger und Selbstverwalter: Begriff und Erscheinungsformen," https://www.verfassungsschutz.de/DE/Themen/Reichsbuerger-und-Selbstverwalter/Begriff-und-Erscheinungsformen/begriff-und-erscheinungsformen_artikel.html.

68 Robert Koch-Institut, "Coronavirus Disease 2019(COVID-19)," Daily Situation Report of the Robert Koch Institute 22 August 2020, UPDATED STATUS FOR GERMANY https://www.rki.de/DE/Content/InfAZ/N/Neuartiges_Coronavirus/Situationsberichte/2020-08-22-en.pdf?__blob=publicationFile

69 Stefan Schaaf, "Vom Umweltanwalt zum Wirrkopf," *TAZ*, 31 August 2020, https://taz.de/Der-Anwalt-Robert-Kennedy-Jr/!5706424/; the full speech, in English and German, is available at: https://youtu.be/zfe__wsmvSY.

70 See the video of the Kennedy speech at https://youtu.be/zfe__wsmvSY

to include the *Reichsbürger* and, according to contemporary accounts, perhaps with the collusion or connivance of AfD members of parliament, to say nothing of Russian fifth column agents, who notoriously frolic in Berlin – attempted to enter the Reichstag illegally and violently while the parliament was in session.[71] In the end, police repelled the attack, and the parliament finished its business, which happened to be Coronavirus-related legislation.

4.4   Is it an Emergency Yet?

Parliamentarians and others expressed their outrage at the assault on the seat of Germany's legislature (and the core of its democracy) – but even with the *Reichsbürger* literally at the door, no one in the Merkel cabinet or the legislature declared a state of emergency. This non-eventuality is important. Objectively, an attempted incursion into the Reichstag certainly sounds like the kind of event that could trigger a "state of defense" in the FRG, as contemporary constitutional argot has it. In the end, however, the attempted breach of the Reichstag really only added another justification or two to the pile of reasons that moved the BfV to observe the AfD as a potential threat to German democracy,[72] just as the state-level office of constitutional protection in Baden-Württemberg (state capital: Stuttgart) initiated an investigation of *Querdenken 711* in early 2021.[73]

No doubt many of the AfD party faithful look at the BfV's decision as more evidence of an iron-fisted FRG government set on silencing all non-adherents of the *multi-kulti* orthodoxy. And without question, there is something bracing about a major democracy retaining the right to ban whole parties from the democratic contest – unless and until Germany's political history is added to the computations – under the banner of lessons of the years 1930–1933 in a twentieth- and now twenty-first-century democracy that aggressively defends itself against threats to its fundamental liberal-democratic constitutional system.[74] In this case, the interwar period of Germany's first democracy witnessed fractured and fracturing of the center-oriented parties that ultimately left the Weimar Republic particularly susceptible to the National Socialist takeover between 1930 and 1933, while other parties preferred to war among themselves, rather than face together what soon enough became clearly the common totalitarian threat.[75] As part of the effort to curtail such unholy effects of splinter parties in the Bonn democracy, the Federal Republic instituted, for one example, its five-percent clause, a threshold of parliamentary participation embedded in

---

71 Deutsche Welle, "'Shameful' attempt to storm the Reichstag," 31 August 2020, https://www.dw.com/en/german-leaders-slam-extremists-who-rushed-reichstag-steps/a-54758246; https://www.dw.com/en/shameful-attempt-to-storm-the-reichstag/av-54774124.

72 Wolf Wiedmann-Schmidt, "Verfassungsschutz beobachtet AfD nun bundesweit," Der Spiegel, 3 March 2021, https://www.spiegel.de/politik/deutschland/rechtsextremismus-verdachtsfall-verfassungsschutz-beobachtet-afd-nun-bundesweit-a-136d80ce-4549-4a23-8174-19ad70f20643. The harder-right faction of the AfD knows as der Flügel ("the Wing") had been listed as a "significant right-extreme" threat in March of 2020. See the announcement of the BfV: https://www.verfassungsschutz.de/SharedDocs/Pressemitteilungen/DE/2020/Pressemitteilung_2020_1.html.

73 Baden-Württemberg Landesamt für Verfassungsschutz, "Die Querdenken-Bewegung – zwischen Verschwörungsmythen und Bürgerprotest," 28 January 2021, https://www.verfassungsschutz-bw.de/,Lde/Vortrag_+_Die+Querdenken-Bewegung+_+zwischen+Verschwoerungsmythen+und+Buergerprotest_.

74 While the whole volume speaks to this point in compelling detail and variety of perspectives, a particularly helpful discussion of this point is Dieter Grimm, "Über den Umgang mit Parteiverboten," in Claus Leggewie and Horst Meier, eds., *Verbot der NPS oder mit Rechtsradikalen leben?* (Frankfurt a.M.: Suhrkamp, 2002), esp. pp. 139–140.

75 See Karl Dietrich Bracher, *Die Auflösung der Weimarer Republik: Eine Studie zum Problem des Machtverfalls in der Demokratie*, Schriften des Instituts für politische Wissenschaft, Vol. 4 (Stuttgart and Düsseldorf: Ring Verlag, 1955); Ursula Büttner, *Weimar, die Überforderte Republik, 1918–1933*, Vol. 18 of Wolfgang Benz and Ursula Büttner, eds., *Gebhardt: Handbuch der deutschen Geschichte*, 10th ed. (Stuttgart: Klett-Cotta, 2010), pp. 608–714.

the Federal Voting Law.[76] Another such measure includes the constitutional provision – Art. 21, especially para. 2 – that allows for the prohibition of parties that "by reason of their aims or the behavior of their adherents, seek to undermine or abolish the free democratic basic order or to endanger the existence of the Federal Republic of Germany …".[77] The ultimate decision about the democratic chops (or not) of any party that errs – or goose-steps – into the realm of extremism belongs to the Federal Constitutional Court, according to the *Grundgesetz*.[78]

In the FRG's first decade, both the self-proclaimed successor party of the Nazis, the Sozialistische Reichspartei (SRP), and the German communist party (KPD) were banned. Resolutely anti-Semitic, anti-American, and antidemocratic, the neo-Nazi SRP won two seats in the first federal parliament and posted some startling results in *Land* elections before it was banned in 1952, along with its paramilitary organization and its youth wing. The KPD only ever cleared the 5-percent hurdle in the first parliamentary election in 1949, but its militancy and resolute rejection of the Bonn Republic's democracy still made it a threat, according to the Constitutional Court. The KPD challenged the ban all the way to the European Commission on Human Rights, which left the party more or less in business, though with negligible effect, until 1956.

Frank Biess evocatively describes this period of early West German history in terms of "democratic angst" – when conservative and liberal intellectuals and politicians worried extensively and often in print about the FRG's future prospects in the shadow of Weimar's failings and the Third Reich, as well as the perceived ill-effects of democratizing.[79] Since 1956, however, the Federal Republic has not outlawed another party – even as variously extreme groups have emerged to some prominence. One thinks in this connection of the so-called National Party of Germany (NPD), which arose in 1964 and which the federal government has sought several times to ban. Another example is the *Republikaner*, a pugnaciously anti-European and anti-immigrant far-right nationalist party that gained visibility and votes through the 1980s and into the early 1990s until its reflexive anti-communism put it on the wrong side of German unification and, thus, largely out of the running for electoral significance. The BfV had the *Reps* under observation from 1992 until 2007, but no further measures were undertaken thereafter.

Indeed, the official confidence in the resilience of Germany's constitutional order seems to have grown significantly over the years. In 2017, the federal Constitutional Court rejected the most recent petition to ban the NPD, mostly because the party had little practical national effect, having never won enough votes in federal elections to seat a member. (It had posted significant results in state elections until 2016, however, and in 2014, the NPD sent its first and last member to the European Parliament.) This latter-day requirement – that the promulgators of an odious and unconstitutional ideology also be in the position to do something meaningful about it in German society – seems to represent a certain relaxation of the FRG's "democratic angst," more of a settling-in to the unsexy but meaningful political stability that Manfred Kuechler has described as the most striking characteristic of postwar Germany.[80]

---

76 Bundesminesterium der Justiz und für Verbraucherschutz, "Bundeswahlgesetz," para. 6, https://www.gesetze-im-internet.de/bwahlg/__6.html

77 Basic Law: https://www.bundesregierung.de/breg-en/chancellor/basic-law-470510

78 The justices on the Federal Constitutional Court are nominated by the houses of parliament for a single 12-year term. See the court's English-language page on "Justices of the Constitutional Court," https://www.bundesverfassungsgericht.de/EN/Richter/richter_node.html.

79 Frank Biess, *German Angst: Fear and Democracy in the Federal Republic of Germany* (Oxford: OUP, 2020), esp. pp. 159–160.

80 Manfred Kuechler, "Political Attitudes and Behavior in Germany: The Making of a Democratic Society," in Michael G. Huelshoff, Andrei S. Markovits, and Simon Reich, eds., *From Bundesrepublik to Deutschland: German Politics after Unification* (Ann Arbor: University of Michigan Press, 1993), p. 35.

Moreover, as the KPD and NPD cases demonstrate, the German court system remained and remains available to all the groups that face listing, observation, or prohibition – as a matter of constitutional requirement (Art. 19). As the eminent scholar of twentieth-century Germany, Karl Dietrich Bracher, pointed out in connection with an earlier request about the NPD, this (due) process, even, or perhaps especially, if the Constitutional Court refuses to ban the party at issue, fulfills the "obligation of democratic self-defense" against forces that would seek to stage another "German catastrophe."[81] In the AfD's case, the party successfully pressed a procedural point in March 2021, which at least delayed any further measures by the BfV, pending some further juridical review.[82] That is to say that allegations of allowing violent protestors into the Reichstag and holding questionable beliefs about the origins and vectors of COVID-19 *do not* suffice by themselves to get the AfD banned as a political party. As Bracher suggests, German democracy comes out the winner whether the process protects a party that advocates a creepy, quasi-totalitarian program but that nonetheless appears to uphold the letter and the spirit of the constitution OR culminates in the prohibition of a dangerously undemocratic party.[83]

The party-ban provision tracks with other language in the German constitution that brings this concern for basic democratic soundness to the individual level. In fact, the *Grundgesetz* stands out among democratic constitutions for its unabashed thou-shalt-not clauses – notably articles 18 and 19, which round out the "Basic Rights" title of the document. The first 17 articles provide for the protection of exactly the fundamental liberties that "Basic Rights" implies – from freedom of expression and association to the guarantee of human dignity and personality development. But Article 18 forms an or-else provision, meant to preserve the democracy against those who would use their liberties against it:

> Whoever abuses the freedom of expression, in particular the freedom of the press (paragraph (1) of Article 5), the freedom of teaching (paragraph (3) of Article 5), the freedom of assembly (Article 8), the freedom of association (Article 9), the privacy of correspondence, posts and telecommunications (Article 10), the rights of property (Article 14), or the right of asylum (Article 16a) in order to combat the free democratic basic order shall forfeit these basic rights. This forfeiture and its extent shall be declared by the Federal Constitutional Court.[84]

Article 19, more relevantly, requires that any law that might restrict the practice of basic rights cannot interfere with the *essence* of the Basic Law (Sec. 2). Moreover, it must apply broadly (rather than singling out an individual case), and it must acknowledge by name and number the right that it means to infringe.[85] Thus, even in temporarily curtailing or limiting basic rights amid a pandemic, the contemporary German constitution requires maximum process and protection of individuals and their liberties. This mechanism is fundamental to the Federal Republic's democratic project – in stark contrast to the National Socialist ideal of, for example, health policy, which emphasized the "health of the nation" over any particular individual's rights.[86]

---

81 Karl Dietrich Bracher, "Pflicht zur Gegenwehr," in Claus Leggewie and Horst Meier, eds., *Verbot der NPS oder mit Rechtsradikalen leben?* (Frankfurt a.M.: Suhrkamp, 2002), p. 151.
82 Deutsche Welle, "Gericht untersagt Verfassungsschutz vorerst AfD-Beobachtung," 5 March 2021, https://www.dw.com/de/gericht-untersagt-verfassungsschutz-vorerst-afd-beobachtung/a-56782227; see also Art. 19 of the *Grundgesetz*: https://www.bundesregierung.de/breg-en/chancellor/basic-law-470510.
83 Karl Dietrich Bracher, "Pflicht zur Gegenwehr," in Claus Leggewie and Horst Meier, eds., *Verbot der NPS oder mit Rechtsradikalen leben?* (Frankfurt a.M.: Suhrkamp, 2002), p. 149.
84 Basic Law: https://www.bundesregierung.de/breg-en/chancellor/basic-law-470510.
85 Basic Law: https://www.bundesregierung.de/breg-en/chancellor/basic-law-470510.
86 See, for example, Hans Günter Hockerts, ed., *Drei Wege deutscher Sozialstaatlichkeit* (Munich: Oldenbourg, 1998), p. 57 and p. 60.

History and language both matter in the German law. Perhaps most noteworthy in this connection is the fact that the term "emergency laws" does not appear in the constitution or even in state-level law. There is mention of measures in response to natural disasters, and there are provisions for a "state of defense" (as in classical national defense) in Title Xa. Here, function follows form; the federal German *Grundgesetz* purposefully avoids both the name and the modality of emergency laws, which occupy a particularly unhappy place in the German political, legal, and cultural discourse. The *Urtrauma*, as it were, dates to the Weimar Constitution and especially the notorious Art. 48, which allowed the Reich President to intervene, up to and including deploying the armed forces domestically, in/against civil society to ensure the sanctity of public order and security. On this basis, the Nazis enacted various presidential executive orders that culminated in the Enabling Laws of 1933 – which expressly excluded the parliament from the institution or repeal of the civil-liberties restrictions (although both houses of parliament approved the act at the time) – in response to a manufactured crisis, which, in fact, involved a mentally ill man who may or may not have tried to set fire to the Reichstag, unless Hermann Goering had his Sturmabteilung (SA) do so.[87] The Nazis refreshed the law every four years, as required – and in the meantime simply disregarded any inconvenient aspects of the Weimar constitution that had not been suspended by the enabling laws, amid an ongoing "state of emergency" and a fairly systematic hollowing out of existing law to enable state terror, generalized war, and mass murder. These developments in the legal domain of the Nazi seizure of power and the ensuing *Gleichschaltung* (the totalitarian "synchronization" of state and society) provided the basis in law of the Third Reich's sudden shift to dictatorship in 1933 – at the cost of parliamentary preeminence, civil liberties, and human rights, among other things.[88]

As such, "emergency" represents a fraught and freighted term in German political and legal discourse. For one important example, the original Basic Law made no mention of national defense – internal or external; practical or procedural – or of the legal issues attendant to crisis and war; the four occupying powers excluded such paragraphs by dint of the principles of denazification, demilitarization, democratization, and decartelization. Nonetheless, the issue swiftly reemerged in the 1950s with the questions of German–German division and the low-intensity conflict that was the early Cold War and their impact on both or either of the postwar German regimes. Here, the issue was the constitutional and legal implications of two new German armies in East and West and the burden of national division amid intense ideological conflict of left and right.

In the case of the FRG, indeed, despite some fairly consistent arguments, especially from conservative leaders in the 1950s and early 1960s, the FRG refused to enact any kind of crisis laws beyond natural-disaster provisions until the pivotal year of 1968. Then, the inter-generational and -class struggles rampant in western Europe at the time of the mature Cold War gave rise, however accurately, to the "broader perception of a crisis of democracy and the potentially destabilizing challenges of a return of the Nazi past," in the words of Biess; suddenly the prevailing angst focused on an over-powerful and increasingly authoritarian, if not totalitarian, Bonn state in the mesmeric sway of a war-crazed United States, carpet-bombing Southeast Asia.[89]

---

87 Benhamin Carter Hett, *Burning the Reichstag: An Investigation Into the Third Reich's Enduring* Mystery (Oxford: OUP, 2014); Michael Gruetter, *Das Dritte Reich, 1933–1945*, Vol. 19 of Gebhardt: Handbuch der deutschen Geschichte, 10th ed. (Stuttgart: Klett-Cotta, 2014) pp. 51–65.
88 See, for example, Michael Stolleis, *The Law under the Swastika* (Chicago and London: University of Chicago Press, 1998), p. 12.
89 Frank Biess, *German Angst: Fear and Democracy in the Federal Republic of* Germany (Oxford: OUP, 2020), p. 184. As always, some context here proves helpful. The FRG went into a recession in the mid-1960s, which begins to explain why and how the NPD emerged in 1964; the war in Vietnam consumed more U.S. attention and resources while arousing tumult in the West while various shades of communist ideology roiled their own crowds. The emergency laws of the 1960s arose when the United States, the United Kingdom, and France still had rights of

Thus, lawmakers were extremely careful to title (and populate) the new section of the *Grundgesetz* in terms of a state of defense. More specifically, the "state of defense," as found in the words and experience of government, law, and arms of the Bonn Republic, concerned a Warsaw Pact or comparable military assault on the FRG from without, rather than generalized unpleasantness.[90] On the other hand, the promulgation of these laws led to multiple protests from the earliest days – ultimately contributing to the formation of the FRG's student movement and the new-left extra-parliamentary opposition[91] – starting around 1965, when such measures were still in the proposal phase, and culminating in the mass demonstrations in May 1968 that give this year its enduring significance in German politics and society … and democracy.

In this context, Karl Dietrich Bracher's principled and cautionary dissent resonates then as now: "Wherever the constitutional order is interrupted to stop-gap a 'crisis,' the danger exists that a limited dictatorship will convert legalistically to an unlimited one."[92] In the end, even the rather circumscribed "state of defense" laws of Title Xa have never been activated in their full measure – even, for example, in the so-called German Autumn of 1977, which saw the kidnapping and murder of prominent industrialist and one-time SS-officer Hanns Martin Schleyer; the hijacking of the *Landshut* (Lufthansa Flight 181); the murder amid a botched kidnapping attempt of Dresdner Bank's head, Jürgen Ponto; and the assassination of Germany's attorney general, Siegfried Buback by the Red Army Fraction (*Rote Armee Fraktion* or RAF). Ultimately, what came out of the bloody events of 1977 was a "contact ban," which in the language of the time allowed the state, in very particular circumstances, to curtail the otherwise unfettered visits between defense attorneys and their clients charged with terrorism under a specific provision (para. 129a of the criminal statute) in light of the actions of the legal representatives of the first generation of RAF members, including smuggling in the firearms with which Jan-Carl Raspe and Andreas Baader committed suicide in their cells on the same night that German authorities stormed the *Landshut* in Mogadishu. Still, as Biess makes very clear, the significance of these events – the passage of or the protests about the state-of-defense laws in the 1960s or the legal response to the German Autumn in 1977, among others – lies mostly in the length and breadth and depth of the emotional charge.[93] Germans have consistently and actively worried about government overreach and illiberal tendencies in policy and politics. Thus, their COVID-era concerns, particularly about the legal framework and safeguards, want serious analysis, especially in the context of this longer record of law, government, and crisis.

4.5 Second Guessing the Second Wave

But how much is too much of a good thing? While the legal system and the legal framework for the COVID response in Germany has performed as designed and as hoped, the discourse about

---

oversight and intervention in the domestic politics of the Bonn Republic connected with the crisis and wartime response to a Warsaw Pact assault or communist fifth-columnists, which, in fact, existed in their number at the time. Today this situation is termed "hybrid war," but such a process is anything but new, and German legal theory practice struggled for a while to confront this phenomenon.

90 Basic Law: https://www.bundesregierung.de/breg-en/chancellor/basic-law-470510; see especially Art. 115a, para. 1.

91 Frank Biess, *German Angst: Fear and Democracy in the Federal Republic of Germany* (Oxford: OUP, 2020), p. 187.

92 Boris Spernol, *Notstand der Demokratie: Der Protest gegen die Notstandgesetze und die Frage der NS-Vergangenheit* (Essen: Klartext, 2008), p. 43, quoting Karl Dietrich Bracher, "Parlamentarische Demokratie und Notstand," in Frankfurter Hefte 20, 1965. This unhappy evolution sounds rather like the distinction that Carl Schmitt makes between commissarial and sovereign dictatorship in his volume by the same name (*Dictatorship*). See William E. Scheuerman, "States of Emergency" in Jens Meierhenrich and Oliver Simons, eds., *The Oxford Handbook of Carl Schmitt* (Oxford: OUP, 2016), p. 534.

93 Frank Biess, *German Angst: Fear and Democracy in the Federal Republic of Germany* (Oxford: OUP, 2020), p. 185.

it – fixated as it is on a nonexistent state of emergency – probably has culminated in "normative disorientation," in Kersten and Rixen's pithy characterization.[94] In real life, no such emergency – nor any surrogate – was declared, and Germans remain secure in their civil liberties as far as the legal system is concerned. Again, there is nothing especially "normal" about the day-to-day affairs in the FRG as the pandemic and the response pass the one-year mark in early 2021. But, legally and practically, it is not an emergency as the term figures in the German constitutional–legal lexicon.

Nonetheless, the turmoil that ensued over the summer and early autumn of 2020 evidently influenced the policies that formed amid the second wave of Coronavirus in the last months of the year 2020. In the face of dramatically increasing infection, illness, and death rates – by mid-October, the FRG was reporting upwards of 10,000 new COVID cases a day and Spahn himself tested positive for the disease on 21 October – the health ministry continued to push its "hot-spot strategy" of highly localized measures, as well as adding more letters to its AHA guidance[95] – a clear indication of the government's reluctance to impose more muscular restrictions and further incite the Corona-skeptics. The initial result was what came to be dubbed "lockdown light," which commenced on 2 November 2020[96] – less restrictive measures than Germany had enacted in the spring, even as the second wave of Coronavirus looked to be much worse in the FRG.

At about this same time – mid-autumn 2020 – the talk turned to the various vaccines that were then in development, notably the Pfizer BioNTech formulation, which was a home-team effort out of Mainz. Immunization represents the third phase, mitigation, of epidemic control. Thus, the Federal Ministry of Health busied itself with mass vaccination plans that, at the time of this writing half a year later, had not eventuated with the breadth or depth that first-wave admirers of the German response might have hoped. In the meantime, the ranks of the Corona-skeptics grew to include COVID vaccine skeptics, if not necessarily skeptics of potential vaccination requirements.[97]

By December 2020, the German government had to shift to a "hard" lockdown amid a precipitous rise in COVID infections – exceeding 25,000 new cases a day just before Christmas. Measures included curfews, limitations on gatherings, and school closures over the holidays. The traditional German Christmas markets and pop-up mulled wine stands – holiday fixtures – were cancelled. By January 2021, the closure of schools and day-care facilities was extended along with the rest of the hard lockdown, ultimately into March.

The dreaded virus mutations, named in the popular press for the states in which they were first recognized ("UK variant," "South African variant") began to appear right around the new year.[98] In these circumstances – a recently approved vaccine roll-out since 26 December, and generally falling but still eye-watering COVID case numbers despite growing – Uwe Volkmann took again to the pages of the *FAZ* to press his point about "hypothetical" overburdening of the public health system versus the "widespread" intrusions on individual liberties, now in terms of the second-wave response.[99] Volkmann's broad implication of overreach, based on the legal assessment of the appropriateness of the Merkel government's belated hard lockdown, still did not address the science

---

94 Jens Kersten and Stephan Rixen, *Der Verfassungsstaat in der Corona-Krise* (Munich: C.H. Beck, 2020), p. 31.
95 Bundesministerium für Gesundheit, "Coronavirus-Pandemie (SARS-CoV-2): Chronik bisheriger Maßnahmen und Ereignisse," https://www.bundesgesundheitsministerium.de/coronavirus/chronik-coronavirus.html.
96 Deutsche Welle, "Coronavirus: Germany to impose one-month partial lockdown," 28 October 2020, https:// www.dw.com/en/coronavirus-germany-to-impose-one-month-partial-lockdown/a-55421241.
97 This important distinction appears in Jens Kersten and Stephan Rixen, *Der Verfassungsstaat in der Corona-Krise* (Munich: C.H. Beck, 2020), pp. 84–85.
98 Bundesministerium für Gesundheit, "Coronavirus-Pandemie (SARS-CoV-2): Chronik bisheriger Maßnahmen und Ereignisse," https://www.bundesgesundheitsministerium.de/coronavirus/chronik-coronavirus.html.
99 Uwe Volkmann, "Wir Verdrängungskünstler," *Frankfurter Allgemeine Zeitung,* 25 January 2021, https://www.faz .net/aktuell/feuilleton/debatten/wie-lassen-sich-die-corona-massnahmen-begruenden-17162587.html?premium.

of such details as the infection rates or any other evidence that might militate for preempting a collapse of the national health-care system.

But by February 2021, with case numbers dropping and popular antipathy toward the anti-Coronavirus measures rising, the mood in parliament and in the public embraced an easing of restrictions for social and political reasons, particularly with a federal election due in September, though not really for legal ones. Thus, in March, with the Easter holiday looming once again and a third wave of COVID infections cresting, the Merkel government initially announced the strictest lockdown yet[100] … then almost immediately retracted the plan and even apologized for it.[101] On the day that Angela Merkel reversed the third-wave lockdown plan – 24 March 2021 – there were nearly 16,000 new cases of COVID-19 in Germany and 248 deaths.[102]

4.6 Happily Ever After?

The protests continued, including a demonstration of 10,000 or so *Querdenker* in Stuttgart on Easter Sunday 2021. By this time, the police, while not condoning the myriad failures to comport with masking and distance rules, intervened only where criminal behavior was at issue – in this case, an assault of a journalist.[103] Evidently, Germany's post-COVID "normal" thus came to include a certain kind of popular if not populist political performance and direct action, the pandemic version of the demonstrations and discussions that have attended all of the inflection points of the FRG's history since 1949 – perhaps the flip-side of Biess' *Ängste* or at least the democratic way through them.

On the one hand, this dynamic of questioning, challenging, reviewing, and revising forms a key "… part of an open democracy – that we explain our political decisions and make them transparent," as Chancellor Angela Merkel said in a rare unscheduled televised speech on 18 March 2020, as the German COVID response began in earnest. [104] On the other hand, it also speaks to what Carl Schmitt might consider a fateful gap between "liberalism's preference for fixed, codified general norms" – like emergency or even disaster provisions – and the need to execute quickly in times of crisis, in Scheuerman's characterization.[105] However questionable the politics or alternate "science" of the hygiene-demonstrators, this significant and persistent protest surely helps the government refine its approach to the pandemic while maintaining its focus on the protection of public health as well as individual rights.

None of the foregoing is meant to minimize the economic and political impacts – probably deeper and broader even than the contemporary critics suggest – of the Coronavirus on and in the FRG or its concept of state, society, economy, and international order that is under general threat from many points of the ideological compass. The RKI's three-step approach ends with mitigation; recovery likely comes next, though these plans exceed the brief and the expertise of the disease-control

---

100 Deutsche Welle, "Germany imposes strict lockdown over Easter," 23 March 2021, https://www.dw.com/en/germany-imposes-strict-lockdown-over-easter/a-56948895.

101 Deutsche Welle, "COVID: Angela Merkel backtracks on Easter lockdown after uproar," 24 March 2021, https://www.dw.com/en/covid-angela-merkel-backtracks-on-easter-lockdown-after-uproar/a-56969820.

102 Robert Koch-Institut, "Coronavirus SARS-CoV-2 – Situationsbericht vom 24.3.2021," https://www.rki.de/DE/Content/InfAZ/N/Neuartiges_Coronavirus/Situationsberichte/Maerz_2021/2021-03-24-de.html.

103 Frankfurter Allgemeine Zeitung, "Angriffe auf Journalisten bei Querdenker-Demonstration in Stuttgart," 4 April 2021.

104 Deutsche Welle, "Merkel: Coronavirus is Germany's greatest challenge since World War II," 18 March 2020, https://www.dw.com/en/merkel-coronavirus-is-germanys-greatest-challenge-since-world-war-ii/a-52830797.

105 William E. Scheuerman, "States of Emergency" in Jens Meierhenrich and Oliver Simons, eds., *The Oxford Handbook of Carl* Schmitt (Oxford: OUP, 2016), p. 560.

agency. And as the pandemic persists, such issues are, in their turn, very well likely to prompt further considerations of proportionality, especially the appropriateness part, in the constitutional sense.

Thus, however, many waves of COVID-19 – and ensuing political, legal, and indeed constitutional ripples – might await Germany and however much angst the disease or the response might provoke, the fundamental legal framework in the FRG asks the right questions and institutes the fitting procedures by which the state and society can derive solid democratic answers. The debate, the process, and the protest ultimately serve, fortify – and, in this case, confirm – Germany's democratic health. In other words, the COVID-19 response may or may not represent a "democratic imposition," as Merkel put it, but it certainly does not herald the demise of the FRG's democracy.[106]

---

106 Deutsche Welle, "Merkel: "Das Virus ist eine demokratische Zumutung," 28 August 2020, https://www.dw .com/de/merkel-das-virus-ist-eine-demokratische-zumutung/a-54729946.

5

The United Kingdom Legislative Response to Coronavirus: Shotgun or Machine Gun

Ronan Cormacain[1] and Duncan Fairgrieve[1,2]

[1] *British Institute of International and Comparative Law, London, England*
[2] *Comparative Law, Université de Paris, Dauphine, France*

5.1 Introduction

The UK's response to the coronavirus pandemic has been rooted in law. Ordinary and emergency powers have been used to enact primary and secondary legislation in relation to coronavirus. The legislation has covered a huge scope of social and commercial life in the UK, from lockdown measures, international travel, financial support, and vaccines. The nature of the legislative response has been rapid, constantly changing and voluminous. This has led to problems around lack of effective scrutiny, conflation of law with guidance, legislation which is hard to understand and apply, and a creep of emergency procedures into everyday lawmaking. Most recently there have been problems of compliance with the law by those charged with making it. This chapter will assess the British response to the pandemic in the context of the UK's legal system and legislative processes. The authors will describe the nature of the legal and institutional frameworks and the legislative response to the pandemic, address the use of emergency powers, assess restrictions on civil liberties and vaccination policy, and conclude with some problems posed by the manner in which the British pandemic response was handled within the framework of British law.

5.2 Reliance Upon Law

One noteworthy aspect of the UK's response to coronavirus is so obvious that it is not often commented upon. It is that the UK's response has been in accordance with, and carried out by, law. Every part of the response has been within the legal order. Not only that, but nearly every part of it has been implemented by means of law. There was no serious attempt to step outside the legal order and for the executive to simply do whatever was necessary, regardless of legal status. The state is so accultured to both the Rule of Law, and to ruling by way of law, that there was no credible argument that it could rule outside the law. Schmitt's argument that states of emergency entitle the government to rule without law never had any traction in the UK during the pandemic.[1] Instead, the UK followed the argument of Dyzenhaus that states of emergency fall within the legal order.[2]

---

1 C. Schmitt, Political Theology: Four Chapters on the Concept of Sovereignty (1922).
2 D. Dyzenhaus and V. Schmitt, Dicey: Are States of Emergency Inside or Outside the Legal Order? (August, 21 2008). *Cardozo Law Review*, Vol 27, p. 2005, 2006, Available at SSRN: https://ssrn.com/abstract=1244562.

As one of us wrote at the start of the pandemic,

> …law is not irrelevant in a public emergency… Whether the threat comes from war, terrorism or a major pandemic, law still has a role to play in ensuring the legitimacy of the Government's response. The Rule of Law requires that we are ruled in accordance with the law, and that we are all subject to the law.[3]

Although the UK at times strayed from the path of the Rule of Law, there was never any serious attempt to act outside the law as a sustained policy. What then was the framework within which this legal response was conducted?

5.3 Nature of the Legal Framework

5.3.1 Machine Gun Legislative Response

Legislation has been the tool of choice for virtually all of the UK's response to coronavirus. The legislative response has been massive. The Hansard Society (a leading research body on the UK Parliament) maintains what it calls a Coronavirus Statutory Instruments Dashboard.[4] As of 28 November 2021, the UK government has laid 533 coronavirus-related statutory instruments before the Westminster Parliament, an average of 6 per week from the start of the pandemic. If anything, this is an underestimate of the total volume of coronavirus legislation produced in the UK as it only counts Westminster/English secondary legislation. It does not count any primary legislation, nor any secondary legislation from any of the devolved administrations in the UK (Scotland, Northern Ireland, or Wales).

This is a machine gun legislative response – it is rapid fire, constantly reloading, aiming at multiple targets in a slightly haphazard fashion. It is not a single shot from a rifle at a single target, nor is it a single shotgun blast hitting multiple targets. It is as if the government is trying to hit multiple targets, which keep popping up again and again. Each of these 533 statutory instruments does something slightly different, aiming at another aspect of the problem, or recalibrating to more effectively hit its target. A huge amount of government resources are devoted toward this legislative response. The Hansard Society estimates that 30% of all legislative output of the government during the pandemic has been coronavirus related.

5.3.2 Devolution and the Legislative Response

There are four separate nations in the UK: England, Scotland, Wales, and Northern Ireland. The Westminster Parliament passes laws for the entirety of the UK, as well as laws for England. The three devolved administrations (Scotland, Wales, and Northern Ireland) each possess their own legislatures: the Scottish Parliament, Senedd Cymru (for Wales), and the Northern Ireland Assembly.

---

3 R. Cormacain, "Does law fall silent in the war against Covid-19?" (18 March 2020) British Institute of International and Comparative Law. Available at https://www.biicl.org/newsitems/16406/does-law-fall-silent-in-the-war-against-covid-19?cookiesset=1&ts=1638131258.
4 Available at https://www.hansardsociety.org.uk/publications/data/coronavirus-statutory-instruments-dashboard.

Health is a devolved matter in Scotland, Wales, and Northern Ireland (the devolved jurisdictions), meaning that each devolved administration is in charge of its coronavirus response, and each devolved legislature is entitled to pass its own coronavirus laws. This means that the Scottish Parliament enacts its own primary legislation on coronavirus, and that the Scottish Government enacts its own secondary legislation on coronavirus (that legislation being authorized by the Scottish Parliament). The same holds true for Wales and Northern Ireland.

The constitutional convention in the UK (known as the Sewel Convention) stipulates that the Westminster Parliament would not pass legislation for which a devolved legislature has competence, without the consent of that devolved legislature. Consequently, the Westminster Parliament could only pass health legislation for Northern Ireland if the Northern Ireland Assembly first passed a legislative consent motion. Although this convention has not always been observed (for example, in relation to Brexit), it has been observed when it comes to coronavirus. This means that each of the devolved jurisdictions has substantial autonomy when it comes to charting its own response to the pandemic.

There is considerable co-ordination between the legislatures and between the devolved administrations and the UK government. When time permits, they discuss with each other what their legal approach will be, and what legislation they are planning on enacting. The legal framework in place (discussed further below) is largely the same in all four nations, which means that the form of legislative response is very similar. In terms of content, the legislative responses are similar, but not the same. The legislation all follows the same format and the same style, but there are variations of substance. A reader of a statute from one devolved jurisdiction would see lots of similar language and similar patterns in the statute of another jurisdiction. There is no obligation to have uniformity throughout the UK, but in practical terms, having similar provisions helps readers of the legislation. Variations can be significant but are not huge. As a broad generalization, Scotland, Wales, and Northern Ireland are slightly more cautious than England and tend to be quicker to impose restrictions and slower to relax them.

Where something relates to a matter which is not devolved (for example, something like taxation or international relations), then the Westminster Parliament will enact UK-wide legislation on that matter.

5.3.3 Overview of the Legislative Framework

Although there are statutes which could be described as "constitutional statutes" in the UK, there is no formal, codified constitution. Therefore, there is no constitutionally prescribed way of declaring an emergency and thus accessing emergency powers. Instead, the government has relied upon ordinary legislation to implement its legal response.

As set out earlier, the legislative response has been massive. Set out in the tables below are the main laws governing the state's response.

England

Primary legislation	Secondary legislation
Coronavirus Act 2020	The Health Protection (Coronavirus, Restrictions) (No. 3) (England) Regulations 2020
Public Health (Control of Disease) Act 1984	The Health Protection (Coronavirus, Restrictions) (Self-Isolation) (England) Regulations 2020
	The Health Protection (Coronavirus, International Travel and Operator Liability) (England) Regulations 2021

Scotland

Primary legislation	Secondary legislation
Coronavirus Act 2020	The Health Protection (Coronavirus) (Requirements) (Scotland) Regulations 2021
Coronavirus (Scotland) Act 2020	The Health Protection (Coronavirus) (International Travel) (Scotland) Regulations 2020
Coronavirus (Scotland) (No. 2) Act 2020	The Health Protection (Coronavirus, Public Health Information for Persons Travelling to Scotland) Regulations 2020
Public Health etc. (Scotland) Act 2008	

Wales

Primary legislation	Secondary legislation
Coronavirus Act 2020	The Health Protection (Coronavirus Restrictions) (No. 5) (Wales) Regulations 2020
Public Health (Control of Disease) Act 1984	The Health Protection (Coronavirus, International Travel) (Wales) Regulations 2020
	The Health Protection (Coronavirus, Public Health Information for Persons Travelling to Wales, etc.) Regulations 2020
	The Health Protection (Coronavirus Restrictions) (Functions of Local Authorities, etc.) (Wales) Regulations 2020

Northern Ireland

Primary legislation	Secondary legislation
Coronavirus Act 2020	The Health Protection (Coronavirus, Restrictions) Regulations (Northern Ireland) 2021
Public Health Act (Northern Ireland) 1967	The Health Protection (Coronavirus, International Travel) Regulations (Northern Ireland) 2021
	The Health Protection (Coronavirus, International Travel, Operator Liability and Information to Passengers) Regulations (Northern Ireland) 2021

This list of secondary legislation is merely a snapshot as of December 2021. They are likely to change many more times.

The Coronavirus Act 2020 was enacted in March 2020, as the pandemic was reaching the UK. It is a collection of provisions on many different subject areas, all connected by being made in response to the pandemic. Overall, the Act had three main aims:

1. to give further powers to the government to slow the spread of the virus,
2. to reduce the resourcing and administrative burden on public bodies, and
3. to limit the impact of potential staffing shortages on the delivery of public services.[5]

---

5 See further, Institute for Government "Coronavirus Act 2020" https://www.instituteforgovernment.org.uk/explainers/coronavirus-act.

For example, it contains provisions on: emergency registration of health professionals and social workers, emergency volunteers, health service indemnification, registration of deaths, investigatory powers, food supply, inquests, disclosure rules, statutory sick pay, pensions, use of video and audio technology in courts, postponement of elections, financial assistance for industry, protections from eviction, and many more subjects. It was a substantial piece of legislation covering a huge amount of detail in a wide range of matters.

The two Scottish Coronavirus Acts make additional provision for Scotland. The other jurisdictions did not enact new primary legislation dealing solely with the pandemic. The various Public Health Acts set out the framework for dealing with public health generally, as well as containing provisions covering public health emergencies. In addition to these key pieces of legislation, other primary legislation sometimes dealt in part with coronavirus. For example, the Corporate Insolvency and Governance Act 2020 contained permanent measures on the insolvency law regime, as well as temporary measures on insolvency and corporate governance which would apply only during the pandemic.

Turning to the secondary legislation, the tables above list two of the main categories: the domestic restrictions on liberty and the restrictions in relation to international travel (including rules on those operating transport to the UK). The first category contains all the restrictions on daily activities. For example: lockdowns, restrictions on gatherings, going outside without excuse, shop closures, bubbling within households, restrictions on visiting other households, etc. The second category introduces requirements for travellers to the UK. Aside from these two categories, there are many more pieces of secondary legislation in specific subject areas.

The technique for enacting the secondary legislation is constant and continuous amendment, followed by occasional consolidation. This means that the original health protection regulations are made, and then amended on a regular basis (from once every few days to once every few weeks). At some point, the amendments are so great that the regulations are revoked in their entirety and then re-enacted in a consolidated form. For example, the regulations governing international travel to Northern Ireland (the Health Protection (Coronavirus, International Travel) Regulations (Northern Ireland) 2020 were amended 37 times. Then, in 2021, these regulations, and all the amending regulations were revoked and a new consolidated set of regulations was made, the Health Protection (Coronavirus, International Travel, Operator Liability and Information to Passengers) Regulations (Northern Ireland) 2021. These new 2021 Regulations are then subject to new amendments on a regular basis.

The regional similarities and differences can be seen from these tables. Each jurisdiction relied upon the Coronavirus Act 2020 and on its own version of a Public Health Act. These Public Health Acts contain very similar provisions, with the appropriate adjustments so that they work in the slightly different structure in each of the devolved jurisdictions. Once again, there is a large degree of overlap. For example, the Public Health Act (Northern Ireland) 1967 did not contain powers to deal with public health emergencies before the pandemic struck. So the Coronavirus Act 2020 amended that Act by introducing emergency powers into it, those powers being the near-exact replica of the emergency powers contained in the Public Health (Control of Disease) Act 1984 already applying in England and Wales. So, the wording of the powers is nearly exactly the same.

Turning next to secondary legislation, the similarities are also striking. The main pieces of secondary legislation were all made under each jurisdiction's Public Health Acts. The powers set out in each of these Public Health Acts are strikingly similar. The naming conventions of the legislation are also strikingly similar. Although the longer the pandemic has gone on, the more variation in content there has been, the pattern of regulation remains similar. The precise requirements and the nature of the exemptions do vary, but the broad thrust is similar.

5.3.4 Pre-existing Laws or New Laws

There has been a combination of reliance upon existing legislation and legislative powers and the enactment of new legislation setting out new legislative powers. The most obvious new law is the Coronavirus Act 2020 itself, made in the midst of the virus reaching the UK. This contained both substantive changes to the regulatory regime (new things that must be done, or new restrictions) as well as empowering further legislative changes by way of secondary legislation.

However, when it came to the key measures which sought to restrict the spread of the virus, most of these pieces of secondary legislation were made under pre-existing powers set out in the various Public Health Acts. These Public Health Acts contained general powers on maintaining public health. They also contained powers that could be exercised in an emergency. It is these general and emergency powers that have been relied upon extensively to make the secondary legislation on coronavirus.

Most, if not all, of the secondary legislation relied upon to deal with coronavirus was made post the arrival of coronavirus in the UK.

The UK had another piece of pre-existing legislation which contained powers to do things during an emergency, the Civil Contingencies Act 2004. The Civil Contingencies Act 2004 has not been used at all during the pandemic. There has been an ongoing debate in constitutional circles over the desirability of this decision.[6] Although there is by no means unanimity on this, the weight of opinion is that the government was right not to use this legislation. There are a number of reasons for this. First, the situation is not so severe that these powers need to be used. Second, regulations made under this Act would apply across the UK, meaning that the devolved jurisdictions would have no power to make their own laws. Third, (and perhaps more cynically) the 2004 Act granted Parliament the power to amend emergency regulation, and the government did not want Parliament to have this power.

5.3.5 Use of Emergency/Urgency Powers and Procedures or Use of Regular Powers and Procedures

The Coronavirus Act 2020 was fast-tracked through Parliament, completing all stages in just 4 sitting days. Other legislation which dealt with coronavirus in some way also had expedited passage through Parliament. For example, the Corporate Insolvency and Governance Act 2020 passed through all stages in approximately one month. By comparison, most legislation takes between six months and two years to get through all its parliamentary stages. It is therefore fair to conclude that primary legislation on coronavirus has been pushed through Parliament at a very high speed.

Turning to secondary legislation. The starting point for England and Wales is the Public Health (Control of Disease) Act 1984 – (analogous provisions apply in Scotland and Northern Ireland). The main power for imposing domestic restrictions is set out in section 45C. Under that section, a minister may make regulations

> for the purpose of preventing, protecting against, controlling or providing a public health response to the incidence or spread of infection or contamination.

When it comes to restrictions on international travel, the source of authority is section 45B of the Act. That section allows a minister to make regulations

---

6 See, for example, the consideration of this Act by a parliamentary committee, House of Commons, Public Administration and Constitutional Affairs Committee, "Parliamentary Scrutiny of the Government's handling of Covid-19" (Fourth Report of Session 2019-2021, HC 377).

(a) for preventing danger to public health from vessels, aircraft, trains, or other conveyances arriving at any place,

(b) for preventing the spread of infection or contamination by means of any vessel, aircraft, train, or other conveyance leaving any place, and

(c) for giving effect to any international agreement or arrangement relating to the spread of infection or contamination.

Under section 45Q, the domestic restriction regulations must not be made unless a draft of them has first been laid before, and approved by a resolution of each House of Parliament. In Westminster, this is referred to as the draft affirmative procedure. The draft affirmative procedure is one of the highest forms of Parliamentary scrutiny there is – appropriate where restrictions on personal freedoms are being introduced on peril of breaking the criminal law.

Also under section 45Q, the international health restrictions must be laid before Parliament, and Parliament has the power to annul them. This is known as the negative procedure. The crucial difference is that with domestic restrictions, there is a requirement for an active vote to authorize it, but with international travel restrictions, there is merely the power to pass a vote to annul it.

Section 45R then sets out what is termed the "emergency procedure." Under S. 45R(2), the obligation to get parliamentary approval before making the regulations does not apply if the regulations

> contain a declaration that the person making it is of the opinion that, by reason of urgency, it is necessary to make the order without a draft being so laid and approved.

Under the emergency procedure, the following then applies:

- The regulations must be laid before Parliament after they are made.
- Regulations will lapse if they are not approved by resolution of each House of Parliament within 28 days.
- In calculating this period of 28 days, no account is taken of days during which Parliament is prorogued or dissolved, or during a period when both Houses are adjourned for more than 4 days.

In Westminster, this is called the made affirmative procedure. It means that lockdown regulations using this procedure can be made and come into force straightaway without first being authorized or debated by Parliament.

It may be thought that the different types of parliamentary procedures used to approve secondary legislation would have an impact upon the effectiveness of the scrutiny that the legislation received. However, in practice, regardless of the type of procedure, all secondary legislation on Covid has invariably been approved by Parliament. Despite persistent concern from within the legislatures about the content and procedure for making these laws, no legislature has ever rejected them.

This is the approach that was taken in practice. It is however worthwhile considering the approach that could have been used, that is to say, by using the Civil Contingencies Act 2004. The 2004 Act applied to emergencies, defined as "an event or situation which threatens serious damage to human welfare in a place in the United Kingdom; an event or situation which threatens serious damage to the environment of a place in the United Kingdom."[7] The most important power in that Act is the power to make emergency regulations.[8] Emergency regulations must be laid before Parliament as soon as is reasonably practicable, and lapse seven days after being laid unless Parliament approves them. Very unusually, Parliament has the power to amend these regulations. Regulations made under this Act apply throughout the UK.

---

7 Sections 1 and 19, Civil Contingencies Act 2004.
8 Section 20.

5.3.6 Sunset Clauses/Expiry Dates

A sunset clause is a provision in legislation that states that it will end or expire on a particular date. There are several variations on this general theme. For example, that the legislation will end unless a particular procedure is followed/vote cast/power invoked. Or, that it will continue indefinitely, but it can be brought to an end more quickly if a particular procedure is followed/vote cast/power invoked.

The Coronavirus Act 2020 contains a number of sunset clauses.

Under section 89(1), the Act expires two years after it is made.

Under section 90, there is a power to alter that expiry date. The government may make regulations to shorten or extend the expiry date, but only by up to six months. This power to extend may be exercised more than once, but each individual extension is still limited to six months. If the expiry date is extended, the regulations must be laid before Parliament. If those extending regulations are not approved by Parliament within 40 days, they lapse.

Under section 98, there is a procedure for a six monthly Parliamentary review. There must be a motion passed by Parliament calling for the Act to continue. If Parliament does not pass this motion, then the government must take action under section 90 to bring forward the expiry date.

There are sunset clauses in the Scottish Coronavirus Acts.

Turning to the secondary legislation, all of the domestic restriction regulations and the international travel regulations have built-in sunset clauses. The nature of these sunset clauses has changed over time. Originally, the regulations were all set to expire six months after they were made, with an obligation to review them every 21 or 28 days. Now, the regulations are more likely to include a definite end date, but that end date is amended by subsequent regulations. The net effect of this is that, despite sunset clauses, these regulations have remained in force, in one guise or another, for the entirety of the pandemic.

5.4 Substance of the Legal Response

5.4.1 Restrictions on Individual Liberties

Coronavirus legislation has imposed substantial restrictions on individual liberties. The nature of the restrictions has not been constant, but has varied over time. As a broad generalization, the harshest measures were imposed at the start of the pandemic, with these measures being relaxed over time. However, whenever the numbers of infections rise, or there is the fear of them rising, then the severity of the restrictions increases.

The most severe restrictions were:

- Restriction on movement – no-one could leave their home without reasonable excuse. Reasonable excuse included things like shopping for essentials, taking exercise alone or with members of your household, providing care, accessing health care, or other critical public services.
- Restriction on overnight stays in other houses – must stay in your own house with your own household, unless a reasonable excuse.
- Restriction on public gatherings – no more than two people could gather in a public place, later relaxed so that larger numbers could gather together.
- Restrictions on close contact between individuals.

These measures were relaxed, so that people were allowed to mix together in "bubbles" of their own household, or one other household. Greater numbers of people could gather indoors or outdoors. Exemptions were widened for specific events (weddings, funerals, etc.).

These restrictions on liberties are enforced by way of the criminal law. The penalties are relatively minor, comprising a financial fine only. The offences do not include the possibility of imprisonment for breach.

5.4.2 Travel Restrictions

Substantial restrictions have been imposed on travel to the UK. As with the restrictions on individual liberties, these have gone up and down in response to different stages of the pandemic. These generally include:

- Prohibition on travellers from certain countries from arriving in the UK.
- Information to be given by passengers arriving in the UK.
- Requirement to have a negative test for coronavirus upon arrival.
- Requirement to book and undertake tests after arrival.
- Requirement to isolate at home or a period of time after arrival.
- Requirement to isolate in a government facility (a quarantine hotel) for a period of time after arrival.

These rules are also enforced by the criminal law, and as with lockdown restrictions, the penalties are relatively minor.

5.4.3 Vaccination Policy

The UK Covid-19 vaccine procurement programme was widely seen as having been a considerable success. Under the leadership of Dame Kate Bingham, chair of the UK Vaccine taskforce, the UK had one of the most rapid rollouts of the Covid-19 vaccination programme. In late 2020, the UK Medicines & Healthcare Regulatory Agency (MHRA) granted temporary authorizations under Regulation 174 of the Human Medicine Regulations 2012 to a vaccine produced by Pfizer/BioNTech and then subsequently in early 2021 to the AstraZeneca and Moderna vaccines. Temporary-use authorizations, rather than the ordinary market authorization route, were sought as this process allows for the emergency supply of unlicensed pharmaceutical products in response to public health threats including pathogenic agents such as Covid-19.

A government minister was appointed in November 2020 with specific responsibility for Covid-19 vaccination deployment. Advice on vaccines was also provided to the government by the Joint Committee of Vaccination and Immunization, a statutory body with a remit to advise on vaccination policy. According to recent government figures, almost 48 million persons as of January 2022 had received 2 doses of a Covid-19 vaccination, representing circa 83% of those over 12 years old in the UK.

The relatively small but significant percentage of those in the general population who remain unvaccinated has however led to discussion about potential mandatory Covid-19 vaccination of the general populace.[9] This has however been on a number of occasions ruled out by ministers as contrary to general policy, though it is to be noted that there have been mandatory immunization in the past in the UK.[10]

---

9 See discussion in L. Edwards and K. Grieman, "No jab, no job?" Employment law and mandatory vaccination requirements in the UK (November 2021), available at: 'No jab, no job'? Employment law and mandatory vaccination requirements in the UK (biicl.org).

10 In reality though, vaccination of infants was actually mandatory in the nineteenth century and parents who failed to immunize their children faced fines or prison terms: see discussion in J. Colgrove, "Immunization and Ethics: Beneficence, Coercion, Public Health, and the State" in A. Mastroianni, J. Kahn, and N. Kass (eds), *The Oxford Handbook of Public Health Ethics* (September 2019) pages 436–437.

The government did however decide that vaccination would be made compulsory for social care staff in England. Regulations were issued whereby it is necessary in order to enter a care home for individuals to demonstrate that they have received a complete course of Covid-19 vaccination.[11] These regulations cover both those directly employed within care homes as well as those coming into care homes as healthcare workers and volunteers. These rules came into force in November 2021. The way in which this legislation was made has attracted criticism by being done by secondary legislation rather than primary legislation, the lack of proper impact assessment, and the low level of scrutiny available.[12]

It has also been recently announced that this would be extended to cover all frontline health and social care workers, including all NHS and independent health care services, and that it is intended that this is to come into force by 1 April 2022. In January 2022, the Health Secretary announced a likely reversal of this policy in light of the "intrinsically less severe" Omicron variant, launching a consultation on ending vaccination as a condition of deployment in health and all social care settings.[13] The minister stated that "it is no longer proportionate to require vaccination as condition of deployment through statute." This change in policy would apply to both health and social care workers.

In recent times with the recent surge in infections due to the Omicron variant, there has again been renewed discussion about the feasibility of recourse to mandatory vaccination for the general populace. This was encouraged also by the fact that a policy of mandatory vaccination was adopted in some European countries such as Italy. Section 45E of the Public Health (Control of Disease) Act 1984 does not include the power to require mandatory vaccination by way of public health regulations, so any change in approach would therefore necessarily require primary legislation.[14]

Another complex and sensitive issue raised by the emergency vaccination programme is the policy in respect of those who suffer vaccine injury. As is well known, vaccines can cause adverse effects, the great majority of which are mild and temporary. In very rare circumstances, vaccine can cause serious adverse effects, and this has alas been the case for Covid-19 vaccines with cases of fatal or life altering blood-clots (known as **VITT** or **CVST**) and inflammation of the heart (myocarditis and pericarditis).

The aforementioned regulations under which the vaccines were authorized were very restrictive in terms of civil liability. Regulation 345(3) of the Human Medicine Regulations 2012 provides in effect for an immunity, whereby marketing authorization holders, manufacturers, and health professionals are not subject to civil or administrative liability for any consequences resulting from the use of an unauthorized medicinal product. The immunity in Regulation 345 is however not absolute. It does not provide complete immunity from civil liability; a carve-out is explicitly provided for in terms of product liability under the Consumer Protection Act 1987 (the CPA) (in Regulation 345(4)).[15] It is thus stated that there is no immunity in relation to a claim under section 2 of the CPA.

A consequence of this is that there is in effect a channeling of liability toward the cause of action based upon product liability under the CPA. The specific regime applicable to clinical trials of medicinal products which would normally apply to the period before a medical product is granted

---

11 The Health and Social Care Act 2008 (Regulated Activities) (Amendment) (Coronavirus) Regulations 2021.
12 B. Fowler, "The care home Covid vaccination Regulations: a case study in problems with the delegated legislation system" (Hansard Society, August 2021).
13 Vaccination: Condition of Deployment: 31 Jan 2022: House of Commons debates - TheyWorkForYou.
14 See comparative law discussion of the legal provisions relating to Mandatory Vaccination on the Lex-Atlas website: Blog Symposium on Mandatory Vaccination - Lex-Atlas: Covid-19 (lexatlas-c19.org).
15 Under Regulation 174A, the immunity is removed where a person who would otherwise be able to claim the immunity is responsible for a sufficiently serious breach of the conditions attached by the licensing authority to the product's supply.

a license in the UK is inapplicable in the current circumstances given the temporary authorization. The immunity under Regulation 345(3) moreover results in an exclusion of claims under the orthodox common law causes of action of contract, tort, and breach of statutory duty.

As a result, great emphasis is placed upon the product liability regime pursuant to the CPA 1987. Restrictions on time and space prevent us from reviewing this regime in detail here. Two points will however be made. First, liability under these provisions requires proof by the claimant that the product was defective, that damage was sustained by the claimant, and that this damage was caused by defect. Making out these elements can often be challenging, particularly so where the product in question is a medicine, especially one which has generally been considered to have successfully saved many lives.[16] Second, it is also to be noted that the success rate of actions under the CPA has not been high, particularly in group actions concerning medicines and medical devices where claims have failed on defect and causation grounds.[17] The development risks defense under the CPA (which does not require a finding of negligence) may still pose significant problems for a claimant as it enables a manufacturer to rely on the fact that the objective state of scientific and technical knowledge, at the time the vaccine was put into circulation, was not such as to enable the existence of the defect to be discovered.

In light of the foregoing, the route to compensation in case of harm deriving from a Covid-19 vaccine under the Regulations is likely to be a challenging one.

There is however a statutory scheme. The Vaccine Damage Payment Scheme, created pursuant to the Vaccine Damage Payment Act 1979, provides an ex-gratia one-off payment for those who suffer serious injury as a result of vaccination. The scheme was created by virtue of the Vaccine Damage Payments Act 1979 and allows for the provision of a lump-sum payment for persons who have been severely disabled as a result of vaccination against a series of specified diseases, which now includes Covid-19.[18] The scheme is premised on no-fault liability, so there is no requirement to show negligence or any other type of fault. The main weakness of the scheme is that the lump sum is £120,000[19] and so awards will often be a great deal less than tort law damages for similar harm. In cases of serious harm or death, the sum is entirely inadequate to cover the impact of the vaccine injury. It also compares very unfavorably with similar schemes in France or Nordic countries, and can be contrasted with an average payment under the US National Childhood Vaccine Injury Act of over half a million dollars (between 2006 and 2016).[20] The current scheme also requires that all eligible applicants in the UK must meet the 60% disablement criteria, which derived from the Industrial Injuries and War Pensions Schemes. This criterion is outdated and unfair as many applicants with significant injuries might not necessarily meet this threshold on the basis of the current scheme and will therefore have no access to funds via the VDPS (Vaccine Damage Payment System).

---

16 See A. Heppinstall, "COVID-19, Vaccines, Brexit and Vaccine Damage Claims" (2020) 2 EPLR 104; D. Fairgrieve, P. Feldschreiber, G. Howells, and M. Pilgerstorfer, "Products in a Pandemic: Liability for Medical Products and the Fight against Covid-19" (2020) *European Journal of Risk Regulation* 1.

17 In the recently published *Report of the Independent Medicines and Medical Devices Safety Review*, which reviewed the case law in respect of healthcare products, it is stated that: "To date, litigation has not served the patient groups we have met well. In the future a more equitable way to deliver redress that truly works for patients must be developed. Even the best pre-market testing will not capture all adverse events that may occur in real world treatment with pharmaceuticals and medical devices. Individuals may be harmed by new products in ways that were not foreseen during development and testing. We must establish an effective redress mechanism for those who suffer avoidable harm or unforeseen drug or device injury." (*The Report of the Independent Medicines and Medical Devices Safety Review* (2020), Appendix 3, para 7, page 213).

18 Vaccine Damage Payments (Specified Disease) Order 2020, SI 2020/1411.

19 Vaccine Damage Payments Act 1979 Statutory Sum Order 2007.

20 Admittedly this under a different damages regime where medical expenses recovery is more significant than in Europe.

Another issue is that of causation: [21] recent figures show that over 65% of claims fail for that very reason.[22] Indeed, there is a more general concern about the low success rate of the scheme. Recent data have suggested that the success rate of award has been reducing markedly in recent times, with in reality very little financial help forthcoming. A report undertaken for the Irish Health Research Board compared the British and US schemes as follows:[23]

> In the USA, from 1989–2017 the average yearly cost of payouts was US$130 million, while in the UK, the average annual cost from 2002–2012 was GB£284,000. It is worth noting that no claims have been paid out for a number of recent years in the UK, and the number of payouts per year has been approaching zero since 2009.

5.4.4 Track and Trace

The UK Government set up a NHS Test and Trace Service in May 2020 as part of their Covid-19 recovery strategy.[24] Under this scheme, people who received a positive Covid-19 result after a PCR test were asked to communicate the details of people with whom they have been in close contact in the preceding days so that they can be contacted by NHS tracing teams.

On the first introduction of Test and Trace, there was no legal obligation to isolate following a notification from the service. As of September 2020, regulations were adopted which created a legal duty for close contacts to self-isolate after receiving a notification from Test and Trace: The Health Protection (Coronavirus, Restrictions) (Self-Isolation) (England) Regulations 2020 (SI 2020/1045). These regulations are still in force, although they have been amended multiple times over the last 11 months. An individual commits an offence if they fail to self-isolate when required to do so, unless they have a "reasonable excuse" for the failure.[25] The maximum penalty upon conviction is a fine, although an individual can pay a fixed penalty notice to avoid prosecution. The sum of the fixed penalty notice will be set at £1,000 in the first instance, but can rise above for repeat offenders.[26]

5.4.5 Support Measures – Furlough Payments, no Evictions

A plethora of support measures were put together by the UK Government in order to soften the financial impact of the pandemic on the general public, including the protection of tenants from eviction,[27] a scheme of mortgage holidays implemented for consumers during the period March–October 2020,[28] and a similar scheme in respect of personal loans and credit card debts. There were also modifications to the UK tax system, with income tax payments being deferred until 31 January 2021, and the possibility of other tax deferrals of payments on request to the tax authorities. VAT (a tax on the sale of goods and services) was also reduced in various areas, such as zero rating for personal protective equipment used for protection from coronavirus.[29]

---

21 R. Goldberg, *Medicinal Product Liability and Regulation* (Oxford: Hart Publishing, 2013), p 11.
22 See generally E. Rajneri, J.-S. Borghetti, D. Fairgrieve, and P. Rott, "Remedies for Damage Caused by Vaccines: A Comparative Study of Four European Legal Systems" (2018) European Review of Private Law 57, at 90.
23 Health Research Board, *Vaccine Injury Redress Programmes: an Evidence Review* (March 2019) page 18.
24 See generally K. Lines, *The Contact Tracing Self-Isolation Regime in England: A Rule of Law Analysis* (Bingham Centre for Rule of Law, October 2021), available at:
120_bingham_centre_-_report_on_self-isolation_regulations.pdf (biicl.org).
25 Regulation 2B and 3(3).
26 Regulation 12(4).
27 See section 81 and Schedule 29 of the Coronavirus Act 2020.
28 See Guidance issued by the Financial Conduct Authority: Mortgages and coronavirus: our guidance for firms (March 2020).
29 The Value Added Tax (Zero Rate for Personal Protective Equipment) (Coronavirus) Order 2020.

There has been a raft of governmental measures undertaken to support businesses during the period of disruption caused by Covid-19. There was also a furlough scheme, the Coronavirus Job Retention Scheme, allowing businesses to place employees on temporary leave of absence and recoup 80% of their usual monthly wage costs from the UK tax authorities. It ended on 30 September 2021. In parallel, there was also governmental support for self-employed persons impacted by the crisis, with the creation of a Self-Employment Income Support Scheme.

There were also a series of government-backed and guaranteed loans and financing facilities. In terms of finance, the government launched a Covid Corporate Finance Facility (CCFF). The CCFF was operated by the Bank of England (BoE) on behalf of HM Treasury. [30] Under this scheme, the BoE was able to buy commercial paper from larger companies, i.e. unsecured, short-term debt instrument issued by a company. For larger businesses, there was also the Coronavirus Large Business Interruption Loan Scheme. This scheme helped medium and large-sized businesses to access loans and other kinds of finance up to £200 million, and was available through British Business Bank-accredited lenders and partners.

5.5 Problems/Analysis of the Legal Response

5.5.1 Reliance upon Emergency Procedures and Processes to Make Law in a Rush

When the Coronavirus Act 2020 was rushed through Parliament at breakneck speed, there was at least a forum for debate, and a mechanism for amending the legislation during the course of its enactment. The urgency of the situation did justify this urgent response, breaching the normal conventions on the time necessary to debate important legislation. When the first set of the domestic restrictions and international travel regulations were made, there was a clear justification for using both the vehicle of secondary legislation, and the urgent procedure – the measures needed to be implemented straightaway.

However, as the pandemic progressed, it is less and less clear that we need the method of law-making to be secondary legislation and for the urgent procedure to be used. This was the point made by Mark Harper MP during the parliamentary debate on approving the first set of English regulations – "I understand why that did not take place when the regulations were first brought in, but any subsequent amendments should be debated by the House."[31] There is a sizeable minority opinion now in Parliament (under the collective name of the Covid Recovery Group) that there should no longer be reliance upon these urgent procedures.

The criteria set out in section 45R for the use of the emergency procedure is that it is necessary, by reason of urgency, to make the regulations without them first being approved by Parliament. After more than a year and a half, it is unclear why it is still necessary by reason of urgency to use the emergency procedure. The twists and turns of the virus are not entirely unpredictable. Even though there are new variants, it is no longer a new disease. We know that, in broad terms, if we relax restrictions the disease will spread more quickly, and if we tighten them, the disease will spread more slowly.

This unjustified reliance upon emergency procedures has contributed to the next problem, the lack of parliamentary scrutiny.

---

30 See Joint HM Treasury and Bank of England Covid Corporate Financing Facility (CCFF) – Consolidated Market Notice 22 June 2020: https://www.bankofengland.co.uk/markets/market-notices/2020/joint-hmt-and-boe-ccff-consolidated-market-notice-may-2020.
31 Hansard 4 May 2020, Vol 675, Column 462.

5.5.2 Lack of Effective Parliamentary Scrutiny

Important legislation, which severely impacts upon the rights of individuals, can be justified in a public health emergency. However, there needs to be a forum in which that justification can be tested, and the measures themselves can be properly scrutinized. With primary legislation enacted through the normal procedures, then that opportunity does exist (at least in theory). If the government wishes to enact laws which curtail civil liberties, then someone needs to stand up in Parliament and explain it, and then parliamentarians have several months of going through the details and debating each individual point in that legislation. If an individual clause is found objectionable, it must be specifically justified, and Parliament has the opportunity to amend it.

This is the standard (perhaps slightly idealistic) procedure for enacting primary legislation. However, coronavirus legislation in the UK does not go through this process. Instead, there is either (a) rushed primary legislation or (b) poorly scrutinized secondary legislation. With rushed primary legislation, there is no time to properly consider the details, and very little in the way of an opportunity to propose meaningful and considered amendments. Furthermore, there is little realistic chance to actually reject that legislation wholesale. In practical terms, if the legislature has one day to consider a 300-page piece of legislation, there is no way this can be done effectively. And it would be political suicide to vote against the law designed to protect the country from coronavirus.

When it comes to secondary legislation, these problems are magnified. First, there is simply not the scrutiny given to secondary legislation that is given to primary legislation. An Act of Parliament may have 20 days of debates, plus additional time spent in committees. A piece of secondary legislation will, if lucky, have a few hours of debate on one occasion.

Second, the use of the urgent procedure means that Parliament will be debating secondary legislation which has already been made and is already in force. This problem has been described as follows:

> The government's casual approach to the scheduling of debates on SIs means they have often been in force for weeks before MPs could consider them. A succession of lockdown regulations saw MPs debating and approving SIs even after they had been amended by a later instrument.[32]

The time delay between it being made and it being debated in both Houses of Parliament has meant that some parliamentary debates have been completely pointless – debating a rule even after that rule has been revoked.

This lack of proper scrutiny causes serious problems.[33]

First, there is not the same opportunity to spot and correct mistakes in legislation. Rushed legislation results in more mistakes. Rushed scrutiny means less chance to catch those mistakes. The Hansard Society characterizes this:

> Some Coronavirus-related SIs (which have not always been immediately withdrawn or revoked) have had omissions, technical mistakes and drafting shortcomings. As a result, others of the Coronavirus-related SIs have been made, at least in part, in order to correct these errors by amending the earlier instruments.[34]

———————

32 M. Russell, R. Fox, R. Cormacain, and J. Tomlinson, "The marginalisation of the House of Commons under Covid has been shocking; a year on, parliament's role must urgently be restored" (April 2021) available at https://constitution-unit.com/.

33 See further R. Cormacain, "Parliamentary Scrutiny of Coronavirus Lockdown Regulations: A Rule of Law Analysis" (Bingham Centre for the Rule of Law, September 2020).

34 Hansard Society, Coronavirus Statutory Instruments Dashboard.

Second, there is not the same opportunity for a wider public dissemination of the rules, leading to a lack of awareness of the rules, and trust in their legitimacy. The Institute for Government made the following observation:

> A willingness to engage with parliament and opposition parties would have allowed the government to hear and address concerns. This could have helped to add clarity, and restore trust, before the regulations were altered.[35]

The public, industry groups, patient organizations, medical staff, etc., are much more likely to engage with Parliament, if Parliament is debating coronavirus rules before they come into force and which they can influence. They are much less likely to engage if Parliament is debating something which was law four weeks ago, but is now no longer law.

Third, there is not the same opportunity to debate the efficacy of coronavirus rules. In the crucible of a debate on primary legislation, there is time, space, and resources to argue about what would be the best legislative response to coronavirus. There is also the opportunity to pass amendments to draft legislation in order to more effectively recalibrate that response. With secondary legislation, these same opportunities simply do not exist. As one of us previously said:

> Government simply presenting the public with the outcome of their decision does not contribute to the most efficacious balance being struck. Parliamentary debate and scrutiny provides a forum in which all voices in this discussion can be heard. The best way to expose a bad policy is if a Minister has to stand up in advance in Parliament and justify it.[36]

Professor Norton, who is also a parliamentarian in the House of Lords in the UK, posed the following set of questions that parliamentarians should consider in considering whether to enact emergency coronavirus legislation:

- How appropriate are the powers sought?
- Are they too extensive and open-ended?
- Should the powers be time-limited or at least amenable to early revocation?
- How are extensive powers to direct the actions of citizens, not least limiting their movements, compatible with individual liberty?[37]

The procedures for making emergency legislation and secondary legislation simply do not give effective opportunities for addressing these points.

5.5.3 Conflation of Law with Guidance

Two of the most obvious ways to deal with the pandemic are to make laws obliging people to do certain things, and to issue guidance advising them to do certain things. One is not automatically better than the other, and both have their place in a public health emergency. Law connotes legal obligation, backed up by sanctions, possibly including criminal penalties. Guidance connotes suggestions and advice, with a greater degree of flexibility and discretion allowed, and for which there

---

35 A. Nice, "The government should stop avoiding parliamentary scrutiny of its coronavirus legislation" (2 June 2020, Institute for Government).
36 R. Cormacain, "Parliamentary Scrutiny of Coronavirus Lockdown Regulations: A Rule of Law Analysis" (Bingham Centre for the Rule of Law, September 2020).
37 Lord Norton of Louth, Foreword – Global Legislative Responses to Coronavirus (2020) 8 Theory and Practice of Legislation 237.

is no punishment for failure to comply. Both can coexist satisfactorily, so long as it is clear what is law and what is guidance.

However, right from the start of the pandemic, the government has conflated law and guidance in a very confusing way. Official summaries of the law also contain guidance. Press conferences and press statements combine both law and guidance together. Hickman's view was that "it was not possible for people to know, without a high level of sophisticated legal knowledge, whether statements contained in the coronavirus guidance were statements of law, interpretations of the law or public health advice."[38] There is insufficient linguistic distinction between "you must do this under the law" and "we are advising you to do this." Lines has said that

> Inaccurate or confusing statements of the law undermine the Rule of Law. They are also likely to damage trust in Government messaging, which may have wider implications for the efficacy of the public health response to the pandemic.[39]

For example, during the first lockdown, the government told people that they could only exercise outside once per day, but the actual regulations placed no limit on the amount of times they could exercise. People were repeatedly told about the 2 meter rule (they must stay 2 meters apart from others), even though this was only ever guidance, and did not appear in the legislation.

This type of confusion undermines public confidence, and the willingness of people to follow the law. But there were even more serious consequences for law enforcement. The rapidity of legislative change meant that the police were grasping to find out what the actual law was. As a consequence, they sometimes relied on what the government was telling people what the law was. This led to individuals being charged and convicted for breach of what was just guidance, not law.

This conflation of law and guidance has continued throughout the pandemic. Even in October 2021, Lines highlighted the example of confusion between law and guidance in contact tracing. The manually based system where individuals were contacted by officials and told them they had to isolate is backed up by law. The mobile phone app is guidance. But they are both portrayed by the government has having the force of law.[40]

5.5.4 Inaccessible and Unintelligible Legislation

Much of the secondary legislation on domestic restrictions and international travel has been difficult to access in a timely fashion, and difficult to understand. This is a result of two practices in the way that these laws are made.

First, the practice of making it, laying it before Parliament, and bringing it into force with very little time between these stages. For example, the Health Protection (Coronavirus, Restriction) (All Tiers and Obligations of Undertakings) (England) (Amendment) Regulations 2020 were

- Made at 6 a.m. on 20 December 2020.
- Came into force at 7 a.m. on 20 December 2020.
- Laid before Parliament on 21 December 2020.

It is very common for new laws to be made and come into force straightaway, or come into force at 4 a.m. the next day. The public have no practical way of knowing the content of these new regulations, which may not even be published online for hours or even days after they have been made.

---

38 T. Hickman, "The use and misuse of guidance during the UK's coronavirus lockdown" (September 2020) https://papers.ssrn.com/sol3/papers.cfm?abstract_id=3686857.
39 K. Lines, "18 months of COVID-19 Legislation in England: A Rule of Law Analysis" (October 2021).
40 K. Lines, "The Contact Tracing Self-Isolation Regime in England: A Rule of Law Analysis" The Bingham Centre for the Rule of Law (7 October 2021).

In the UK, the official rule is that ignorance of the law is no defense. However, it is difficult to see the fairness of prosecuting someone for a law which has not yet been published.

The second practice which makes legislation difficult to access and understand is the practice of rapid amendments. Legislative changes are normally measured in terms of years, but with coronavirus, the law can change every week. This makes it nearly impossible for people to know what the current law is. The technique for making new regulations is by way of textual amendment to the old text. This makes the amending legislation almost indecipherable to the casual reader. For example, regulation 4 of the Health Protection (Coronavirus, International Travel and Restrictions) (Wales) (Miscellaneous Amendments) Regulations 2021 reads:

(1) Regulation 2A (exemptions for vaccinated travellers and others) is amended as follows.
(2) In paragraph (3)—
    (a) omit sub-paragraph (b);
    (b) omit sub-paragraph (ba);
    (c) in sub-paragraph (c)—
        (i) after paragraph (ii) insert—
            (ia) a certificate of COVID-19 records issued by an approved third country or territory;
            (ib) a North American Certificate;
        (ii) at the end, insert "and";
    (d) omit sub-paragraph (ca).
(3) In paragraph (4A)—
    (a) at the end of sub-paragraph (b), insert "and";
    (b) after sub-paragraph (c), omit "and";
    (c) omit sub-paragraph (d).

The regulations are technically correct, but very hard for anyone to see how the law is changing. This is however ameliorated by the practice of incorporating the amendments into the legislation within a very short period of time. This means that, within a few days, a revised version of the legislation appears online.

5.5.5 Risk of Creep of Emergency Practices into Normal Lawmaking

There was a risk that government would get used to the relaxed procedures for lawmaking during the pandemic and start to apply these to ordinary lawmaking. One of us previously suggested that we ought to keep coronavirus legislation "socially distanced" from ordinary legislation.[41] That risk is still present and has manifested itself in a number of ways. This has not happened so much with the content of normal legislation, which does by and large follow what happened before the pandemic. However, the main problem has been with the lawmaking process more generally. Six months into the pandemic, there was a claim that Parliament had been "sidelined."[42] This was followed up 18 months into the pandemic by a detailed critique of the marginalization of Parliament by a joint paper from a number of institutions.[43] This listed 5 major problem areas:

- Erosion of parliamentary control: emergency legislation.
- Erosion of parliamentary control: regulations.

---

41 R. Cormacain, "Keeping Covid-19 emergency legislation socially distant from ordinary legislation: principles for the structure of emergency legislation" (2020) 8 Theory and Practice of Legislation 245.
42 M. Russell and L. James, "MPs are right. Parliament has been sidelined" (The Constitution Unit, 28 September 2020) available at https://constitution-unit.com/2020/09/28/mps-are-right-parliament-has-been-sidelined.
43 M. Russell, R. Fox, R. Cormacain and J. Tomlinson, "The marginalisation of the House of Commons under Covid has been shocking; a year on, parliament's role must urgently be restored" (April 2021) available at https://constitution-unit.com/.

- Erosion of parliamentary control: money.
- Denial of MPs' equal participation rights.
- Wholesale and unnecessary use of proxy votes.

Some of these problem areas related only to coronavirus legislation, but some of them have diminished the quality of parliamentary engagement and scrutiny more generally.

5.5.6 Compliance with the Rules by Those in Power

The final problem has been not so much the rules themselves, but compliance with those rules by those in power. There have been occasional instances of breaches of the various lockdown rules by those in power across the UK and in the devolved jurisdictions, but these have been relatively minor, and the breaches have been followed by legal or political accountability (meaning fines, or people losing their jobs).

However, Boris Johnson, the UK Prime Minister, would appear to have led a culture of disregard for the rules at the highest level. His most senior special adviser, Dominic Cummings, undertook a long-distance car journey at a time when a strict lockdown was in operation. One excuse he offered for a road trip was that he wanted to "test his eyesight" by going for a drive. This apparently brazen breach of the rules, combined with the farcical excuse did not result in either a legal nor a criminal penalty.[44] There have been widespread allegations of rule-breaking by the Prime Minister himself at various parties in 10 Downing Street, his official residence, during lockdown.[45] Although this has been subject to an internal civil service investigation,[46] a police investigation and multiple allegations of rule-breaking by parliamentarians, at time of writing, there has been no legal or political penalty.

If those who make the rules do not follow the rules, there is a clear breakdown in trust, and a reduced likelihood that individuals will follow those rules.

5.6 Conclusion

Although the legal response to the pandemic in the UK has not been ideal, it has, by and large, been in accordance with the Rule of Law. The majority of the official response has been by way of primary and secondary legislation, generally made at breathtaking pace, and regularly amended. Each of the four nations in the UK has followed a similar approach, although there have been regional variations. Legislative powers that pre-existed coronavirus have been used, along with newly enacted powers. Most of the secondary legislation to deal with the pandemic has been made during the pandemic. There has been a reliance on both emergency powers and ordinary powers. Coronavirus legislation generally contains a sunset clause, although expiry dates are regularly extended.

There has been too much reliance on these emergency powers and rushed lawmaking and this has caused problems. There are insufficient opportunities for the legislatures to properly do their job and scrutinize the vast amount of coronavirus legislation. The government has regularly

---

44 R. Cormacain, "Instinct or rules: making moral decisions in the Cummings scandal," U.K. Const. L. Blog (28th May 2020) available at https://ukconstitutionallaw.org.
45 BBC News, "Police to investigate Downing Street lockdown parties" (26 January 2022) available at https://www .bbc.co.uk/news/uk-politics-60123850.
46 See update published on 31 January 2022: Investigation into alleged gatherings on government premises during Covid restrictions: Update (publishing.service.gov.uk)

conflated law with guidance, leading the public and officials to be ensure what is a legal obligation with criminal law sanctions for failure to comply, and what is merely a suggestion. The volume of legislation and rapidity of its change have made it difficult to access and understand it. Some bad practices around lawmaking processes have crept into the system, and now also apply to regular lawmaking. There has been a perception that those at the highest level who made the rules are not complying with the rules.

Section 2

Countries making Extensive use of Emergency Laws and Securitization

6

The State of Exception and its Effects on Civil Liberties in Italy During the COVID-19 Crisis

Anna Malandrino[1,2], Margherita Paola Poto[3,4]*, and Elena Demichelis[5]

[1] *Department of Political and Social Sciences, University of Bologna, Bologna, Italy*
[2] *KPM Center for Public Management, University of Bern, Bern, Switzerland*
[3] *Department of Management, University of Turin, Turin, Italy*
[4] *Faculty of Law, UiT The Arctic University of Norway, Tromsø, Norway*
[5] *PhD in Administrative Law, University of Turin, and Lawyer in Turin, Italy*

6.1   Introduction

The ongoing global pandemic represents an unprecedented challenge for contemporary political systems. The novel coronavirus SARS-CoV-2 was identified as the source of a series of atypical respiratory diseases in the Hubei Province of Wuhan, China, in December 2019 (hence the term COVID-19). On 30 January 2020, following the recommendations of the Emergency Committee, the WHO Director-General declared COVID-19 a Public Health Emergency of International Concern (PHEIC) and exhorted the international community to find ways to significantly accelerate intervention and containment measures. The declaration of COVID-19 as a global pandemic was not late in coming. On 11 March 2020, Dr. Tedros Adhanom Ghebreyesus, the WHO Director-General declared COVID-19 a pandemic: "This is not just a public health crisis, it is a crisis that will touch every sector; so every sector and every individual must be involved in the fights" (WHO 2020; see also Cucinotta and Vanelli 2020).

Governments invoked states of emergency, or states of exception (SoE) (Agamben 2005), with an observable expansion of their power, which – at least from the perspective of the Western world – deeply shook the basic structural principles of democratic societies, and first and foremost the principle of separation of powers. Hence, the scholarship has critically observed the oscillation between states of normality (hereinafter the term *normality* is understood in its etymological meaning of "conform to a norm or standard"[1]) and SoE, and the consequent delicate operation of rights' weighing (life and health vis-à-vis other fundamental rights and liberties, such as freedom of movement, privacy, and education). The way SoE affected or jeopardized the foundations of democracy has been increasingly evident in several delicate moments for Western democracies. One example of this is in the aftermaths of the two world wars, when democratic regimes were transformed by the gradual expansion of executive powers and the subsequent SoE. Another example comes from international human rights law, where the approach is known as a State of Derogation, and implies that, in emergency situations, a state is allowed to suspend and restrict

---

* *Margherita Paola Poto co-wrote sections 6.1 and 6.7 and wrote sections 6.2.1 and 6.2.2 (excluding Table 6.1).*

1 https://www.merriam-webster.com/words-at-play/normalize-normalization-meaning (accessed 29 July 2021).

Impacts of the Covid-19 Pandemic: International Laws, Policies, and Civil Liberties, First Edition. Edited by Nadav Morag.
© 2023 John Wiley & Sons, Inc. Published 2023 by John Wiley & Sons, Inc.

certain treaty rights.[2] In case of a public emergency that threatens the societal security of a nation, international human rights treaties allow the states to suspend the protection of certain fundamental rights. Agamben (2005) lists the cases of the International Covenant on Civil and Political Rights (ICCPR; entered into force in 1976), Art. 4; the European Convention on Human Rights (ECHR; entered into force in 1950), Art. 15; the American Convention on Human Rights (ACHR; entered into force in 1978), Art. 27. The SoE ignited as a response to the global pandemic seems to stem from this latter case. In an article of early 2020, Agamben raised his criticism on the SoE established in Italy, claiming that the (then) epidemic was conjured up by the Italian authorities and exacerbated by national media (Agamben 2020). For the Italian philosopher Agamben, there was an instrumentalization of the virus as a form of mass panic and as a pretext to extend emergency executive powers (Agamben 2020). Agamben's provocative statement stimulates a debate on the definition of SoE, its legitimacy, and its impact on the limitation of rights and liberties of a democratic state.

Research for this chapter focuses on the impacts of the pandemic containment measures and the consequent considerable restrictions to constitutional rights and civil liberties (Cercel et al. 2020). Little research has been conducted to assess whether these containment measures qualify as SoE, as well as on the risks of continuous oscillations between SoE and states of normality. Our contribution addresses this gap by answering the following overarching research questions: What are the constituent elements and principles governing SoE? And, how have they been impacting the system of civil liberties in Italy? By tackling these questions, we also address how the SoE and its containment measures have been impacting the system of civil liberties in Italy, and what the constituent elements (*content*) and effects of containment measures have been in Italy. We address the issue of parliamentary control over the measures adopted in times of emergency (*oscillations between SoE and states of normality*), and finally, we reflect on how democracies can respond to the current global health crisis effectively, while protecting the democratic values of rule of law, human rights, and civil liberties.

To answer our research questions, we develop a conceptual definition of SoE, looking into its foundations (justification), limits (temporal, objectives), and scrutinizing the domestic attempts to regulate, limit, mitigate, and control the oscillations between SoE and states of normality. We test our application on the case of Italy, looking into the containment measures adopted throughout the three pandemic waves, and examining our results through the lens of both SoE regulation and implementation. Our method involves a critical analysis of legislation, administrative acts, and case law, together with a literature review from both the public policy area and the legal domain.

Following this Introduction, in Section 6.2, we define the essential elements of SoE both in general and in the Italian context; in Section 6.3, we explore some of the features that characterize the declaration and implementation of SoE on a global level with a focus on the COVID-19 emergency; in Sections 6.4 and 6.5, we analyze, respectively, the regulation and implementation of SoE and containment measures in Italy during the COVID-19 pandemic; in Section 6.6, we highlight the effects of SoE and containment measures on civil liberties. Finally, in Section 6.7, we draw some conclusions regarding the main critical aspects of SoE in Italy and some implications relevant to both research and policymaking.

---

2 See for example Art. 5 Fourth Geneva Convention: https://www.un.org/en/genocideprevention/documents/atrocity-crimes/Doc.33_GC-IV-EN.pdf (accessed 7 September 2021).

6.2 Defining the Elements of States of Exception (SoE)

6.2.1 States of Exception in the General Context

SoE are justified in democratic societies by *ad hoc* constitutional provisions allowing the adoption of emergency measures in specific cases, such as the state of siege or war, public security, or safety (Cercel et al. 2020). The central element of SoE is the exception to the normal legislative operation of the law, which is not adopted through parliamentary acts but through decisions of the executive, and that has to be restored once the emergency has been resolved (Cercel et al. 2020).

It is understood that the emergency is a temporally limited phenomenon and therefore the continuing SoE is no longer justified beyond the time frame of the emergency. As a consequence, the exceptional measures adopted by the executive are justified only within the scope of the emergency. If the emergency is caused by a matter of public safety, as is the case with the current global pandemic, the emergency law strikes a balance between the fundamental right to (individual and collective) health, and other rights or liberties (including privacy, movement, and education).

The continuing crisis, as well as the oscillations of states of crisis and states of normality, run the risk of producing the following ripple effects on the good functioning of a democracy:

1. the measures may become embedded in the normal legislative system, enacting long-lasting transformations in the system (Cercel et al. 2020);
2. the balancing of rights protection and freedom restrictions may lack a valid, continuous justification; and in the worst-case scenarios,
3. the socioeconomic fabric might be threatened, and civil harmony risks being undermined.

6.2.2 Italy

The first Italian response to the COVID-19 emergency came on 31 January 2020, when the Council of Ministers adopted a resolution declaring a national health emergency for six months due to the spread of the related infectious disease (cf. **Table** 6.1). This provision was justified by the constitutional framework and in particular under Art. 120, para 2, of the Italian Constitution: "The government can act for bodies of the regions, metropolitan cities, provinces and municipalities if the latter fail to comply with international rules and treaties or EU legislation, or in the case of grave danger to public safety and security, or whenever such action is necessary to preserve legal or economic unity and in particular to guarantee the basic level of benefits relating to civil and social entitlements, regardless of the geographic borders of local authorities."

The resolution stated that the emergency could not be addressed with ordinary means and powers and that it was thus necessary to promptly issue extraordinary measures aimed at coping with the serious international situation that had arisen. Since then, the then President of the Council of Ministers issued numerous decrees to curb the spread of the pandemic (see **Table** 6.1), following its evolution and the oscillation of COVID-19 cases (waves). Meanwhile, political pressure led to a change in government and leadership. The containment measures continued to be adopted by the executive power after this change, as well. Not only political parties but also parts of the public opinion questioned the legitimacy of the state of emergency continuation, especially raising their concerns on the justification of liberties' restrictions (Biolcati et al. 2021).

Table 6.1 Public policy measures adopted in Italy to contain and manage the COVID-19 emergency.

Date	Measure
Jan-20	Deliberation of Council of Ministers, 31 January 2020. Declaration of the state of emergency as a result of the health risk related to the outbreak of diseases resulting from viral transmissible agents.
Feb-20	DL No. 6 of 23 February 2020. Urgent measures regarding the containment and management of the epidemiological emergency from COVID-19.
	DPCM 25 February 2020. Further implementing provisions of DL No. 6 of 23 February 2020.
Mar-20	DPCM 1 March 2020. Further implementing provisions of DL No. 6 of 23 February 2020.
	DL 2 March 2020, No. 9. Urgent support measures for families, workers, and businesses related to the epidemiological emergency from COVID-19.
	DPCM 4 March 2020. Further implementing provisions of DL No. 6 of 23 February 2020, applicable throughout the country.
	Deliberation of Council of Ministers, 5 March 2020. Additional appropriation for the implementation of interventions as a result of the health risk related to the outbreak of diseases resulting from viral transmissible agents.
	DPCM 8 March 2020. Further implementing provisions of DL No. 6 of 23 February 2020.
	DL 8 March 2020, n. 11. Extraordinary and urgent measures to counter the COVID-19 epidemiological emergency and contain the negative effects on judicial activity.
	L. No. 13 of 5 March 2020. Conversion into law, with amendments, of DL No. 6 of 23 February 2020.
	DPCM 9 March 2020. Further implementing provisions of DL No. 6 of 23 February 2020, applicable throughout the country.
	DL 9 March 2020, No. 14. Urgent provisions for the strengthening of the National Health Service in relation to the COVID-19 emergency.
	DPCM 11 March 2020. Further implementing provisions of DL No. 6 of 23 February 2020, applicable throughout the country.
	DL 17 March 2020, No. 18. Measures to strengthen the National Health Service and economic support for families, workers, and businesses related to the COVID-19 epidemiological emergency.
	DPCM 22 March 2020. Further implementing provisions of DL No. 6 of 23 February 2020, applicable throughout the country.
	DL 25 March 2020, No. 19. Urgent measures to cope with the COVID-19 epidemiological emergency.
Apr-20	DPCM 1 April 2020. Provisions implementing DL No. 19 of 25 March 2020, applicable throughout the country.
	DL 8 April 2020, no. 22. Urgent measures on the regular conclusion and orderly start of the school year and on state examinations.
	DL 8 April 2020, no. 23. Urgent measures on access to credit and tax compliance for companies, special powers in strategic sectors, as well as interventions on health and work, extension of administrative and procedural terms.
	DPR 9 April 2020. Extraordinary annulment of Ordinance No. 105 of 5 April 2020 of the Mayor of the City of Messina.
	DPCM 10 April 2020. Further implementing provisions of DL No. 19 of 25 March 2020, applicable throughout the country.
	Deliberation of Council of Ministers, 6 April 2020. Additional appropriation for the implementation of interventions as a result of the health risk related to the outbreak of diseases resulting from viral transmissible agents.

Table 6.1 (Continued)

Date	Measure
	DL 20 April 2020, no. 26. Urgent provisions on electoral consultations for the year 2020.
	Deliberation of Council of Ministers, 20 April 2020. Additional appropriation for the implementation of interventions as a result of the health risk related to the outbreak of diseases resulting from viral transmissible agents.
	DPCM 26 April 2020. Further implementing provisions of DL No. 6 of 23 February 2020, applicable throughout the country.
	L. No. 27 of 24 April 2020. Conversion into law, with amendments, of DL No. 18 of 17 March 2020. Extending deadlines for the adoption of legislative decrees.
	DL 30 April 2020, no. 28. Urgent measures for the functionality of the systems of interception of conversations and communications, further urgent measures in the field of penitentiary order, as well as supplementary and coordinating provisions in the field of civil, administrative, and accounting justice and urgent measures for the introduction of the COVID-19 alert system.
May-20	DL 10 May 2020, no. 29. Urgent measures on home detention or deferment of the execution of the sentence, as well as on the replacement of pretrial detention in prison with the measure of home arrest, for reasons related to the COVID-19 health emergency, of persons detained or interned for crimes of terrorist and mafia-type organized crime, or for crimes of criminal association related to drug trafficking or for crimes committed by taking advantage of the conditions or in order to facilitate the mafia association, as well as inmates and internees subjected to the regime provided by Article 41-bis of L. 26 July 1975, no. 354, as well as for reasons related to the COVID-19 health emergency, as well as, finally, in the matter of meetings with relatives or other persons to which convicted persons, internees, and defendants are entitled.
	DL 10 May 2020, No. 30. Urgent measures on epidemiological studies and statistics on SARS-COV-2.
	DL 16 May 2020, No. 33. Additional urgent measures to cope with the COVID-19 epidemiological emergency.
	DPCM 17 May 2020. Provisions implementing DL No. 19 of 25 March 2020 and DL No. 33 of 16 May 2020.
	DPCM 18 May 2020. Amendments to Art. 1, para 1, letter cc), of the DPCM of 17 May 2020.
	DL 19 May 2020, No. 34. Urgent measures on health, support to work and economy, as well as social policies related to the COVID-19 epidemiological emergency.
	L. No. 35 of 22 May 2020. Conversion into law, with amendments, of DL No. 19 of 25 March 2020.
Jun-20	L. No. 40 of 5 June 2020. Conversion into law, with amendments, of DL no. 23 of 8 April 2020.
	L. 6 June 2020, No. 41. Conversion into law, with amendments, of DL no. 22 of 8 April 2020.
	DPCM of 11 June 2020. Further provisions implementing DL No. 19 of 25 March 2020 and DL No. 33 of 16 May 2020.
	DL 16 June 2020, no. 52. Further urgent measures on wage supplementation treatment, as well as extension of terms on emergency income and emergence of labor relations.
	L. 19 June 2020, No. 59. Conversion into law, with amendments, of DL no. 26 of 20 April 2020.
	L. No. 70 of 25 June 2020. Conversion into law, with amendments, of DL no. 28 of 30 April 2020.
Jul-20	L. No. 72 of 2 July 2020. Conversion into law, with amendments, of DL No. 30 of 10 May 2020.
	DPCM 14 July 2020. Further provisions implementing DL No. 19 of 25 March 2020 and DL No. 33 of 16 May 2020.

(Continued)

Table 6.1 (Continued)

Date	Measure
	L. No. 74 of 14 July 2020. Conversion into law, with amendments, of DL No 33 of 16 May 2020.
	L. No. 77 of 17 July 2020. Conversion into law, with amendments, of DL no. 34 of 19 May 2020.
	Coordinated Text of DL 19 May 2020, No. 34.
	Deliberation of Council of Ministers, 29 July 2020. Extension of the state of emergency as a result of the health risk related to the outbreak of diseases resulting from viral transmissible agents.
	DL No. 83 of 30 July 2020. Urgent measures related to the expiration of the declaration of COVID-19 epidemiological emergency of 31 January 2020.
Aug-20	DPCM of 7 August 2020. Further provisions implementing DL No. 19 of 25 March 2020 and DL No. 33 of 16 May 2020.
	DL 14 August 2020, no. 104. Urgent measures for the support and revitalization of the economy.
Sep-20	DPCM 7 September 2020. Further provisions implementing DL No. 19 of 25 March 2020 and DL No. 33 of 16 May 2020.
	DL 8 September 2020, No. 111. Urgent provisions to address urgent financial and support needs for the start of the school year, related to the COVID-19 epidemiological emergency.
	L. 25 September 2020, No. 124. Conversion into law, with amendments, of DL No 83 of 30 July 2020.
Oct-20	Deliberation of Council of Ministers, 7 October 2020. Extension of the state of emergency as a result of the health risk related to the outbreak of diseases resulting from viral transmissible agents.
	DL No. 125 of 7 October 2020. Urgent measures related to the extension of the declaration of the state of COVID-19 epidemiological emergency and for the operational continuity of the COVID alert system, as well as for the implementation of Directive (EU) 2020/739 of 3 June 2020.
	DPCM 13 October 2020. Further provisions implementing DL No. 19 of 25 March 2020, converted, with amendments, by L. No. 35 of 25 May 2020, and DL No. 33 of 16 May 2020, converted, with amendments, by L. No. 74 of 14 July 2020.
	L. No. 126 of 13 October 2020. Conversion into law, with amendments, of DL No. 104 of 14 August 2020.
	DPCM 18 October 2020. Further provisions implementing DL No. 19 of 25 March 2020, converted, with amendments, by L. No. 35 of 25 May 2020, and DL No. 33 of 16 May 2020, converted, with amendments, by L. No. 74 of 14 July 2020.
	DL 20 October 2020, No. 129. Urgent provisions on tax collection.
	DPCM 24 October 2020. Further provisions implementing DL No. 19 of 25 March 2020, converted, with amendments, by L. No. 35 of 25 May 2020, and DL No. 33 of 16 May 2020, converted, with amendments, by L. No. 74 of 14 July 2020.
	DL 28 October 2020, No. 137. Additional urgent measures on health protection, support to workers and businesses, justice and security, related to the COVID-19 epidemiological emergency.
Nov-20	DPCM of 3 November 2020. Further provisions implementing DL No. 19 of 25 March 2020, converted, with amendments, by L. No. 35 of 25 May 2020, and DL No. 33 of 16 May 2020, converted, with amendments, by L. No. 74 of 14 July 2020.
	DL 9 November 2020, No. 149. Additional urgent measures regarding health protection, support for workers and businesses and justice, related to the COVID-19 epidemiological emergency.

Table 6.1 (Continued)

Date	Measure
	DL 23 November 2020, No. 154. Urgent financial measures related to the COVID-19 epidemiological emergency.
	L. No. 159 of 27 November 2020. Conversion into law, with amendments, of DL No 125 of 7 October 2020.
	DL No. 157 of 30 November 2020. Additional urgent measures related to the COVID-19 epidemiological emergency.
Dec-20	DL No. 158 of 2 December 2020. Urgent provisions to cope with health risks related to the spread of the COVID-19 virus.
	DPCM of 3 December 2020. Further provisions implementing DL No. 19 of 25 March 2020, converted, with amendments, by L. No. 35 of 22 May 2020, and DL No. 33 of 16 May 2020, converted, with amendments, by L. No. 74, as well as DL No. 158 of 2 December 2020.
	DL 18 December 2020, No. 172. Additional urgent provisions to address health risks related to the spread of the COVID-19 virus.
	L. 18 December 2020, No. 176. Conversion into law, with amendments, of DL No. 137 of 28 October 2020.
Jan-21	DL 5 January 2021, No. 1. Additional urgent provisions regarding containment and management of the COVID-19 epidemiological emergency.
	Deliberation of Council of Ministers, 13 January 2021. Extension of the state of emergency as a result of the health risk related to the outbreak of diseases resulting from viral transmissible agents.
	DL 14 January 2021, No. 2. Additional urgent provisions regarding the containment and prevention of the COVID-19 epidemiological emergency and the elections for the year 2021.
	DPCM 14 January 2021. Further implementing provisions of DL No. 19 of 25 March 2020, converted, with amendments, by Law No. 35 of 22 May 2020, of DL No. 33 of 16 May 2020, converted, with amendments, by Law No. 74, and of DL No. 2 of 14 January 2021.
	L. No. 6 of 29 January 2021. Conversion into law, with amendments, of DL No 172 of 18 December 2020.
	DL 30 January 2021, no. 7. Extension of terms in the field of tax fulfillments, assessment, collection and payments, as well as methods of execution of penalties as a result of the COVID-19 epidemiological emergency.
Feb-21	DL No. 12 of 12 February 2021. Further urgent provisions on the containment of the COVID-19 epidemiological emergency.
	DL 23 February 2021, No. 15. Additional urgent provisions on national movement of people for the containment of the COVID-19 epidemiological emergency.
Mar-21	DPCM of 2 March 2021. Further implementing provisions of DL No. 19 of 25 March 2020, converted, with amendments, by Law No. 35 of 22 May 2020, of DL No. 33 of 16 May 2020, converted, with amendments, by Law No. 74, and of DL No. 15 of 23 February 2021.
	DL 5 March 2021, no. 25. Urgent provisions for the postponement of electoral consultations for the year 2021.
	L. 12 March 2021, No. 29. Conversion into law, with amendments, of DL No. 2 of 14 January 2021.
	DL 13 March 2021, No. 30. Urgent measures to cope with the spread of COVID-19 and support measures for workers with minor children in distance learning or quarantine.
	L. 18 March 2021, No. 35. Establishment of the National Day in memory of the victims of the coronavirus epidemic.
	DL 22 March 2021, No. 41. Urgent measures regarding support to businesses and economic operators, labor, health, and territorial services, related to the COVID-19 emergency.

(Continued)

Table 6.1 (Continued)

Date	Measure
Apr-21	DL 1 April 2021, No. 44. Urgent measures for the containment of the COVID-19 epidemic, on SARS-CoV-2 vaccinations, justice, and public competitions.
	DL 22 April 2021, no. 52. Urgent measures for the gradual resumption of economic and social activities in compliance with the requirements for containing the spread of the COVID-19 epidemic.
	Deliberation of Council of Ministers, 21 April 2021. Extension of the state of emergency as a result of the health risk related to the outbreak of diseases resulting from viral transmissible agents.
	DL 30 April 2021, no. 56. Urgent provisions regarding legislative deadlines.
May-21	L. No. 58 of 3 May 2021. Conversion into law, with amendments, of DL No. 25 of 5 March 2021.
	L. 6 May 2021, No. 61. Conversion into law, with amendments, of DL No. 30 of 13 March 2021.
	DL No. 59 of 6 May 2021, containing urgent measures relating to the Supplementary Fund to the National Recovery and Resilience Plan and other urgent measures for investments.
	DL 18 May 2021, No. 65. Urgent measures relating to the COVID-19 epidemiological emergency.
	L. No. 69 of 21 May 2021. Conversion into law, with amendments, of DL no. 41 of 22 March 2021.
	DL 25 May 2021, No. 73. Urgent measures related to the COVID-19 emergency, for businesses, work, youth, health, and territorial services.
	L. No. 76 of 28 May 2021. Conversion into law, with amendments, of DL No. 44 of 1 April 2021.
Jun-21	L. No. 87 of 17 June 2021. Conversion into law, with amendments, of DL No. 52 of 22 April 2021.
	DPCM of 17 June 2021. Implementing provisions of Art. 9, para 10, of DL No. 52 of 22 April 2021.
Jul-21	L. No. 101 of 1 July 2021. Conversion into law, with amendments, of DL No. 59 of 6 May 2021.
	DL no. 105 of 23 July 2021. Urgent measures to cope with the COVID-19 epidemiological emergency and for the safe exercise of social and economic activities.
	L. No. 106 of 23 July 2021. Conversion into law, with amendments, of DL No. 73 of 25 May 2021.

Source: Official Gazette of the Italian Republic/Ministero della Giustizia/Public Domain. Latest update: 29 July 2021.

6.3 States of Exception During the Pandemic: Declaration, Implementation, and Effects

Before analyzing the peculiarities of the Italian experience with the SoE during the COVID-19 pandemic, it is important to understand some general features of the declaration, implementation, and effects on civil liberties of the SoE according to its political definition as well as within the context of the pandemic in the rest of the world, in order to contextualize the Italian case study.

6.3.1 Establishing and Implementing the States of Exception

According to Schmitt, "Sovereign is he who decides on the state of exception" (Schmitt 1985, p. 5). The SoE represents an exception to the principle of people's sovereignty in democratic societies because the executive temporarily exerts that sovereignty, even though within the limits of constitutional provisions (emergency in case of war, public security, or safety). Dangers of autocratic deviations can indeed hide in a *de jure* or *de facto* "permanent" SoE (Whiting and Kaya 2021). While a healthy democracy only employs the SoE to face extraordinary and/or temporary circumstances and, therefore, sets a time limit within which they can produce effects, an autocracy – whether it is consolidated or aspiring – will be less likely to grant the time limit guarantee to its ruled people.

Different national contexts envisage different configurations of subnational autonomy in the implementation of SoE decisions (Kettl 2020). Variations in the implementation of central government measures can arise both between and within national contexts also due to the absence of national leadership and a lack of coordination between public authorities (Sadiq et al. 2020). During the COVID-19 pandemic, these phenomena were detected in several political systems in Europe (for an overview, cf. Colfer 2020; about, e.g. Spain, cf. Royo 2020; about Belgium and the Netherlands, Van Overbeke and Stadig 2020) and the United States (Bowling et al. 2020; Rozell and Wilcox 2020). In this panorama, the Italian case has not represented an exception. National decisions have sometimes sparked uncertainty regarding the allocation of decision-making powers among local, regional, and national authorities, thus producing a diverse set of policy responses and policy-delivery processes (Malandrino and Demichelis 2020).

Another major consequence of the unexpectedness of the pandemic and of the difficulties in crafting policy responses throughout the world has been the greater role of discretion, in the absence of clear and stable directives from governments, in the implementation of the SoE by street-level bureaucrats (SLBs), defined as "public service workers who interact directly with citizens in the course of their jobs" (Lipsky 1980, p. 3). If discretionary powers are expected to be exerted within the limits of the law, in times of unexpected emergencies, their exercise risks to be subject to individual perceptions. In such a scenario, SLBs may exercise their discretionary power according to their perception of the individual policy client's values and preferences (Brodkin 2011; Tummers et al. 2015; Thomann and Rapp 2018; Lotta and Pires 2019; Gofen and Lotta 2021). Policy clients are, in turn, "subjected to street-level decisions and framed as the powerless side of the interaction" (Gofen et al. 2019, p. 198). In times of crisis, the higher number of tasks SLBs are assigned as well as policy ambiguity might contribute to the expansion of their discretion (Davidovitz et al. 2021; Gofen and Lotta 2021; Lotta et al. 2021; Malandrino and Sager 2021). While the exercise of discretionary powers can on one hand leave room for the beneficial effects of administrative creativity, on the other hand it can undermine the rule of law (Lienhard et al. 2022), and, ultimately, threaten the civil rights and liberties of a democratic state.

6.3.2 The Potential Effects of States of Exception on Civil Liberties

In relation to the COVID-19 pandemic, citizens have been found to be willing to accept limitations of their civil liberties in exchange for improved control of risks (Zweifel 2020). However, the asymmetries in the implementation of the SoE might result in unequal limitations of civil liberties. For instance, the right to receive educational services might not be ensured equally across school levels and geographical locations (SVIMEZ 2020). On the one hand, the higher level of teachers' discretion might bring about positive consequences in terms of the time dedicated to students by teachers themselves, which in turn can contribute to their professionalism (Malandrino and Sager 2021). On the other hand, an indirect consequence of that discretion is that students might not always receive the same amount of time and attention at all ages as well as throughout a country (SVIMEZ 2020). A potential problem with student assessment also arose across the globe, since teachers in both schools and universities had to understand how to evaluate effectively and fairly in online learning scenarios (Prenkaj et al. 2020), as well as to deal with the privacy-related implications of new education delivery modes.

In another key policy sector, i.e. healthcare, the spread of the virus and the consequent containment measures incentivizing the usage of online services rather than physical presence in clinics and hospitals have been argued to represent possible threats to privacy and cybersecurity (cf. Bassan 2020; Sardi et al. 2020). This, of course, might in turn give rise to an increase in the already-existing asymmetries in the protection of the right to privacy depending on the emergency usage of telemedicine (Gabbrielli et al. 2020). Not least, the SoE and the consequent activation of contact-tracing procedures under government surveillance also posed issues for individual privacy. Although a correlation has been found in several countries between the usage of contact-tracing apps and a reduction in the spread of COVID-19, the ethical implications of these technologies for individual liberties have been the subject of much discussion (Urbaczewski and Young 2020). Efforts have been made to start issuing guidelines for ethical use of these apps, which inter alia should arguably involve review and exit strategies for apps that are no longer beneficial, with assessments made by independent bodies rather than by app designers or governments (Morley et al. 2020).

6.4 States of Exception and Containment Measures during the COVID-19 Pandemic in Italy: Regulatory Aspects

As a general concept, regulating means to adopt rules that discipline aspects of human life, in principle for their well-being (Braithwaite 2017). This section illustrates the most important rules that governed the COVID-19 SoE in Italy, while the next two sections are, respectively, devoted to policy implementation and policy effects on civil liberties.

In Italy, the pandemic seems to have accelerated pre-existing processes of transformation concerning institutional and legal aspects (Fantigrossi 2021), thus exposing fragilities in the institutional and governance framework. The most critical dimensions concerned the allocation of powers between parliament and the executive, as well as along the central–local government continuum, and the restriction of some fundamental liberties also due to the incorrect use of regulatory sources (Chiti 2020).

The Italian Constitution does not contain any general provision on the SoE that may be applicable whenever an emergency arises, unlike constitutions in other jurisdictions in Europe (e.g. Spain and France). There are, however, specific provisions on extraordinary events, allowing a temporary derogation of the democratic separation of powers. Among these, Art. 120, para. 2, of the Italian Constitution establishes the state's faculty to exercise subsidiary powers vis-à-vis subnational units in the event of serious danger to public safety and security (Accademia Nazionale dei Lincei, hereinafter "ANL," 2020).

In cases of atypical state of emergency – which is outside the cases expressly provided for by the Constitutional framework – the constitutional case law has long established the application of a principle according to which in the face of an emergency situation, parliament and government have not only the right and power but also the precise and unavoidable duty of providing for the adoption of appropriate emergency legislation (Italian Constitutional Court, judgment no. 15 of 1982).

More specifically, the Civil Protection Code (namely Artt. 7 and 24, DLgs no. 1/2018) establishes that for emergencies of national importance, the Council of Ministers is entrusted with the power to deliberate on a state of emergency, provided that its duration and territorial extension are also determined. This does not exclude – in compliance with the Italian constitutional framework – parliamentary involvement in the decision-making process, particularly when the national emergency requires restrictions to liberties and rights, as has happened in the current pandemic.

If the need for and urgency of the emergency does not allow an early intervention of parliament, the executive will still be able to take action by adopting a legally binding act such as the decree-law (DL), which provisionally enters into force but requires the enactment of parliament to gain definitive force, which must intervene within 60 days since the adoption of the DL itself.

From the initial phase of the state of emergency, in institutional terms, confusion arose because parliament was not involved in the decision-making process. This is because the executive initially intervened with administrative acts of a regulatory nature, rather than a legislative act that requires legislation from parliament. As noted above, following the WHO declaration, on 31 January 2020, the Council of Ministers issued a six-month state of emergency, which was then extended several times until 31 December 2021. Minor emergency measures were taken by the national executive until the first national lockdown which took place in March 2020 when the central government was joined by local governments (20 Italian regions and two autonomous provinces) in the crisis management, with the consequent coordination and allocation-of-power problems (see Section 6.5).

The emergency response in Italy was basically guided by the data regarding the spread of the infection: it began from the areas mainly affected by the epidemic and then extended throughout the national territory (Ronga 2020). Only after the first case of second-level transmission of the virus had been reported (on 18 February 2020 in Codogno, a municipality in Lombardy), the Council of Ministers adopted a first DL (no. 6/2020) in February 2020 – and converted it into L. no. 13/2020 in March 2020. DL no. 6/2020 authorized the executive or other "competent authorities" to manage the crisis. Thus, the executive adopted numerous measures by means of different regulatory sources other than DLs (including DPCMs and decrees of sectoral ministries) and in relation to countless subject matters (cf. **Table** 6.1). Such a plethora of prescriptions made it difficult even to learn about the existence of certain rules as well as to interpret them, thus undermining legal certainty (Ronga 2020). In addition to this, several authoritative scholars (Azzariti 2020), as well as public opinion and some parliamentarians questioned whether – at least at the beginning of the pandemic – parliament would be able to meet its constitutional decision-making and control role vis-à-vis the emergency measures. In March 2020, parliament decided to partially suspend its activity: the parliamentary agenda shows that, at the beginning of the crisis, the number of sessions significantly decreased to an almost weekly deadline, and the subject matters under discussion were reduced and focused only on the issues concerning the coronavirus (Grisolia 2020).

In order to cope with the danger of contagion, it was proposed to allow remote participation of parliamentarians in the discussion and vote of containment measures. However, the proposal was dropped because many argued that the Italian Constitution requires "physical" presence in parliament to calculate the deliberative quorum and presupposes a strict conception of political representation which is necessarily linked to the parliamentary dialectic that allows serving the public interest amidst dialogue, argumentation, and negotiation between various political forces (Grisolia 2020). At the level of the political debate, it was proposed to amend the Italian Constitution to strengthen the role of parliament in states of emergency, providing that, after deliberation of the state of crisis by Parliament, a special commission would take up parliamentary duties (Constituent Assembly, XVIII Legislature, Proposal for a constitutional law no. 2452). However, scholars agree that a constitutional reform of this type does not seem necessary, but would nonetheless be desirable in order to make proper use of the rules and instruments that the existing Italian Constitution is already able to offer, as well as to extend and strengthen the powers of control over the executive that are vested in parliament. An example of this is the use of general guidelines on emergency management (ANL 2020). In this sense, only at the end of May 2020, the legislator (L. no. 35/2020) planned the involvement of parliament in the enactment of governmental measures relating to emergency management. The President of the Council of Ministers, or a minister delegated by him, is now obliged to inform parliament in advance about the content of the measures to be adopted, in order to take into account any guidelines formulated by it (Art. 2, para. 1, DL no. 19/2020, converted into L. no. 35/2020). Thus, parliament can take action to guide the executive in the implementation of the choices made, also by way of proposing necessary changes (Grisolia 2020).

6.5 States of Exception and Containment Measures During the COVID-19 Pandemic in Italy: Implementation

Policy implementation refers to "the way policies are actually applied by the targeted addressees [and] transformed into concrete actions" (Newig and Koontz 2014).

In the Italian experience, the COVID-19 crisis management has been characterized by oscillations between the government's initial will to play an incisive role (Mandato 2020) and the interinstitutional conflicts along the central–local government continuum that stemmed from the subnational units' competence to take further measures (Malandrino and Demichelis 2020). The Italian republic is divided into 20 Regions that roughly correspond to the historical territorial articulation. Italian Regions have legislative power and administrative autonomy, to be exercised in compliance with the limits set by the Constitution, providing that local acts should not conflict with national interest. The regional councils can also adopt legislation for the enforcement of national law when it contains the adequate provisions. During the pandemic, in Italy, many regional governments considerably limited citizens' liberties more restrictively than the central government (Giorgio 2020). The measures adopted in this sense included the closure of schools, universities, and museums, as well as the prohibition of any public events, and triggered a normative intervention with DL 19/2020 (Art. 3), which established that the policies adopted by regions must (i) operate in the absence of measures adopted by the central government; (ii) be justified by the supervening worsening of the health risk in the region concerned; (iii) consist in measures further restricting social and productive activities in the region concerned.

However, even after this intervention, new conflicts arose regarding the limitations on economic activities and involving both the central government and regions and municipalities. These conflicts were finally brought before an administrative court (TAR Catanzaro, judgment of 9 May 2020, no. 841). The judges ruled that it is the Italian President of the Council of Ministers who decides on the necessary measures to counteract the spread of the COVID-19 virus in compliance with the subsidiarity principle. Moreover, similar limitations concern municipalities, as DL 19/2020 states that mayors cannot adopt emergency measures in conflict with state prescriptions, while normally a mayor can adopt ordinances departing from the law to face urgent local issues (Malandrino and Demichelis 2020).

At the street-level bureaucracy level, a degree of uncertainty and variation could be observed especially in the field of justice administration throughout the country. In Italy, some judges are in charge of scheduling judicial hearings and adopting guidelines concerning the operation of trials in accordance with the law. During the COVID-19 epidemic, organizational measures in the justice administration system were dynamically adapted to the evolution of the emergency in order to prevent essential and nonessential activities from undergoing paralysis (Malandrino and Demichelis 2020; Veltri 2020). To regulate the operation of the administrative justice system, there was an overproduction of legislative interventions in only two months (DL no. 9 of 2 March 2020; DL no. 11 of 8 March 2020; DL no. 18 of 17 March 2020; DL no. 23 of 8 April 2020; DL no. 27 of 24 April 2020; DL no. 28 of 30 April 2020). However, in spite of this, the resulting legal framework was still partially obscure and patchy. Nonlegislative acts were adopted to clarify the legal framework, but this sometimes resulted in additional burdens for justice administrators, which complicated the operation of trials (Volpe 2020). While the early crisis management stage was characterized by the postponement of hearings and procedural deadlines, subsequently the legislator imposed "written hearings" to be conducted exclusively through an exchange of written notes (DL 18/2020) and "videoconference hearings" to be attended by counsels and parties only (DL 28/2020), which were conducted even by the Constitutional Court (decree of the President of the Constitutional Court of 20 April 2020).

However, significant variation can be observed concerning the practical measures adopted by the individual judicial offices for the resumption of justice-related activities, with e.g. some courts trying to avoid videoconference hearings and other courts choosing to arrange those kinds of hearings, provided that they had the express consent of the parties (Altieri and Blasi 2020). This variation, in turn, produced uncertainty vis-à-vis the operational modes of trials and triggered the criticism of both judges (Italian Council of State, court order of 21 April 2020, no. 2539; for a different view, however, cf. TAR Napoli, judgment of 29 May 2020, no. 2074) and lawyers (Giunta UCPI 2020) regarding the compatibility of both written and videoconference hearings with the existing legal framework.

6.6 The Effects of States of Exception Measures on Civil Liberties

Policy effects can be defined as the ultimate outcomes of deliberation (Baur 2012). In this regard, one of the most debated issues in Italy concerns the constitutional conformity of the containment measures where they restrict fundamental liberties without the control of parliament or the judiciary.

The Italian Constitution establishes that limitations to fundamental liberties (such as personal freedom and freedom of movement, respectively, Art. 13 and Art. 16) can be established solely by law, in order to protect other constitutionally relevant interests and following the proportionality criterion (ANL 2020). The protection of constitutional rights and freedom is provided by parliament through political control, both of a preventive and an *ex post* nature, on the work of the executive, and, ultimately, through the exercise of judiciary power (at the constitutional, ordinary, and administrative level). As mentioned, during the initial phase of the pandemic, administrative acts, i.e. sub-legislative acts with a regulatory nature, were adopted to manage the crisis, with the consequence that their impact has been removed from the control of parliament and courts. It has therefore been debated whether these kinds of acts have been adopted in compliance with the rule of law and constitutional provisions. A much-debated issue concerned whether the first act adopted by the government after the emergency declaration (DL no. 6/2020 of February 2020) adequately met the constitutional principles of legality and proportionality, since it granted the administrative authority the power to adopt "further measures" for emergency management without defining its content and limits and, consequently, allowing restrictions to liberties without adequate coverage by the law, as would be required by the Italian Constitution (ANL 2020).

To contain the spread of the epidemic, in late February, the Minister of Health and the regional governments jointly established the "red zones" (*zone rosse*) in two of the twenty Italian Regions (Lombardy and Veneto), where lockdown measures were therefore adopted: schools and businesses were closed and people were not allowed to exit from those zones. The first national lockdown measure – extended throughout the Italian territory – was adopted in March 2020, and the government continued to manage the crisis by using sub-legislative acts (emergency decrees) throughout the "first wave," which resulted in an abundant normative production compared to the following two waves covered in this chapter (see **Table** 6.1). Those emergency measures frequently overlapped with each other, and it seemed that their adoption responded to the "perception of the inadequacy of sector regulations established to manage different types of emergency (civil protection- and health-related) in the face of an epidemic that, in terms of aggressiveness and spread, had never been experienced in the Republican era" (Pinelli 2020, p. 6; Ronga 2020, p. 7, translations).

The foundations for the limitation of civil liberties due to the COVID-19 emergency were laid during this first wave and subsequently extended or lifted in response to epidemiological trends. The measures adopted gave rise to the first lockdown, at first limited to high-risk zones and then extended to the rest of the country. These measures involved movement restrictions except for duly self-declared work or health reasons, as well as bans on sporting events and gatherings in general, school and university closure, and limitations on bar and restaurant opening (DPCM of 8 March 2020). In the event of a police check, it was necessary to show a self-certification in which the declarer certified the reasons for movement, under penalty of forgery in the event of an untruthful declaration (DPCM 8 March 2020). Restrictions were further strengthened with the closure of all nonessential businesses and the encouragement of home-work arrangements (DPCM of 11 March). Finally, further restrictions concerned the movement of people (within 200 m from home) and the operation of business activities (DPCM 22 March; cf. Mattei 2021).

The Italian Constitution allows restrictions on the right to congregate in public places (Art. 17, para 3). The emergency measures adopted in Italy also strictly forbade all meetings in private places, to the point that public religious services were no longer allowed (there is copious literature on this issue; among others, Montesano 2020).

Freedom of movement and, consequently, personal freedom in general, were also limited through both "the application of the precautionary quarantine measure to persons who have had close contact with confirmed cases of infectious disease or returning from areas located outside the Italian territory" (Art. 1, para 1(d) of DL no. 19/2020, translation), and "a total ban on persons who have been quarantined for being found to be virus-positive to leave their homes or dwellings" (Art. 1, para 1(e) of DL no. 19/2020, translation).

In summer 2020, most restrictive measures were lifted due to the improvement in the general epidemiological indicators. During the "second wave," in autumn 2020, the color-based system was introduced, ensuring that containment measures would not be identical throughout the national territory due to the different impact the pandemic was having in terms of both epidemiological indicators and healthcare system overload. Emergency measures were jointly adopted by the Ministry of Health and the Local Authorities (DPCM of 3 November 2020), sharing political responsibilities in decision-making. However, within the political debate at the national level, some of the restrictions on businesses and social services were no longer perceived as tolerable, such as the closing of bars and restaurants after 10 p.m. or distance learning at school. Distance learning, in particular, was the subject of a political battle (Malandrino and Capano, 2022) due to the damage that some have argued it creates in terms of isolation, depression, and poorer educational outcomes for thousands of young people.

After the second wave, the color-based system was progressively updated and modified: based on epidemiological data (including the Rt transmissibility index and the incidence of infections) and data relating to the overload of healthcare facilities (among which the hospitalization rate), regions and autonomous provinces were classified into risk areas identified by different colors (white, yellow, orange, and red). For each of these risk areas, specific restrictive measures were established. The classification of subnational units into risk areas took place through DLs or Ordinances of the Ministry of Health.

In Italy, the restrictions imposed in the first phase of the pandemic and their compatibility with the Constitutional freedom of movement have been widely debated (DPCM 8 March 2020). Amidst this debate, a court declared the inapplicability of the prohibition to leave the place of residency (DPCM 8 March 2020), because according to Italian law, such a measure can only be issued by a judge in a context where the right of defense is guaranteed (Court of Reggio Emilia, decision n. 54 of 27 January 2021). However, this judgment has been criticized on grounds of the fact that the Constitution itself establishes the possibility of restrictions on the freedom of movement for health or safety reasons (Gigliotti 2020). In this sense, it has been pointed out that the numerous exceptions to the emergency restriction exclude its classification as a sanction restricting personal freedom since people were still allowed to leave their homes for work or medical reasons as well as for basic needs (Gigliotti 2020). Thus, the emergency ban on people's movement from home imposed in the first phase of the pandemic cannot be considered as a measure implying liberty deprivation.

Considering that – according to part of the Italian constitutional case law (*inter alia*, Italian Constitutional Court, judgment no. 23 of 1975, judgment no. 30 of 1962 and judgment no. 99 of 1980) – personal freedom is affected by measures that, regardless of the degree of coercion, devalue the individual's personality and degrade social dignity, it has been concluded that "[n]one of the measures adopted [so far during the pandemic] seems to go in this direction, since they are general measures, formulated in specific terms, which affect the community as a whole and are justified by the need to protect the health of its components" (De Stefano 2020, translation). Such a conclusion is also confirmed by the fluctuating policy stringency curve, which followed the epidemiological trends and was justified in light of the need for health protection (cf. **Figure** 6.1).

Notwithstanding the above argument, it has been claimed that an impairment of individual liberties by reason of the precautionary principle – which, as such, could prevail over any competing interest – does not comply with the Italian legal framework, since the constitutional principle of measure proportionality itself prevents it; moreover, that principle would tend to produce unsustainable outcomes in today's risk society (De Stefano 2020; Pitruzzella 2020). In addition, it has been argued that the Italian legal system does not seem to recognize a general hierarchy of constitutional values: in this sense, the Constitutional Court specified that "all fundamental rights

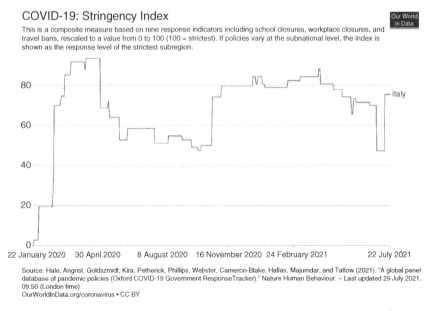

Figure 6.1 Evolution of policy stringency index in Italy during the COVID-19 pandemic.

protected by the Constitution are in a relationship of mutual integration and it is not possible to identify one of them that has absolute primacy over others. Protection must always be 'systemic and not divided into a set of uncoordinated rules that are in potential conflict with each other' […]. If this were not the case, there would be the unlimited exercise of one of the rights, which would become 'tyrant' towards the other constitutionally recognized and protected legal situations, which constitute, as a whole, an expression of the dignity of the person" (judgment no. 85 of 2013, translation).

6.7 Conclusions

The chapter illustrates the essential features of the SoE in response to the COVID-19 crisis and with specific regard to its impacts on civil liberties in Italy. It is based on an analytical understanding of public policy that, while keeping in mind the artificiality of any heuristics, distinguishes between regulatory and implementation-related aspects and looks at the effects produced by regulatory interventions. It sets the Italian case study in a broader context that considers the general features of SoE and of the COVID-19 response worldwide since both states of emergencies and the liberties they impact on are themes of relevance for all democracies. It then employs analytical tools such as the examination of case law and legal literature to assess the Italian case.

The use of concepts and categories borrowed from both legal and policy sciences enables the provision of a multifaceted picture that goes beyond the normative datum and at the same time enriches the policy perspective with juridical knowledge, while allowing us to present some of the potential criticalities in terms of the limitation of democratic principles and liberties. In this light, it analyzes the impact of the SoE on civil liberties in Italy, distinguishing between the regulatory phase of the SoE and its implementation, in order to account for the role of various actors, including legislators, courts, the executive, and SLBs.

The analysis of the regulatory phase shows the importance of legal certainty and clarity in the definition of the interinstitutional relationships between the parliament and the executive. From the scrutiny of the SoE implementation, it emerges how the rule of law and, once again, legal certainty are essential to limit the misuse of power by the bureaucracy and ultimately to prevent unequal treatment and the violation of the equality principle. Finally, the analysis of the SoE's effects on civil liberties highlights how the public debate – involving both scholars and public opinion – can be inflamed by issues concerning personal liberties and how positions change based on the alleged legitimacy of restrictive measures for the public interest (represented by health, in this case). We conclude that careful consideration must be given to all the elements of the SoE to evaluate its impact on fundamental rights and civil liberties.

Further research is needed to identify and map the institutional mechanisms that allow the preservation of the rule of law in times of emergency. In the Italian context, the complexity of interinstitutional dynamics (overlap of responsibilities, regulatory overproduction, and ambiguities of ad-hoc normative acts) calls for greater simplification and clarity in the definition of the institutional responsibilities in times of emergency.

References

Accademia dei Lincei. 2020. Problemi di ordine costituzionale determinati dall'emergenza della pandemia da COVID-19. www.giustizia-amministrativa.it (accessed 11 May 2022).

Agamben, G. 2005. *State of Exception*. Belgrade: Nova srpska politička misao.

Agamben, G. 2020. The state of exception provoked by an unmotivated emergency. *Positions Politics.* http://positionswebsite.org/giorgio-agamben-the-state-of-exception-provoked-by-an-unmotivated-emergency/ (accessed 20 April 2021).

Altieri, G. and Blasi, I. 2020. *Emergenza COVID-19 – Procedimenti da remoto: il processo penale non può rinunciare al dibattimento in aula*, Guida al Diritto – Il Sole 24 Ore. https://www.diritto24.ilsole24ore .com/art/guidaAlDiritto/dirittoPenale/2020-04-24/procedimenti-remoto-processo-penale-non-puo-rinunciare-dibattimento-aula-104003.php?refresh_ce=1.

Azzariti, G. 2020. Editoriale. Il diritto costituzionale d'eccezione, *Costituzionalismo.it*, Fascicolo 1.

Bassan, S. 2020. Data privacy considerations for telehealth consumers amid COVID-19, *Journal of Law and the Biosciences*, 7(1): lsaa075.

Baur, D. 2012. *NGOs as Legitimate Partners of Corporations*. Issues in Business Ethics, vol. 36. Dordrecht: Springer.

Biolcati, F., Vezzoni, C., Ladini, R., Chiesi, A.M., Dotti Sani, G.M., Guglielmi, S., and Segatti, P. 2021. Come monitorare la risposta dell'opinione pubblica a eventi imprevisti? Il progetto ResPOnsE COVID-19. *Polis*, 36(1): 165–177.

Bowling, C.J., Fisk, J.M., and Morris, J.C. 2020. Seeking patterns in chaos: transactional federalism in the Trump administration's response to the COVID-19 pandemic, *The American Review of Public Administration*, 506–7: 512–518.

Braithwaite, V. 2017 Closing the gap between regulation and the community. In *Regulatory Theory: Foundations and Applications*, edited by P. Drahos. Acton ACT, Australia: ANU Press, pp. 25–42.

Brodkin, E.Z. 2011. Policy work: street-level organizations under new managerialism. *Journal of Public Administration Research and Theory*, 21(suppl_2): i253–i277.

Cercel, C., Fusco, G.G., and Lavis, S. (Eds.). 2020. *States of Exception: Law, History, Theory*. London: Routledge.

Chiti, E. 2020. Questi sono i nodi. Pandemia e strumenti di regolazione: spunti per un dibattito. *laCostituzione.info*.

Colfer, B. 2020. Public policy responses to COVID-19 in Europe. *European Policy Analysis* 6: 126–137.

Cucinotta D., and Vanelli M. 2020. WHO declares COVID-19 a pandemic. *Acta Bio-Medica* 91(1): 157–160.

Davidovitz, M., Cohen, N., and Gofen, A. 2021. Governmental response to crises and its implications for street-level implementation: policy ambiguity, risk, and discretion during the COVID-19 pandemic. *Journal of Comparative Policy Analysis: Research and Practice*, 231: 120–130.

De Stefano, F. 2020. La pandemia aggredisce anche il diritto? Intervista a Corrado Caruso, Giorgio Lattanzi, Gabriella Luccioli e Massimo Luciani. *Giustizia Insieme*.

Fantigrossi, U. 2021. Il diritto della pandemia: libertà di circolazione e trasporti nel governo dell'emergenza COVID-19. www.giustizia-amministrativa.it (accessed 11 May 2022).

Gabbrielli, F., Bertinato, L., De Filippis G., Bonomini, M., and Cipolla M. 2020. Interim provisions on telemedicine healthcare services during COVID-19 health emergency. Version of 13 April 2020. *Rapporti ISS COVID-19* n. 12/2020.

Gigliotti, A. 2020. Sulla illegittimità dei DPCM in una recente sentenza del Tribunale di Reggio Emilia. *laCostituzione.info*.

Giorgio, M. 2020. Il controverso rapporto Stato-Regioni nella gestione dell'emergenza sanitaria. *iusinitinere.it*, 2020: 1–6.

Giunta UCPI. 2020. Disciplina emergenziale per la celebrazione delle udienze penali. Le osservazioni della Giunta UCPI. www.camerepenali.it (accessed 11 May 2022).

Gofen A., and Lotta G. 2021. Street-level bureaucrats at the forefront of pandemic response: a comparative perspective *Journal of Comparative Policy Analysis: Research and Practice*, 23(1): 3–15.

Gofen, A., Blomqvist, P., Needham, C.E., Warren, K., and Winblad, U. 2019. Negotiated compliance at the street level: personalizing immunization in England, Israel and Sweden. *Public Administration*, 97(1): 195–209.

Grisolia, M.C. 2020. Il rapporto Governo-Parlamento nell'esercizio della funzione normativa durante l'emergenza COVID-19. *Osservatorio sulle fonti*, fasc. speciale, 2020.

Kettl, D.F. 2020. States divided: the implications of American Federalism for COVID-19. *Public Administration Review*, 80: 595–602.

Lienhard A., Bieri P., and Malandrino A. 2022. The role of constitutional and administrative law in the politics of public administration, *Edward Elgar Handbook on the Politics of Public Administration*, edited by Andreas Ladner and Fritz Sager. Edward Elgar Publishing. https://www.e-elgar.com/shop/gbp/handbook-on-the-politics-of-public-administration-9781839109430.html.

Lipsky, M. 1980. *Street level Bureaucracy: Dilemmas of the Individual in Public Service* (30th Anniversary Expanded edn in 2010). New York: Russell Sage Foundation.

Lotta, G., and Pires, R. 2019. Street-level bureaucracy research and social inequality. In *Research Handbook on Street-Level Bureaucracy* edited by Peter Hupe. Cheltenham: Edward Elgar Publishing.

Lotta, G., Coelho, V.S., and Brage, E. 2021. How COVID-19 has affected frontline workers in Brazil: a comparative analysis of nurses and community health workers. *Journal of Comparative Policy Analysis: Research and Practice*, 23(1): 63–73.

Malandrino, A., and Capano, G. 2022. Institutional Mayhem as Usual: Intergovernmental Relations between the Central Government and the Regions in Italy during the Early Stages of the COVID-19 Pandemic. In *COVID-19 in Europe and North America: policy responses and multi-level governance*, edited by Veronique Molinari and Pierre-Alexandre Beylier, Berlin, Boston: De Gruyter Oldenbourg, pp. 167–190. https://doi.org/10.1515/9783110745085-008 (accessed 11 May 2022)

Malandrino, A., and Demichelis, E. 2020. Conflict in decision-making and variation in public administration outcomes in Italy during the COVID-19 crisis. *European Policy Analysis*, 6(2): 138–146.

Malandrino, A., and Sager, F. 2021. Can teachers' discretion enhance the role of professionalism in times of crisis? A comparative policy analysis of distance teaching in Italy and Switzerland during the COVID-19 pandemic. *Journal of Comparative Policy Analysis: Research and Practice*, 23(1): 74–84.

Mandato, M. 2020. Il rapporto Stato-Regioni nella gestione del Covid-19. *Nomos*, 2020(1): 1–8.

Mattei, P. 2021. Coordination and health policy responses to the first wave of COVID-19 in Italy and Spain. *Journal of Comparative Policy Analysis: Research and Practice*, 23(2): 274–281. Special Issue on The COVID -19 Crisis: Policies, Outcomes, and Lesson Drawing.

Montesano, S. 2020. Libertà di culto ed emergenza sanitaria: sintesi ragionata delle limitazioni introdotte in Italia per contrastare la diffusione del COVID-19. *Quaderni di diritto e politica ecclesiastica*, 2/2020.

Morley, J., Cowls, J., Taddeo, M., and Floridi, L. 2020. Ethical guidelines for COVID-19 tracing apps *Nature*, 582(7810): 29–31.

Newig, J., and Koontz, T.M. 2014. Multi-level governance, policy implementation and participation: the EU's mandated participatory planning approach to implementing environmental policy. *Journal of European Public Policy,* 21(2): 248–267.

Van Overbeke T., and Stadig, D. 2020. High politics in the Low Countries: COVID-19 and the politics of strained multi-level policy cooperation in Belgium and the Netherlands. *European Policy Analysis*, 6: 305–317.

Pinelli C. 2020. Il precario assetto delle fonti impiegate nell'emergenza sanitaria e gli squilibrati rapporti fra Stato e Regioni. *Astrid*, 5: 1–8.

Pitruzzella, G. 2020. La società globale del rischio e i limiti alle libertà costituzionali. Brevi riflessioni a partire dal divieto di sport e attività motorie all'aperto. *Giustizia Insieme*.

Prenkaj, B., Stilo, G., and Madeddu, L. 2020. Challenges and solutions to the student dropout prediction problem in online courses. In *Proceedings of the 29th ACM International Conference on Information & Knowledge Management* (CIKM '20) (19–23 October 2020). New York, NY, USA: Association for Computing Machinery, pp. 3513–3514.

Ronga, U. 2020. Il Governo nell'emergenza (permanente). Sistema delle fonti e modello legislativo a partire dal caso COVID-19. *Nomos*, 1: 1–34.

Royo, S. 2020. Responding to COVID-19. The case of Spain. *European Policy Analysis*, 6(2): 180–190.

Rozell, M.J., and Wilcox, C. 2020. Federalism in a time of plague: how federal systems cope with pandemic, *The American Review of Public Administration*, 50(6–7): 519–525.

Sadiq, A.-A., Kapucu, N., and Hu, Q. 2020. Crisis leadership during COVID-19: the role of governors in the United States. *International Journal of Public Leadership*, 17(1): 65–80.

Sardi, A., Rizzi, A., Sorano, E., and Guerrieri, A. 2020. Cyber risk in health facilities: a systematic literature review. *Sustainability*, 12(17): 7002.

Schmitt, C. 1985. *Political Theology: Four Chapters on the Concept of Sovereignty*. Cambridge, MA: MIT Press.

SVIMEZ 2020. L'Italia diseguale di fronte all'emergenza pandemica: il contributo del Sud alla ricostruzione. https://ot11ot2.it/notizie/rapporto-svimez-2020-litalia-diseguale-di-fronte-allemergenza-e-il-contributo-del-sud-alla (accessed 11 May 2022).

Thomann, E., and Rapp, C. 2018. Who deserves solidarity? Unequal treatment of immigrants in Swiss welfare policy delivery. *Policy Studies Journal*, 46(3): 531–552.

Tummers, L., Bekkers, V., Vink, E., and Musheno, M. 2015. Coping during public service delivery: a conceptualization and systematic review of the literature. *Journal of Public Administration Research and Theory*, 25(4): 1099–1126.

Urbaczewski, A., and Young J.L. 2020. Information Technology and the pandemic: a preliminary multinational analysis of the impact of mobile tracking technology on the COVID-19 contagion control. *European Journal of Information Systems*, 29(4): 405–414.

Veltri, G. 2020. Il processo amministrativo. L'oralità e le sue modalità in fase emergenziale: "tutto andrà bene". *Il Diritto Amministrativo*, 2020(6). https://www.giustizia-amministrativa.it/web/guest/-/veltri-il-processo-amministrativo-l-oralita-e-le-sue-modalita-in-fase-emergenziale-tutto-andra-bene-2022-05-11 (accessed 11 May 2022).

Volpe, C. 2020. Pronti, partenza, via! Il nuovo processo amministrativo da remoto ai nastri di partenza, Giustamm – Rivista di Diritto Amministrativo, XVII. https://www.giustizia-amministrativa.it/web/guest/-/volpe-c-pronti-partenza-via-il-nuovo-processo-amministrativo-da-remoto-ai-nastri-di-partenza (accessed 11 May 2022).

Whiting, M., Kaya, Z.N. 2021. Autocratization, permanent emergency rule and local politics: lessons from the Kurds in Turkey. *Democratization*, 28(4): 821–839. https://doi.org/10.1080/13510347.2021.1871602.

WHO. 2020. Virtual Press Release. https://www.who.int/director-general/speeches/detail/who-director-general-s-opening-remarks-at-the-media-briefing-on-COVID-19---11-march-2020 (accessed 25 July 2021).

Zweifel, P. 2020. The COVID-19 crisis: a public choice view. *Economic Affairs*, 40: 395–405.

7

Praise the Alarm: Spain's Coronavirus Approach

Carolyn Halladay[1], Florina C. Matei[2], and Andres de Castro[3]

[1] National Security Affairs Department, Naval Postgraduate School, Monterey, CA, USA
[2] Center for Homeland Defense and Security, Naval Postgraduate School, Monterey, CA, USA
[3] Universidad Nacional de Educación a Distancia – Enseñanza Online, Madrid, Spain

There was dancing in the streets in Spain at midnight, as 9 May turned into 10 May 2021, and the state of emergency lapsed – in the official argot, a "state of alarm," under which the Spanish government had imposed nationwide Coronavirus restrictions. Actually, the *estado de alarma* that expired on 9 May was, in fact, the second one that Spain's central government effected during the crisis. The first COVID-19 lockdown lasted 94 days. The second one went on for nearly seven months. In both cases, such measures as curfews, internal and international travel limits, and closures of or capacity caps for indoor venues ranging from restaurants to churches had kept Spaniards home. They also emptied Spain's beaches and other tourist sites and dealt a formidable blow to the Spanish economy, while Spain paid a horrible human cost in terms of infections and deaths. Hence, the late-night impromptu jubilations on 9 May, which the English-language Reuters news agency deemed "freedom fiestas,"[1] portending the end of many miseries.

At one level, the two state-of-alarm declarations represent an almost unprecedented development in Spain's democratic history, much like the pandemic that prompted them. Since 1978, the central government had only once before invoked this emergency power – amid an air-traffic controller's strike in December 2010 and January 2011. Such highly centralized authority is unusual in contemporary Spain, with its cherished territorial order as a unified but decentralized regional

The ideas and views expressed in this chapter are the authors' only, and do not represent the official view or policies of the U.S. government, the U.S. Department of the Navy, or the Government of Spain. The authors would like to thank Prof. Dr. Donald Abenheim and Mr. Santiago Arca Henon for their insights and suggestions for improving this chapter.

1 Reuters, "'Freedom' fiestas: Spaniards celebrate end of COVID curfew," 10 May 2021, https://www.reuters.com/world/europe/freedom-fiestas-spaniards-celebrate-end-covid-curfew-2021-05-09/.

state,[2] – in which the 17 Comunidades Autónomas ("autonomous communities" or regions) retain significant self-rule vis-à-vis the central/national government.

Still, Spaniards largely complied with the requirements – especially in the second lockdown, which allowed more regional tailoring of response measures.[3] And there was rather less conspiracy theorizing and anti-mask hysteria in Spain than other European Union member states witnessed.[4] In this aspect, the vaunted "indissoluble unity" of Spain – enshrined in Art. 2 of the Spanish constitution – was on full display during the states of alarm; the Spanish stuck together and weathered the pandemic and the response as a nation.[5]

For one thing, a state of alarm represents the least onerous of the three levels of emergency that the Spanish constitution sets out – alarm, exception, and siege (martial law) – in Art. 116.[6] According to Organic Law 4/1981, the central government may declare an *estado de alarma* for up to 15 days, with extensions possible in increments of the same 15 days, in case of:[7]

- Natural disasters or "public misfortunes," including earthquakes, floods, fires, or major accidents.
- Health crises, including epidemics.
- Disruption of essential public services.
- Shortages of basic necessities.

---

2 Spain's territorial organization defies easy description, as it does not fit the conventional definition of a federal state. For example, the autonomous communities/regions have no role in the upper house of parliament; most of the Senate is elected at the provincial level. And while the autonomous communities have regional superior courts, they do not adjudicate regional law on its own terms; rather, the regional courts are meant to effect the unified judicial power of the Spanish state. See Art. 117, sec. 5 of the Spanish Constitution, https://www.boe.es/legislacion/documentos/ConstitucionINGLES.pdf and the preamble of the Organic Law on the Judiciary of 1 July 1985, *Ley Orgánica 6/1985, de 1 de julio, del Poder Judicial*, https://www.boe.es/eli/es/lo/1985/07/01/6/con; see also Ferran Requejo, "Is Spain a Federal Country?" 50 Shades of Federalism, 2017, http://50shadesoffederalism.com/case-studies/spain-federal-country/. Art. 2 of the constitution specifies the "the indissoluble unity of the Spanish Nation"; while the Comunidades Autónomas are enshrined in Part VIII of the constitution, particularly Art. 137, Art. 138 goes on to reaffirm the "the principle of solidarity proclaimed in [Art.] 2." Many authors deem Spain as a "quasi-federal" model of decentralization; Andrea Bonime-Blanc suggests the cumbersome but highly descriptive term "regionizable unitary state." See Andrea Bonime-Blanc, *Spain's Transition to Democracy: The Politics of Constitution-Making*, 3rd ed., part of the series Studies of the Research Institute on International Change, Colombia University (New York: El Torcal Press, 2013), p. 72.
3 See, for example, Conor Stewart, "How often have you worn a face mask outside your home to protect yourself or others from coronavirus (COVID-19)?" Statista, 12 January 2021, https://www.statista.com/statistics/1114375/wearing-a-face-mask-outside-in-european-countries/.
4 Kristjan Archer and Ilana Ron Levey, "Trust in Government Lacking on COVID-19's Frontlines," Gallup Blog, 20 March 2020, https://news.gallup.com/opinion/gallup/296594/trust-government-lacking-frontlines-covid.aspx. The 77% of Spaniards who went into the Coronavirus crisis with some or a lot of trust in the government – a significant higher rate of confidence than, for example, in the United States at the same time – seemed to set the tone for the fairly unified popular reaction in Spain.
5 Spain, The Spanish Constitution, 31 October 1978, https://www.boe.es/legislacion/documentos/ConstitucionINGLES.pdf.
6 Spain, The Spanish Constitution, 31 October 1978, https://www.boe.es/legislacion/documentos/ConstitucionINGLES.pdf; the Spanish-language version appears in Spain's official register, the Boletín Oficial del Estado (BOE) here: https://www.boe.es/boe/dias/1978/12/29/pdfs/A29313-29424.pdf.
7 Spain, *Ley Orgánica 4/1981 de 1 de junio, de los estados de alarma, excepción y sitio*, 5 June 1981, https://www.boe.es/buscar/act.php?id=BOE-A-1981-12774. Chapter II of the law deals specifically with the state of alarm; the list of appropriate emergency situations appears in Art. 4. The Spanish constitution (Art. 81) requires the passage of such an organic law to operationalize constitutional requirements.

The same law specifies that a state of alarm allows the central government to limit but not suspend certain civil liberties, including the movement of people and vehicles but only "at certain times and places."[8]

For another thing, Spain, much like the Federal Republic of Germany and Italy after World War II, created in its democratic transition – and these decades later still relies on – its firmly Kelsenian constitutional court (Tribunal Constitucional), a "pure" rather than politicized institution[9] separate from ordinary judicial power that remains essential to Spain's political stability.[10] In this sense, the court is meant to tackle such questions as the necessity or appropriateness of various Coronavirus-related restrictions, even while the crisis is ongoing, to ensure that Spain's constitution and the individual and civil liberties it protects remain healthy.

This chapter examines the challenge and the response of Spanish law, government, and society to the unprecedented global pandemic in 2020–2021, especially in the aspect of the state of emergency as government in the extreme. As a nation with a legacy of civil war and dictatorship, as well as an exemplary democratic recovery in the past half century, Spain actively balanced – and rebalanced – the restrictions of certain rights in the name of thwarting COVID-19, while preserving fundamental constitutional freedoms and other virtues of due process of law. This study explores these developments, the relevant sources of constitutional legitimacy, and the deeds of the government(s) in an extraordinary crisis, and it finds that Spain is likely to emerge from the pandemic healthy in all of these respects.

7.1 *Quien aprisa juzgó, despacio se arrepintió*: The Early Days of COVID and the Spanish Response

The first confirmed instance of COVID-19 in Spain, the so-called index case of the disease caused by the SARS-CoV-2 virus, was diagnosed on 31 January 2020 – in a German tourist visiting the Canary Islands. More than a week passed before a second case was reported, this time involving a Briton in Mallorca, who seems to have contracted the virus "after coming into contact with someone in France."[11] Spain's first COVID fatality – on 13 February 2020 – was a 69-year-old man from Valencia who had recently returned from a trip to Nepal; his death was not reported until early March, as the determination came only after his autopsy.[12] Many of the early cases involved visitors to Spain

---

8 Spain, *Ley Orgánica 4/1981 de 1 de junio, de los estados de alarma, excepción y sitio*, 5 June 1981, https://www.boe .es/buscar/act.php?id=BOE-A-1981-12774. See especially Art. 11.

9 Hans Kelsen, *Pure Theory of Law*, trans. Max Knight (Berkeley: University of California Press, 1967).

10 Enrique Guillen Lopez, "Judicial Review in Spain: The Constitutional Court," *Loyola of Los Angeles Law Review*, Vol. 41 (2008), p. 530. https://digitalcommons.lmu.edu/llr/vol41/iss2/3

11 Reuters, "Spanish authorities confirm Briton is country's second coronavirus case," 9 February 2020, https:// www.reuters.com/article/us-china-health-spain-idUSKBN20309T.

12 Reuters, "Spain reports first coronavirus death in Valencia," 3 March 2020, https://www.reuters.com/article/us-health-coronavirus-spain-death/spain-reports-first-coronavirus-death-in-valencia-idUSKBN20Q2TG. The note that the victim had recently been to Nepal appears in Jacobo Alcutén, "Valencia confirma el primer muerto con coronavirus en España: un hombre de 69 años que falleció el 13 de febrero," 20 Minutos, 3 March 2020, https:// www.20minutos.es/noticia/4174137/0/primer-muerto-coronavirus-espana/. (A month later, Reuters also cited the man's foreign travel: Reuters, "TIMELINE-How the coronavirus spread in Spain," 1 April 2020, https://www.reuters .com/article/health-coronavirus-spain-factbox/timeline-how-the-coronavirus-spread-in-spain-idUSL8N2BO4TL.) The 20 Minutos piece also speculates that the Valencia death might be Europe's first COVID-19 fatality, as it predated by a couple of days the well-publicized COVID-related death in France of a Chinese tourist. See, for example, BBC.com, "Coronavirus: First death confirmed in Europe," 15 February 2020, https://www.bbc.com/ news/world-europe-51514837.

or Spaniards who had traveled outside Spain, especially to Italy.[13] On 3 March, the Spanish Health Ministry, in a Twitter post, urged that sports events be cancelled or played without spectators if they were likely to attract crowds from areas that were deemed then to be at high risk for Coronavirus, including most pointedly northern Italy.[14] For a few more days, it seemed that the prediction a month earlier by Dr. Fernando Simón, the head of the Medical Emergencies System in the Spanish Ministry of Health – that "Spain will only have a handful of cases" – would pan out.[15] Indeed, on 5 March, the country reported about 150 cases of Coronavirus, albeit with a troubling cluster in Madrid and another in the Basque Country; there had been just three deaths so far.[16]

By 13 March, however, the virus had appeared in all 50 Spanish provinces, and it was spreading exponentially. Just days after the World Health Organization (WHO) proclaimed Coronavirus as an international pandemic (11 March), Spain was suddenly closing in on 5,000 cases of COVID-19 – and nearly 1,000 deaths.[17] At the national level, a growing number of prominent politicians tested positive for Coronavirus, including Minister of Equality Irene Montero (but only after she had met with H.M. the Queen, who then had to be tested), a senator from the conservative People's Party, several top members of the right-wing Vox party, and former Secretary General of NATO and former High Representative of the Union for Foreign Affairs and Security Policy Javier Solana. With the eye-watering rise in infections, the Spanish legislature, the Cortes Generales, suspended its activity for a period of 15 days. Spain's top football league, La Liga, announced suspended operations for at least two weeks.[18]

Under normal circumstances, responsibility for health law and enforcement falls first to the Comunidades Autónomas. Thus, region by region, Spain's schools were shuttered, initially for two-week intervals. Some regional governments suspended operations, as did some regional court systems, at least for most business, according to Royal Decree 463/2020 of 14 March 2020. The world-renowned Sagrada Familia basilica in Barcelona closed its doors to tourists and construction workers alike on this day. The Basque Country announced a state of emergency, heralding a regional lockdown, on 13 March 2020. (Ultimately, the Basque and Galician elections, scheduled for 5 April, were postponed until July.) Other communities promulgated their own restrictions, particularly concerning the movement of people within and between the regions.

---

13 Nuria Oliver, Xavier Barber, Kirsten Roomp, and Kristof Roomp, "Assessing the Impact of the COVID-19 Pandemic in Spain: Large-Scale, Online, Self-Reported Population Survey," *Journal of Medicine Internet Research*, Sept. 2020, DOI: 10.2196/21319, https://www.ncbi.nlm.nih.gov/pmc/articles/PMC7485997/. See especially the Background section.
14 At the time, there was some confusion as to the nature of the Health Ministry's guidance – and the extent to which bound policy. *El País*, for one, reported the announcement as a recommendation. See Pablo Linde, Pedro Gorospe, Oriol Güell, "Spain recommends sports matches be played behind closed doors over coronavirus fears," *El País*, 3 March 2020, https://english.elpais.com/society/2020-03-03/coronavirus-spreads-to-health-workers-in-spains-basque-country.html. The same day, however, Reuters reported the Ministry's tweet as more directive: Reuters, "Spain reports first coronavirus death in Valencia," 3 March 2020, https://www.reuters.com/article/us-health-coronavirus-spain-death/spain-reports-first-coronavirus-death-in-valencia-idUSKBN20Q2TG.
15 Giles Tremlett, "How did Spain get its coronavirus response so wrong?" The Guardian, 26 March 2020, https://www.theguardian.com/world/2020/mar/26/spain-coronavirus-response-analysis. Economía Digital, 26 March 2020. https://www.economiadigital.es/politica/coronavirus-los-errores-del-gobierno-en-la-gestion-de-la-crisis-sanitaria-the-guardian_20047665_102.html.
16 Reuters, "Spain reports first coronavirus death in Valencia," 3 March 2020, https://www.reuters.com/article/us-health-coronavirus-spain-death/spain-reports-first-coronavirus-death-in-valencia-idUSKBN20Q2TG.
17 See especially Table 1 in Working group for the surveillance and control of COVID-19 in Spain, "The first wave of the COVID-19 pandemic in Spain: characterisation of cases and risk factors for severe outcomes, as at 27 April 2020," *Euro Surveillance*, 2020 Dec 17; 25(50): 2001431, https://www.ncbi.nlm.nih.gov/pmc/articles/PMC7812423/
18 Sam Marsden, "Coronavirus crisis: La Liga suspended indefinitely," ESPN, 23 March 2020, https://www.espn.com/soccer/spanish-primera-division/story/4077753/coronavirus-crisis-la-liga-suspended-indefinitely.

By the end of March 2020, Spain's COVID-19 death toll (7,424 on 30 March alone) exceeded the official number of fatalities in mainland China, where the virus reportedly first broke out.[19] By the end of April 2020, Spain had outstripped even Italy in terms of virus victims. With 24,543 deaths and nearly a quarter million total infections on 30 April, Spain was second only to the United States in absolute numbers.[20] The emergency was well underway.

7.2 *Culpa no tiene, quien hace lo que debe:* The First Wave and the First Lockdown

The first lockdown came up quickly, amid the fast-rising infection rates and the fast-changing guidance from national, European, and world health leaders. On 14 March 2020, the central government enacted Royal Decree 463/2020, which inaugurated the first COVID-related state of alarm in Spain and, thus, the so-called first lockdown. (Art. 116.1 of the Spanish Constitution requires an Organic Law – specifically Organic Law 4/1981 – for the establishment of the legal details, just as the same article of the Constitution requires a decree to effect a state of alarm.[21]) Contemporary critics lambasted Prime Minister Pedro Sánchez for announcing the measures a full day in advance of them taking legal effect,[22] arguably encouraging people to scatter through the country to shelter in place more comfortably, even if they were leaving hot-spot areas to do so.[23] But the decree represented a major interruption of Spanish social and economic life – and a significant deviation from Spain's decentralized political/legal order. Presumably, the socialist leader felt that the extreme situation and the response warranted a bit of fore-warning.

Articles 1 and 2 of RD 463/2020 established the state of alarm and applied it to the entirety of Spain, respectively.[24] Art. 3 fixed a 15-day period for the state of alarm, a limit that appears in Art. 116, sec. 2 of the Spanish constitution. (Thus, although the "first lockdown" in Spain is said to have run from 14 March to 21 June 2020, the restrictions actually entailed six extensions of the state of alarm.[25]) Art. 4 identifies the central government as the competent authority during the state of alarm, and Art. 8 lays the legal foundation for effectively nationalizing the regional security forces. The communities remained responsible for the day-to-day governance of the regions, guided by relevant instructions that the central government issued.

---

19 Nuria Oliver, Xavier Barber, Kirsten Roomp, and Kristof Roomp, "Assessing the Impact of the COVID-19 Pandemic in Spain: Large-Scale, Online, Self-Reported Population Survey," *Journal of Medicine Internet Research*, Sept. 2020, https://doi.org/10.2196/21319, https://www.ncbi.nlm.nih.gov/pmc/articles/PMC7485997/. See especially the Background section.
20 See the study by the Madrid-based University Institute of Studies on Migration, prepared for the European Union Agency for Fundamental Rights (FRA), "Coronavirus pandemic in the EU – Fundamental Rights Implications," 4 May 2020, https://fra.europa.eu/sites/default/files/fra_uploads/es_report_on_coronavirus_pandemic-_may_2020.pdf.
21 The Kelsen's pyramid of Spanish laws, from the top down, goes: Constitution, Organic Law (which regulates fundamental rights), Law, *Real Decreto Ley* (law decrees), *Reales Decretos legislativos* (legal decrees), and *Reglamentos* (with the central government's regulations coming before the regions').
22 Government of Spain, "Government will declare state of emergency due to coronavirus on Saturday," 13 March 2020, https://www.lamoncloa.gob.es/lang/en/presidente/news/Paginas/2020/20200313_emergency.aspx.
23 Giles Tremlett, "How did Spain get its coronavirus response so wrong?" The Guardian, 26 March 2020, https://www.theguardian.com/world/2020/mar/26/spain-coronavirus-response-analysis. Economía Digital, 26 March 2020. https://www.economiadigital.es/politica/coronavirus-los-errores-del-gobierno-en-la-gestion-de-la-crisis-sanitaria-the-guardian_20047665_102.html.
24 All references to RD 463/2020 can be substantiated by the published text in the Official State Gazette (Boletín Oficial del Estado or BOE) at https://www.boe.es/boe/dias/2020/03/14/pdfs/BOE-A-2020-3692.pdf.
25 The extensions may be found at: RD 476/2020, of 27 March 2020; RD 487/2020 of 10 April; RD 492/2020 of 25 April.

The restrictions that RD 463/2020 imposed on the Spanish public came in several broad categories: Limitations on the movements of people (Art. 7); suspension of all in-person education and training (Art. 9); closures in the commercial, cultural, and recreational sectors (Arts. 10) as well as limitations on religious ceremonies and services (Art. 11), a matter of some urgency with the Easter holidays nearing. (Other measures included provisions for capacity restrictions on public transit, rationalizing and fortifying the Spanish national healthcare system, and suspending certain administrative and legal deadlines. The decree also guaranteed the continuation of public utilities and the operation of "critical services.") Still, at least one expert has described the first state of alarm as more of a "lock-in" than a lockdown.[26]

One of the earliest global – and, indeed, viral in the social-media sense, thanks in part to a retweet from Ivanka Trump – impressions of Spain's first COVID lockdown, particularly its "containment" provisions, involved the crooning cops of Mallorca. More than a week into the initial state of alarm, five police officers in Algaida, led by Pedro Adrover (who, in his spare time, is also a body-builder and a singer in the Latin-ska-punk fusion band Ses Bubotes) and accompanied by a guitar and the light bars on their official vehicles, spent three hours on Saturday, 21 March, going street to street in an effort to bring happy children's music – *Un, dos, tres. En Joan Petit quan balla…* (One, two, three. Little Joan dances) – to the entire municipality.[27]

Little else could have alleviated the youngsters' boredom at this point, as they were inescapably stuck at home. Spain's initial state of alarm, according to Art. 7, only allowed individual adults outside of their dwellings for such circumscribed and specific purposes as grocery shopping or going to the pharmacy; seeking medical care; caring for the elderly or disabled; going to the bank; or amid "force majeure or a situation of need." Children fit none of the excepted categories, so minors could not go outdoors in the first six or so weeks of the lockdown unless they had to accompany a parent on the few allowed activities. Eventually, the Ministry of Health published an order that eased these strictures somewhat: As of 26 April 2020, children under the age of 14 were permitted to move around in the fresh air for one hour a day, not more than one kilometer from home, in the company of one parent or guardian. The usual social distancing rules still applied, even to Spaniards who were too young to read them.[28] Cebada and Dominguez make a particular point of the disproportionate burden that the first state of alarm placed on children "without any reasoning enshrined in law."[29] Similarly, the Spanish Ombudsman (*Defensor del Pueblo*) called attention to the potentially harmful effects of keeping children strictly indoors, particularly "when the number of members of the family unit is high and the dwellings are small."[30]

RD 463/2020 was purposefully fuzzy on people going to work, not least because the Spanish economy remained broadly in recovery mode since the Spanish economic crisis from 2008 to 2014, wrought of the European sovereign debt crisis starting in 2008. On the one hand, traveling to or from a place of employment formed one of the specified reasons that an individual adult could

---

26 Miguel Ángel Presno Linera, "Beyond the State of Alarm: COVID-19 in Spain," VerfBlog, 13 May 2020, https://verfassungsblog.de/beyond-the-state-of-alarm-covid-19-in-spain/, https://doi.org/10.17176/20200513-133803-0.
27 Lucía Bohórquez, "Spanish police sing and dance to entertain children in lockdown," *El País*, 25 March 2020, https://english.elpais.com/society/2020-03-25/spanish-police-sing-and-dance-to-entertain-children-in-lockdown.html.
28 Spain, Order on the conditions in which children should be displaced during the health crisis caused by COVID-19 (Orden sobre las condiciones en las que deben desarrollarse los desplazamientos por parte de la población infantil durante la situación de crisis sanitaria ocasionada por el COVID-19), 25 April 2020, https://www.boe.es/buscar/act.php?id=BOE-A-2020-4665.
29 Alicia Cebada Romero and Elvira Dominguez Redondo, "Spain: One Pandemic and Two Versions of the State of Alarm," VerfBlog, 26 February 2021, https://doi.org/10.17176/20210226-154142-0, https://verfassungsblog.de/spain-one-pandemic-and-two-versions-of-the-state-of-alarm/.
30 Defensor del Pueblo, "Actuaciones por la crisis del Covid-19," 17 April 2020, https://www.defensordelpueblo.es/noticias/defensor-crisis-covid/.

be on the streets during the first state of alarm. On the other hand, the decree closed down whole sectors, notably tourism (which alone accounts for 12%–15% of the Spanish economy, depending on who crunches the numbers) and entertainment, mostly to keep people from congregating. Indeed, the annex to RD 463/2020 lists 10 broad subsectors of facilities and businesses, mostly in these sectors, subject to temporary closure amid the larger effort to curtail COVID-19 in Spain.[31] At the same time, the Spanish government was pushing tele-work and a Royal Decree was issued on 23 September 2020 regulating tele-work. By 29 March, however, when Royal Decree-Law 10/2020 ("regulating recoverable paid leave for employees who do not provide essential services, in order to reduce population mobility in the context of the fight against COVID-19") mandated that most of the working public should remain at home, albeit with some financial relief, the line between "essential" and "non-essential" workers and sectors has been pretty clearly drawn.[32]

The Spanish central government understood the dilemma facing the country. Without question, "containment," in the words of the law enacting the state of alarm, would save lives and preserve capacity in hospitals so that the sickest Spaniards could count on timely treatment. (A couple of days in April 2020 saw some 900 deaths in a single 24-hour period, a gruesome record in Spain and Europe at the time.[33]) On the other hand, closing down whole sectors threatened Spain's economic recovery, particularly in the realm of small business.[34] Even as the first lockdown was extended, the government passed five laws by 30 April that sought to mitigate the economic damage:

- Royal Decree-Law 8/2020, 17 March on the economic impact of COVID-19.
- Royal Decree-Law 9/2020, of 27 March, which adopts complementary measures, in the field of employment, to mitigate the effects of COVID-19.
- Royal Decree-Law10/2020 of 29 March, regulating recoverable paid leave for employees who do not provide essential services, in order to reduce population mobility in the context of the fight against COVID-19.
- Royal Decree-Law 13/2020 of 7 April, adopting certain urgent measures in the field of agricultural employment.
- Royal Decree-Law 15/2020 of 21 April on urgent complementary measures to support the economy and employment.

Moreover, at the end of June, the Spanish social security agency effected its first and long-awaited payment of the "minimum vital income" (*Ingreso Mínimo Vital*) of between €462 and €1015 to households bereft of earnings in this period. (The exact amount depended on how many people formed the family unit.[35]) Nonetheless, the economic damage was considerable: Spain posted its

---

31 The annex appears in the text of the decree in the BOE. The categorization of the enterprises subject to closure appears in an employment alert published by the law firm of Baker McKenzie, "Main Aspects of Royal Decree 463/2020, dated 14 March, Declaiming a State of Emergency in Spain to Manage the Health Crisis Caused by COVID-19," March 2020, https://www.lexology.com/library/detail.aspx?g=4be6a7f7-665e-40df-ba25-9e30291f6277.
32 Spain, Real Decreto-ley 10/2020, "… por el que se regula un permiso retribuido recuperable para las personas trabajadoras por cuenta ajena que no presten servicios esenciales, con el fin de reducir la movilidad de la población en el contexto de la lucha contra el COVID-19," 29 March 2020, https://www.boe.es/buscar/act.php?id=BOE-A-2020-4166.
33 "Spain records over 900 coronavirus deaths for second day," The Local, 3 April 2020, https://www.thelocal.es/20200403/spain-records-over-900-coronavirus-deaths-for-second-day/. El País, "Más de 900 muertos por segundo día consecutivo," 3 April 2020. https://elpais.com/sociedad/2020/04/03/actualidad/1585928862_406154.html.
34 Nuria Oliver, Xavier Barber, Kirsten Roomp, and Kristof Roomp, "Assessing the Impact of the COVID-19 Pandemic in Spain: Large-Scale, Online, Self-Reported Population Survey," *Journal of Medicine Internet Research*, Sept. 2020, https://doi.org/10.2196/21319, https://www.ncbi.nlm.nih.gov/pmc/articles/PMC7485997/. See, for example, the Results section.
35 Ingreso Mínimo Vital https://www.citizensadvice.org.es/faq/ingreso-minimo-minimum-vital-income-update/.

biggest economic contraction since the Civil War (1936–1939) – some 11% overall for 2020 and nearly 18% in the second quarter of the year, that is, during the 94-day first lockdown.[36]

In all, the first state of alarm was a hard lockdown, more restrictive than many operating elsewhere in Europe. Still, even as the Spanish government extended the state of alarm in 15-day increments until mid-June 2020 and successively tightened restrictions on mobility and social interactions, the Spanish public proclaimed its abiding support for the response measures – and, to a significant extent, complied with the orders.[37] Spanish and global media took note of the "balcony police" and "window cops," citizens who hurled insults or even eggs at presumptive scofflaws who were seen in the streets in defiance of the COVID rules.[38]

Even with the overwhelming (and sometimes ovate) force of popular approval for the Spanish government's measures, citizens and legal experts alike had – and voiced – concerns about the first lock-down. For example, during the early weeks of the initial lockdown, the central government conducted its press conferences with journalists participating remotely – and with questions submitted in advance to Miguel Ángel Oliver, the Deputy Minister for Communication. Some alleged that the government "filtered" the inquiries.[39] A manifesto that became a hashtag – "the freedom to ask"/ *#laLibertaddePreguntar* – circulated in early April 2020; amid such pressure and an evolving understanding of how Coronavirus is (and is not) communicated, the government returned to formats that allowed journalists to pose their questions without intermediaries.[40]

Around the same time, on 3 April 2020, the Spanish Ombudsman, Francisco Fernández Marugán, claimed already to have fielded 1,000 complaints about COVID-19 measures in the scant three weeks since the state of alarm took effect.[41] In this period, for example, law enforcement personnel had arrested more than 2,800 people for flouting various lockdown provisions and issued

---

36 Antonio Maqueda, "Spain's economy shrank 11% in 2020, in biggest drop since Civil War," *El País*, 29 January 2021, https://english.elpais.com/economy_and_business/2021-01-29/spains-economy-shrank-11-in-2020-in-biggest-drop-since-civil-war.html.

37 Nuria Oliver, Xavier Barber, Kirsten Roomp, and Kristof Roomp, "Assessing the Impact of the COVID-19 Pandemic in Spain: Large-Scale, Online, Self-Reported Population Survey," *Journal of Medicine Internet Research*, Sept. 2020, https://doi.org/10.2196/21319, https://www.ncbi.nlm.nih.gov/pmc/articles/PMC7485997/.

38 Noor Mathani, "Los 'policías de balcón' que insultan a discapacitados y sanitarios por estar en la calle," El País, 26 March 2020, https://elpais.com/sociedad/2020-03-26/los-policias-de-balcon-que-insultan-a-discapacitados-y-sanitarios-por-estar-en-la-calle.html; Marta Borraz, "Justicieros de balcón en tiempos de cuarentena: 'Me han insultado y deseado la muerte por salir con mi hijo con autism'," El Diario, 24 March 2020, https://www.eldiario.es/sociedad/justicieros-cuarentena-deseado-ventanas-autista_1_1006614.html; Giles Tremlett, "How a small Spanish town became one of Europe's worst Covid-19 hotspots," The Guardian, 4 June 2020, https://www.theguardian.com/world/2020/jun/04/spain-la-rioja-small-town-one-of-europes-worst-covid-19-hotspots.

39 "Cientos de periodistas rechazan el control de las preguntas en las ruedas de prensa en La Moncloa," ABC España, 6 April 2020, https://www.abc.es/espana/abci-medio-centenar-periodistas-rechazan-control-preguntas-ruedas-prensa-moncloa-202003312101_noticia.html. See also Dolores Utrilla, Manuel Antonio García-Muñoz, and Teresa Pareja Sánchez, "Spain: Legal Response to Covid-19," *Oxford Constitutional Law*, April 2021, https://doi.org/10.1093/law-occ19/e10.013.1, https://oxcon.ouplaw.com/view/10.1093/law-occ19/law-occ19-e10#law-occ19-e10-note-21.

40 Council of Europe, "Addendum to the Report: Press freedom suffers in Council of Europe member states under COVID-19," 29 April 2020, https://www.coe.int/en/web/media-freedom/covid-19-addendum. Among the Chapter 1 constitutional articulations of "fundamental rights and public freedoms," Art. 20 of the Spanish constitution protects the freedom of expression in all forms and modalities (sec. 1[a]) and expressly forbids any prior restraint (sec. 2). Moreover, sec. 3 of the same article guarantees access "to truthful information" – inclusive of the journalists and other critics who pressed their "freedom to ask" in April 2020. There are no exceptions to this roomy liberty in the Spain, except those cases that are subject to a court order or measures that protect "youth and childhood."

41 Defensor del Pueblo, "Más de un millar de quejas por el Covid-19," 3 April 2020, https://www.defensordelpueblo.es/noticias/mas-millar-quejas-covid-19/.

more than 330,000 sanctions,[42] which prompted the Ombudsman to request any information on disciplinary proceedings that might indicate police misconduct in this regard.[43] (Fines for breaking curfew or other infractions could run as high as €600,000, a mild fortune in a country where the average annual income among people still employed during the pandemic was less than €50,000.[44]) On 17 April,[45] the Ombudsman – who is, according to the official website, "the High Commissioner of Parliament responsible for defending citizens' fundamental rights and civil liberties by monitoring the activity of the Administration and public authorities"[46] – reported that he had, two weeks earlier, presented three recommendations to the Deputy Minister of Internal Affairs in connection with the state of alarm:[47]

- Improve official communications and outreach "so that citizens know the limits and restrictions of their fundamental rights that have been affected by the state of alarm."
- Instruct the police and the gendarmerie (Guardia Civil) about the limits of enforcement, particularly sanctions, of citizen activities that Art. 7 of RD 463/2020 expressly permits.
- Urge provincial and regional entities not to impose stricter limits than RD 463/2020 already entails in the interest of consistent and equitable treatment of citizens across Spain.

In mid-June 2020, Spain's constitutional court heard a case against the state of alarm brought by 52 parliamentarians.[48] On 11 June, one of the members of the Constitutional Court, Pedro González-Trevijano proposed that the Court nullify the state of alarm as unconstitutional; he argued that given the circumstances in 2020, the government should have, instead opted for a declaration of a state of exception or stage of siege.[49] No decision has been forthcoming as of July 2021. If the Constitutional Court ultimately rules the state of alarm to be unconstitutional, then citizens who were fined for violating its provisions will have the right to be refunded. And all the sanctions will be left without effect.

---

42 "Medio millón de sanciones y detenciones por violar el confinamiento en un mes," La Vanguardia, 12 April 2020, https://www.lavanguardia.com/vida/20200412/48447581790/sanciones-detenciones-policia-confinamiento-violacion-incumplimiento-policia-nacional-guardia-civil-espana-coronavirus.html.

43 Defensor del Pueblo, "Actuaciones por la crisis del Covid-19," 17 April 2020, https://www.defensordelpueblo.es/noticias/defensor-crisis-covid/.

44 Alicia Cebada Romero and Elvira Dominguez Redondo, "Spain: One Pandemic and Two Versions of the State of Alarm," VerfBlog, 26 February 2021, https://doi.org/10.17176/20210226-154142-0, https://verfassungsblog.de/spain-one-pandemic-and-two-versions-of-the-state-of-alarm/. See also Table 1 in Dolores Utrilla, Manuel Antonio García-Muñoz, and Teresa Pareja Sánchez, "Spain: Legal Response to Covid-19," *Oxford Constitutional Law*, April 2021, https://doi.org/10.1093/law-occ19/e10.013.1, https://oxcon.ouplaw.com/view/10.1093/law-occ19/law-occ19-e10#law-occ19-e10-note-21.

45 Defensor del Pueblo, "Actuaciones por la crisis del Covid-19," 17 April 2020, https://www.defensordelpueblo.es/noticias/defensor-crisis-covid/.

46 Defensor del Pueblo, "What is the Defensor del Pueblo?" https://www.defensordelpueblo.es/en/who-we-are/what-is-the-defensor/.

47 Defensor del Pueblo, "Restricciones durante el estado de alarma," https://www.defensordelpueblo.es/resoluciones/restricciones-durante-el-estado-de-alarma/.

48 Like many populist parties in Europe, Vox had initially supported the broad project of a state of alarm and a lockdown – particularly where closing the borders was concerned. Its late-June machinations – coming just days before the first state of alarm ended – seemed largely demonstrative, rather than substantial. See "El Tribunal Constitucional estudiará el recurso de Vox contra el estado de alarma," europapress, https://www.europapress.es/nacional/noticia-cvirus-tribunal-constitucional-admite-tramite-recurso-vox-contra-estado-alarma-20200506130005.html and Graham Keeley, "Spain's Right Wing Party Supporters Rebel Against Socialist Government's COVID Restrictions," Voice of America, 17 June 2020, https://www.voanews.com/europe/spains-right-wing-party-supporters-rebel-against-socialist-governments-covid-restrictions.

49 "El magistrado ponente del recurso de Vox propone al Constitucional declarar ilegal el primer estado de alarma," La Voz de Galicia, 20 June 2021, https://www.lavozdegalicia.es/noticia/sociedad/2021/06/10/magistrado-ponente-recurso-vox-propone-constitucional-declarar-ilegal-primer-estado-alarma/00031623347937264874782.htm.

By this time, however, the first lockdown had ended, and all of Spain looked forward to a relatively normal summer of recovery, reconstruction, and recreation – international, domestic, and regional.

7.3 *Cada uno quiere justiciar, mas no por su casa:* The Second Wave and the Second Lockdown

Sensitive to the unusual centralization of power and authority under the state of alarm, even before the first lockdown ended, the central government pronounced a "de-escalation plan" by which leaders meant to wind down the first COVID-related state of alarm. To this end, the government published five "general dispositions" on Sunday, 3 May 2020, that refined the state of alarm.[50] The titles and, in fact, the details are fairly technical; one of the five orders establishes a mask mandate on public transportation. Another focuses on "co-governance" with the autonomous communities and cities of Ceuta and Melilla. But taken together and in context, these five orders marked real, legal, and practical progress toward an easing of COVID-19 restrictions and a shift of control and authority back to the regions.

The plan, which resulted from extensive consultations with the regional authorities, actually had been in the works for some weeks before these measures took effect. Indeed, on 28 April 2020, the central government released the official De-Escalation Plan, which set out a gradual and systematic approach to life after the state of alarm.[51] Specifically, the plan proposed the following phases:

- Phase 0: Preparation – entailing modest reopenings, more or less on the individual level, for example: restaurants offering take-away-only service or personal training sessions for national-level athletes. The key function of the government at this stage would be to prepare public spaces with signage and other protection measures.
- Phase 1: Initial – allowing certain facilities (notably hotels and churches, as well as agricultural fields) to reopen with a capacity cap of 30%.
- Phase 2: Intermediate – permitting more businesses to open at 30% capacity and foreseeing a return to in-person education in September 2020.
- Phase 3: Advanced – upping the capacity limits to 50% in many venues, provided masking and social distancing requirements can be maintained. This phase also foresaw much more personal mobility, even for recreational purposes.
- New Normality: – ending the formal restrictions but retaining "epidemiological surveillance" and urging a certain amount of "self-protection of citizens."

Of signal importance in the de-escalation: The provinces and regions saw some flexibility restored in the implementation of these phases. So, for example, the new rules imposed a curfew (*toque de queda*) from 2,300 to 0600. Depending on local circumstances, however, the regions could add an hour to the curfew period, or, under very special conditions, dispense with it altogether.[52] As Prime Minister Pedro Sánchez noted on 28 April 2020, "The process will not be uniform; it will be asymmetric and at different speeds, but coordinated, whereby it is governed by the same rules."[53] In

---

50 Boletín Oficial del Estado: domingo 3 de mayo de 2020, Núm. 123, "I. Disposiciones generals," 3 May 2020, https://www.boe.es/boe/dias/2020/05/03/.
51 Spain, "Plan de desescalada," 28 April 2020, https://www.lamoncloa.gob.es/consejodeministros/Paginas/enlaces/280420-enlace-desescalada.aspx.
52 See, for example, the map and explanation of the different curfews at "Toque de queda en España por comunidades," ABC, 2 March 2021, https://www.abc.es/sociedad/abci-toque-queda-hora-empieza-termina-comunidad-nsv-202103021613_noticia.html.
53 Government of Spain, "Government approves de-escalation plan which will gradually be implemented until end of June," 28 April 2020, https://www.lamoncloa.gob.es/lang/en/gobierno/councilministers/Paginas/2020/20200428council.aspx.

the Spanish context, nonuniformity and asymmetry among the regions are desirable characteristics of national-level policy; the decentralization is healthy again.[54]

With the new normality breaking out all over, the summer of 2020 shaped up reasonably well. Much of Spain's tourism infrastructure was open for some semblance of business amid capacity restrictions and distancing and masking requirements. The land border with France was reopened, and international air travel resumed. The numbers of Coronavirus infections started rising almost as soon as Spain's first lockdown ended, but initially, the summer's COVID patients mostly reported mild symptoms, if any; only about 3% of patients required hospitalization at all, and only 0.5% needed intensive care. But with the advent of autumn and cooler temperatures – and amid a steady rumble of grousing about the "social irresponsibility" of young people, who continued to congregate in "pubs, discos, and private parties"[55] – a second wave began to crest in Spain. By 7 September 2020, Spain could count more than 500,000 COVID-19 cases since the pandemic began – and 29,500 deaths.[56]

In late September 2020, the regional government of Madrid – the locus of 25%–30% of the new Coronavirus cases in the country – imposed mobility restrictions on several areas of the city where the infection rate had exceeded 1,000 per 100,000 people. As it happened, these areas were among Madrid's poorer postal codes, which reignited debate about inequality in the pandemic response.[57] But Madrid's Regional President Isabel Díaz Ayuso of the center-right People's Party (Partido Popular) framed the move as a tailored measure meant to avoid a total lockdown of the Spanish capital and the economic damage that surely would follow.[58] The opposition to Ayuso's government tried to claim that the partial closure of certain neighborhoods was targeting some of the poorest areas in Madrid.[59] The central government found these measures insufficient and sought, through an order from the national Ministry of Health,[60] to effect stricter limits across the city, notably a "perimetral confinement,"[61] curtailing nonessential travel outside or across the affected areas – in this case, the

---

54 As a run-up to de-escalation, on 8 June, the several regions became competent to lessen COVID-related strictures, even before the state of alarm ended. "Coronavirus: España vuelve a reportar una jornada sin muertos," DW, 8 June 2020, https://www.dw.com/es/coronavirus-espa%C3%B1a-vuelve-a-reportar-una-jornada-sin-muertos/a-53733155.

55 The quoted phrases appear in: Maria Teresa Murillo-Llorente and Marcelino Perez-Bermejo, "COVID-19: Social Irresponsibility of Teenagers Towards the Second Wave in Spain," *Journal of Epidemiology*, 2020; 30(10): 483. Published online 5 October 2020. Prepublished online 8 August 2020. https://doi.org/10.2188/jea.JE20200360, https://www.ncbi.nlm.nih.gov/pmc/articles/PMC7492708/. The allegations echoed in many sources at the time, however – and not just in Spain. Certainly, the second wave saw much higher infection rates among young Spaniards in its early phases.

56 Spanish Government, "Estado de situación del COVID-19," 7 September 2020, https://www.lamoncloa.gob.es/serviciosdeprensa/notasprensa/sanidad14/Paginas/2020/07092020_datoscovid19.aspx.

57 Silvio Castellanos and Clara-Laeila Laudette, "Madrid region orders partial lockdown in poorer areas hit by COVID-19," Reuters, 18 September 2020, https://www.reuters.com/article/us-health-coronavirus-spain-madrid/madrid-region-orders-partial-lockdown-in-poorer-areas-hit-by-covid-19-idUSKBN26927C.

58 Silvio Castellanos and Clara-Laeila Laudette, "Madrid region orders partial lockdown in poorer areas hit by COVID-19," Reuters, 18 September 2020, https://www.reuters.com/article/us-health-coronavirus-spain-madrid/madrid-region-orders-partial-lockdown-in-poorer-areas-hit-by-covid-19-idUSKBN26927C.

59 "Vecinos de Madrid obligados a recluirse dicen que se estigmatiza a los barrios humildes," La Vanguardia, 19 September 2020. https://www.lavanguardia.com/vida/20200919/483560548027/madrid-confinamiento-barrios-humildes-estigmatizacion.html.

60 Government of the Autonomous Community of Madrid, "Aplicamos la Orden del ministro de Sanidad y mantenemos algunas zonas básicas de salud," 2 October 2020, https://www.comunidad.madrid/noticias/2020/10/02/aplicamos-orden-ministro-sanidad-mantenemos-algunas-zonas-basicas-salud.

61 This turn of phrase – "perimetral confinement" – appears in many sources translated, probably by computer, from Spanish to English. See, for example, "The Madrid cities under the state of alarm: What you can and can't do," *El Pais*, 9 October 2020, https://english.elpais.com/spanish_news/2020-10-09/the-madrid-cities-under-the-state-of-alarm-what-you-can-and-cant-do.html. In its essence, it means making a bubble out of an area with a particularly high infection rate, limiting traffic in and out in an effort to contain the spread of the disease.

capital city and its environs, with a combined population of some 4.5 million. Ultimately, the matter went to the Tribunal Superior de Justicia de Madrid, and the regional high court quashed the order on 8 October.[62] The next day, the central government declared a state of alarm for Madrid, reviving the restrictions, by way of Royal Decree 900/2020.[63] Only the constitutional court can review or overturn such a law.

To be sure, the state of alarm for Madrid outlined a rather less burdensome lockdown than Spain had experienced in the spring. Its main provisions included a ban on leaving or entering Madrid for nonessential travel (which category expressly excluded work, business, or school trips); capacity limits of 50% in hotels, restaurants, and other business; required closing times of 2200 for most business or 2300 for hospitality venues; a 30% occupancy cap for churches; and a ban on gatherings of more than six people in public or private.[64] At the same time, however, the decree that activated the state of alarm also sent 7,000 additional law enforcement personnel to Madrid to enforce the provisions, though even this show of force might not have proven terribly effective with Spain's national day holiday pending on 12 October – and with it the customary exodus of *Madrileños* from the city for the long weekend. More to the constitutional point, the entire episode struck many observers as a potential threat to Spain's cherished regional autonomy.

To some extent, the muddle about jurisdiction and authority in Madrid amid the second wave of infection prompted the second COVID state of alarm in Spain – a clear response in unclear times.[65] In addition, though, more than a million Spaniards had been infected with Coronavirus by the end of October 2020, the highest rate in western Europe. So amid some protest and somewhat more concern, the central government announced Royal Decree 926/2020, which imposed the state of alarm across all of Spain on 25 October 2020.[66] The requirements largely mirrored the strictures of the Madrid state of alarm – curfews, restrictions on nonessential travel, etc. But this decree also goes on at some length about the roles and competencies of the regions – and not just to extend the central government's authority.[67] Even the prefatory material acknowledges the divergent COVID

---

62 The actual situation with the order in Madrid was somewhat more complicated than most contemporary media reports had it. Technically, the Madrid high court overturned the health order that the regional government issued to effect the central government's requirements; the court had jurisdiction especially because of the fundamental civil rights involved in a curfew or travel ban. (See Art. 74 of the Organic Law on the Judiciary, *Ley Orgánica 6/1985, de 1 de julio, del Poder Judicial*, 1 July 1985, https://www.boe.es/eli/es/lo/1985/07/01/6/con.) Thus, "the limiting … of fundamental rights established by Order 1273/2020, of 1 October, of the [Madrid] Ministry of Health, merely in execution of the communicated [central government] Order of September 30, 2020, constitutes an interference in the fundamental rights of citizens without legal authorization …" Comunicación Poder Judicial, "El TSJ de Madrid deniega la ratificación de las 'medidas Covid' al afectar la Orden comunicada del ministro de Sanidad derechos fundamentals," 8 October 2020, https://www.poderjudicial.es/cgpj/es/Poder-Judicial/Noticias-Judiciales/El-TSJ-de-Madrid-deniega-la-ratificacion-de-las--medidas-Covid--al-afectar-la-Orden-comunicada-del-ministro-de-Sanidad-derechos-fundamentales. Still, the effect of this decision was to curtail the restrictions for infringing on fundamental civil liberties, which measures require a formal, declared state of alarm.

63 Spain, *Real Decreto 900/2020, de 9 de octubre, por el que se declara el estado de alarma para responder ante situaciones de especial riesgo por transmisión no controlada de infecciones causadas por el SARS-CoV-2*, 9 October 2020, https://www.boe.es/boe/dias/2020/10/09/pdfs/BOE-A-2020-12109.pdf.

64 Government of Spain, "El Consejo de Ministros decreta el estado de alarma para controlar la pandemia en los territorios más afectados," 9 October 2020, https://www.lamoncloa.gob.es/consejodeministros/resumenes/Paginas/2020/091020-cministros_extra.aspx.

65 Alicia Cebada Romero and Elvira Dominguez Redondo, "Spain: One Pandemic and Two Versions of the State of Alarm," VerfBlog, 26 February 2021, https://doi.org/10.17176/20210226-154142-0, https://verfassungsblog.de/spain-one-pandemic-and-two-versions-of-the-state-of-alarm/.

66 Government of Spain, *Real Decreto 926/2020, de 25 de octubre, por el que se declara el estado de alarma para contener la propagación de infecciones causadas por el SARS-CoV-2*, 25 October 2020, https://www.boe.es/buscar/act.php?id=BOE-A-2020-12898.

67 Government of Spain, *Real Decreto 926/2020, de 25 de octubre, por el que se declara el estado de alarma para contener la propagación de infecciones causadas por el SARS-CoV-2*, 25 October 2020, https://www.boe.es/buscar/act.php?id=BOE-A-2020-12898; see especially Ch. III.

situations in some communities, noting, for example, the significantly lower infection rate on the (relatively isolated) Canary Islands.[68] And, in the end, it gives a great deal of latitude to the regions as far as which measures to enact and to which extent.[69] Specifically, it allows the regions to exceed national-level measures within certain tolerances without seeking judicial approval. For example, Castilla y León established a stricter curfew, starting from 2200 as opposed to 2300 hours; to be sure, the original plan from the regional government had sought to start the curfew at 2000 was refused by the judiciary.[70]

Thus, the second COVID state of alarm in Spain spoke to several of the concerns that the first state of alarm had raised, even if it failed to address the length and breadth and depth of the issues in detail: proportionality, regional autonomy, and local experience. Perhaps the most striking thing about the second state of alarm was the language that suggested – and later justified – that it could be extended for up to six months, rather than every 15 days, with a "pre-approval" from the legislature.[71] Specifically, the 9 November 2020 extension of the second state of alarm did, in fact, fix its expiry for half a year out, namely 9 May 2021.[72] Cebada and Dominquez suggest that this accommodation owes something to the awkwardness of the first Coronavirus state of alarm, whereby the fortnightly parliamentary oversight became "a scrutiny that progressively undermined a minority government within a climate of enormous tension between political parties and within society at large."[73] The six-month clock on the extension of the second state of alarm thus bought the central government some peace and quiet to consider the situation at hand. But what did it do for/to the Spanish democracy, particularly its unified but decentralized, regional order?

7.4 *Con necesidad, no hay ley?* States of Emergency in Spain and Beyond

Spain – as in: Spanish law and society – maintains a peculiar or perhaps peculiarly Spanish relationship to emergency laws, which, broadly speaking, prove troublesome in other democracies, particularly those with totalitarian or authoritarian legacies within a human memory. (On the one hand, Germany resists a declaration of emergency as a matter of democratic principle; on the other hand, Italy almost instantly made its COVID response a matter of national emergency.) To no small extent, this circumstance owes to Spanish confidence in the legal system – meaning

---

68 Government of Spain, *Real Decreto 926/2020, de 25 de octubre, por el que se declara el estado de alarma para contener la propagación de infecciones causadas por el SARS-CoV-2,* 25 October 2020, https://www.boe.es/buscar/act .php?id=BOE-A-2020-12898; see Ch. II.

69 Dolores Utrilla, Manuel Antonio García-Muñoz, and Teresa Pareja Sánchez, "Spain: Legal Response to Covid-19," *Oxford Constitutional Law,* April 2021, https://doi.org/10.1093/law-occ19/e10.013.1, https://oxcon .ouplaw.com/view/10.1093/law-occ19/law-occ19-e10#law-occ19-e10-note-21, para 57.

70 "El Supremo suspende el toque de queda a las 20:00 de Castilla y León, que vuelve a las 22:00," Radio Televisión Española, 16 February 2021, https://www.rtve.es/alacarta/audios/24-horas/toque-queda-castilla-leon-vuelve-2200/ 5794529/.

71 Royal Decree 926/2020, 25 October 2020. https://www.boe.es/boe/dias/2020/10/25/pdfs/BOE-A-2020-12898 .pdf.

72 Government of Spain, *Real Decreto 926/2020, de 25 de octubre, por el que se declara el estado de alarma para contener la propagación de infecciones causadas por el SARS-CoV-2,* 25 October 2020, https://www.boe.es/buscar/act .php?id=BOE-A-2020-12898 as modified by Royal Decree 956/2020 (Government of Spain, *Real Decreto 956/2020, de 3 de noviembre, por el que se prorroga el estado de alarma declarado por el Real Decreto 926/2020, de 25 de octubre, por el que se declara el estado de alarma para contener la propagación de infecciones causadas por el SARS-CoV-2,* 9 November 2020, https://www.boe.es/eli/es/rd/2020/11/03/956/con).

73 Alicia Cebada Romero and Elvira Dominguez Redondo, "Spain: One Pandemic and Two Versions of the State of Alarm," VerfBlog, 26 February 2021, https://doi.org/10.17176/20210226-154142-0, https://verfassungsblog.de/ spain-one-pandemic-and-two-versions-of-the-state-of-alarm/.

the Kelsen-inflected system of laws that sustain and affirm Spain's democracy. In other words, Spaniards believed (and believe) that the legal system would work out an end to the states of alarm, preserving order and stability with minimal damage to their civil liberties. This faith in juridical institutions is not a self-evident outgrowth of Spain's modern history, however, particularly in the twentieth century.

In the last 300 years – that is, for as long as modern Europeans have drafted such charters – Spain has had seven constitutions[74] plus an *Estatuto Real,* which served the same purpose even if it was not formally a constitution, beginning with the influential though interrupted Constitution of Cádiz (1812).[75] *La Pepa*, as this first document is known more popularly,[76] marked a high point of nineteenth-century liberalism (in the sense of "liberty") and stands out as one of the three "functional democratic constitutions" in Spanish history.[77] The second democratic Spanish constitution, according to Christiansen, was the short-lived Constitution of 1931, a modernizing, secularizing, and ultimately highly controversial, if not divisive, document that arguably helped stoke the passions and politics that fed Spain's brutal Civil War (1936–1939).[78] Indeed, Christiansen characterizes this charter as the "no-compromise, imposition-by-the-victors model."[79] In fact, in 1935, constitutional reform or revision occupied leaders on the left (for example, then-Prime Minister Alejandro Lerroux, of the Partido Radical, who set up a parliamentary commission to review 41 articles to advance the party's preferences on religion, regionalism, and property) and on the right (when conservative War Minister José María Gil-Robles y Quiñones de León announced his desire for a "complete revision") all the way up to the collapse of the republic.[80]

Even the most liberal-minded lawmakers of the time retained the repressive emergency powers from the old regime in the republic period, where political violence was already prevalent.[81] From the very beginning, the new government declared itself to be a "regime of full powers" (*régimen de plenos poderes*); it promulgated the Defense of the Republic Law on 21 October 1931, which predated the constitution by eight days.[82] (The law's express intention to suspend civil liberties in times of turmoil actually contradicted the rights guaranteed in the new charter, but the law was simply "tacked onto" the constitution, as Payne writes, contradictions and all.[83]) As it happened,

74 Spanish Parliament, 11 June 2021, https://www.congreso.es/cem/constesp1812-1978.
75 Spain, CONSTITUCIÓN DE CÁDIZ [Constitution of Cádiz], 19 March 1812, http://www.cervantesvirtual.com/servlet/SirveObras/c1812/12159396448091522976624/index.htm.
76 The nickname owes to the diminutive form of Joseph (Jose), or in this case St. Joseph; the Cortes of Cádiz ratified the constitution on San Jose's saint's day, 19 March 1812.
77 Eric C. Christiansen, "Forty Years from Fascism: Democratic Constitutionalism and the Spanish Model of National Transformation," *Oregon Review of International Law*, Vol. 20 (2018), https://digitalcommons.law.ggu.edu/cgi/viewcontent.cgi?article=1836&context=pubs, p. 7.
78 The drafters and backers of the 1931 Constitution were particularly resolute in their anti-clericalism and, in some cases, anti-Catholicism, which issue rapidly became politicized in the fissile social circumstances of this period in Spain. The class conflict, which also manifested in the progressive provisions of the 1931 Constitution, proved to be just as polarizing and just as prevalent in the violence that ensued. See, for example, Julián Casanova and Carlos Gil Andrés, *Twentieth Century Spain: A History*, trans. Martin Douch, (Cambridge: Cambridge University Press, 2014), pp. 127–140. See also Paul Preston, *The Spanish Civil War: Reaction, Revolution, and Revenge* (New York: WW. Norton & Co., 2006), pp. 87–88.
79 Eric C. Christiansen, "Forty Years from Fascism: Democratic Constitutionalism and the Spanish Model of National Transformation," *Oregon Review of International Law*, Vol. 20 (2018), p. 30, https://digitalcommons.law.ggu.edu/cgi/viewcontent.cgi?article=1836&context=pubs.
80 Julián Casanova and Carlos Gil Andrés, *Twentieth Century Spain: A History*, trans. Martin Douch, (Cambridge: Cambridge University Press, 2014), pp. 142–143.
81 Stanley G. Payne, "Political Violence During the Spanish Second Republic," *Journal of Contemporary History*, Vol. 25, No. 2/3 (May–June, 1990), pp. 269–288, esp. p. 272.
82 Spanish Constitution 1931. https://www.congreso.es/cem/const1931.
83 Stanley G. Payne, "Political Violence During the Spanish Second Republic," *Journal of Contemporary History*, Vol. 25, No. 2/3 (May–June, 1990), p. 273.

the Civil Guard and other security forces authored much of the violence upon orders from the government – for example, the "Revolución de Asturias" in 1934 when Lerroux was the President of the Council of Ministers.[84] Amid increasingly contentious election results, armed rebellions, and coup threats, leaders often called for the declaration of a state of emergency even as late as the *coup d'etat* that initiated the Civil War in the summer of 1936.

The dictatorship of Francisco Franco, which followed the Civil War, abolished the 1931 Constitution very shortly after the Falange Española seized power in Spain. Instead, the Franco regime proceeded on the basis of seven "Fundamental Laws of the Kingdom" (*Leyes Fundamentales del Reino*), articulated between 1936 and 1967 to govern the basic operations of Spain while concentrating all power in the head of state, namely Franco himself.[85] One of these "fundamental laws" was the so-called *Fuero de los Españoles*,[86] passed in 1945, ostensibly to establish a semblance of civil rights protection in Franco's dictatorship, but mostly created as "window dressing" to assuage the western allies that Francoism somehow encompassed their norms and values.[87] The name of the law itself provides important insights into Franco's quasi-constitutional aspirations. For one thing, the word *fuero* in this context connotes a feudal privilege, something granted to a loyal or at least obedient subject by a liege or ruler, rather than an inalienable right inherent in all people. In this regard, it based such rights on "the Spanish" – *los españoles* – pointedly eliding the regions in favor of the principles of Falange Española that prioritized the national interests, broadly understood.

Moreover, Art. 33 of the law states: "The exercise of the rights recognized in this *fuero* may not undermine the spiritual, national, and social unity of Spain."[88] Such a violation of Spanish unity lies largely in the eye of the beholder – in this case, the *Generalísimo* himself. As Christiansen notes, "The nature of authoritarian governance is the substitution of the wishes of a single ruler for actual rule of law."[89] Art. 33 of the *Fuero de los Españoles* also fairly drips with the implied "or else." A lone person flouting Spanish unity, in accordance with the law, would not have the right to free speech or assembly – or personal liberty. Given these circumstances, individuals or groups of people would face the kinds of repression that, in other circumstances, might be categorized as martial law, with no judicial recourse. In other words, the ill-defined and undeclared but often experienced state of emergency remained close to the surface of Spanish legal and political affairs for the entirety of the Franco regime.

Signally, when Spain transitioned to democracy, starting with Franco's death in 1975, the prevailing political and popular concern was not a backslide into fascism or even authoritarianism but rather a return to the devastating chaos of the Civil War. For example, Julián Casanovas and Carlos Gil Andrés point to the Amnesty Act of 15 October 1975 – which covered "all politically

---

84 Casanova and Gil Andrés note tartly: "The Civil Guard, as events proved time and again during those years, was incapable of maintaining order without opening fire." Julián Casanova and Carlos Gil Andrés, *Twentieth Century Spain: A History*, trans. Martin Douch, (Cambridge: Cambridge University Press, 2014), p. 120.

85 See President of the Government of Spain, *Decreto 779/1967, de 20 de abril, por el que se aprueban, los textos retundidos de las Leyes Fundamentales del Reino*, 20 April 1967, https://www.boe.es/boe/dias/1967/04/21/pdfs/A05250-05272.pdf. An eighth "fundamental law" was passed during the political transition (though after Franco's death), enabling free elections.

86 Spain, *Fuero de los Españoles de 17 de julio de 1945*, 17 July 1945, http://www.cervantesvirtual.com/nd/ark:/59851/bmc127t0.

87 Eric C. Christiansen, "Forty Years from Fascism: Democratic Constitutionalism and the Spanish Model of National Transformation," *Oregon Review of International Law*, Vol. 20 (2018), https://digitalcommons.law.ggu.edu/cgi/viewcontent.cgi?article=1836&context=pubs, p. 14, n. 66, quoting Raymond Carr and Juan Pablo Fusi Aizpurúa, *Spain: Dictatorship to Democracy* (Boston & London: Allen Unwin, 1979), p. 45.

88 Spain, *Fuero de los Españoles de 17 de julio de 1945*, 17 July 1945, http://www.cervantesvirtual.com/nd/ark:/59851/bmc127t0. Art. 33 appears in Chapter II.

89 Eric C. Christiansen, "Forty Years from Fascism: Democratic Constitutionalism and the Spanish Model of National Transformation," *Oregon Review of International Law*, Vol. 20 (2018), https://digitalcommons.law.ggu.edu/cgi/viewcontent.cgi?article=1836&context=pubs, p. 14.

motivated acts, 'whatever their result,' and also 'any crimes or offences which might have been committed by the authorities, public servants, and agents of public order during the investigation and prosecution of the acts included in this law'."[90] They write further: "The political culture of the people and public discourse of the parliamentarians were influenced by the traumatic memory of the war and the fear that a similar situation would be repeated in the middle of a process dominated by the uncertainty caused by the economic crisis, social conflict, terrorism, and anxiety about threats of military involvement."[91] Spanish unity and stability in Spain thus remain closely linked.

Against this backdrop, it is hardly surprising that the third democratic Spanish constitution – the current one, which dates from 1978 – still expressly allows for a state of emergency, all with an eye toward keeping order and unity. Importantly, however, the Spanish constitution also classifies emergency responses into the three levels laid out in Art. 116 – alarm, exception, and siege (martial law) – essentially a tiered approach to limitations on certain (but not all) civil liberties. In this way, the current Spanish constitution reveals its origins amid a so-called pacted transition model, in which, as Michel Rosenfeld describes, "[n]egotiation and an eventual pact leading to a new constitution depending on both the leadership of the *ancient régime* … and the proponents of a new constitutional order …."[92] In other words, conversation and compromise among the leaders of even very divergent political groupings came together to make this constitution, which is also very much a creature of compromise. Take, for example, Art. 166, with its insistence on the sanctity of fundamental civil liberties, even amid dire emergencies.[93]

Casanovas and Gil Andrés spend most of a chapter on "the long period of drafting and discussion the Constitution" of 1978.[94] It sounds like an arduous process. Such is the nature of a pacted transition. (Christiansen similarly reports in some detail on the 36-member Committee for Constitutional Affairs and Public Liberties – which ultimately appointed a seven-member drafting committee to get the job done.[95]) The finished product was made – on purpose and quite successfully – of compromises, including give-and-take on the state(s) of emergency provisions. As Andrea Bonime-Blanc writes, "In a surprise coalitional victory … a measure protecting all liberties under any circumstance was passed."[96] The result was Art. 116, which specifies that the bodies of state and government necessary to safeguard citizens' rights must remain in operation, irrespective of which level of emergency prevails as it is later developed in the Organic Law 4/1981.

Whatever else eventuated, Art. 33 of the *Fuero de los Españoles* became a thing of the past with these developments. At the same time, though, the idea and the particulars of states of emergency

90 Julián Casanova and Carlos Gil Andrés, *Twentieth Century Spain: A History*, trans. Martin Douch, (Cambridge: Cambridge University Press, 2014), p. 310. Ley 46/1977, de 15 de octubre, de Amnistía BOE de 17 de octubre de 1977.
91 Julián Casanova and Carlos Gil Andrés, *Twentieth Century Spain: A History*, trans. Martin Douch, (Cambridge: Cambridge University Press, 2014), p. 310.
92 Michel Rosenfeld, "Constitutional Identity," Ch. 35 in Michel Rosenfeld and András Sajó, *The Oxford Handbook of Comparative Constitutional Law* (Oxford: Oxford University Press, 2012), p. 769. For a detailed account on pacted transitions in general, and Spain's transition in particular, see: Juan J. Linz, and Alfred C. Stepan. *Problems of Democratic Transition and Consolidation: Southern Europe, South America, and Post-communist Europe* (Baltimore: Johns Hopkins University Press, 1996).
93 Andrea Bonime-Blanc, *Spain's Transition to Democracy: The Politics of Constitution-Making*, 3rd ed., part of the series Studies of the Research Institute on International Change, Colombia University (New York: El Torcal Press, 2013), p. 99.
94 Julián Casanova and Carlos Gil Andrés, *Twentieth Century Spain: A History*, trans. Martin Douch, (Cambridge: Cambridge University Press, 2014), p. 314.
95 Eric C. Christiansen, "Forty Years from Fascism: Democratic Constitutionalism and the Spanish Model of National Transformation," *Oregon Review of International Law*, Vol. 20 (2018), https://digitalcommons.law.ggu.edu/cgi/viewcontent.cgi?article=1836&context=pubs, p. 20.
96 Andrea Bonime-Blanc, *Spain's Transition to Democracy: The Politics of Constitution-Making*, 3rd ed., part of the series Studies of the Research Institute on International Change, Colombia University (New York: El Torcal Press, 2013), p. 79.

remained a fixture of Spanish law into the democratic age. The persistence of this preference, as well as the broad compliance with the COVID-era states of alarm, suggest that, with an eye more toward the upheaval of Civil War than to the repressions of Franco's dictatorship, the Spanish would like to retain their civil-rights protections at the highest level possible under the prevailing circumstances, but they prize stability and order, as well.

In this context, then, it is not surprising that, in December 2020, the Spanish constitutional court denied a petition – a *recurso de amparo*[97] – from an individual who sought to have the lockdown travel restrictions, at least over the Christmas holidays, declared a violation of his fundamental rights.[98] This suit was brought by Curro Nicolau Castellanos, a lawyer who had made something of an avocation of suing for clarifications and limits to the state of alarm amid Spanish constitutional theory and practice.[99] In the end, the decision hinged on technicalities of legal procedure, but the spirit was clear: The states of alarm in 2020–2021 accorded with the letter and the spirit of Spain's constitution.

7.5 *Hasta que pruebes, no absuelvas ni condenes:* COVID and the Law Amid Spanish Tensions

Perhaps this same preference for stability and order helps explain or at least contextualize, for instance, the Ombudsman's rejection of some 617 requests for intervention in or about the first state of alarm, particularly from the commercial sector.[100] In his finding, Fernández Marugán alludes to his obligation especially to protect the rights of disadvantaged groups in Spain, but he seems to suggest that even very grave interruptions of an individual's business may not implicate a fundamental right as the constitution means it.[101] In all, this question – and various other legal issues leftover from the COVID-19 response – can only gain in currency and complexity as Spain returns its attention to other pressing matters of law and politics.

The question of the length and breadth and depth of regional autonomy has not come much clearer since the states of alarm. Officially, Spain's new normality restores regional preeminence in health matters. Websites discuss the various COVID-related restrictions; on 3 June 2021, for example, the Spanish Supreme Court (Tribunal Supremo) overturned curfews and limits on social gatherings that the regional government of the Balearic Islands sought to impose after the lapse of the national (second) state of alarm.[102] Most narrowly, the argument hinged on the necessity

---

97 The Spanish constitution, in Art. 53, sec. 2, specifies the *amparo* appeal as one of the two remedies that citizens have to press for the protection of their core civil and political rights through the judiciary.

98 José María Brunet, "El Constitucional deniega el amparo a un particular que recurrió el estado de alarma," El País, 23 December 2020, https://elpais.com/espana/2020-12-23/el-constitucional-deniega-el-amparo-a-un-particular-que-recurrio-el-estado-de-alarma.html.

99 See more broadly Eric C. Christiansen, "Forty Years from Fascism: Democratic Constitutionalism and the Spanish Model of National Transformation," *Oregon Review of International Law*, Vol. 20 (2018), https://digitalcommons.law.ggu.edu/cgi/viewcontent.cgi?article=1836&context=pubs, p. 59: "Chapter 2 rights bind all government entities, and legislation that limits those rights is substantively constrained by the essential content requirement."

100 Defensor del Pueblo, "Resolución adoptada por el Defensor del Pueblo (e.f.), en relación con las solicitudes de recurso de inconstitucionalidad contra el Real Decreto 463/2020, de 14 de marzo …," 3 September 2020, https://www.defensordelpueblo.es/wp-content/uploads/2020/09/resolucion_estado_alarma.pdf.

101 Defensor del Pueblo, "Resolución adoptada por el Defensor del Pueblo (e.f.), en relación con las solicitudes de recurso de inconstitucionalidad contra el Real Decreto 463/2020, de 14 de marzo …," 3 September 2020, https://www.defensordelpueblo.es/wp-content/uploads/2020/09/resolucion_estado_alarma.pdf, see especially p. 25.

102 A.L.S, "El Supremo dicta que las autonomías no pueden imponer toques de queda con las leyes sanitarias," *La Rázon*, 3 June 2020, https://www.larazon.es/sociedad/20210603/4fxrrvta3jbrlowpvyimkb3ezm.html.

of these measures, but the decision also seems to pit national civil liberties against regional jurisdiction over health.

The 1978 Constitution created or, in some ways, re-created the contemporary Spanish territorial order, notably reviving the Comunidades Autónomas. The process spanned from December 1979, with the fast-track autonomy granted to the Basque Country and Catalonia, to February 1983, when Madrid and Castilla y León rounded out the roster of 17 regions following the constitutionally pre-scribed five-year provisional stage. And the characteristically "pacted" compromise/tension – here between stabilizing the public order and protecting civil liberties – prevails. As Bonime-Blanc sum-marizes: "While the Autonomous Community can exercise certain restricted rights and powers, the central state maintains a tight grip on such activities."[103] She points to the muscular language in the constitution that delineates the authority of the central government – versus the conditional wording ("may have jurisdiction") that attends the roles and responsibilities of the regions.[104] In many ways, the legal and legalistic disputes about Spain's COVID-19 response reflect this unsettled discursive situation.

In other ways, the Coronavirus debates may have distracted, but not deterred, proponents of greater regional independence – or, in the case of Catalán, secession. The specter of national dis-solution in the form of Catalonian secession had formed a feature of Spanish politics for some decades.[105] Indeed, mere months before COVID-19 overwhelmed Spanish politics and society, in October 2019, the Tribunal Supremo, the highest court in the land in all matters except for con-stitutional questions, announced nine unanimous guilty verdicts and prison terms in the sedition trials of 12 prominent figures in the Catalonian separatist movement. The defendants, among other things, had championed a secret 2017 ballot that called for Cataluña/Catalunya, with its capital in Barcelona, to secede from Spain, and they continued to advocate for referenda and other measures in this connection, even though the Tribunal Constitucional had already declared it unconstitu-tional for failing to follow the appropriate process to call for a referendum, contravening articles 23, 81, and 92 as well as against articles 1, 2, and 168 of the Spanish Constitution.[106] Catalonia erupted in mass demonstrations, counter-protests, and shutdowns of such public infrastructure as Barcelona's main train station and airport though the autumn. The COVID-19 lockdowns cur-tailed the popular unrest to some extent, though in between waves of infection, the popular actions continued. For instance, tens of thousands took to the streets on 11 September 2020 to mark the national day of Catalonia, "La Diada," the day in 1714 that the Siege of Barcelona, as part of the War of Spanish Succession, ended with victory for Philip V of Spain.[107] Strikingly, the crowd was mostly masked and distanced, a kind of unity amid central-government health guidance, despite the sepa-ratist messages that some of the demonstrators brought with them. In mid-2021, it is unclear how or whether the Coronavirus experience might affect the legal or political circumstances in Catalonia.

Another contentious political issue – migration – took an unexpected legal turn during the pan-demic when, in March 2020, the Spanish government closed its eight migrant detention centers

---

103 Andrea Bonime-Blanc, *Spain's Transition to Democracy: The Politics of Constitution-Making*, 3rd ed., part of the series Studies of the Research Institute on International Change, Colombia University (New York: El Torcal Press, 2013), p. 86.

104 Andrea Bonime-Blanc, *Spain's Transition to Democracy: The Politics of Constitution-Making*, 3rd ed., part of the series Studies of the Research Institute on International Change, Colombia University (New York: El Torcal Press, 2013), p. 87.

105 A quick and handy synthesis of this matter appears in Arlo Ardon, *The Return of the Radical Right in Spain*, NPS master's thesis, March 2020, https://calhoun.nps.edu/handle/10945/64861, esp. pp. 52–55.

106 Spanish Constitutional Court, 11 June 2021.
https://www.tribunalconstitucional.es/NotasDePrensaDocumentos/NP_2017_083/2017-4335STC.pdf.

107 Joan Faus, "Catalans rally for independence despite health warnings," Reuters, 11 September 2020, https://www.reuters.com/article/us-spain-politics-catalonia/catalans-rally-for-independence-despite-health-warnings-idUSKBN26213J.

(Centros de Internamiento de Extranjeros or CIEs), releasing some 450 people who had been held while they awaited the adjudication of their cases in certain criminal or administrative matters that might result in their deportation. Indeed, just after the first state of alarm went into effect, the Defensor del Pueblo had asked for the closures in the face of rising first-wave infection rates in the crowded facilities.[108] In addition, border closures in Spain and elsewhere left the CIEs with little prospect of repatriating any of the internees.[109] Organic Law 4/2000 of 11 January had created the CIEs – actually as part of a sweeping reform of immigration to Spain that gave significant rights and protections to migrants.[110] Even before the pandemic, however, many activists and nongovernmental organizations had come to call for the reform or closure of the CIEs, even as public attitudes toward migration and especially illegal migration hardened and the influx of migrants, particularly from Morocco, grew precipitously.[111] Critics slammed the CIEs for their lack of transparency and for gaps in oversight that allowed for abuses; others complained that the system was ineffective, with fewer than half of the internees ultimately being deported after spending up to 60 days in poor conditions.[112] As one scholar noted in 2017, "Nobody – not even the government – publicly defends maintaining the current situation."[113]

And yet, the CIEs and the controversy persisted until 19 March 2020, when the detention centers were closed. Dorothy Estrada-Trank captured the hope that this development seemed to portend for opponents of the CIEs: "Thus, alternatives to migratory detention are now a reality and the possibility of ending migratory detention as a structural and permanent option in the aftermath of the lockdown is now a prospect within reach."[114] In the end, the Spanish Interior Ministry reopened the CIEs in late September 2020, even with the second state of alarm (and lockdown) clearly in the offing.[115] Clearly, the popular mood toward migration remained grim. Still, the Spanish legal/constitutional preference for protecting at-risk populations found a surprising half-year of expression amid the pandemic in the closure of the CIEs. However temporary, the closures proved that it could be done – and in the event, without imperiling Spanish law, order, or unity.

7.6 *El fin veremos; hasta entonces no hablemos:* Conclusion

Even as the "freedom fiestas" broke up on 10 May 2021 or so, Spain continued to battle the pandemic, and many health-related restrictions remained in place. But with the end of the second

108 Defensor del Pueblo, Actuaciones ante la pandemia de COVID-19. https://www.defensordelpueblo.es/wp-content/uploads/2020/12/Documento_COVID-19.pdf.
109 European Commission, "Spain: Migrant detention centres re-opened following COVID-19," European Website on Integration, 24 September 2020, https://ec.europa.eu/migrant-integration/news/spain-migrant-detention-centres-re-opened-following-covid-19.
110 Note that it was amended by Organic Laws 8/2000 December 22, 11/2003 September 29, 14/2003 November 20, 2/2009 December 11 and 10/2011 July 27. See also: https://www.boe.es/boe/dias/2011/04/30/pdfs/BOE-A-2011-7703.pdf.
111 Arlo Ardon, *The Return of the Radical Right in Spain*, NPS master's thesis, March 2020, https://calhoun.nps.edu/handle/10945/64861, esp. pp. 38–40.
112 Markus Gonzáles Beilfuss, "Los Cie: Una Realidad Controvertida y Compleja," Anuario CIDOB de la Inmigración 2017 (December 2017), p. 300. https://www.cidob.org/en/articulos/anuario_cidob_de_la_inmigracion/2017/spanish_migrant_detention_centres_cie_a_complex_and_controversial_reality.
113 Markus Gonzáles Beilfuss, "Los Cie: Una Realidad Controvertida y Compleja," Anuario CIDOB de la Inmigración 2017 (December 2017), pp. 310–311. https://www.cidob.org/en/articulos/anuario_cidob_de_la_inmigracion/2017/spanish_migrant_detention_centres_cie_a_complex_and_controversial_reality.
114 Dorothy Estrada-Tranck, "COVID-19 and the State of Alarm vis-à-vis Human Rights in Spain," Bill of Health (Harvard Law), 21 May 2020, https://blog.petrieflom.law.harvard.edu/2020/05/21/spain-global-responses-covid19/.
115 European Commission, "Spain: Migrant detention centres re-opened following COVID-19," European Website on Integration, 24 September 2020, https://ec.europa.eu/migrant-integration/news/spain-migrant-detention-centres-re-opened-following-covid-19.

state of alarm, the nation's several regions could, in principle, mount their own responses as befit their particular circumstances and concerns, subject to the constitutional requirements that preserve Spanish civil liberties and Spanish unity. In this regard, the end of the second *estado de alarma* marked a welcome return to normal legal/constitutional circumstances, if not an overnight restoration of full social normality.

"Normality" has figured in most plans for emerging from lockdown, but what might post-pandemic normality look like in Spain? Without question, the human toll of COVID-19 in Spain has been staggering. As of July 2021, more than 80,000 Spaniards have died and some 3.7 million have been infected. The economic impact of the pandemic will ramify for some time, although the Bank of Spain currently predicts a strong recovery, at least in 2021.[116]

Spain's legal response to the COVID-19 crisis, particularly the states of alarm, shaped the experience of life under lockdown but also informs expectations about what should happen next. For example, in May 2021, more sober observers, in every sense, worried that the "freedom fiestas" would give way to a crush of cases brought to the Tribunal Constitucional.[117] As of July 2021, such an onslaught has not eventuated. One lone region, Galicia, attempted to effect legislation to mandate vaccination, which effort the court rejected.[118] Some peri-pandemic cases are still working their way through deliberations, but the courts – especially the constitutional court – are hardly incapacitated. Rather, they are working as well as the drafters (or pacters) of the 1978 constitution could have hoped. Indeed, even if Spain's constitutional court had been buried, literally or figuratively, in *amparo* petitions and business from the regions, Spaniards may remain secure in the knowledge that their independent judiciary was and is making decisions to maintain the order and stability of the Spanish nation – to include the preservation and protection of Spanish civil liberties.

116 Teresa Romero, "Forecast of the impact of the coronavirus on GDP in Spain in different scenarios between 2020 and 2023," Statista, 10 February 2021, https://www.statista.com/statistics/1167959/covid-19-impact-in-he-gdp-spanish-provided-by-stage/.
117 See, for example, Jessica Mouzo, "After the state of alarm: Which coronavirus restrictions are in place in each Spanish region?" El País, 10 May 2021, https://english.elpais.com/society/2021-05-10/after-the-state-of-alarm-which-coronavirus-restrictions-are-in-place-in-each-spanish-region.html.
118 "El Tribunal Constitucional suspende la vacunación obligatoria que recoge la ley de salud de Galicia," ABC, 20 April 2021, https://www.abc.es/espana/galicia/abci-tribunal-constitucional-suspende-vacunacion-obligatoria-recoge-ley-salud-galicia-202104201749_noticia.html; see also, Government of Spain, "Ley 8/2021, de 25 de febrero, de modificación de la Ley 8/2008, de 10 de julio, de salud de Galicia," 2 April 2021, https://www.boe.es/buscar/doc.php?id=BOE-A-2021-5209.

8

Pandemic Pangs and Fangs: Romania's Public Safety and Civil Liberties in the COVID-19 Era[1]

Florina C. Matei

Center for Homeland Defense and Security, Naval Postgraduate School, Monterey, CA, USA

Since 20 February 2020, when the first case of COVID-19 was recorded, till June 2021, Romania applied some of the most restrictive anti-COVID measures in Europe.[2] Such measures – implemented during an initial two-month State of Emergency (SOE), followed by an ongoing State of Alert (SOA) – ranged from mandatory facemask and social distancing, to obligatory quarantine, to restrictions of movement, to total lockdown. In May 2020, the Constitutional Court invalidated sanctions for lockdown while in June 2020, it ruled unconstitutional specific restrictions for some Romanians who returned home from European Union (EU) countries. It was not until June 2021, following a significant decrease in infection rates, that the authorities in Bucharest lifted some of these restrictions. This chapter discusses Romania's COVID-19 journey through the lens of the trade-off between health security and civil liberties. It finds that the Romanian Government's response to the pandemic was less than perfect, partly because of the inadequate legal framework on emergency situations, and partly because of political crises and clashes that plagued Romania since the outbreak of the pandemic. As such, while some of the measures imposed by the government helped preventing the spread of the coronavirus, others resulted in unwarranted infections and unnecessary infringements on human rights and freedoms.

8.1 Legal Framework and Policy Approaches Vis-À-Vis Quarantine, Isolation, and Other Social Distancing Measures

Romania's Constitution – adopted in 1991 and amended in 2003 by Law 429 of 2003 – is the law of the land, which establishes the structure and roles of the country's government, its citizens'

1 The views expressed in this chapter do not reflect the policy or view of the U.S. Government, Department of Defense, or Department of Navy. The author would like to acknowledge Dr. Irena Chiru and Mr. Nicolae Vâjdea's assistance in conducting this research.

2 The first case was a man who contracted the virus from an Italian traveler. "Primul caz de coronavirus în România. Raed Arafat a dat detalii despre starea lui de sănătate: Nu prezintă simptome," *Digi24*, 26 February 2028, https://www.digi24.ro/stiri/actualitate/primul-caz-de-coronavirus-in-romania-1266806?__ grsc=cookieIsUndef0&__grts=54236491&__grua=7f65ff317c237641f7aace3b7dac03d6&__grrn=1; Caroline Kantis, Samantha Kiernan and Jason Socrates Bardi, "UPDATED: Timeline of the Coronavirus. A frequently updated tracker of emerging developments from the beginning of the COVID-19 outbreak," *ThinkGlobalHealth*, 1 July 2021, https://www.thinkglobalhealth.org/article/updated-timeline-coronavirus; Daniela Budu, "Ombudsman's report on pandemic," *Radio Romania International*, 17 September 2020, https://www.rri.ro/en_gb/ombudsmans_report_on_ pandemic-2623368. At the time of the writing, August 2021, Romania reported over 1,083,000 cases and 34,278 COVID-19-related deaths. https://www.digi24.ro/stiri/informatii-oficiale-despre-coronavirus-in-romania-126626.

rights and responsibilities, and the country's manner of enacting laws.[3] The Constitution stipulates that the President can issue a Presidential Decree to declare a State of Exception – which involves the declaration of a State of Siege or a SOE on the entirety of Romanian territory, or, alternatively, in specific regions or zones in the country, as well as the conditions under which the President can declare a State of Exception. [4] The State of Siege involves adopting exceptional political, military, economic, and social measures throughout the country or in specific locations, in response to serious, current, or imminent threats; the SOE is similar to State of Siege but imposes nonmilitary measures involving threats to national security, the functioning of government, and natural disasters.[5] A SOE must not exceed 30 days at a time, but can be extended indefinitely by Presidential Decree, subject, in each instance, to the approval of the legislature. The President needs the Parliament's approval within five days of a declaration of a State of Siege or SOE, and, in order to be legally valid, the executive order declaring a State of Siege or SOE must be countersigned by the Prime Minister and published in the Romanian Official Gazette. In line with the Constitution, the Parliament must function – and cannot be dissolved – during the entire State of Siege or SOE. If the Parliament is not in session, it needs to meet within 48 hours from the initiation of the State of Exception, and operate during the SOE. The Presidential Decree enables the Minister of Internal Affairs to adopt specific regulations that deal with public order – called "Military Ordinances" – and temporarily limit certain rights immediately.[6] The legal basis for emergency situations also allows the armed forces to take over responsibilities of public administration throughout the crisis.[7] Law 453 of 2004, however, does not provide stipulations related to epidemic crises.[8]

The legal framework for emergencies is completed by the SOA – defined as a "response to an emergency of particular magnitude and intensity" – which is regulated by Government Emergency

---

3 http://www.cdep.ro/pls/dic/site.page?id=339.

4 http://www.cdep.ro/pls/dic/site.page?id=339. The State of Siege or Emergency is further regulated by Law 453 of 2004 that approved the Government Emergency Ordinance on the State of Siege and Emergency 1 of 1999. http://legislatie.just.ro/Public/DetaliiDocument/16739; and https://lege5.ro/Gratuit/gu3dinbw/legea-nr-453-2004-pentru-aprobarea-ordonantei-de-urgenta-a-guvernului-nr-1-1999-privind-regimul-starii-de-asediu-si-regimul-starii-de-urgenta. In 2004, the Government issued Emergency Ordinance 21 on the National System of Management of Emergency Situations, which set up a system of coordination during emergency situations. https://lege5.ro/Gratuit/gu3dgmby/ordonanta-de-urgenta-nr-21-2004-privind-sistemul-national-de-management-al-situatiilor-de-urgenta. Romania has 42 districts. Each district coordinates and organizes – administratively – all events related to public life, including health-related courses of actions. Mariana Cernicova-Buca and Adina Palea, "An Appraisal of Communication Practices Demonstrated by Romanian District Public Health Authorities at the Outbreak of the COVID-19 Pandemic," *Sustainability* 2021, 13, 2500, pp. 1–19, https://doi.org/10.3390/su13052500.

5 Florina Cristiana Matei, "Romania," in Leonard Weinberg, Elizabeth Francis, Eliot Assoudeh eds., *Routledge Handbook of Democracy and Security*, London: Routledge 2020, 251–263; and Thomas C. Bruneau and Florina Cristiana Matei (eds.) *The Routledge Handbook of Civil Military Relations* (London: Routledge, 2012).

6 "Coronavirus COVID-19 outbreak in the EU. Fundamental Rights Implications," Country report, Romania, Human European Consultancy, 23 March 2020, https://fra.europa.eu/sites/default/files/fra_uploads/romania-report-covid-19-april-2020_en.pdf. The term "military" is not related to the military institution or military rule.

7 Florina Cristiana Matei, "Romania," in Leonard Weinberg, Elizabeth Francis, Eliot Assoudeh eds., *Routledge Handbook of Democracy and Security*, London: Routledge 2020, 251–263; Florina Cristiana (Cris) Matei (2009).

8 However, OUG 21 of 2004 on the organization and the functioning of the National System of Management of the Emergency Situations includes "the risk of mass sickness" in the same category of risk as disasters, which allows the government to declare a SOE based on OUG 1 of 1999. "Coronavirus COVID-19 outbreak in the EU. Fundamental Rights Implications," Country report, Romania, Human European Consultancy, 23 March 2020, https://fra.europa.eu/sites/default/files/fra_uploads/romania-report-covid-19-april-2020_en.pdf.

Ordinance (OUG) 21 of 2004 (reviewed in 2014),[9] OUG 68 of 2020, and Law 55 of 2020.[10] Both the SOE and the SOA empower the National Committee for Special Emergency Situations (CNSSU), an interagency forum chaired by the Minister of Internal Affairs – upon approval by the Prime Minister – to establish temporary and gradual measures aimed at combating specific threats to citizens' life and health.[11] The SOA can be declared at local, county, or national level, when the analysis of risk factors indicate the need to augment the response to an emergency situation, for a limited period of time, which cannot exceed 30 days. But it can be extended any time – though no more than 30 days at once – when warranted by the risk analysis. The SOA can end before the declared deadline, when the risk analysis indicates that such a state is no longer required.[12] When the SOA applies to at least half of the administrative-territorial units across Romania, the measure requires parliamentary approval; and the parliament is required to provide its approval of or denial within five days since the request. If the parliament refuses to approve a SOA, the SOE must cease.[13]

In Romania, only laws can limit civil rights and liberties; Emergency Orders, Government Decisions, or Ministerial Orders cannot restrict these freedoms.[14] While the legal framework permits restrictions of rights and liberties during the SOE,[15] a few rights are exempt from any limitation, such as: "the right to life, the right not to be subjected to torture and other inhuman or degrading treatments, the principle nulla poena sine lege, access to justice."[16]

Romania declared its first SOE from 21 to 22 January 1999 during the strikes initiated by Romanian miners who protested against harsh political and work conditions; its second SOE on 6 August 2018, in the aftermath of the outbreak of African swine flu; and the third (and last) SOE between 16 March 2020 and 15 May 2020, amid the outbreak of the COVID-19 pandemic.[17]

---

9 The Romanian constitution does not include provisions related to the SOA. OUG 21 of 2004 was adopted after the terrorist attacks in EU/NATO countries, to combat risks and threats to national security. Elena-Simina Tănăsescu and Bogdan Dima, "The Parliament in the time of coronavirus. The Role of the Romanian Parliament during the COVID-19 Sanitary Crisis. A diminishment of the executive decision-making power," 101–111, https://www.robert-schuman.eu/en/doc/ouvrages/FRS_Parliament.pdf.

10 Both OUG 68 of 2020 and Law 55 of 2020 modified OUG 21 of 2004, to specifically deal with the coronavirus pandemic. Law 55 of 2020 provides for the establishment of specific – temporary and gradual – measures specifically aimed at preventing and combatting COVID-19 pandemic effects; to safeguard the right to life, physical integrity, and health protection (including limiting physical activity and exercise and other fundamental rights and liberties). https://www2.deloitte.com/ro/en/pages/business-continuity/articles/COVID-19-legislative-tracker.html.

11 Bianca Selejan-Gutan, "Romania in the Covid Era: Between Corona Crisis and Constitutional Crisis," verfassungsblog, 21 May 2020, https://verfassungsblog.de/romania-in-the-covid-era-between-corona-crisis-and-constitutional-crisis.

12 http://legislatie.just.ro/Public/DetaliiDocument/225620; https://www2.deloitte.com/ro/en/pages/business-continuity/articles/COVID-19-legislative-tracker.html.

13 https://www2.deloitte.com/ro/en/pages/business-continuity/articles/COVID-19-legislative-tracker.html.

14 Daniela Budu, "Ombudsman's report on pandemic," Radio Romania International, 17 September 2020, https://www.rri.ro/en_gb/ombudsmans_report_on_pandemic-2623368.

15 The Presidential Decree must clearly list which rights will be restricted.

16 Bianca Selejan-Gutan, "Romania in the Covid Era: Between Corona Crisis and Constitutional Crisis," verfassungsblog, 21 May 2020, https://verfassungsblog.de/romania-in-the-covid-era-between-corona-crisis-and-constitutional-crisis/.

17 Florina Cristiana Matei, "Romania," in Leonard Weinberg, Elizabeth Francis, Eliot Assoudeh eds., *Routledge Handbook of Democracy and Security*, London: Routledge 2020, 251–263; Florina Cristiana (Cris) Matei (2009). The SOE was replaced by a SOA, which continued until the time of writing of this chapter.

8.2 Quarantine, Isolation, and Other Social Distancing Measures During the Covid-19 Pandemic

The public health crisis caused by the SARS-COV-2 pandemic began in March 2020 in the midst of an unrelated political crisis.[18] Nevertheless, Romania's first official response to the COVID-19 outbreak occurred on 29 January 2020, immediately after the World Health Organization (WHO) declared it an international emergency, when CNSSU held its first pandemic-related meeting, which addressed possible courses of action to combat the disease.[19] Specifically, the government imposed stricter border controls to limit travel to and from most affected countries (such as China and Italy); enforced isolation and testing of all persons coming from high-risk countries; recommended social isolation measures for everybody; banned gatherings of more than 100 persons, and later of more than 50 persons, and limiting the export of medical supplies. More stringent restrictions were subsequently implemented after March 2020, under the SOE and SOA measures.

8.2.1 From a State of Emergency amidst a Political Crisis...

On 16 March 2020, when the official cases reached 168, President Klaus Iohannis declared a 30-day SOE throughout Romania's entire territory, via Presidential Decree 195 of 2020.[20] The Decree restricted the following freedoms and rights: "a) Freedom of movement; b) Right to intimate, family and private life; c) Inviolability of home; d) Right to education; e) Freedom of assembly; f) Right of private property; g) Right to strike; h) Economic freedom." [21] In this context, the government's first actions aimed at boosting the capabilities of the agencies tasked with public health and strengthening national emergency response, including closure of all education institutions, economic stimulus measures for businesses affected by the SOE, and providing social benefits for workers affected by the SOE. [22] In addition, 12 Military Ordinances issued by

---

18 On 5 February 2020, the majority in the legislature, comprised of political parties that formed a social–democrat political coalition, adopted a motion of censure against the minority liberal Government, to force early Parliamentary elections. On 9 March 2020, Romania had a minority Interim Government, under the dismissed Prime Minister Ludovic Orban. Because the President could not obtain a vote of confidence (as the nominated candidate withdrew on 12 March), the President nominated Orban again, whose Government received the Parliament's approval on 14 March 2020. "Coronavirus COVID-19 outbreak in the EU. Fundamental Rights Implications," Country report, Romania, Human European Consultancy, 23 March 2020, https://fra.europa.eu/sites/default/files/fra_uploads/romania-report-covid-19-april-2020_en.pdf.

19 "Coronavirus COVID-19 outbreak in the EU. Fundamental Rights Implications," Country report, Romania, Human European Consultancy, 23 March 2020, https://fra.europa.eu/sites/default/files/fra_uploads/romania-report-covid-19-april-2020_en.pdf.

20 http://legislatie.just.ro/Public/DetaliiDocumentAfis/223831. On 17 March, the Romanian authorities informed the Council of Europe that Romania activated the State of Emergency clause of the European Convention on Human Rights. Bianca Selejan-Gutan, "Romania in the Covid Era: Between Corona Crisis and Constitutional Crisis," verfassungsblog, 21 May 2020, https://verfassungsblog.de/romania-in-the-covid-era-between-corona-crisis-and-constitutional-crisis/.

21 http://legislatie.just.ro/Public/DetaliiDocumentAfis/223831; and "Coronavirus COVID-19 outbreak in the EU. Fundamental Rights Implications," Country report, Romania, Human European Consultancy, 23 March 2020, https://fra.europa.eu/sites/default/files/fra_uploads/romania-report-covid-19-april-2020_en.pdf.

22 Bianca Selejan-Gutan, "Romania in the Covid Era: Between Corona Crisis and Constitutional Crisis," verfassungsblog, 21 May 2020, https://verfassungsblog.de/romania-in-the-covid-era-between-corona-crisis-and-constitutional-crisis/. "Coronavirus COVID-19 outbreak in the EU. Fundamental Rights Implications," Country report, Romania, Human European Consultancy, 23 March 2020, https://fra.europa.eu/sites/default/files/fra_uploads/romania-report-covid-19-april-2020_en.pdf. "2020 Country Reports on Human Rights Practices: Romania," Department of State's Bureau of Democracy, Human Rights, and Labor Report, 30 March 2021, https://www.state.gov/reports/2020-country-reports-on-human-rights-practices/romania/.

the Minister of Internal Affairs, upon approval by the Prime Minister, mandated supplementary "gradually applicable" isolation, quarantine, and lockdown measures.

On 16 March 2020, Military Ordinance 1 banned dine-in service in restaurants, bars, and coffee-shops (while allowing home delivery), as well as public gatherings.[23] On 19 March 2020, the government amended the Criminal Code (via OUG 28 of 2020) to allow applying harsher penalties for violators of quarantine or self-isolation orders, or for people who deliberately concealed travel information.[24] Military Ordinance 1 directed local public authorities to help persons over 65 or disabled people without any support during quarantine.[25] Military Ordinance 2, issued on 21 March, banned nonessential movement from 10 pm to 6 am and recommended – not mandated – that the population stay indoors during the day.[26] Military Ordinance 2 also suspended commercial activities in malls,[27] reduced public transportation, and restricted religious services.[28] All individuals who failed to respect these restrictions were prosecuted based on the Criminal Code and forcefully placed in quarantine centers by law enforcement agencies.[29]

In March 2020, the government closed Romania's borders to foreign citizens, except for the following categories: relatives of Romanian citizens or family members of citizens of the EU or EEA member states; citizens of Switzerland who live in Romania; diplomats or persons possessing valid business or work-related visas; refugees; humanitarian groups representatives; military members; representatives of international organizations; and persons who travel for family or health-related emergencies.[30] Yet, the authorities in Bucharest failed to devise a clear plan for the safety of Romanian citizens who returned from countries that reported high infection rates.[31] On the one hand, when the government decided to ground all commercial flights between the red zone countries and Romania, it left these citizens stranded in these countries.[32] Similarly, seasonal workers who were forced to return to Romania because they lost their jobs in the EU member country where

---

23 At that time, the government did not ban any nonessential movement. "Coronavirus COVID-19 outbreak in the EU. Fundamental Rights Implications," Country report, Romania, Human European Consultancy, 23 March 2020, https://fra.europa.eu/sites/default/files/fra_uploads/romania-report-covid-19-april-2020_en.pdf.
24 If such violations result in medical staff being infected, the penalty included up to 15 years imprisonment. http://legislatie.just.ro/Public/DetaliiDocument/224258.
25 Some local authorities, for instance, made available a phone line for elderly or incapacitated individuals to request support in purchasing food and medicine, or to report an emergency. "Coronavirus COVID-19 outbreak in the EU. Fundamental Rights Implications," Country report, Romania, Human European Consultancy, 23 March 2020, https://fra.europa.eu/sites/default/files/fra_uploads/romania-report-covid-19-april-2020_en.pdf.
26 Only essential movement was permitted/recommended, including, for example, traveling to/from work, when teleworking was impossible; traveling for emergency health situations; leaving home for grocery and medicine purchases or to assist family members in an emergency; and walking pets in areas very close to home. Meeting in groups larger than three nonfamily members was forbidden. http://www.cdep.ro/pls/legis/legis_pck.htp_act?ida=164484.
27 Except for grocery stores, home utility stores, and pharmacies. "Coronavirus COVID-19 outbreak in the EU. Fundamental Rights Implications," Country report, Romania, Human European Consultancy, 23 March 2020, https://fra.europa.eu/sites/default/files/fra_uploads/romania-report-covid-19-april-2020_en.pdf.
28 Priests were allowed to perform these services in churches, but virtually. Private religious events, including baptism or funerals were also allowed in churches, but with no more than nine people. "Coronavirus COVID-19 outbreak in the EU. Fundamental Rights Implications," Country report, Romania, Human European Consultancy, 23 March 2020, https://fra.europa.eu/sites/default/files/fra_uploads/romania-report-covid-19-april-2020_en.pdf.
29 "Coronavirus COVID-19 outbreak in the EU. Fundamental Rights Implications," Country report, Romania, Human European Consultancy, 23 March 2020, https://fra.europa.eu/sites/default/files/fra_uploads/romania-report-covid-19-april-2020_en.pdf.
30 "Coronavirus COVID-19 outbreak in the EU. Fundamental Rights Implications," Country report, Romania, Human European Consultancy, 23 March 2020, https://fra.europa.eu/sites/default/files/fra_uploads/romania-report-covid-19-april-2020_en.pdf.
31 Dubbed "red zone" countries. Examples include France, Italy, and Spain.
32 For example, Romanians who were in passage or on vacation in Italy could not return to Romania for days, thanks to the Romanian authorities' grounding of all commercial flights between Italy and Romania in February

they were working were also unable to return to Romania.[33] On the other hand, the government lacked a standardized quarantine plan for all citizens who returned from red zone countries. For instance, while the government forced the citizens who were on vacation abroad to quarantine for 14 days in government-approved institutions,[34] it, paradoxically, did not mandate quarantine for seasonal workers; nor did the Romanian authorities issue any guidance on what to do in case that the returned seasonal workers contracted the virus.[35]

The beginning – and very rapid surge – of confirmed coronavirus-related deaths in late March 2020, among citizens and medical personnel, triggered additional restrictions.[36] On 23 March 2020, the Minister of Internal Affairs issued Order 487 of 2020, which suspended the treatment of

----

2020. Sandra Mantu, "EU Citizenship, Free Movement, and Covid-19 in Romania," *frontiersin*, 9 December 2020, https://www.frontiersin.org/articles/10.3389/fhumd.2020.594987/full.

33 These seasonal workers were Romanians between 20 and 64 years of age, who traveled to EU countries for labor purposes (based on prior approval from the Romanian Government). Sandra Mantu, "EU Citizenship, Free Movement, and Covid-19 in Romania," *frontiersin*, 9 December 2020, https://www.frontiersin.org/articles/10.3389/fhumd.2020.594987/full.

34 Failure to observe these restrictions would result in fines mounting to 20,000 RON (approximately $5,000)—a rather high fine, considering that the net minimum salary in Romania is $500) – and criminal cases. Cristina Lupu, "Romania," in Bican Sahin and Ivaylo Tsonev eds., *Expressing Civil and Political Liberties in Times of Crisis. COVID-19 first wave as a case study: Bulgaria, Greece, North Macedonia, and Romania*, Sofia, Bulgaria: Friedrich Naumann Foundation for Freedom, 2021, 20–25, https://www.freiheit.org/sites/default/files/2021-04/expressing-civil-and-political-liberties-in-times-of-crisis.pdf.

35 While further measures added requirements for transportation, these measures did not clarify how compliance with the regulation was going to be monitored. Sandra Mantu, "EU Citizenship, Free Movement, and Covid-19 in Romania," *frontiersin*, 9 December 2020, https://www.frontiersin.org/articles/10.3389/fhumd.2020.594987/full.

36 On 22 March 2020, three Romanian citizens with pre-existing medical conditions – like diabetes, cancer, and kidney failures – died because of the virus. Then, on 23 March, some 70 medical personnel of the main hospital in the county of Suceava contracted the virus, and two patients died. The infection within medical facilities should not come as a surprise, considering that Romania is the EU country that invests the least in health care as compared to any other member states (for instance, the authorities only built one new hospital since the end of the communist regime), has the highest mortality rate among EU countries from curable illnesses; one of the lowest life expectancies within the EU. This neglect of health care on the part of authorities is the legacy of the Ceausescu regime, which enabled bribery in the delivery of medical services, corruption related to healthcare procurement, and abuse of leadership and management positions. Ultimately, years of corruption and healthcare mismanagement resulted in precarious medical facilities and limited access to protective equipment for the medical personnel – which, in turn, not only hindered the medical staff's readiness to respond to the pandemic effectively, but also endangered their lives. All these challenges caused a rapid rise in infections among doctors and nurses, who then infected patients who were hospitalized with other illnesses—which is exactly what happened in Suceava county. The Romanian authorities swiftly fired the director of the hospital in Suceava after the surge. For more details, see: "Încă un român a murit din cauza conoravirusului. Trei decese confirmate în România," *Digi24*, 22 March 2020, https://www.digi24.ro/stiri/actualitate/inca-un-roman-a-murit-din-cauza-conoravirusului-trei-decese-confirmate-in-romania-1279526; Andra Timu and Irina Vilcu, "Romania Drafts in Army to Run More Hospitals Amid Virus," *Bloomberg News*, 14 April 2020, https://www.bnnbloomberg.ca/romania-drafts-in-army-to-run-more-hospitals-amid-virus-1.1421197; "Thousands rally in Romania against coronavirus curfew, defy gathering ban," *Reuters*, 30 March 2021, https://www.reuters.com/article/health-coronavirus-romania-protests/thousands-rally-in-romania-against-coronavirus-curfew-defy-gathering-ban-idUSL8N2LS5O6; "Update: At least 70 doctors and nurses infected with Coronavirus at Suceava County Hospital. Medical staff blame the hospital management," *The Romania Journal*, 25 March 2020, https://www.romaniajournal.ro/society-people/update-at-least-70-doctors-and-nurses-infected-with-coronavirus-at-suceava-county-hospital-medical-staff-blame-the-hospital-management/; "Suceava County Hospital shuts down following high number of COVID-19 infections. Suceava – the biggest coronavirus hot zone in Romania," *The Romania Journal*, 25 March 2020, https://www.romaniajournal.ro/society-people/suceava-county-hospital-shuts-down-following-high-number-of-covid-19-infections-suceava-the-biggest-coronavirus-hot-zone-in-romania/; "2020 Country Reports on Human Rights Practices: Romania," Department of State's Bureau of Democracy, Human Rights, and Labor Report, 30 March 2021, https://www.state.gov/reports/2020-country-reports-on-human-rights-practices/romania/; and Stephen Thomson and Eric C Ip, "COVID-19 emergency measures and the impending authoritarian pandemic," *Journal of Law and the Biosciences* 2020 Jan-Dec; 7(1): lsaa064. Published online 2020 Sep 29. https://doi.org/10.1093/jlb/lsaa064.

nonemergency medical cases in both public and private hospitals. [37] On 24 March, the government issued Military Ordinance 3, which mandated a national lockdown, placed the armed forces in charge of hospitals, and tasked the military to support police and Gendarmerie personnel in enforcing these new SOE-related measures.[38] The authorities banned movement outside the home or household, unless it was for work, or purchase of basic needs items (like, for example, food or medicine).[39] A new OUG – 34 of 2020 – adopted by the authorities on 26 March 2020 increased the amount of fines for violators of the provisions of the Decree and of the associated military ordinances, and provided for harsher penalties for certain criminal offences related to the SOE (like, for example, obstructing the efforts to combat the diseases).[40]

Six additional Military Ordinances were issued between 29 March and 16 April 2020, further strengthening previously imposed fines and restrictions: extending the ban on international travel; placing the city of Suceava, along with eight adjacent communes, under total quarantine; further extending the national lockdown period; banning the export of some basic foods; recommending that residential buildings be equipped with sanitary products and that their stairways and elevators be periodically disinfected, and the like. In parallel, local authorities made wearing protection masks mandatory.[41] During this time, the government authorized Romanian seasonal workers to travel to other states using charter flights. However, the authorities – again – lacked a plan for the health of these citizens, which resulted in additional crises. For instance, initially, the Romanian authorities failed to require the recruitment companies to provide the Romanian Government the number and state of health of the seasonal workers expected to travel for labor to EU countries, and the exact venue where they would work – which left some 1,800 Romanians who were supposed to fly to Germany stranded in the parking lot of an airport in Transylvania, without any respect for

---

37 https://stirioficiale.ro/informatii/informare-de-presa-23-martie-2020-ora-2-13pm; "Coronavirus COVID-19 outbreak in the EU. Fundamental Rights Implications," Country report, Romania, Human European Consultancy, 23 March 2020, https://fra.europa.eu/sites/default/files/fra_uploads/romania-report-covid-19-april-2020_en.pdf.
38 http://www.cdep.ro/pls/legis/legis_pck.htp_act?ida=164533. In this context, the Romanian military executed such logistical and medical tasks in support to the authorities as providing transport for medical personnel, supplies, and bodies of the deceased; cleaning public places; facilitating testing; deploying military hospitals next to civilian medical facilities; and enforcing lockdown restrictions by patrolling the streets. Some medical staff refused to obey the restrictions imposed by the armed forces, while some doctors even quit. http://euromil.org/armed-forces-and-covid-19/; "Coronavirus in Romania: Army deploys mobile hospital near Bucharest to treat Covid-19 patients. Authorities prepare for spike in the number of cases," *Romania Insider*, 18 March 2020, https://www.romania-insider.com/coronavirus-romania-military-hospital; Craig Turp-Balazs, "Coronavirus: Yes, it's serious, but do we really need the army on the streets?," *Emerging Europe*, 25 March 2020, https://emerging-europe.com/from-the-editor/coronavirus-yes-its-serious-but-do-we-really-need-the-army-on-the-streets/; and Andra Timu and Irina Vilcu, "Romania Drafts in Army to Run More Hospitals Amid Virus," *Bloomberg News*, 14 April 2020, https://www.bnnbloomberg.ca/romania-drafts-in-army-to-run-more-hospitals-amid-virus-1.1421197.
39 Citizens older than 65 were only permitted to leave their homes between 11 a.m. and 1 p.m. Walker S, Davies C., "Lack of testing raises fears of coronavirus surge in eastern Europe," *The Guardian*, 29 March 2020, https://www.theguardian.com/world/2020/mar/29/lack-of-testing-raises-fears-of-coronavirus-surge-in-eastern-europe.
40 These fines thus became more substantial for the average Romanian. http://legislatie.just.ro/Public/DetaliiDocument/224526.
41 http://www.cdep.ro/pls/legis/legis_pck.lista_anuala?an=2020&emi=5,133&tip=120&rep=0. On 26 March 2020, the Romania's airline company TAROM suspended all internal flights. Walker S, Davies C, "Lack of testing raises fears of coronavirus surge in Eastern Europe," *The Guardian*, 29 March 2020, https://www.theguardian.com/world/2020/mar/29/lack-of-testing-raises-fears-of-coronavirus-surge-in-eastern-europe. "Révolte des soignants en Roumanie: 'Envoyés à la mort les mains nues'," *7sur7.be*, 1 April 2020, https://www.7sur7.be/monde/revolte-des-soignants-en-roumanie-envoyes-a-la-mort-les-mains-nues~ae35ffaf/?referrer=https%3A%2F%2Fwww.google.com%2F; Bianca Selejan-Gutan, "Romania: COVID-19 Response in an Electoral Year. Overview of Legal and Political Response and Adaptation to COVID-19," *verfassiungblog.de*, 26 March 2021, https://verfassungsblog.de/romania-covid-19-response-in-an-electoral-year/; and Sandra Mantu, "EU Citizenship, Free Movement, and Covid-19 in Romania," *frontiersin*, 9 December 2020, https://www.frontiersin.org/articles/10.3389/fhumd.2020.594987/full.

social distancing measures.[42] As a corrective measure, Military Ordinance 8 of 9 April mandated prior government approval for the transportation – using charter flights – of seasonal workers from Romania to other countries.[43]

On 14 April 2020, the President of Romania extended the SOE for 30 more days, via Decree 240 of 2020.[44] Between 27 April and 13 May 2020, three more military ordinances were issued, which stipulated that except for reasons related to work and medical emergency, people over 65 could only leave their homes between 7 a.m. and 11 a.m. and between 7 p.m and 10 p.m.[45] These Ordinances also lifted the quarantine previously imposed in two counties.[46]

These measures also imposed upon Romanians a requirement to complete an official form prior to leaving their home, detailing the reason for going out, which would be presented along with proper identification to law enforcement or armed forces personnel, upon request.[47] Failure to do so would result in fines ranging from 2,000 Romanian lei (RON) (approximately $450) up to 20,000 (approximately $4,500).[48] As a result, the government budgeted millions of U.S. dollars in RON from fines.[49] These strict restrictions did not discourage some quite inventive Romanians from leaving their homes. As the regulations allowed Romanians to walk their pets, some of them would go out holding a fish in a plastic bag, telling the law enforcement officers that they were actually "walking" their pet, while others would "drive" a cat for some 30 km away from their home, on the back seat of their personal vehicle.[50] Finally, the SOE did not discourage Romanians from protesting, even if the price paid was high fines.[51]

---

42 Sandra Mantu, "EU Citizenship, Free Movement, and Covid-19 in Romania," *frontiersin*, 9 December 2020, https://www.frontiersin.org/articles/10.3389/fhumd.2020.594987/full.

43 http://www.cdep.ro/pls/legis/legis_pck.htp_act?ida=164898; and Sandra Mantu, "EU Citizenship, Free Movement, and Covid-19 in Romania," *frontiersin*, 9 December 2020, https://www.frontiersin.org/articles/10.3389/fhumd.2020.594987/full.

44 The new Decree preserved the previous Decree's stipulations. On 6 April 2020, the Government issued OUG 44 of 2020, which stipulated that local elections would be postponed to an undetermined date in 2020. The Ordinance also extended the decision-making mandate of the local authorities. http://legislatie.just.ro/Public/DetaliiDocument/224731; Bianca Selejan-Gutan, "Romania in the Covid Era: Between Corona Crisis and Constitutional Crisis," *verfassungsblog*, 21 May 2020, https://verfassungsblog.de/romania-in-the-covid-era-between-corona-crisis-and-constitutional-crisis/.

45 http://www.cdep.ro/pls/legis/legis_pck.lista_anuala?an=2020&emi=5,133&tip=120&rep=0.

46 Elena-Simina Tănăsescu and Bogdan Dima, "The Parliament in the time of coronavirus. The Role of the Romanian Parliament during the COVID-19 Sanitary Crisis. A diminishment of the executive decision-making power," 101–111, https://www.robert-schuman.eu/en/doc/ouvrages/FRS_Parliament.pdf; and Bianca Selejan-Gutan, "Romania in the Covid Era: Between Corona Crisis and Constitutional Crisis," *verfassungsblog*, 21 May 2020, https://verfassungsblog.de/romania-in-the-covid-era-between-corona-crisis-and-constitutional-crisis/.

47 "COVID-19 has served as the pretext for widespread surveillance," https://www.europeandatajournalism.eu/eng/News/Data-news/COVID-19-has-served-as-the-pretext-for-widespread-surveillance.

48 These fines were quite high, considering that the net minimum salary in Romania is approximately $500. During the State of Emergency, the Romanian authorities applied over 300,000 fines and warnings, amounting to some 600,000,000 lei (approximately $130 million). Cristina Lupu, "Romania," in Bican Sahin and Ivaylo Tsonev eds., *Expressing Civil and Political Liberties in Times of Crisis. COVID-19 first wave as a case study: Bulgaria, Greece, North Macedonia, and Romania*, Sofia, Bulgaria: Friedrich Naumann Foundation for Freedom, 2021, 20–25, https://www.freiheit.org/sites/default/files/2021-04/expressing-civil-and-political-liberties-in-times-of-crisis.pdf; Chris Irvine, "Romania makes millions from handing out strict coronavirus fines," *New York Post*, 22 April 2020, https://nypost.com/2020/04/22/romania-makes-millions-from-handing-out-strict-coronavirus-fines/.

49 From 24 March to 19 April 2020, for instance, the police issued 200,000 fines were issued, totaling approximately $85 million. "COVID-19 has served as the pretext for widespread surveillance," https://www.europeandatajournalism.eu/eng/News/Data-news/COVID-19-has-served-as-the-pretext-for-widespread-surveillance.

50 Chris Irvine, "Romania makes millions from handing out strict coronavirus fines," *New York Post*, 22 April 2020, https://nypost.com/2020/04/22/romania-makes-millions-from-handing-out-strict-coronavirus-fines/.

51 For example, in April 2020, activist Mihail Bumbes protested against lockdown-caused pollution in Bucharest, for clean air, while in May he protested in front of the MAI against policy abuses. In April, Bumbeș was not fined,

Several state and private institutions continued to operate uninterrupted throughout the SOE. The Parliament, for example, initially worked remotely, but after five weeks, on 23 April 2020, it returned to in-person mode.[52] Similarly, while the majority of Courts limited their in-person program with the public, and some courts even suspended their activity with the public, the extreme emergency court trial procedures continued.[53] Nevertheless, the Decree on the SOE placed limits on the right to receive visits and goods on hold for all convicted persons, along with permits for leaving the penitentiary.[54] In addition, the SOE indirectly obstructed access to justice and to a fair trial in Romania, because it reduced the number of available personnel, and thus limited the judiciary to act promptly and effectively, which in turn resulted in "excessively long trials," as the State Department experts note.[55] Also, problematic was the fact that the impacted citizens were virtually deprived of any legal way to protest the decisions in court – which was, arguably, yet another "deprivation of liberty," as the state did not allow these citizens the opportunity for an urgent appeal in front of a judge. [56] Interestingly, Romania's ski resorts remained open throughout the winter, in contrast to the resorts in the rest of the European countries – arguably because some influential Romanians sought to keep profiting.[57] The SOE ended on 14 May 2020, when the authorities decided to impose more relaxed anti-COVID measures.

---

but in May he was fined 3,000 lei (approximately $650) on administrative grounds, and his statement was improperly filed. Cristina Lupu, "Romania," in Bican Sahin and Ivaylo Tsonev eds., *Expressing Civil and Political Liberties in Times of Crisis. COVID-19 first wave as a case study: Bulgaria, Greece, North Macedonia, and Romania*, Sofia, Bulgaria: Friedrich Naumann Foundation for Freedom, 2021, 20–25, https://www.freiheit.org/sites/default/files/2021-04/expressing-civil-and-political-liberties-in-times-of-crisis.pdf.

52 Elena-Simina Tănăsescu and Bogdan Dima, "The Parliament in the time of coronavirus. The Role of the Romanian Parliament during the COVID-19 Sanitary Crisis. A diminishment of the executive decision-making power," 101–111, https://www.robert-schuman.eu/en/doc/ouvrages/FRS_Parliament.pdf; and Bianca Selejan-Gutan, "Romania in the Covid Era: Between Corona Crisis and Constitutional Crisis," verfassungsblog, 21 May 2020, https://verfassungsblog.de/romania-in-the-covid-era-between-corona-crisis-and-constitutional-crisis/.

53 Right to access to justice: OUG 1/1999 provides for access to justice based on a list provided by either the Leadership Collective of the High Court of Cassation and Justice, or the Leadership Collectives of the appeal courts – based on which cases fall under which court's jurisdiction. "Coronavirus COVID-19 outbreak in the EU. Fundamental Rights Implications," Country report, Romania, Human European Consultancy, 23 March 2020, https://fra.europa.eu/sites/default/files/fra_uploads/romania-report-covid-19-april-2020_en.pdf; https://verfassungsblog.de/romania-in-the-covid-era-between-corona-crisis-and-constitutional-crisis/.

54 However, the Decree increased the length and the number of conversations for convicts, and granted detainees the right to online conversations (based on the number of visits to which they were legally entitled to in a non-State of Emergency situation). "Coronavirus COVID-19 outbreak in the EU. Fundamental Rights Implications," Country report, Romania, Human European Consultancy, 23 March 2020, https://fra.europa.eu/sites/default/files/fra_uploads/romania-report-covid-19-april-2020_en.pdf.

55 "2020 Country Reports on Human Rights Practices: Romania," Department of State's Bureau of Democracy, Human Rights, and Labor Report, 30 March 2021, https://www.state.gov/reports/2020-country-reports-on-human-rights-practices/romania/. Additionally, these personnel had limited access to technology to allow them to carry out their activity effectively in the virtual space. Also, see: Cristian Gherasim, "Covid-19: Democracy and rule of law under pressure in EU," *EU Observer*, 29 March 2020, https://euobserver.com/coronavirus/151376.

56 Cristina Lupu, "Romania," in Bican Sahin and Ivaylo Tsonev eds., *Expressing Civil and Political Liberties in Times of Crisis. COVID-19 First Wave as a Case Study: Bulgaria, Greece, North Macedonia, and Romania*, Sofia, Bulgaria: Friedrich Naumann Foundation for Freedom, 2021, 20–25, https://www.freiheit.org/sites/default/files/2021-04/expressing-civil-and-political-liberties-in-times-of-crisis.pdf.

57 Craig Turp-Balazs, "Romania, where Covid-19 restrictions are modest, but people protest anyway," *Emerging Europe*, 30 March 2021, https://emerging-europe.com/from-the-editor/romania-where-covid-19-restrictions-are-modest-but-people-protest-anyway/.

8.2.2 …To a State of Alert: Anachronistic Legislation Meets Ebbing and Flowing Restrictions

On 3 May 2020, the Ombudsman challenged the OUG 21 of 2004, which regulates the SOE, before the Constitutional Court.[58] As an exit strategy, on 15 May 2020, the Romanian Government replaced the SOE with a SOA and notified the European Court of Human Rights (ECHR) on the suspension.[59] In this context, two days before the issuing of the SOA, on 13 May 2020, the Parliament adopted Law 55 of 2020 on the SOA, yet which could not legally enter in effect until 18 May 2020.[60] However, as the State of Exception expired on 14 May 2021, the CNSSU was forced to issue a 30-day SOA using OUG 34 of 2020 – to give the SOA a veneer of legality.[61] On 18 May 2020, when the law on SOA entered into force, a new SOA was issued by the government for entire country for 30 days, via Government Resolution HG 394 of 2020 on the SOA.[62] The measures imposed by the SOA included the following: restrictions of movement outside of the city of

---

58 One of the claims presented by the Ombudsman was that the OUG stipulations pertaining to restrictions imposed during the state of alert (Article 4) were ambiguous and hence could violate fundamental rights. On 13 May 2020, the Court ruled that the disputed act is constitutional as long as the actions and measures implemented did not limit fundamental rights. The Court, nevertheless, indicated that some of the stipulations of the EGO – like, for example, possible evacuation from the affected area – were infringing upon fundamental rights, hence violating Article 115(6) of the Romanian Constitution. Bianca Selejan-Gutan, "Romania in the Covid Era: Between Corona Crisis and Constitutional Crisis," *verfassungsblog*, 21 May 2020, https://verfassungsblog.de/romania-in-the-covid-era-between-corona-crisis-and-constitutional-crisis/; Elena-Simina Tănăsescu and Bogdan Dima, "The Parliament in the time of coronavirus. The Role of the Romanian Parliament during the COVID-19 Sanitary Crisis. A diminishment of the executive decision-making power," 101–111, https://www.robert-schuman.eu/en/doc/ouvrages/FRS_Parliament.pdf; Constitution…Bianca Selejan-Gutan, "Romania in the Covid Era: Between Corona Crisis and Constitutional Crisis," *verfassungsblog*, 21 May 2020, https://verfassungsblog.de/romania-in-the-covid-era-between-corona-crisis-and-constitutional-crisis/.
59 Bianca Selejan-Gutan, "Romania in the Covid Era: Between Corona Crisis and Constitutional Crisis," *verfassungsblog*, 21 May 2020, https://verfassungsblog.de/romania-in-the-covid-era-between-corona-crisis-and-constitutional-crisis/; Cristina Lupu, "Romania," in Bican Sahin and Ivaylo Tsonev eds., *Expressing Civil and Political Liberties in Times of Crisis. COVID-19 First Wave as a Case Study: Bulgaria, Greece, North Macedonia, and Romania*, Sofia, Bulgaria: Friedrich Naumann Foundation for Freedom, 2021, 20–25, https://www.freiheit.org/sites/default/files/2021-04/expressing-civil-and-political-liberties-in-times-of-crisis.pdf.
60 The legal framework requires "two days to allow a request for constitutional review before promulgation and another three days after the publication in the official journal in order to enter into force." Although Law no. 55/2020 was published in the Official Gazette on 15 May, it entered into force on 18 May 2020. Elena-Simina Tănăsescu and Bogdan Dima, "The Parliament in the time of coronavirus. The Role of the Romanian Parliament during the COVID-19 Sanitary Crisis. A diminishment of the executive decision-making power," 101–111, https://www.robert-schuman.eu/en/doc/ouvrages/FRS_Parliament.pdf.
61 Thus, on 15 May 2020, the authorities issued OUG 68 of 2020, which modified OUG 21 of 2020, to allow the government to implement the state of alert until Law 55 of 2020 would enter into force. In line with OUG 68 of 2020, the National Committee for Emergency Situations Decision number 24 on 15 May 2020, which declared a nationwide state of alert; which remained valid until 18 May 2020, when Law 55 of 2020 came into force. On 18 May, the Government issued Decision 394 of 2020 declaring the state of alert at national level for 30 days, which was approved by the Parliament two days later, with minor changes. Elena-Simina Tănăsescu and Bogdan Dima, "The Parliament in the time of coronavirus. The Role of the Romanian Parliament during the COVID-19 Sanitary Crisis. A diminishment of the executive decision-making power," 101–111, https://www.robert-schuman.eu/en/doc/ouvrages/FRS_Parliament.pdf.
62 The Parliament approved it on 20 May 2020. Bianca Selejan-Gutan, "Romania in the Covid Era: Between Corona Crisis and Constitutional Crisis," *verfassungsblog*, 21 May 2020, https://verfassungsblog.de/romania-in-the-covid-era-between-corona-crisis-and-constitutional-crisis/.

residence, mandatory mask wearing in indoor public spaces, and limitations of public gatherings of large[63] group.[64]

The SOA has been renewed every month since May 2020, with several modifications based on the severity of the pandemic. For instance, as cases appeared to plateau by the end of the summer, on 15 September 2020, the government allowed public gatherings of up to 100 persons.[65] In September 2020, schools also reopened.[66] However, on 26 October 2020, as a surge in infection rate occurred once again at the national level,[67] the authorities in Bucharest mandated a second, indefinite, closure of all schools and universities.[68] On 9 November 2020, as new infections, hospitalizations, and deaths continued, the Romanian Government mandated new restrictions. These restrictions

---

63 The government did not forbid all types of public gatherings; concerts, for example, with up to 500 participants, were not banned. "Romania wants to reopen schools after three-month closure – president," *Reuters*, 14 January 2021, https://www.reuters.com/article/us-health-coronavirus-romania/romania-wants-to-reopen-schools-after-three-month-closure-president-idUSKBN29J2AD.

64 The Decree lifted some of the restrictions issued during the SOE. For example, the lockdown was suspended, hair salons and dental practices were allowed to operate, religious services were allowed outdoors, and some hotels, museums, and shopping malls were reopened. Nevertheless, schools were still closed while both indoor and outdoor dining was still not allowed. Access to public and private institutions was permitted only upon a health check, which included a questionnaire and the measurement of the body temperature. Leaving the city of residence was permitted only with a reasonable justification and a signed statement. Individual returning to Romania had to self-quarantine. Bianca Selejan-Gutan, "Romania in the Covid Era: Between Corona Crisis and Constitutional Crisis," *verfassungsblog*, 21 May 2020, https://verfassungsblog.de/romania-in-the-covid-era-between-corona-crisis-and-constitutional-crisis/.

65 "2020 Country Reports on Human Rights Practices: Romania," Department of State's Bureau of Democracy, Human Rights, and Labor Report, 30 March 2021, https://www.state.gov/reports/2020-country-reports-on-human-rights-practices/romania/.

66 "Romania wants to reopen schools after three-month closure – president," *Reuters*, 14 January 2021, https://www.reuters.com/article/us-health-coronavirus-romania/romania-wants-to-reopen-schools-after-three-month-closure-president-idUSKBN29J2AD.

67 Some of these surges occurred due to violations of imposed restrictions. For example, some Orthodox priests kept using the same teaspoon and the same chalice to serve children communion – a common practice pre-pandemic, yet which was banned by the Romanian government and the Holy Synod during the state of alert. Other examples of such violations include frequent participation of citizens – including politicians – in large gatherings, without masks and social distancing. A couple of Parliamentarians ended up fighting with the law enforcement officers, which resulted in the Parliamentarians being subjected to fines. In addition, local state agencies did not impose quarantine equally in other cities, even if the infection rates were equal. The government did not come up with a suitable plan for the winter holidays either. "Arhiepiscopul Teodosie al Tomisului a împărtășit mai mulți copii folosind aceeași linguriță și același potir, sfidând regulile impuse de autorități și de Sfântul Sinod," *HotNews.ro*, 16 May 2020, https://www.hotnews.ro/stiri-coronavirus-24000098-video-arhiepiscoul-teodosie-tomisului-impartasit-mai-multi-copii-folosind-aceeasi-lingurita-acelasi-potir-sfidand-regulile-impuse-autoritati-sfantul-sinod.htm; "Distracție și aglomerație în Vama Veche / Administratorul unei terase, amendat cu 2.000 de lei," *HotNews.ro*, 6 July 2020, https://www.hotnews.ro/stiri-coronavirus-24155738-video-distractie-aglomeratie-vama-veche-administratorul-unei-terase-amendat-2-000-lei.htm; and "Imaginile cu scandalul provocat de cei doi deputați PSD care s-au certat cu polițiștii într-un fast-food din Capitală / Au fost amendați cu 4000 de lei și pentru nepurtarea măștii," HotNews.ro, 7 July 2020, https://www.hotnews.ro/stiri-coronavirus-24158471-cei-doi-deputati-psd-care-certat-politia-intr-fast-food-din-capitala-amendati-4000-lei-pentru-nepurtarea-mastii-initial-fost-amendati-pentru-scandal.htm. On 1 September 2020, indoor dining was allowed, and the number of people who could take part in private events increased to 50 for indoor and 100 for outdoor events. Indoor clubs remained closed. Bianca Selejan-Gutan, "Romania: COVID-19 Response in an Electoral Year. Overview of Legal and Political Response and Adaptation to COVID-19," *verfassiungblog.de*, 26 March 2021, https://verfassungsblog.de/romania-covid-19-response-in-an-electoral-year/.

68 Bianca Selejan-Gutan, "Romania: COVID-19 Response in an Electoral Year. Overview of Legal and Political Response and Adaptation to COVID-19," *verfassiungblog.de*, 26 March 2021, https://verfassungsblog.de/romania-covid-19-response-in-an-electoral-year/.

included a curfew between 11 p.m. and 5 a.m. (with the exception of citizens who were purchasing gas or medicine or authorized home delivery workers), mandatory face masks in both open and closed venues, and the closure of indoor farmers' markets. While not mandated, remote working was encouraged.[69] Schools reopened on 8 February 2021 for the second time during the pandemic, which, along with other causes,[70] resulted in a new soar of infections by early March, and prompted the government to impose stricter measures between 8 March and 13 May 2021. The government imposed a nationwide curfew from 8 p.m. (changed a few time, from the initial 11 pm in early March) until 5 a.m.; mandated store closure at 6 p.m. from Friday to Sunday, in all locations where more than 4 coronavirus cases per 1,000 inhabitants were reported; required restaurants, cafes, movie theaters, and concert halls to operate indoors at 50% capacity; authorized partial opening/closure of schools, based on the number of infections; and required face masks in all public spaces, irrespective of the number of COVID cases.[71]

The government eased several restrictions on 15 May and 1 June 2021, including increasing the number of people who can attend outdoor cultural and entertainment activities from 500 to 1,000 (based on either proof of vaccination or a negative COVID-19 test; or proof of recovery from the

---

69 "DOCUMENT CNSU. Noile restricţii care se aplică în România începând de luni, 9 noiembrie," *Digi24*, 9 November 2020, https://www.digi24.ro/stiri/actualitate/document-cnsu-noile-restrictii-care-se-aplica-in-romania-incepand-de-luni-9-noiembrie-1397314. The government did not postpone the legislative elections that were scheduled for 6 December 2020, which triggered criticism. "Amânarea alegerilor parlamentare. Miză mare şi Covid 19, pretext," *Radio Europa Liberă România*, 6 December 2021, https://romania.europalibera.org/a/amanare-alegeri-parlamentare-2020-6-decembrie/30868508.html; "Iohannis, pledoarie pentru alegeri: 'Democraţia nu poate fi pusă în paranteză, trebuie garantată prin alegeri libere. Ce exemplu mai bun decât SUA?'" *HotNews.ro*, 5 November 2020. https://www.hotnews.ro/stiri-politic-24399834-iohannis-pledoarie-pentru-alegeri-democratia-nu-poate-pusa-paranteza-trebuie-garantata-prin-alegeri-libere-exemplu-mai-bun-decat-sua.htm.
70 The authorities refused to impose stricter restrictions for political and electoral reasons: fear that they would lose both in the local and general elections (on 27 September and, respectively, on 6 December 2020). They delegated restriction-decision-making responsibilities to local authorities, whose response was ineffective. Bianca Selejan-Gutan, "Romania: COVID-19 Response in an Electoral Year. Overview of Legal and Political Response and Adaptation to COVID-19," *verfassiungblog.de*, 26 March 2021, https://verfassungsblog.de/romania-covid-19-response-in-an-electoral-year/.
71 Exceptions included relatives of EEA citizens and residents, persons traveling for essential work or study, transiting travelers, and persons who traveled for emergencies. Individuals arriving from high-risk countries were mandated to provide a negative COVID-19 test taken no more than 72 hours before arrival, followed by 14-day self-quarantine (or 10 days if testing negative eight days after self-quarantine). Persons who had proof of full course of immunization against COVID-19 no less than 10 days prior to their arrival in Romania or tested positive for COVID-19 and recovered in the previous 90 days were also exempt from isolation. The curfew was lifted between 1 and 2 May and 8 and 9 May 2021, to allow Romanians to attend Easter-related services. Despite these restrictions, opposition-run anti-restriction and anti-vaccination protests occurred in the capital and Romania's major cities throughout March 2021. On 30 March 2021, one of the protests in Bucharest became violent as police were attacked by demonstrators defying a curfew – resulting in some 12 injured policemen. Nicoleta Banila, "Romania tightens Covid-19 restrictions to tame surge in Covid-19 cases," *SeeNews*, 26 March 2021, https://seenews.com/news/romania-tightens-covid-19-restrictions-to-tame-surge-in-covid-19-cases-735894; "Romania: Authorities extend COVID-19-related state of alert and constituent restrictions until at least May 12 /update 17," 12 April 2021, https://www.garda.com/crisis24/news-alerts/465801/romania-authorities-extend-covid-19-related-state-of-alert-and-constituent-restrictions-until-at-least-may-12-update-17; "Anti-restriction protests held in Romania as virus surges Anti-restriction protesters have taken to the streets in several Romanian cities against new pandemic measures that came into force a day earlier amid rising COVID-19 infections," *AP*, 29 March 2021, https://abcnews.go.com/International/wireStory/anti-restriction-protests-held-romania-virus-surges-76754456; Bianca Selejan-Gutan, "Romania: COVID-19 Response in an Electoral Year. Overview of Legal and Political Response and Adaptation to COVID-19," *verfassiungblog.de*, 26 March 2021, https://verfassungsblog.de/romania-covid-19-response-in-an-electoral-year/; https://abcnews.go.com/Health/wireStory/latest-sri-lanka-banned-travel-country-77662565; and Craig Turp-Balazs, "Romania, where Covid-19 restrictions are modest, but people protest anyway," *Emerging Europe*, 30 March 2021, https://emerging-europe.com/from-the-editor/romania-where-covid-19-restrictions-are-modest-but-people-protest-anyway/.

disease); permitting events with more than 1,000 people if everybody is showing proof of vaccination; allowing private events such as weddings or baptisms for up to 50 people (indoors) or 70 people (outdoors), and even more if all people are vaccinated; increased the allowed restaurants' indoor seating capacity from 50 to 70% (and more if everybody is vaccinated); allowed the bars and clubs to operate between 05:00 and 24:00, but at a limited capacity of 50% and only for vaccinated people.[72]

8.2.2.1 Vaccination Campaign: Needles for Fangs

Romania started its anti-COVID-19 vaccination on 27 December 2020, and underwent three phases: the first phase (27 December 2020–15 January 2021), for all medical personnel and other health care employees, including pharmacists, and psychologists; the second phase (15 January 2021–15 March 2021), for individuals of 65 and older or persons with grave chronic illnesses, as well as essential workers and first responders (from the education, armed forces employees, law enforcement, and firefighting agencies); and the third phase (15 March 2021-present), for the general population 16 and older.[73] By August 2021, approximately 4.8 million people have been vaccinated with a least one dose.[74]

To boost the vaccination campaign and incentivize the reluctant population to get vaccinated, the central and local government authorities, in collaboration with family doctors, developed several options for vaccination, including online appointments on the government-run platform "Programare.vaccinare-covid.gov.ro," as well as mobile and drive-through vaccination centers, or vaccination events (known as "vaccination marathons") organized at major venues (such as the National Library in Bucharest) in the capital and other big cities.[75] One of the most inventive endeavors to boost immunizations comes from the local government and management of the Bran Castle – associated with Dracula – who tried to lure visitors with a free trip to the "torture chamber" in return for accepting to be vaccinated (also for free). [76] In this connection, Ilie explains: "Doctors and nurses with fang stickers on their scrubs are offering free Pfizer…shots to all-comers at…Bran Castle."[77]

---

72 Irina Marica, "COVID-19: Romania further eases restrictions from June 1," *Romania Insider*, 28 May 2021, https://www.romania-insider.com/romania-further-eases-covid-restrictions.
73 Andrei Chirileasa, "Romania starts anti-COVID vaccination campaign," *Romania Insider*. 28 December 2020, https://www.romania-insider.com/romania-first-vaccines-anti-covid. Since 18 January, individuals who traveled to Romania from red zones became exempt, if they received their second COVID-19 vaccine shot at least 10 days prior to their arrival in Romania; unless they travel to Romania with their unvaccinated children. "Persoanele care au făcut și a doua doză de vaccin nu mai intră în carantină la sosirea în România," 18 January 2021, *Digi24*, https://www.digi24.ro/stiri/actualitate/persoanele-care-au-facut-si-a-doua-doza-de-vaccin-nu-mai-intra-in-carantina-la-sosirea-in-romania-1436300.
74 https://vaccinare-covid.gov.ro/actualizare-zilnica-31-07-evidenta-persoanelor-vaccinate-impotriva-covid-19/. The Romanian authorities sought to vaccinate 5 million people by June 2021 and 10 million by September 2021. According to a survey released in April 2021, Romanians were the most reluctant people of the EU's new members toward getting inoculated with anti-COVID-19 vaccines. "'Dracula's castle' offers tourists Covid shots. Visitors to Bran Castle in Romania offered vaccines – with a free trip to the 'torture chamber' thrown in," *The Guardian*, 10 May 2021, https://www.theguardian.com/world/2021/may/10/dracula-castle-offers-tourists-covid-shots.
75 Irina Marica, "COVID-19: Bucharest has the highest vaccination rate in Romania," *Romania Insider*, 5 May 2021, https://www.romania-insider.com/bucharest-vaccination-rate-may-2021; Luiza Ilie, "Vlad the vaccinator: Dracula's castle lures visitors with COVID-19 jabs," *Reuters*, 8 May 2021, https://www.reuters.com/world/europe/vlad-vaccinator-draculas-castle-lures-visitors-with-covid-19-jabs-2021-05-08/.
76 According to Ilie, "Those who receive the vaccine are handed a certificate hailing their 'boldness and responsibility' promising they will be welcome at the castle 'for the coming 100 years'." Luiza Ilie, "Vlad the vaccinator: Dracula's castle lures visitors with COVID-19 jabs," *Reuters*, 8 May 2021, https://www.reuters.com/world/europe/vlad-vaccinator-draculas-castle-lures-visitors-with-covid-19-jabs-2021-05-08/.
77 Luiza Ilie, "Vlad the vaccinator: Dracula's castle lures visitors with COVID-19 jabs," *Reuters*, 8 May 2021, https://www.reuters.com/world/europe/vlad-vaccinator-draculas-castle-lures-visitors-with-covid-19-jabs-2021-05-08/.

8.2.3 Transparency During the Pandemic: Between Thought Police, Strategic "Mis" Communications, and Conspiracy Theories

Although freedom of expression was not restricted by the government during the SOE, scattered actions by either authorities or some public institutions to silence their personnel or citizens resulted in violations of these freedoms. First, public institutions – such as law enforcement agencies and hospitals – made several attempts to curb their personnel's freedom of speech, and, in turn, citizens' access to information.[78] For instance, as early as March 2020, the central government prohibited local authorities and public health officials from informing the public on the number of completed COVID-19 tests and/or the number of infections in each county.[79] Similarly, after the change of leadership in the Suceava hospital, the hospital issued an administrative order that banned employees, under criminal law, to provide any information to the press.[80]

In parallel, the Romanian Government, along with some public institutions, also banned media's access to information and intimidated journalists and whistle-blowers violated the ban, using penal sanctions for disobedience.[81] Indeed, the Ministry of Internal Affairs (MAI) fired a whistle-blower after he informed the public about the law enforcement agencies' lack of equipment, as well as on the pressure on police officers to give out large amounts of fines during the SOE.[82] Additionally, authorities significantly fined citizens that provided their opinions either through social media platforms, or by placing banners in their windows or balconies that showed that they were against the restrictions.[83] Moreover, the Romanian Government provided unclear or conflicting messaging to the media and ultimately the public. For example, while the Romanian authorities did not

---

78 Cristina Lupu, "Romania," in Bican Sahin and Ivaylo Tsonev eds., *Expressing Civil and Political Liberties in Times of Crisis. COVID-19 first wave as a case study: Bulgaria, Greece, North Macedonia, and Romania*, Sofia, Bulgaria: Friedrich Naumann Foundation for Freedom, 2021, 20-25, https://www.freiheit.org/sites/default/files/2021-04/expressing-civil-and-political-liberties-in-times-of-crisis.pdf.
79 "2020 Country Reports on Human Rights Practices: Romania," Department of State's Bureau of Democracy, Human Rights, and Labor Report, 30 March 2021, https://www.state.gov/reports/2020-country-reports-on-human-rights-practices/romania/. Whistle-blowers would were to be fined or fired. Yet, oddly, some officials posted personal data of self-quarantined persons in their area (including their names and addresses) on their social media networks; like, for example, the mayor of a village in Vaslui county who posted on his Facebook page such information. Cristina Lupu, "Romania," in Bican Sahin and Ivaylo Tsonev eds., *Expressing Civil and Political Liberties in Times of Crisis. COVID-19 first wave as a case study: Bulgaria, Greece, North Macedonia, and Romania*, Sofia, Bulgaria: Friedrich Naumann Foundation for Freedom, 2021, 20–25, https://www.freiheit.org/sites/default/files/2021-04/expressing-civil-and-political-liberties-in-times-of-crisis.pdf; Sandra Mantu, "EU Citizenship, Free Movement, and Covid-19 in Romania," *frontiersin*, 9 December 2020, https://www.frontiersin.org/articles/10.3389/fhumd.2020.594987/full; "Coronavirus COVID-19 outbreak in the EU. Fundamental Rights Implications," Country report, Romania, Human European Consultancy, 23 March 2020, https://fra.europa.eu/sites/default/files/fra_uploads/romania-report-covid-19-april-2020_en.pdf.
80 "2020 Country Reports on Human Rights Practices: Romania," Department of State's Bureau of Democracy, Human Rights, and Labor Report, 30 March 2021, https://www.state.gov/reports/2020-country-reports-on-human-rights-practices/romania/; Cristina Lupu, "Romania," in Bican Sahin and Ivaylo Tsonev eds., *Expressing Civil and Political Liberties in Times of Crisis. COVID-19 first wave as a case study: Bulgaria, Greece, North Macedonia, and Romania*, Sofia, Bulgaria: Friedrich Naumann Foundation for Freedom, 2021, 20–25, https://www.freiheit.org/sites/default/files/2021-04/expressing-civil-and-political-liberties-in-times-of-crisis.pdf.
81 Cristina Lupu, "Romania," in Bican Sahin and Ivaylo Tsonev eds., *Expressing Civil and Political Liberties in Times of Crisis. COVID-19 first wave as a case study: Bulgaria, Greece, North Macedonia, and Romania*, Sofia, Bulgaria: Friedrich Naumann Foundation for Freedom, 2021, 20–25, https://www.freiheit.org/sites/default/files/2021-04/expressing-civil-and-political-liberties-in-times-of-crisis.pdf.
82 MAI would later reconsider the decision. Cristina Lupu, "Romania," in Bican Sahin and Ivaylo Tsonev eds., *Expressing Civil and Political Liberties in Times of Crisis. COVID-19 first wave as a case study: Bulgaria, Greece, North Macedonia, and Romania*, Sofia, Bulgaria: Friedrich Naumann Foundation for Freedom, 2021, 20–25, https://www.freiheit.org/sites/default/files/2021-04/expressing-civil-and-political-liberties-in-times-of-crisis.pdf.
83 A student from Cluj received a 1,000 RON fine (approximately $210) for complaining about the way her mayor managed the COVID-19 pandemic. "2020 Country Reports on Human Rights Practices: Romania," Department of

suspend the right of protest during the SOE, the government did not clearly inform the citizens on the right of protest, and consequently many Romanians thought that the right of assembly and of protest was suspended.[84] Likewise, while the government decided to – and announced that it would – postpone elections,[85] it did not provide clear information on how coronavirus-infected patients or quarantined citizens would actually vote.[86] On 5 April 2020, the Prime Minister publically contradicted the Deputy Minister of Health Raed Arafat, who used his official Facebook page to raise awareness on the need to use masks, including the homemade types.[87] Additionally, despite vaccination campaigns, outreach to citizens who did not know how to access information related to immunization against COVID-19, or lack access to vaccination information altogether, was minimal.[88] Occasionally, the Romanian authorities simply failed to inform the citizens on imposing COVID-19-related restrictions.[89]

Following carping criticism from civil society groups, in April 2020, the government established a Strategic Communications Task Force to manage strategic communications, including expanding daily reports to include county-level breakdowns.[90] Yet, the situation did not improve. The Task

---

State's Bureau of Democracy, Human Rights, and Labor Report, 30 March 2021, https://www.state.gov/reports/2020-country-reports-on-human-rights-practices/romania/.

84 Cristina Lupu, "Romania," in Bican Sahin and Ivaylo Tsonev eds., *Expressing Civil and Political Liberties in Times of Crisis. COVID-19 first wave as a case study: Bulgaria, Greece, North Macedonia, and Romania*, Sofia, Bulgaria: Friedrich Naumann Foundation for Freedom, 2021, 20–25, https://www.freiheit.org/sites/default/files/2021-04/expressing-civil-and-political-liberties-in-times-of-crisis.pdf.

85 The Parliament adopted specific measures regarding the upcoming elections, like, for example, delaying local elections that were supposed to be held in June 2020. Bianca Selejan-Gutan, "Romania: COVID-19 Response in an Electoral Year. Overview of Legal and Political Response and Adaptation to COVID-19," *verfassiungblog.de*, 26 March 2021, https://verfassungsblog.de/romania-covid-19-response-in-an-electoral-year/.

86 In a non-pandemic context, hospitalized patients would vote via a mobile voting booth. Cristina Lupu, "Romania," in Bican Sahin and Ivaylo Tsonev eds., *Expressing Civil and Political Liberties in Times of Crisis. COVID-19 first wave as a case study: Bulgaria, Greece, North Macedonia, and Romania*, Sofia, Bulgaria: Friedrich Naumann Foundation for Freedom, 2021, 20–25, https://www.freiheit.org/sites/default/files/2021-04/expressing-civil-and-political-liberties-in-times-of-crisis.pdf.

87 Prime Minister Orban contradicted Arafat, casting doubts on the hygiene of these masks. "Arafat: Nu este nevoie de masca medicală că să va protejați, puteți improviza," *HotNews.ro*, 5 April 2020, https://www.hotnews.ro/stiri-coronavirus-23790826-arafat-masca-medicala-protejare-coronavirus.htm; "Orban, despre legile cu privire la purtarea măştilor: Nu poţi să impui obligativitate cât timp nu sunt accesibile pentru cetăţeni," *Digi24*, 5 April 2020, https://www.digi24.ro/stiri/actualitate/sanatate/orban-despre-legile-cu-privire-la-purtarea-mastilor-nu-poti-sa-impui-obligativitate-cat-timp-nu-sunt-accesibile-pentru-cetateni-1287155.

88 Like, for example, Maria Coanda, an 81-year-old woman from a southern Romanian village who suffered from a heart illness, who, after three months since she became eligible for vaccination, was not vaccinated, because she was not aware how to register for it online. Nor did she get any assistance or guidance from her doctor. Many older people with medical conditions were in her situation. Luiza Ilie, "Vulnerable Romanians left behind in COVID-19 vaccine push," *Reuters*, 30 March 2021, https://www.reuters.com/article/us-health-coronavirus-romania-vaccine/vulnerable-romanians-left-behind-in-covid-19-vaccine-push-idUSKBN2BM0ZC.

89 For instance, the government informed the Council of Europe on the activation of ECHR State of Emergency clause, but not the Romanian public, which only learned about it on 19 March 2020, from *France Press*. Similarly, authorities failed to consider – and properly communicate – the psychological effects of the pandemic. For example, advising population on medical issues was not accompanied by a psychological component, which would inform the citizens on how to accept advice and how to implement advice in their day-to-day behavior. Also, some recommendations, like, for instance, pleas to remain calm, were wrong, as they invalidated normal psychological reactions (worry, sadness, and unhappiness) in these circumstances. Bianca Selejan-Gutan, "Romania in the Covid Era: Between Corona Crisis and Constitutional Crisis," *verfassungsblog*, 21 May 2020, https://verfassungsblog.de/romania-in-the-covid-era-between-corona-crisis-and-constitutional-crisis/; "Un an de pandemie în România. O analiză psihologică de Daniel David: Lipsa componentei de psihologie în demersurile publice – o mare greșeală," *Revistasinteza*, 3 March 2021, https://www.revistasinteza.ro/un-an-de-pandemie-in-romania-o-analiza-psihologica-de-daniel-david-lipsa-componentei-de-psihologie-in-demersurile-publice-o-mare-greseala.

90 "2020 Country Reports on Human Rights Practices: Romania," Department of State's Bureau of Democracy, Human Rights, and Labor Report, 30 March 2021, https://www.state.gov/reports/2020-country-reports-on-human-rights-practices/romania/.

Force, for one – whose membership remained shrouded in secrecy – was the only body that could inform the public on any COVID-19 pandemic-related issues.[91] In addition, during the SOE, most of the communication still occurred via press statements, without any questions allowed from the media.[92]

Furthermore, the Romanian authorities did not effectively fight fake news, conspiracy theories, misinformation, and disinformation – which Romanians tend to fall victim to all too easily. Some of these campaigns were domestic in nature, mostly targeting members of the Romanian diaspora who returned home. As Mantu notes, "Fear of a mass exodus of Romanians returning from Italy and bringing with them the virus started to influence public opinion leading to a wave of hate towards them."[93] In the immediate aftermath of the pandemic outbreak, news providing false information on potential restrictions, school closing or reopening, or deaths – which were eventually debunked – were quite common.[94] Some of these campaigns were developed by external actors (including Russia), aimed at instilling distrust in Romania's government institutions.[95] While the government attempted to limit access to webpages or websites that transmitted false COVID-19-related data and information, it was not entirely successful in this effort. For example, while in March 2020 the country's telecommunications regulator limited access to 15 websites, it reinstated access by May.[96]

---

91 Cristina Lupu, "Romania," in Bican Sahin and Ivaylo Tsonev eds., *Expressing Civil and Political Liberties in Times of Crisis. COVID-19 first wave as a case study: Bulgaria, Greece, North Macedonia, and Romania*, Sofia, Bulgaria: Friedrich Naumann Foundation for Freedom, 2021, 20–25, https://www.freiheit.org/sites/default/files/2021-04/expressing-civil-and-political-liberties-in-times-of-crisis.pdf.
92 Local press thus was virtually unable to corroborate the received data and provide the public with accurate information. Cristina Lupu, "Romania," in Bican Sahin and Ivaylo Tsonev eds., *Expressing Civil and Political Liberties in Times of Crisis. COVID-19 first wave as a case study: Bulgaria, Greece, North Macedonia, and Romania*, Sofia, Bulgaria: Friedrich Naumann Foundation for Freedom, 2021, 20–25, https://www.freiheit.org/sites/default/files/2021-04/expressing-civil-and-political-liberties-in-times-of-crisis.pdf.
93 Sandra Mantu, "EU Citizenship, Free Movement, and Covid-19 in Romania," *frontiersin*, 9 December 2020, https://www.frontiersin.org/articles/10.3389/fhumd.2020.594987/full; "Coronavirus COVID-19 outbreak in the EU. Fundamental Rights Implications," Country report, Romania, Human European Consultancy, 23 March 2020, https://fra.europa.eu/sites/default/files/fra_uploads/romania-report-covid-19-april-2020_en.pdf;"2020 Country Reports on Human Rights Practices: Romania," Department of State's Bureau of Democracy, Human Rights, and Labor Report, 30 March 2021, https://www.state.gov/reports/2020-country-reports-on-human-rights-practices/romania/.
94 On 16 March 2020, the President issued an Emergency Decree that empowered authorities to eliminate, report, or close websites spreading fake news about the pandemic, with no possibility to appeal. "The struggle with coronavirus and Russian disinformation in Romania," *Warsaw Institute*, 25 April 2020, https://warsawinstitute .review/interviews/romania-a-struggle-with-coronavirus-and-russian-disinformation/; Amnesty International Report 2020/21 (PDF). London: Amnesty International. 2021. p. 301. ISBN 978-0-86210-501-3; "COVID-19 has served as the pretext for widespread surveillance," https://www.europeandatajournalism.eu/eng/News/Data-news/COVID-19-has-served-as-the-pretext-for-widespread-surveillance; Sanja Jovičić, "COVID-19 restrictions on human rights in the light of the case-law of the European Court of Human Rights." *ERA Forum* 21, 545–560 (2021). https://doi.org/10.1007/s12027-020-00630-w, https://link.springer.com/article/10.1007/s12027-020-00630-w; Daniela Budu, "Ombudsman's report on pandemic," Radio Romania International, 17 September 2020, https://www.rri.ro/en_gb/ombudsmans_report_on_pandemic-2623368; and Cristina Buzașu and Pawel Marczewski, "Confrontation Versus Cooperation in Polish and Romanian Civil Society," *Carnegie Europe*, 7 December 2020, https://carnegieeurope.eu/2020/12/07/confrontation-versus-cooperation-in-polish-and-romanian-civil-society-pub-83146.
95 In this connection, Walkowicz notes: "Coronavirus is just a simple flu and should be ignored" – one example is a video that was posted online of a presumed "professor" explaining how the current crisis is nothing more than unjustified panic, as there are already a lot of annual deaths resulting from seasonal flus… [and]…You can treat "coronavirus using x and y products." All this information was false and easily debunked. "The struggle with coronavirus and Russian disinformation in Romania," *Warsaw Institute*, 25 April 2020, https://warsawinstitute .review/interviews/romania-a-struggle-with-coronavirus-and-russian-disinformation/.
96 https://freedomhouse.org/country/romania/freedom-world/2021.

Overall, the pandemic did not justify the authorities' attempts to limit access to information and/or freedom of expression; rather, these limitations negatively affected the trade-off between health security and democracy, because these limitations "prevented the public from learning about the problems in due time and thus stripped them of the opportunity to ask their government to solve them."[97] These perfunctory decisions and measures further diminished the already very limited public trust in government.

8.2.3.1 Civil Society: A Tamed yet Clamorous Cerberus?

The pandemic seems to have brought the government and civil society closer together. On the one hand, the government conducted numerous public consultations with employee associations, think tanks, and nongovernmental organizations (NGOs), thus capitalizing on civil society's input and buy-in in the development and implementation of socioeconomic measures and in creating a comprehensive plan to relaunch the economy.[98] To this end, in February 2020, the government's reinstated the Department for Cooperation with the Associative Environment, which is the government's liaison institution with civil society.[99] On the other hand, unlike the situation in some other countries, Romania's civil society was very keen in collaborating[100] with the local and central authorities not only by providing feedback to authorities' proposed measures, but also by carrying out humanitarian assistance and disaster relief actions. Indeed, according to Cristina Buzașu and Pawel Marczewski, "Many nongovernmental organizations…, including those that focus on democracy and governance issues…redirected their activities to service delivery to help provide medical supplies and a wide variety of social services, particularly for disadvantaged and vulnerable people."[101] In this connection, various NGOs and think tanks conducted fundraising campaigns aimed at purchasing medical equipment and supplies, including protective gear for the health-care personnel. For example, Red Cross Romania organized fundraisers and campaigns aimed at raising COVID awareness-related campaigns among citizens and fighting disinformation

---

97 "2020 Country Reports on Human Rights Practices: Romania," Department of State's Bureau of Democracy, Human Rights, and Labor Report, 30 March 2021, https://www.state.gov/reports/2020-country-reports-on-human-rights-practices/romania/.
98 Cristina Buzașu and Pawel Marczewski, "Confrontation Versus Cooperation in Polish and Romanian Civil Society," *Carnegie Europe*, 7 December 2020, https://carnegieeurope.eu/2020/12/07/confrontation-versus-cooperation-in-polish-and-romanian-civil-society-pub-83146.
99 https://sgg.gov.ro/1/despre-serviciul-politici-de-cooperare-cu-mediul-asociativ/; "Serviciul Politici de Cooperare cu Mediul Asociativ înființat prin Ordinul 410/2020 în cadrul Secretariatului General al Guvernului," *stiri.org*, 20 April 2020, https://www.stiri.ong/institutii-si-legislatie/romania/serviciul-politici-de-cooperare-cu-mediul-asociativ-infiintat-prin-ordinul-4102020-in-cadrul-secretariatului-general-al-guvernului; and Cristina Buzașu and Pawel Marczewski, "Confrontation Versus Cooperation in Polish and Romanian Civil Society," *Carnegie Europe*, 7 December 2020, https://carnegieeurope.eu/2020/12/07/confrontation-versus-cooperation-in-polish-and-romanian-civil-society-pub-83146.
100 This spirit of collaboration was an abrupt departure, Buzașu and Marczewski note, "from the confrontational relationship between Romania's previous social democratic government and civil society, which focused during much of the 2010s on fighting corruption and upholding the rule of law and the independence of the justice system. ..[Even if] some watchdog organizations have drawn attention to the corruption that lies at the root of the poor functioning of the medical system and insufficient sanitary supplies and hospital staff in the context of the pandemic …[everybody more or less agreed that the situation was the result of] three decades of poor governance in the country." Cristina Buzașu and Pawel Marczewski, "Confrontation Versus Cooperation in Polish and Romanian Civil Society," *Carnegie Europe*, 7 December 2020, https://carnegieeurope.eu/2020/12/07/confrontation-versus-cooperation-in-polish-and-romanian-civil-society-pub-83146.
101 Cristina Buzașu and Pawel Marczewski, "Confrontation Versus Cooperation in Polish and Romanian Civil Society," *Carnegie Europe*, 7 December 2020, https://carnegieeurope.eu/2020/12/07/confrontation-versus-cooperation-in-polish-and-romanian-civil-society-pub-83146.

and misinformation related to the virus.[102] The NGO donated all collected funds toward procurement of equipment for hospitals and personnel, and toward the construction of a modular hospital dedicated to severe COVID cases.[103] In addition, civil society organizations informally offered psychological support to citizens.[104] Civil society organizations also supported the government's delay of elections from June 2020 to 27 September 2020. Specifically, civil society components provided explicit recommendations on how to conduct elections during the pandemic – including "increasing the number of days for voting, introducing additional hygiene measures, and reorganizing polling stations" – which the authorities used.[105] In sum, the network of networks of civil society groups, which acted as a bridge between the government and the people, helped improve first responders and medical staff's capabilities to respond to the COVID-19 crisis.[106]

Nonetheless, civil society organizations did not neglect their watchdog function. The Ombudsman and several Human Rights Groups, in particular, sounded alarms with regard to allegations of restrictions of fundamental rights and liberties during the states of emergency and alert. These organizations brought their allegations before the Constitutional Court, which had to exercise its judicial review role several times. One of the first examples of this was the Ombudsman's challenge of the legal framework pertaining to the SOE, and of the Presidential Decree and the emergency measures before the Constitutional Court, which the Ombudsman viewed as violating the principles of separation of powers and of the rule of law provided by the Romanian Constitution, as well as of citizens' fundamental rights.[107] Indeed, on 6 May 2020, upon a request forwarded by the Ombudsman, the Constitutional Court ruled via Decision no. 152 of 2020 that OUG 34 of 2020, which raised the fines for the administrative offences against the government restrictions committed during the SOE was "wholly unconstitutional."[108] Similarly, the Ombudsman notified the

---

102 Cristina Buzașu and Pawel Marczewski, "Confrontation Versus Cooperation in Polish and Romanian Civil Society," *Carnegie Europe*, 7 December 2020, https://carnegieeurope.eu/2020/12/07/confrontation-versus-cooperation-in-polish-and-romanian-civil-society-pub-83146.

103 According to Buzașu and Pawel Marczewski, civil society organizations "provided hospitals with medical equipment worth over $16 million." Cristina Buzașu and Pawel Marczewski, "Confrontation Versus Cooperation in Polish and Romanian Civil Society," *Carnegie Europe*, 7 December 2020, https://carnegieeurope.eu/2020/12/07/confrontation-versus-cooperation-in-polish-and-romanian-civil-society-pub-83146. "The groups raised money to buy more than 115 ventilators, 21 polymerase chain reaction (PCR) testing devices, 30,000 PCR tests, seventy monitors, and another 60,000 medical devices. More than 1.5 million surgical masks and almost 500,000 filter masks have reached medical units throughout Romania." Cristina Buzașu and Pawel Marczewski, "Confrontation Versus Cooperation in Polish and Romanian Civil Society," *Carnegie Europe*, 7 December 2020, https://carnegieeurope.eu/2020/12/07/confrontation-versus-cooperation-in-polish-and-romanian-civil-society-pub-83146.

104 The Association of Psychologists of Romania offered psychological guidance via their website throughout the pandemic. "Un an de pandemie în România. O analiză psihologică de Daniel David: Lipsa componentei de psihologie în demersurile publice – o mare greșeală," *Revistasinteza*, 3 March 2021, https://www.revistasinteza.ro/un-an-de-pandemie-in-romania-o-analiza-psihologica-de-daniel-david-lipsa-componentei-de-psihologie-in-demersurile-publice-o-mare-greseala.

105 Cristina Buzașu and Pawel Marczewski, "Confrontation Versus Cooperation in Polish and Romanian Civil Society," *Carnegie Europe*, 7 December 2020, https://carnegieeurope.eu/2020/12/07/confrontation-versus-cooperation-in-polish-and-romanian-civil-society-pub-83146.

106 It should be noted that civil society groups were not supporting the opposition in their attempts to discredit government's Cristina Buzașu and Pawel Marczewski, "Confrontation Versus Cooperation in Polish and Romanian Civil Society," *Carnegie Europe*, 7 December 2020, https://carnegieeurope.eu/2020/12/07/confrontation-versus-cooperation-in-polish-and-romanian-civil-society-pub-83146.

107 The Constitutional Court dismissed the claims of unconstitutionality, noting that the majority of the restrictions were imposed in line with the law. Bianca Selejan-Gutan, "Romania in the Covid Era: Between Corona Crisis and Constitutional Crisis," *verfassungsblog*, 21 May 2020, https://verfassungsblog.de/romania-in-the-covid-era-between-corona-crisis-and-constitutional-crisis/.

108 The Court opined that the government has violated the "'constitutional limits of legislative delegation,' i.e. the impugned ordinance 'affected' fundamental rights, which is expressly prohibited by Article 115(6) of the Constitution." Critics argued that the Constitutional Court's decision was excessive, noting that while some of OUG

Constitutional Court that the Parliament could not approve or review Law 55 of 2020 – "a legally adopted administrative act issued by the Government" – because it would violate separation of powers principle; on 25 June 2020, the Constitutional Court issued Decision 457, which eliminated the obligatory approval within three days by Parliament of a Government's Decision enforcing the Law 55 of 2020, so all ensuing Government's Decisions that extended the SOA for consecutive 30-day periods were no longer approved by Parliament.[109] Likewise, upon a request put forward on 18 June 2020 by the Ombudsman, the Constitutional Court ruled on 25 June 2020, via Decision 458 that the Decision that empowered the Minister of Health to authorize "preventive" mandatory hospitalization and quarantines – a measure that only Romania took among the rest of the EU members – was unconstitutional.[110] In sum, both the Ombudsman and the Judicial Branch did their best to act as checks on the Executive Branch.

8.2.4 A "Plagued" Executive–Legislative–Judiciary Trifecta

The relationship between the three branches of government was more adversarial than collaborative. The executive–legislative relationship suffered from political squabbling. Hoping to win the upcoming elections, the opposition, which had a majority in the legislature, left the government more or less alone in the fight against coronavirus, while scolding the executive branch in the Parliament, and challenging several decisions to the Constitutional Court.[111] In parallel, the government, the President, and the opposition in the legislature did not miss any opportunity to obstruct or delay the laws adopted by the majority in the Parliament.[112] Occasionally, however, extreme circumstances prompted both branches of the government to reach a compromise. For example, the legislative branch approval of regulations pertaining to the SOE Decree of the President (of March and, respectively, April 2020); and reviewed and adopted Law 55 of 2020, and Law 136 of 2020

34/2020's stipulations failed to observe the principle of proportionality (like, for example, the maximum amount of the fines), it should not have been declared fully unconstitutional. On the other hand, the Court would rule some administrative fines established by emergency ordinances as constitutional. Bianca Selejan-Gutan, "Romania in the Covid Era: Between Corona Crisis and Constitutional Crisis," *verfassungsblog*, 21 May 2020, https://verfassungsblog .de/romania-in-the-covid-era-between-corona-crisis-and-constitutional-crisis/.

109 http://legislatie.just.ro/Public/DetaliiDocumentAfis/227535; Elena-Simina Tănăsescu and Bogdan Dima, "The Parliament in the time of coronavirus. The Role of the Romanian Parliament during the COVID-19 Sanitary Crisis. A diminishment of the executive decision-making power," 101–111, https://www.robert-schuman.eu/en/doc/ ouvrages/FRS_Parliament.pdf.

110 http://legislatie.just.ro/Public/DetaliiDocumentAfis/227548. The Constitutional Court argued that compulsory hospitalization and quarantine deprived Romanians of freedom, while the courses of actions lacked clarity and predictability, which violated the law. Consequently, hospitals started to discharge patients – with or without symptoms – upon request. "2020 Country Reports on Human Rights Practices: Romania," Department of State's Bureau of Democracy, Human Rights, and Labor Report, 30 March 2021, https://www.state.gov/reports/2020-country-reports-on-human-rights-practices/romania/; and Cristina Lupu, "Romania," in Bican Sahin and Ivaylo Tsonev eds., *Expressing Civil and Political Liberties in Times of Crisis. COVID-19 first wave as a case study: Bulgaria, Greece, North Macedonia, and Romania*, Sofia, Bulgaria: Friedrich Naumann Foundation for Freedom, 2021, 20–25, https://www.freiheit.org/sites/default/files/2021-04/expressing-civil-and-political-liberties-in-times-of-crisis.pdf. https://freedomhouse.org/country/romania/freedom-world/2021.

111 Not always did the Constitutional Court rule to increase legislative oversight on government decisions. For example, the Constitutional Court ruled in June 2020 that that the government could extend the SOA without legislative approval. Cristina Lupu, "Romania," in Bican Sahin and Ivaylo Tsonev eds., *Expressing Civil and Political Liberties in Times of Crisis. COVID-19 first wave as a case study: Bulgaria, Greece, North Macedonia, and Romania*, Sofia, Bulgaria: Friedrich Naumann Foundation for Freedom, 2021, 20–25, https://www.freiheit.org/sites/default/ files/2021-04/expressing-civil-and-political-liberties-in-times-of-crisis.pdf.

112 Elena-Simina Tănăsescu and Bogdan Dima, "The Parliament in the time of coronavirus. The Role of the Romanian Parliament during the COVID-19 Sanitary Crisis. A diminishment of the executive decision-making power," 101–111, https://www.robert-schuman.eu/en/doc/ouvrages/FRS_Parliament.pdf.

on public health measures.[113] Yet, ultimately, as Tănăsescu and Dima note, "The power relations between the executive and the legislative branches of government during the State of Emergency and the State of Alert could be characterized as a mutual gridlock."[114]

The relationship between the executive and judicial branches was also tense during the pandemic. On the one hand, the Constitutional Court ruled unconstitutional either parts or whole decisions issued during the pandemic. On the other hand, tensions between the Executive and Judicial branches also emerged because executive branch leadership would disagree with the Court's decisions. For example, the Prime Minister publicly blasted all of the decisions made by the Constitutional Court, while occasionally "suggesting" that Romanians disregard the Court – a direct affront to the checks-and-balances principles and processes of democratic consolidation.[115] In addition, politicization of the Constitutional Court occurred during the pandemic. For example, occasionally, the Court would become involved in conflicts between political opponents and took decisions on "legal" matters that had a high political importance. For example, the Constitutional Court's decision on the administrative fines, etc., reduced the effectiveness of the measures taken by the government to combat the pandemic. In parallel, after its adoption, the law enforcement personnel became less inclined to fine people, after the ruling of Constitutional Court on fines in June 2020 – which unfortunately emboldened Romanians to defy the existing restrictions.[116] In addition, occasionally, the Constitutional Court appears to have used and abused "the Constitution in interpretations that blatantly contradict the previous case-law."[117]

The relationship between the central government and the local authorities was in general good. What was challenging in this relationship is the fact that the central government more often than not put the pandemic decision-making burden on the local governments (like, for example, closing public spaces, banning movement, and mandating mask wearing) – which resulted in inadequate measures, which occasionally resulted in unnecessary infections.[118] Had the central government

---

113 Bianca Selejan-Gutan, "Romania: COVID-19 Response in an Electoral Year. Overview of Legal and Political Response and Adaptation to COVID-19," *verfassiungblog.de*, 26 March 2021, https://verfassungsblog.de/romania-covid-19-response-in-an-electoral-year/; Elena-Simina Tănăsescu and Bogdan Dima, "The Parliament in the time of coronavirus. The Role of the Romanian Parliament during the COVID-19 Sanitary Crisis. A diminishment of the executive decision-making power," 101–111, https://www.robert-schuman.eu/en/doc/ouvrages/FRS_Parliament .pdf.
114 Elena-Simina Tănăsescu and Bogdan Dima, "The Parliament in the time of coronavirus. The Role of the Romanian Parliament during the COVID-19 Sanitary Crisis. A diminishment of the executive decision-making power," 101–111, https://www.robert-schuman.eu/en/doc/ouvrages/FRS_Parliament.pdf.
115 Cristina Lupu, "Romania," in Bican Sahin and Ivaylo Tsonev eds., *Expressing Civil and Political Liberties in Times of Crisis. COVID-19 first wave as a case study: Bulgaria, Greece, North Macedonia, and Romania*, Sofia, Bulgaria: Friedrich Naumann Foundation for Freedom, 2021, 20–25, https://www.freiheit.org/sites/default/files/ 2021-04/expressing-civil-and-political-liberties-in-times-of-crisis.pdf.
116 Bianca Selejan-Gutan, "Romania in the Covid Era: Between Corona Crisis and Constitutional Crisis," *verfassungsblog*, 21 May 2020, https://verfassungsblog.de/romania-in-the-covid-era-between-corona-crisis-and-constitutional-crisis/.
117 Bianca Selejan-Gutan, "Romania in the Covid Era: Between Corona Crisis and Constitutional Crisis," *verfassungsblog*, 21 May 2020, https://verfassungsblog.de/romania-in-the-covid-era-between-corona-crisis-and-constitutional-crisis/.
118 The local authorities based their decisions on testing results. However, not all counties conducted the same number of tests daily. For example, the authorities of those counties that tested a higher number of citizens (like, for example, Cluj and Alba) imposed stricter movement restrictions, while those in counties that did less tests (like, for example, Olt and Călărași), did not. As a result, some citizens of the counties with less testing who worked in other counties and were allowed to commute for work (including in counties with high risk of infection), became infected. Dan Tăpălagă, "Schimbați urgent mecanismul defect prin care autoritățile locale impun restricții / Guvernul Orban trebuie să-și asume decizia politică în plină criză sanitară," 29 October 2020, https://www.g4media .ro/schimbati-urgent-mecanismul-defect-prin-care-autoritatile-locale-impun-restrictii-guvernul-orban-trebuie-sa-si-asume-decizia-politica-in-plina-criza-sanitara.html.

been more assertive in imposing similar standards to local governments for their decision-making process, the number of infections may have been reduced. In this connection, what Cernicova-Buca and Palea emphasized vis-à-vis the post-Communist central–local government relationship in general, applies to the pandemic: "The reform of public services in Romania, carried out in the post-communist period, shifted competencies from the central government towards local/regional bodies, but studies show that the burden is perceived at times as overwhelming."[119]

In sum, relationship between the three democratic pillars was plagued by political infighting and politicization of the Constitutional Court, and affected the freedoms and rights of citizens.

8.3 Conclusion: Civil Liberties and Freedoms

Romania implemented long-lasting and very restrictive anti-COVID measures, which constrained such human rights and liberties as freedom of association, freedom of movement, right of education, and freedom/right to vote.[120] While the majority was justified by the severity of the pandemic effects throughout the country, several instances of infringement upon civil liberties and rights were caused by questionable or confusing – or even controversial – decision-making.[121]

To begin with, the first COVID-19 measures took place on a background of political uncertainty amid political turmoil, coupled with a state of confusion vis-à-vis the magnitude of the pandemic threat to public health and human security. In this connection, Selejan-Gutan notes that "In February-March 2020, the government and the President were looking for a solution in order to initiate the procedure for early elections and at the very first moments of the pandemic the country had an interim government after a motion of censure had passed."[122] On the other hand, concerned with the possibility of losing the upcoming elections, the authorities preferred not to impose strict measures when they should have, which led to in a rapid soaring in the number of infections.[123] For example the Government eased some restrictions during the SOE (allowing protests) but, paradoxically, imposed unnecessary restrictions during the SOA (banning protests).[124] In sum, as Selejan-Gutan highlights, "the restrictions, based on the Presidential Decree, of the access to justice; the confusion on the State of Alert and the adoption of a new

---

119 Mariana Cernicova-Buca and Adina Palea, "An Appraisal of Communication Practices Demonstrated by Romanian District Public Health Authorities at the Outbreak of the COVID-19 Pandemic," *Sustainability* 2021, 13, 2500, pp. 1–19, https://doi.org/10.3390/su13052500.
120 Due to the lack of possibility to vote by mail or electronically.
121 The constitution only permits the constraining of rights and liberties for a limited period of time. Daniela Budu, "Ombudsman's report on pandemic," *Radio Romania International*, 17 September 2020, https://www.rri.ro/en_gb/ombudsmans_report_on_pandemic-2623368; Bianca Selejan-Gutan, "Romania: COVID-19 Response in an Electoral Year. Overview of Legal and Political Response and Adaptation to COVID-19," *verfassiungblog.de*, 26 March 2021, https://verfassungsblog.de/romania-covid-19-response-in-an-electoral-year/; https://link.springer.com/article/10.1007/s12027-020-00630-w.
122 Bianca Selejan-Gutan, "Romania: COVID-19 Response in an Electoral Year. Overview of Legal and Political Response and Adaptation to COVID-19," *verfassiungblog.de*, 26 March 2021, https://verfassungsblog.de/romania-covid-19-response-in-an-electoral-year/.
123 Cristina Lupu, "Romania," in Bican Sahin and Ivaylo Tsonev eds., *Expressing Civil and Political Liberties in Times of Crisis. COVID-19 first wave as a case study: Bulgaria, Greece, North Macedonia, and Romania*, Sofia, Bulgaria: Friedrich Naumann Foundation for Freedom, 2021, 20–25, https://www.freiheit.org/sites/default/files/2021-04/expressing-civil-and-political-liberties-in-times-of-crisis.pdf.
124 Cristina Lupu, "Romania," in Bican Sahin and Ivaylo Tsonev eds., *Expressing Civil and Political Liberties in Times of Crisis. COVID-19 first wave as a case study: Bulgaria, Greece, North Macedonia, and Romania*, Sofia, Bulgaria: Friedrich Naumann Foundation for Freedom, 2021, 20–25, https://www.freiheit.org/sites/default/files/2021-04/expressing-civil-and-political-liberties-in-times-of-crisis.pdf.

law as a 'last resort,' thus transforming the State of Alert into a 'parallel' State of Emergency, not provided by the Constitution…"[125]

Additionally, some of the government's decisions lacked a clear roadmap or plan. The closure/opening of schools is a clear example. The first school closure was sudden, and occurred in a vacuum – without any strategic vision or plan. For instance, the Ministry of Education urged teachers and professors to teach virtually, but did not provide any guidance or support to education institutions across the country – which negatively affected students from vulnerable groups, in particular students from low-income families, who could not afford internet access.[126] The return to school decision also took place without a plan – to include, at the minimum, ensuring that regular COVID testing takes place. The lack of testing capacity coupled with a strained medical system throughout the country resulted in additional unnecessary restrictions – which, in turn, limited the right to education.[127] Another example of lack of vision or plan involves the right to access to justice. Despite the fact that Presidential Decrees allowed cases referring to the SOE to continue, the government did not change the legal framework that allowed citizens to seek justice or expedite the existing processes or trials. As Lupu notes, "These limitations affected the right to justice of citizens, making the justice process even longer than normal in Romania, where trials are already considered too slow."[128]

Unsurprisingly, the government's contradictory regulations affected human rights and freedoms. For instance, Presidential Decree 195 of 16 March 2020, and the ensuing military ordinances infringed upon the right of liberty, as the Decree did not differentiate between the two separate rights – the freedom of movement and the right of liberty – and, therefore, everybody was virtually banned from leaving their homes.[129] Likewise, several measures adopted by the Romanian government – such as, for example, forced admission into hospitals – violated the right to personal liberty, stipulated by Article 5 of the European Convention for Human Rights.[130] Similarly, measures related to freedom of assembly were faulty. For example, interdiction of protests during the SOA was inconsistent and unjustified – because, on the one hand, these demonstrations happened in open areas and during which protesters observe the social distancing measures; and, on the other hand, other types of public gatherings like open air concerts of less than 500 people were not

---

125 Bianca Selejan-Gutan, "Romania in the Covid Era: Between Corona Crisis and Constitutional Crisis," *verfassungsblog*, 21 May 2020, https://verfassungsblog.de/romania-in-the-covid-era-between-corona-crisis-and-constitutional-crisis/.
126 "Coronavirus COVID-19 outbreak in the EU. Fundamental Rights Implications," Country report, Romania, Human European Consultancy, 23 March 2020, https://fra.europa.eu/sites/default/files/fra_uploads/romania-report-covid-19-april-2020_en.pdf.
127 In addition, the quality of education plummeted since 2019. "Romania wants to reopen schools after three-month closure – president," *Reuters*, 14 January 2021, https://www.reuters.com/article/us-health-coronavirus-romania/romania-wants-to-reopen-schools-after-three-month-closure-president-idUSKBN29J2AD.
128 Cristina Lupu, "Romania," in Bican Sahin and Ivaylo Tsonev eds., *Expressing Civil and Political Liberties in Times of Crisis. COVID-19 first wave as a case study: Bulgaria, Greece, North Macedonia, and Romania*, Sofia, Bulgaria: Friedrich Naumann Foundation for Freedom, 2021, 20–25, https://www.freiheit.org/sites/default/files/2021-04/expressing-civil-and-political-liberties-in-times-of-crisis.pdf.
129 Cristina Lupu, "Romania," in Bican Sahin and Ivaylo Tsonev eds., *Expressing Civil and Political Liberties in Times of Crisis. COVID-19 first wave as a case study: Bulgaria, Greece, North Macedonia, and Romania*, Sofia, Bulgaria: Friedrich Naumann Foundation for Freedom, 2021, 20–25, https://www.freiheit.org/sites/default/files/2021-04/expressing-civil-and-political-liberties-in-times-of-crisis.pdf.
130 COVID-infected individuals underwent forced hospitalization during both the SOE and the SOA, although they had no coronavirus symptoms. https://www.freiheit.org/sites/default/files/2021-04/expressing-civil-and-political-liberties-in-times-of-crisis.pdf; Daniela Budu, "Ombudsman's report on pandemic," *Radio Romania International*, 17 September 2020, https://www.rri.ro/en_gb/ombudsmans_report_on_pandemic-2623368.

banned.[131] Ultimately, Romania stumbled in striking a reasonable balance between safeguarding public health and freedom of association.[132] In this connection, Selejan-Gutan stresses: "The authorities were caught insufficiently prepared. The legislation on emergency situations was unclear and incomplete. In these circumstances, the response was strong, but far from being perfect."[133]

Overall, Romania's response to COVID-19 pandemic is a cautionary tale of pandemic, mostly due to the government's haphazard response. To be sure, while most restrictions of rights and freedoms were in line with the Constitution, unclear and incomplete regulations, rushed, ambivalent, and arbitrary decision-making (often motivated by political crises and political gain) and faulty coordination and cooperation with the local authorities resulted in some infringements on human rights and freedoms.

---

131 Critics of protests noted that Romania's anti-restriction protests were rather perplexing because the restrictions were not extreme, but rather poorly communicated. Critics noted that anti-restriction protests were politically motivated, because, while the mask remained compulsory indoor in public spaces, all restaurants, bars, and cafes remained fully functional outdoors, with no mandatory mask wearing. Cristina Lupu, "Romania," in Bican Sahin and Ivaylo Tsonev eds., *Expressing Civil and Political Liberties in Times of Crisis. COVID-19 first wave as a case study: Bulgaria, Greece, North Macedonia, and Romania*, Sofia, Bulgaria: Friedrich Naumann Foundation for Freedom, 2021, 20–25, https://www.freiheit.org/sites/default/files/2021-04/expressing-civil-and-political-liberties-in-times-of-crisis.pdf; and Craig Turp-Balazs, "Romania, where Covid-19 restrictions are modest, but people protest anyway," *Emerging Europe*, 30 March 2021, https://emerging-europe.com/from-the-editor/romania-where-covid-19-restrictions-are-modest-but-people-protest-anyway/.
132 Cristina Lupu, "Romania," in Bican Sahin and Ivaylo Tsonev eds., *Expressing Civil and Political Liberties in Times of Crisis. COVID-19 first wave as a case study: Bulgaria, Greece, North Macedonia, and Romania*, Sofia, Bulgaria: Friedrich Naumann Foundation for Freedom, 2021, 20–25, https://www.freiheit.org/sites/default/files/2021-04/expressing-civil-and-political-liberties-in-times-of-crisis.pdf.
133 Bianca Selejan-Gutan, "Romania in the Covid Era: Between Corona Crisis and Constitutional Crisis," *verfassungsblog*, 21 May 2020, https://verfassungsblog.de/romania-in-the-covid-era-between-corona-crisis-and-constitutional-crisis/.

9

Policymaking and Liberty Restrictions in the Covid-19 Crisis, the Case of France

Angelique Palle[1], Lisa Carayon[2], François Delerue[3], Florian Opillard[4], and Christelle Chidiac[5]

[1] *Research fellow, Institut de recherche stratégique de l'Ecole militaire, Paris, France*
[2] *Assistant Professor, Sorbonne Paris Nord University, IRIS department, Bobigny, France*
[3] *Assistant Professor in Law, IE University, Madrid, Spain*
[4] *Research fellow, Institut de recherche stratégique de l'Ecole militaire, Paris, France*
[5] *Ph.D candidate in Law, Paris Nanterre University, Nanterre, France*

Disclaimer

The results presented in this chapter originate from two research projects financed by the French National Research Agency: ANR Army and ANR Localex.

Our warmest thanks go to the members of these teams who, as students or colleagues contributed to data collection and analysis or provided insights, Julie Arroyo, Laura Bellec, Mileva Boulestreau, Valentin Caro, Léonard Dannoux, Estelle Dantan, Caroline Faure, Yasmin Fernandez, Juliette Frigot, Shirley Gasse, Antonin Gelblat, Célia Gourzones, Stéphanie Hennette-Vauchez, Nicolas Kada, Nicolas Klausser, Fanny Lange, Vincent Louis, Aurèle Pawlotsky, Laurene Pezron, Pénélope Schuwer, Serge Slama, and Julien Verstraete.

9.1   Introduction

This chapter analyzes the legislative and policy response to the Covid-19 pandemic in France. On 12 March 2020, the French President called for a "war against the virus" which was followed by the first lockdown in France on 17 March, and the launch of a military operation called "Opération Resilience" (Bergeron et al. 2020). Unprecedented in French modern history, this set of restrictions to civil liberties taken in the name of collective health security and their association with a strong martial discourse raises questions in a context where other European leaders such as the German chancellor, explicitly refused to associate the restrictions to civil liberties with a warlike discourse (Opillard et al. 2020). This chapter aims at assessing how the French policymakers adapted to the pandemic in terms of regulation and policymaking. The chapter will address questions such as: which administrative level was in charge of taking measures? What were the justifications for them? How were health security and civil liberties balanced? The point here is not to assess the success or failure of these regulations but to understand their design and aim, how they fit in the French legislative framework, and how the balance between civil liberties and health security has been managed. The chapter relies on the cross-referencing of ongoing findings from two research projects financed by the French National research Agency, the first one, "ANR Army," on the role of the armies in the "war" against the coronavirus and its perception by the population The second research project, "ANR Localex" focuses on local and regional normative dynamics.

Elaborating on the results of these two projects, this chapter first presents the context of French policymaking and governance during the Covid-19 crisis, providing background on the country's tradition. We then analyze the nature of the exceptional legislative framework in place at the national level, in light of the use by the French government of the armed forces to help manage the crisis, in a context where the involvement of military forces domestically is extremely regulated. The role of the military involvement in crisis management and its use as a symbol by the French government is questioned, in light of the perception the French population has of this military involvement in crisis management. We thus question the discrepancy existing between the media's perception of the symbolic aspect of the use of the military domestically and the armed forces' ability to carry out missions effectively. In the second part, this chapter analyzes the normative dynamics at other levels of legislative and policymaking. Relying on a review of normative texts issued in the framework of the "état d'urgence sanitaire" (state of emergency related to the sanitary situation) at a prefectorial and municipal level, we question the existence of a governance framework between these different authorities (who is entitled to do what?) focusing on the case of the freedom to come and go (*liberté d'aller et venir*). We then explore the motives[1] (whereas and explanatory statement) preceding the set of regulations passed at the prefectorial and local level through the comparison of the municipalities of Rennes and Nice two, cities of similar size but opposite political ideologies, and their respective prefectures: Alpes-Maritimes and Ille-et-Vilaine. Thus, postulating that the rationale behind civil liberties restrictions at a local level is in certain cases of a political nature more than of a health-related one.

9.2 Policymaking and Liberty Restrictions in France During Covid-19 Crisis, Research Questions and Methodology

This section aims at analyzing how the French government reacted to the pandemic in terms of regulation and policymaking. Which administrative level was in charge of taking measures? What were the justifications for them? How were health security and civil liberties balanced?

The objective of this analysis is threefold. The first objective is to examine the legislative response at the national level by the French government and the recourse to an exceptional legal framework. We then analyze the use of the military in this context as an example of the balance the French government tried to strike between civil liberties and health security, before assessing the perception the population had of this military use and what it says of the seriousness of the crisis.

The second objective concerns the local and regional levels of decision-making. We quantitatively assess the number of texts issued by local authorities, then, through a more detailed reading of the decisions, we focus on the motivations of the texts, looking for the different "influences" of the public decision, between health constraints, scientific data, and the desire to respond to the supposed aspirations of the population. Finally, this cross-analysis allows us to consider the possible circulation of norms by observing the way in which certain normative practices emerge in certain territories before spreading to other areas.

This chapter combines the results of two research projects financed by the French National Research Agency. The first one, "ANR Army" (ending in June 2022) explores "The role of the

---

1 Indicated in the texts under the label "whereas" or "explanatory statements."

armies in the 'war' against the coronavirus and its perception by the population." Led by an inter-disciplinary group of French scholars (geography, sociology, political science, philosophy, and law). This project analyzes the role played by European armies in the Covid-19 crisis, their use by civil power, and the reception by the population of these military intervention (Opillard et al. 2020).

The second project, "ANR Localex" (ending April 2022) focuses on "Local regulation and the COVID-19 epidemic: dynamics of normative actions." It analyzes the local regulations (prefectures–regions–municipalities) taken in France for the management of the Covid-19 crisis. It consists of a systematic census of the measures taken at the prefectoral level, regional level, and a reasoned census of communal decisions (by representative sampling of communes). This project focuses on the measures taken during the first year of the pandemic (2020) (Boulestreau et al. 2020).

This chapter crosses the results of these two projects to aim at a multiscalar analysis of the reaction of the French government and local and regional authorities during the first year of the pandemic (2020). It also draws from the results of both projects to explore the reaction of the population to the restriction measures enforced during this period. The use of the military by the French government, the symbolic aspect of this resort, the analysis of the discourse built around it as well as its reception by the French population is here used as a proxy to understand how the crisis is perceived by both policymakers and citizens.

9.3 Regulation and Policymaking in France During Covid-19, Context and Background

The first cases of Covid-19 were confirmed by the end of December 2019 in France, which is early regarding the international dynamic of the pandemic. The country has been one of the most affected of the European states and ranks sixth in the list of the most affected countries in the world in terms of number of cases in relation to the population and 12 in terms of number of deaths at the time of the writing.[2]

France has a mandatory social health insurance system which is funded through general and earmarked taxation. Healthcare is a national centralized responsibility where the national public health institution (Santé Publique France) designs health strategies while regional authorities only have a small delegated role and implement measures chosen at the national level (Desson et al. 2020).

The management of intensive care units (ICU) has played a major role in the first waves of Covid-19 outbreak in France. Indeed, their sudden overload has been a trigger in the government's decision to enforce the first lockdown, from the 17March to the 10 May 2020. Two-thirds of ICU beds belong to public or nonprofit facilities, the rest being privately owned. The Court of Auditors has pointed out in a 2020 report[3] several issues concerning the ICU management system, one of them being the lack of resort to the private sectors' ICU beds. There is no rise in their share of case management over 2020 and some patients have been taken in charge in public hospitals in emergency conditions while beds were still available in the private sector.

France's crisis management governance structures are inherited from the 2000s. Following the Lothar and Martin storms of 1999, the heat wave of 2003 and with the background of the 11 September attacks in the United States, the French government had designed instruments to face major crisis (Borraz and Cabane 2017). The white papers on national defense and security

---

2 See Worldometer, https://www.worldometers.info/coronavirus/country/france/
3 Réanimation et soins critiques en général: un modèle à repenser après la crise, 2021, Rapport public de la cour des comptes, https://www.ccomptes.fr/sites/default/files/2021-03/20210318-04-TomeI-reanimation-et-soins-critiques-en-general.pdf

of 2008 and 2013 laid the basis of this dispositive, while regular government's regulations had defined its organization (Bergeron et al. 2020).

One of the most striking aspect underlined by both the literature on the pandemic management in France and interviews conducted by the two teams of writers, is the fact that despite France had designed response structures and organizational plans to face this type of crisis, the government decided to create new ones and to rely on them to manage the crisis. This resulting into what Bergeron, Castel, Borraz, and Dedieu call "an organisational crisis" (Bergeron et al. 2020). A specific plan for flu outbreaks (Plan pandémie grippale) had been designed in 2003 after the outbreak of SARS and regularly tested up to 2011, which is its last update, it was not activated. The interministerial crisis unit, on which relies an important part of the governmental organization[4] was set up and activated only on 17 March 2020, which is the date of the first lockdown. This crisis unit (the CIC, Cellule interministérielle de crise) was also a subject of dispute between the ministry of health and the ministry of interior affairs, resulting in significant tensions in the crisis management at the government level.[5] Last, a "scientific council" (Conseil scientifique) is created on 10 March 2020, to advise the French President. Composed of 11 members, mostly medical experts and some academics in sociology, social anthropology, and information technology (Atlani-Duault et al. 2020), it has played a significant role in the crisis management, providing open access advices to the government which have been very commented by the French media.

Relying on this organizational structure, the French policymaking to manage the Covid-19 crisis has been heavily centralized at the national level, in line with the country's heritage and tradition of a state-provided, universal, and free health coverage (Atlani-Duault et al. 2020). In the first waves of the pandemic, all the French national territory has been submitted to the same rules in terms of lockdown measures decided at the national level regardless of the severity of the pandemic in the regions (number of cases and occupation rate of ICU). At the regional and local level, as for general administrative police powers, the rule is that, when specific local circumstances justify it, the local authority may aggravate the national rule[6] (but not lighten it). In fact, they may even be obliged to do so, as the Conseil d'État recalled in the first order it issued concerning the confinement of the population decreed on 16 March 2020: "the representatives of the State in the departments, like the mayors by virtue of their general police powers, are obliged to adopt, when such measures are necessary, more severe prohibitions when justified by local circumstances."[7] Even before the adoption of the first national measures, some of these authorities were able, when confronted with local "clusters," to prohibit, for example, large gatherings or decide to close schools before equivalent national measures were taken. To give full measure of how these powers were used, between March and April 2020 the prefects of the 101 French departments (as well as New Caledonia and French Polynesia) issued more than 1,200 prefectoral decrees related to the state of emergency related to the sanitary situation on their territory, in addition to the measures taken at the national level. In order to fully appreciate the density of the regulatory texts or individual measures (requisitions) that are currently restricting freedom in the fight against the pandemic, it would be necessary to add to these 1,200 prefectoral decrees a very large number of municipal decrees adopted by the 36,000 French municipalities – a census of which has been so far too long and complex to be carried out.

---

4 See the ministerial circular n°6095/SG of 1 July 2019.
5 Interviews with two CIC members from the French Ministry of Armed Forces and the French Ministry of Interior Affairs, March 2021 and June 2021.
6 CE, Sect., 18 avril 1902, *Commune de Néris-les-Bains*, n° 04749.
7 CE, réf., 22 mars 2020, *Synd. Jeunes Médecins*, n° 439674.

9.4 "State of Emergency Related to the Sanitary Situation/Etat d'Urgence Sanitaire": The Recourse to an Exceptional Legal Framework

The very first measures to deal with the epidemic crisis were taken under the special administrative police powers held by the Minister of Health, in particular under articles L. 3131-1 et seq. of the Public Health Code (Boulestreau et al. 2020). On 16 March 2020, in a notable manner both with regard to the rarity of the legal basis invoked and the importance of the measure with regard to rights and freedoms, the Prime Minister relied on his general police power and on the theory of exceptional circumstances to decree the general confinement of the population. On 23 March 2020, the Parliament voted the law n° 2020-290 proclaiming a state of emergency related to the sanitary situation, which was created at the same time, which confers mainly to the Prime Minister and secondarily to the Minister of Health and at the local level to the representative of the State in the department new powers, and in particular

> *For the first: the power to restrict or prohibit the movement of people, to quarantine, to order the temporary closure of establishments open to the public, to requisition goods or services or to take any regulatory measure limiting the freedom of enterprise;*

> *For the second, to take "any regulatory measure relating to the organization and operation of the health system";*

> *For the third, to "take all general or individual measures to apply these provisions."*

On 25 March 2020, the French President, Emmanuel Macron, began to employ a martial discourse comparing the situation to a warlike situation.[8] Beyond the discourses and recourse to a martial vocabulary to mobilize the population, the French government rapidly considered the option of mobilizing the armed forces to manage the crisis. Yet, such a mobilization of the armed forces falls outside the traditional missions assigned to the military. It was thus necessary to invoke an exceptional legal framework allowing for such a mobilization.

In France, military intervention on national territory remains strictly regulated by law. The French Constitution allows for the mobilization of the armed forces in two situations: the state of siege (*état de siège*) and the state of war (*état de guerre*). The Covid-19 crisis falls outside of these two situations which thus cannot be invoked. Apart from these two exceptional cases provided by the Constitution, the use of the armed forces on the national territory can take place on the basis of two distinct legal frameworks: military defense (*défense militaire*) and internal security (*sécurité intérieure*). The first framework, the military defense of the national territory, is strictly regulated by articles R1421-1 à R1422-4 of the French Defense Code. It aims at "contributing to the preservation of the freedom and continuity of action of the Government, as well as to the safeguarding of the organs essential to the defense of the nation."[9] In other words, it concerns mainly the defense of military installations, notably those involved in the French nuclear dissuasion. Moreover, in the event of external threat or invasion, it could be implemented by governmental decision, but this has never been done. In regards to the state of siege and the state of war, it appears that military defense cannot be invoked in the context of the Covid-19 crisis.

The use of the armed forces within the framework of internal security, also known as civil defense, is the relevant framework for our study. The law provides that it is only possible to

---

8 Speech by the French President, Emmanuel Macron, on 'the mobilization to face the Covid-19 outbreak, in particular the role of medical personnel, and the launch of military Operation Resilience to support the fight against the spread of the coronavirus', Mulhouse, France, 25 March 2020.
9 Article R 1421-1 of the Defence Code (our translation).

mobilize the armed forces upon administrative request by the civil authority. This request for requisition or assistance can only intervene in case of a state of necessity, that is to say when the means of the Ministry of the Interior, which is in charge of internal security, are "inexistent, insufficient, unsuitable or unavailable" (« *inexistants, insuffisants, inadaptés ou indisponibles* »), called the "4i" rule.[10] One of the most known examples is the "Opération Sentinelle." Created in 2015 after the terrorist attacks in Paris, it mobilizes about 10,000 militaries on the French territory in complement to the police forces.[11] The decision to declare the Ministry of the Interior's resources inexistent, insufficient, unsuitable, or unavailable is the result of a dialogue between the civilian authorities and the military. In fact, the French army is regularly called upon to provide the civilian authorities with human and material resources, particularly during natural disasters. "Opération Resilience" is part of the operational contract for the protection of the national territory and therefore for internal security. In application of the "4i" rule, the civil authority deemed it necessary to requisition the armed forces to deal with the sanitary crisis.[12]

9.5 The Involvement of the Armed Forces in France in the Covid-19 Crisis Management, Between Political Display and Response to the Crisis

The use of the war metaphor by the President of the French Republic during his speech of 25 March 2020 represented a political momentum for the French executive. Its function was to generate public support for the use of the army on national territory, by emphasizing the exceptional nature of the health situation. Although this martial metaphor is controversial (Opillard et al. 2020), it shows once again the importance of the armies in regard to political power, which convokes war-like narrative when faced with an "invisible enemy." During this mobilization of the armed forces, the French executive has thus relied on the very high level of confidence that the French population has in the armed forces, since nearly 78% of the French population declare they trust the armed forces (Baromètre annuel de la confiance politique, CEVIPOF).[13] Moreover, the quantitative

---

10 Interministerial instruction relating to the engagement of the armed forces on national territory when they intervene on the request of the civil authority/Instruction interministérielle relative à l'engagement des armées sur le territoire national lorsqu'elles interviennent sur réquisition de l'autorité civile, n° 10100/SGDSN/PSE/PSN/NP (NOR : PRMD1733529J), 14 November 2017.

11 On "Opération Sentinelle," see generally: Information report tabled pursuant to Article 145 of the Rules of Procedure by the Committee on National Defence and the Armed Forces in conclusion of the work of a fact-finding mission on the presence and use of the armed forces on national territory' (Committee on National Defence and the Armed Forces of the National Assembly 2016) n° 3864, p. 14 / 'Rapport d'information déposé en application de l'article 145 du Règlement par la Commission de la Défense nationale et des Forces armées en conclusion des travaux d'une mission d'information sur la présence et l'emploi des forces armées sur le territoire national' (Commission de la Défense nationale et des Forces armées de l'Assemblée nationale 2016) n° 3864, p. 14 https://www.assemblee-nationale.fr/14/pdf/rap-info/i3864.pdf

12 'Information report tabled pursuant to Article 145 of the Rules of Procedure by the Committee on National Defence and the Armed Forces on the impact, management, and consequences of the Covid-19 pandemic' (Committee on National Defence and the Armed Forces of the National Assembly 2020) n° 3088, p. 14 / 'Rapport d'information déposé en application de l'article 145 du règlement par la commission de la défense nationale et des forces armées portant restitution des travaux de la commission de la défense nationale et des forces armées sur l'impact, la gestion et les conséquences de la pandémie covid-19' (Commission de la défense nationale et des forces armées de l'Assemblée nationale 2020) n° 3088, p. 14

13 The "Political Confidence Barometer" is an academic survey let by the Centre for Studies on the French Political Life (Centre d'études de la vie politique française) that has become the French benchmark survey on the question of French people's confidence in politics. The database, which has been built up over 11 years, allows for longitudinal monitoring of dimensions such as confidence in oneself, in others, in institutions, and in political personnel, as well as the relationship with democracy, its principles, and its functioning in France. Results can be found online at this address: https://www.sciencespo.fr/cevipof/fr/content/le-barometre-de-la-confiance-politique.html

survey that the ANR Army project conducted on a sample of nearly 3,000 people in February 2021 (Opinionway 2021) allows us to evaluate the appreciation of a representative panel of the French population concerning this intervention: in this panel, nearly 91% of the people interviewed considered that the military intervention was a good thing, a sign that the civilian requisition of military resources has generated strong support.

This being said, it seems necessary not to remain at the mere content of the political speeches around the intervention, as these have masked the reality of the investment of the military on the ground. The announcement of the French military intervention took place in a context, in March 2020, of the mobilization of several armies from European countries (Opillard et al. 2020), and of the saturation of the health systems in several French regions. In this context, Operation Resilience was a health operation on French territory, which, with a few exceptions, did not involve a security mission. From the very first days following the launch of Operation Resilience, several dozen senior French officers were deployed to the crisis units of the Ministry of Health and the Ministry of the Armed Forces, as well as to the Center for Planning and Coordination of Operations (CPCO) of the Ministry of the Armed Forces. Often not mentioned in research on the military response to the health crisis, these highly qualified military personnel filled the staffing gaps in ministerial agencies, often taking on menial tasks that allowed the operating protocols of understaffed administrations to be adapted in a very short time. This influx of high-ranking military officers into civilian administrations sometimes took civilian personnel by surprise, as they saw the arrival of the army and realized the seriousness of the situation. The arrival of several officers in the crisis unit of the Ministry of Health was interpreted as a takeover in the first days of the crisis by the civil staff and was eventually normalized by their integration into existing teams.

At the same time, the mobilization of the Armed Forces Health Service, a joint military organization, represented the largest contingent of the Ministry of the Armed Forces in this health crisis. The SSA was thus mandated to build a military hospital (called "Military Intensive Care Unit") on the parking lot of the Mulhouse hospital, in the Eastern part of France close to the Franco-German border, whose ICU services were saturated. In one week, the SSA built a hospital from materials and protocols that no longer existed in the logistics protocols, repatriating and assembling materials scattered throughout the country to provide 30 ICU beds. By way of comparison, other European countries that also set up military hospitals did not offer ICU care, but only served as relief areas for civilian hospitals. The most important investment of military personnel during the first wave of March–June 2020 concerned health measures, including the care of patients in the eight other military hospitals spread over the French territory, as well as the transfer of patients by military aircraft or by military ships from French hospitals to Germany, or internally, to less affected regions. Although Operation Resilience officially ended in June 2020 and represented the mobilization of just over 3,000 military personnel, the succession of epidemic waves required the continued reception of covid-infected patients in military hospitals in metropolitan France, and the reinstallation of the Military Intensive Care Unit in the ultramarine territories. Finally, the SSA continues to participate in the military response through the vaccination of the population.

Interestingly enough, the use of the military in the management of the Covid-19 pandemic in France has served a symbolic purpose, trying to politically unite the population behind a common "enemy," a logistical and sanitary purpose, but had not much to do with civil liberty restrictions. Compared to other European countries where armed forced reinforced borders (Switzerland, Poland, Czech Republic, and Hungary) or controlled population movement (Germany, Italy, Spain, Bulgaria, Lithuania, and Slovakia), the French armed forces were not involved in the enforcement of civil liberties restrictions (Delerue et al. 2020). However, the perception by the

French population of their actions and duties does not necessarily align with what the armed forces actually received as a mission.

9.6 Perception by the French Population of the Missions Performed by the Armed Forces and of the Nature of the Covid-19 Crisis

The Armed Forces have escaped the deficit of institutional trust that has been undermining the French people's relationship with the classic bodies of political mediation and the workings of representative democracy. Surveys and measurements conducted on this subject in the recent period remind us of the persistence of the favorable image developed by citizens of the French military. Thus, the annual Barometer of Political Confidence carried out by Cevipof measured that nearly eight out of ten French people (78%) acknowledge having confidence in the armed forces. In comparison, the executive branch of government and Parliament get the same level of confidence from four out of ten French people in the best of cases (respectively, 42% for members of parliament, 36% for the President of the Republic, and 35% for the Prime Minister). Despite this set of favorable provisions and these indications of recognition or proximity, there is a limited interest for the military. On a personal level, nearly two-thirds of the French (64%) admit to having little or no interest in military issues (Opinionway 2021). This distance raises questions when compared with the good image of the armed forces and the high level of trust in them.

The pandemic comes in this context as an interesting case study. First of all, the good image of the armed forces maintained, with 54% of the population declaring they felt reassured by the army's intervention during Operation Resilience to face the pandemic while 31% were indifferent and only 14% felt worried (Opinionway 2021).

However, if they approve of the military intervention, the French seem to have little sympathy for the use of a warlike tone to describe this crisis and the means to counter it. Indeed, 58% of them believe that this health crisis and the fight against the virus are not comparable to a war and in the collective imagination, the Covid-19 crisis is closer to major epidemics (40% spontaneously evoke diseases such as the Spanish flu, or the plague...) than to episodes of war (13%) in the history of France.

In terms of balance between civil liberties and health security, at the time of study (February 2021), the French strongly supported the principle of limiting civil liberties to enhance health security. Thus, 82% supported the idea that borders should be closed and controlled with countries outside the European Union. Two-thirds of French people also believe that the restrictions on freedoms imposed in the context of the health crisis are justified. Among the set of measures tested in the survey (lockdown, social distancing, closure of borders, and health requirements such as veering masks) it is the curfew that is most debated, with only 58% of French people believing it is justified (versus 39%). The most divided on the subject are the French under 35 years old (47 vs. 46%), supporters of the leftist "France Insoumise" party (47 vs. 52%), and of the far right party "Le Rassemblement National" (48 vs. 51%).

In this context of approval of the use of the army by the French combined with a high level of trust in its actions and a support in the restriction of civil liberties to fight the pandemic, the French population, however, seemed to be rather unaware of what were the actual missions performed by the armed forces. 64% of the people surveyed knew the armed forces were involved in the Covid-19 crisis management. If the medical and logistical role played by the armed forces is widely known among this population, 51% of them consider it was among the armed forces' missions to enforce confinement and 40% that they were instructed to block the roads to control the movements of the population, missions they never carried out. Indeed, France's policymakers have a specific relation to the armed forces partly shaped by the heritage of the 1962 coup attempted in the context of the Algerian independence (Cohen 2008). As shown in part 4, the legislative context of the use of the armed forces mostly prevents them from carrying missions of civil liberties restrictions on the national territory.

If they approve of the use of the military, the French are critical of the government's management of the crisis: 59% of them do not agree with the idea that "on the whole, the government is managing the current health crisis well" (Opinionway 2021); however, mayors and local elected officials are considered by a majority of the French people to have been effective in the crisis management (58 vs. 39%). We explore in the following section how the local and regional levels of policymaking have been dealing with civil liberties restriction and their multilevel governance.

9.7 Analyzing Local and Regional Measures of Civil Liberties's Restrictions in the Context of the "State of Emergency Related to the Sanitary Situation" (*état d'urgence sanitaire*), the Case of the Freedom of Movement throughout the First to the Second Confinement

The objective of this analysis at local and regional levels of decision-making and regulation is three-fold. First of all, it is a question of quantitatively assessing the number of texts issued by local authorities; this quantitative assessment also makes it possible, through a more detailed reading of the decisions, to assess the normative strategies of local authorities (few decrees with diverse contents or, on the contrary, precise texts for each situation encountered). The analysis then focuses on the motivations of the texts, allowing to see the different "influences" of the public decision, between health constraints, scientific data, and the desire to respond to the supposed aspirations of the population. Finally, this cross-fertilization allows us to consider the possible circulation of norms by observing the way in which certain normative practices emerge in certain territories before spreading to other areas.

Among the many freedoms that have been impacted by policies to combat the Covid-19 pandemic, analysis of the decrees collected has shown that, consistent with a policy of restricting interactions and travel, the freedom to come and go is one of the most restricted by prefectural and municipal measures, in a logic of local aggravation of national norms.[14] These restrictions are all the more important if we take this freedom in a broad sense, in terms of space, time, and materials.

In this section, we take the specific case of freedom of movement and aim more precisely to study how decisions to restrict freedoms are translated into public space in France. We thus question the different types of spaces targeted by the restriction measures and the temporality of these measures according to the evolution of the epidemic (are they preventive? corrective?). The question of the

———

14 Although freedom of movement is central to the regulations adopted to combat the virus, other forms of freedom are at stake through the implementation of these restrictive measures. The freedom of persons is restricted with the placement in quarantine, confinement, and curfew, as well as "the freedom of worship, assembly, demonstration and enterprise" have been limited. See Opinion of the Defender of Rights n°20-10 of 3 December 2020.

articulation and governance between the municipal and prefectural levels of decision-making is also raised: who regulates, according to what time frame, is there a sharing of competence or competition between the levels of decision-making? Finally, the question of the inequalities induced by these measures is explored, particularly concerning where people live and, in particular, regarding access to certain types of leisure areas.

In the primary sense of freedom of movement, many local ordinances have massively restricted the spaces to which people usually have access – in addition to the travel restrictions in force at the national level. Thus, a large number of urban spaces of access to nature (parks, public gardens, etc.) have been completely closed.[15] More broadly, access to certain natural areas outside the urban area and less exposed to leisure activities involving a high population density, but located on the territory of the municipality, has sometimes been prohibited (lakes, beaches, forests, etc.).[16] This spatial limitation of freedom of movement was the work of both municipal and prefectural regulations. However, from the selections of municipalities and prefectures that we have made, it would appear from the initial analyses that the municipalities have made more regulations in this area.

The "freedom to come and go" dimension was then affected in its temporal dimension through the implementation of local curfews.[17] This specific measure deserves to be examined because it illustrates both a phenomenon of "circulation" of norms – which originate in a particular territory before spreading – and a phenomenon of experimentation with measures by certain local authorities, even before these authorities were "seized" by the national legislature.

As the action of mayors in the implementation of these curfews has been questioned by the administrative jurisdictions (Caille 2020; Le Chatelier 2020), it is the prefectures that have multiplied the measures prohibiting night-time movements on the territory of municipalities where it was noted that the confinement measures were not respected; or at least that this respect was considered locally as insufficient. In doing so, about 30 municipalities in France were affected by these bans, which were then extended to the entire territory of the overseas municipalities. It should be noted that it did not appear, at the time, that the local curfew measures were correlated to the health situation in each of the territories.[18] It should also be noted that it is only starting on the 16 October that the curfew is expressly included in the prefects' repertoire of contention to face the pandemic, which was previously developing in a blur of legal norms.[19] In this second phase, the measure is limited to departments where the epidemic pressure is high: the decree lists in an annex the departments in which it applies. In these districts, the prefects therefore proceed to list the municipalities in which a curfew will be applied from 9 p.m. to 6 a.m. For example, 49 communes in Grenoble-Alpes-Métropole are concerned by this measure as of the 17 October 2020.[20] Similarly, 44 communes of Haute-Garonne are targeted by these measures,[21] but the measure is gradually hardened, the curfew being advanced to 8 p.m., then 6 p.m. Once again, the prefectures have preceded the central government: the prefect

---

15 Example: Essonne prefectoral decree n°2020-426, which came into force on 20 March 2020.

16 Example: Sanary-Sur-Mer municipal decree n°20-665-PM, which came into effect on 18 March 2020: prohibition of the Massif du Gros Cerveau, of the Pointe de la Cridé, of the Victorin Blanc area.

17 Example: Mayotte Prefectural Order No. 2020/CAB/490, effective 25 July 2020, in force until 8 August 2020.

18 For example, for 20 March 2020, if the incidence rate is greater than or equal to 10 in the Hérault department, it is between 5 and 10 in the Gard department, and between 1 and 5 in the Tarn department (data: Santé Publique France, COVID-19: Weekly Epidemiological Update of 24 March 2020).

19 Decree no. 2020-1262 of 16 October 2020 prescribing the general measures necessary to deal with the Covid-19 epidemic in the context of the state of emergency related to the sanitary situation, article 51.

20 Prefecture of Isère order n° 38-2020-10-17-001.

21 Prefecture of Haute-Garonne order n°31-2020-10-18-001.

of the Alpes-Maritimes has brought forward the curfew to 6 p.m. starting on the 2 January 2021, considering that the department is more affected by the crisis and that it is therefore necessary to further tighten the national provisions,[22] nearly two weeks before the measure is generalized on the 15 January to the entire national territory regardless of the local health situation.[23]

Last, the ways to circulate have also been regulated. For example, the mayor of Versailles has issued regulation removing bus lanes and replacing them with bicycle lanes to encourage people to travel by bicycle.[24] These decisions, which aim to limit the gathering of people on public transport, have the dual impact of modifying urban organization and, potentially, modifying the uses of these spaces according to the types of population concerned.

9.8 Legitimizing Civil Liberties Restrictions and Shaping the Governance of Policymaking, Comparison of the Two Cities of Rennes and Nice

To the question as to how the restrictions to civil liberties have been managed by local and regional levels, both in terms of legitimation and in terms of governance between the different levels of decision-making, we will compare the cases of the two cities of Rennes and Nice and their respective prefectures: Alpes-Maritimes and Ille-et-Vilaine. The choice of this comparison, taken from the abovementioned data sample, was based on a political criterion: the two agglomerations of comparable size and population, from a political perspective they are historically opposed, Rennes being traditionally a left-wing city while Nice being a right-wing one. The underlying hypothesis was that this political difference could lead to differences in the management and legitimization of restrictions on freedom of movement and in the territorial governance set up with the prefectures. Several questions arise here concerning the measures studied: At what administrative and territorial scale were they taken? At what stages of the health crisis did they intervene? What impact did these measures have on the city's spaces?

In the case of Rennes, from a spatial point of view, the prefecture of Ille-et-Vilaine adopted regulations applicable to the entire concerned municipality (curfew, prohibition of gatherings, etc.), but also specific regulations applicable to specific places that were individualized (and named) in time and space, which could be esplanades or public infrastructures (prohibition or authorization of access to very localized demonstration spaces). The municipality of Rennes, on the other hand, does not take any measures to restrict access at the municipal level during the period studied (March–November 2020), but restricts or authorizes access to certain types of places (parks and gardens, certain large markets, swimming pools, and the area around the stadium). The case of swimming pools is interesting here: closed by the prefecture and then reopened by the municipality, they raise questions about the respective areas of competence of the two and the existing dialogue between them.

---

22 Prefecture of Alpes-Maritimes, decree n° 2021-003 concerning police measures applicable in the department of Alpes-Maritimes in order to slow down the spread of the Covid-19 virus.
23 Decree n° 2021-31 of 15 January 2021 modifying decrees n° 2020-1262 of 16 October 2020 and n° 2020-1310 of 29 October 2020 prescribing the general measures necessary to face the epidemic of Covid-19 within the framework of the state of emergency related to the sanitary situation.
24 Example. Executive Order A-2020-568, effective 6 May 2020.

In the case of Nice, this distribution of areas of competence seems particularly blurred. The prefecture of the Alpes-Maritimes, like the prefecture of Ille-et-Vilaine, regulates either on the scale of the municipality (prohibition of gatherings) or on specific places (bars that have violated the rules of reception of the public, schools with cases), but it also restricts the opening of certain types of places on a permanent basis (bars, shops during certain time slots). The municipality of Nice, like that of Rennes, restricts or prohibits access to certain types of spaces (parks and gardens, markets) but, unlike Rennes, it regulates access to the public space on a municipal scale (restricted authorization to go out and circulate on the public highway from 6 a.m. to noon and then from 6 to 10 p.m. for individual physical activity and walking with only people grouped together in the same home) as well as to individualized places (certain hypermarkets, paths, or avenues). The municipality of Nice issues many more regulations than in the case of Rennes, and the restrictions on access to the same place evolve and harden over time in what seems to be an attempt to adapt the norm to the practices of the public space by the population (as in the case of the *Promenade des Anglais*, which is the subject of several successive access restriction measures). The restrictions also affect more types of spaces than in Rennes (certain portions of streets, hotels, and the entire seafront).

The difference in the treatment of restrictions on movement and access to certain areas under the state of emergency related to the sanitary situation by the municipalities of Nice and Rennes and their respective regional prefectures raises questions: about the division of competences between the municipality and the prefecture, about the motivations behind the implementation of restrictions on certain types of areas, places, or time slots in Nice and not in Rennes, and about the reasons for the legitimacy of these restrictions and their differences.

Faced with these questions, we first explored the question of the health motivation of local measures. The distribution of these different measures over the time of the crisis was analyzed through the following two graphs, for which we tried to understand the relationship between the restrictions of access to certain spaces and the time of aggravation or retreat of the crisis in the spaces concerned. The daily number of people newly hospitalized in the prefecture concerned was represented to give an overview of the regional temporality of the crisis.[25] A distinction was made between orders corresponding to restrictions and those corresponding to the lifting of restrictions.

In the case of Rennes, the municipality regulates mainly during the first confinement, the prefecture of Ille-et-Vilaine then takes over during the deconfinement period when restriction orders as well as lifting of restrictions are taken, then during the rise of the cases which precedes the second confinement, until this one is decided on the national scale. Thus, a dynamic emerges in which the municipality regulates in addition to the national measures while the prefecture acts outside the containment measures taken at the national level. In the case of Nice, this logic is less clear. The municipality of Nice, like that of Rennes, regulates very extensively during the first containment, but unlike Rennes, it does so even after the number of hospitalizations in the department has fallen. The prefecture of the Alpes-Maritimes, on the other hand, regulated very little during the deconfinement period, unlike that of Ille-et-Vilaine. It then acts largely during the rise of cases leading to the second containment but continues during this one, with also decrees of lifting of restrictions (relating in particular to the opening of truck stops). The logic of "handing over" visible in the case of Rennes and the prefecture of Ille-et-Vilaine is less visible in the case of Nice and the Alpes-Maritimes.

---

25 We remind here the dates of "national" confinement during which the measures of establishment closures were national: from 17 March to 11 May 2020 as well as from 30 October to 15 December 2020.

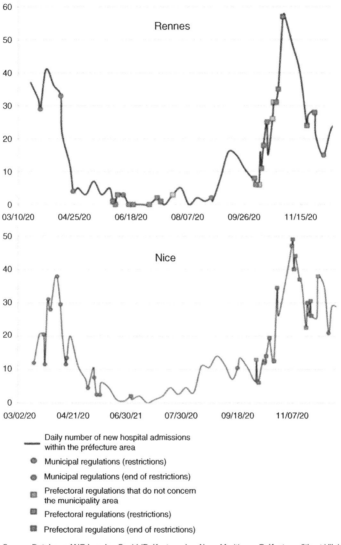

Restriction measures to the freedom to come and go (liberté d'`aller et de venir) comparative analysis of the municipalities of Rennes and Nice

Source: Database ANR Localex Covid (Préfecture des Alpes Maritimes, Préfecture d'Ile et Vilaine, municipalities of Rennes and Nice)

Credit: Pénélope Schuwer @ANR Localex

The comparative example of the municipalities of Rennes and Nice suggests that the trend of the health crisis is not the only possible element of legitimization for local measures to adapt the system of restrictions on freedom of movement. It is therefore useful to study whereas and explanatory statements for the restrictive orders issued during the period.

If the precise description of the health situation, taking into account the incidence rates, the situation of the hospitals or the scientific uncertainties about the transmission of the virus, appear quite early in the whereas and explanatory statement of the prefecture of the

Alpes-Maritimes,[26] the decrees of the municipality of Nice show that certain additional restrictions could be put in place because of more political local factors. Some decisions show that health "risks" can be assessed not only through objective approaches (e.g. incidence rates) or direct observations by public officials, but also through the numerous and repeated complaints of residents regarding the noncompliance with certain health measures.[27] The municipality, taking into account these complaints, considers that it is necessary to go toward more severity. It has gone so far as to prohibit access to certain streets, except for those necessary for residents,[28] and even to prohibit access to the entire public space at certain times of the day and night.[29] This type of prohibition, which is more severe than the national or prefectural rules, raises the question of the differentiated protection of public liberties with regard to the type of space considered and therefore also with regard to the population concerned. It is in this sense that the League for Human Rights attacked the city of Nice for its regulation imposing a curfew at 8 p.m., instead of the 10 p.m. curfew imposed by the prefecture, specifically in the working-class neighborhoods of the city.[30] According to the LDH, this decision was discriminatory and stigmatizing for the inhabitants[31] and went against the words of the President of the Republic held two days earlier, warning the elected officials not to reinforce the rules in place at that time.[32] However, the Nice Administrative Court refused to suspend the decision in summary proceedings by an order of the 22 April 2020,[33] considering that the measure only affected a small fraction of the territory (1.3%) and that the statistics on fines showed frequent violations of the confinement in this zone, but without formally pronouncing on the question of socio-spatial discrimination. It simply stated that "the only circumstance, alleged at the hearing by the applicant association, according to which the delimitation of the sectors thus concerned would constitute a social discrimination of the population residing there is without incidence on the legality of the decree."

---

26 See, for example, the series of decrees on the areas where wearing a mask will be mandatory in June 2020 (decrees n° 2020-689 et seq.) in which the prefecture justifies its decision by the precise incidence rate at the time of the decision as well as by information "brought up" by the mayors of the municipalities concerned regarding population gatherings. In most decisions, the "concern for coherence and legibility" of the measures is noted. It is also possible to mention the cases in which the orders are motivated by scientific uncertainty about the methods of contamination, for example, with regard to swimming and the risk of contamination by fecal matter (order no. 2020-357).

27 See the same whereas for municipal order no. 2020-01132 prohibiting the public from circulating and/or moving on the southern sidewalk of the Promenade Corniglion Molinier, the southern sidewalk of the Promenade des Anglais, the southern sidewalk of the Quai des Etats-Unis, the southern sidewalk of the Quai Rauba Capeu and this, up to the Place Guynemer, for reasons of public safety and health; for municipal by-law no. 2020-01133 prohibiting the public from circulating on Jean Médecin Avenue for reasons of public safety and health, and for municipal by-law no. 2020-01134 restricting individual physical activity and public walking for reasons of public safety and health: "Considering that following numerous telephone complaints, also sent by e-mail by many concerned citizens, received in the various municipal services (. …), it is noted that there are many people who do not have a derogatory certificate").

28 By-law n° 2020-01133.

29 By-law n° 2020-01134 prohibits any individual physical activity or walk outside of the hours determined in Article 1.

30 Municipal by-law n° 2020-01135 ordering hourly restrictions for the public to circulate and/or move around the sectors of Trachel, Jean Vigo, Notre-Dame, Saint-Charles, Bon Voyage, Maccario, Pasteur, Las Planas, and Les Moulins, for reasons of public safety and health.

31 France Bleu, April 18, 2020, "Coronavirus and human rights : The League of Human Rights attacks the city of Nice in justice." https://www.francebleu.fr/infos/politique/coronavirus-et-confinement-la-ligue-des-droits-de-l-homme-va-attaquer-la-ville-de-nice-en-justice-1587205969.

32 The rules planned by the government must continue to be respected. They (…) must be neither reinforced nor reduced, but fully applied. I ask all our elected officials (…) to help ensure that these rules are the same everywhere on our soil", speech by the President of the Republic at his address to the French on 13 April 2020.

33 N° 2001782, v. "Can the mayor impose a curfew to fight against the epidemic?", M.-Chr. de Montecler, Dalloz Actualité, 24 April 2020.

9.9 Conclusion

The study of policymaking and legal framework put in place in France during the first year of the Covid-19 pandemic (2020) raise many questions regarding (i) the discrepancy between the aims and effects of policymaking and regulation and their perception by the population; (ii) the balance between the political expectations of the population and the sanitary measures required; (iii) the governance of regulation at the different levels of local, regional, and national authorities.

At the national level, the French context of balance between the preservation of civil liberties and the enforcement of measures of restrictions aimed at preserving health security is rather complex in light of the military involvement. On the one hand, the French government took a strong martial stance and quite dramatically called upon the army to help with the crisis management, thus using it a symbol to qualify both the seriousness of the situation and the strong involvement of the government relying on the values of courage, leadership, and resilience associated with the military. However, the effective army's missions focused on medical and logistical help, far from the "war" announced against the virus. The French armed forces did not carry any missions of civil liberty restrictions enforcement, contrary to other European countries.

On the other hand, however, if the population seems to have rejected the martial discourse of its government, refusing to associate the Covid-19 crisis to a war or a military event in its history, it welcomed the intervention of the army. Thus, keeping up with the high level of trust that the French army maintains among the French population, but wrongly associating it with missions of civil liberties restriction enforcement that the armed forces did not carry out. This shows a strong discrepancy between the message that is sent by the French government, the one that is received by the population and what actually happens on the ground within the ties of the French legal framework which is very restrictive when it comes to the use of the army on the national territory.

At regional and local levels of regulation and decision-making, the spatialized study of local restrictions on the freedom of movement of people reveals the way in which the regulatory management of the health crisis has profoundly affected the distribution of public space within the population. The exclusion of certain spaces, sometimes to the point of privatization, combined, in times of confinement, with restrictions on the sphere of movement of individuals, was able to achieve its objective of avoiding the mixing of populations, but also at the cost of a form of segregation of the public. The motivation of the decrees also reveals a consideration of the fears of the population, which is not necessarily correlated to the reality of the epidemic, and whose management is therefore intimately political, in the literal sense of the relationship of elected officials with their electorate. This observation invites reflection on the question of whether the most local level is really the most relevant for decision-making adapted to the local health situation.

References

Atlani-Duault, L., Chauvin, F., Yazdanpanah, Y., Lina, B., Benamouzig, D., Bouadma, L., Druais, P. L., Hoang, A., Grard, M.-A., Malvy, D., & Delfraissy, J.-F. (2020). France's COVID-19 response: balancing conflicting public health traditions. *The Lancet*, 396(10246), 219–221. https://doi.org/10.1016/S0140-6736(20)31599-3

Bergeron, H., Borraz, O., Castel, P., & Dedieu, F. (2020). *Covid-19: Une crise organisationnelle*. Sciences Po Les Presses.

Borraz, O., & Cabane, L. (2017). States of crisis. In *Reconfiguring European States in Crisis*, D. King and P. Le Galès (p. 394–412). Oxford University Press.

Boulestreau, M., Caro, V., Dantan, E., Fernandez, Y., Gasse, S., Gourzones, C., Lange, F., Louis, V., Pawlotsky, A., & Pezron, L. (2020). Les mesures locales d'aggravation de l'état d'urgence sanitaire. *La Revue des droits de l'homme. Revue du Centre de recherches et d'études sur les droits fondamentaux.* https://doi.org/10.4000/revdh.9189.

Caille, P. (2020). Présentation du dossier thématique Covid-19 / Thematic presentation of the Covid-19 issue. *Civitas Europa*, 45(2), 5–8.

Cohen, S. 2008). Le pouvoir politique et l'armée. *Pouvoirs,* 125(2), 19. https://doi.org/10.3917/pouv.125 .0019.

Delerue, F., Jolly, E., Michelis, L., Muxel, A., Opillard, F., & Palle, A. (2020). COVID-19 and the Mobilization of the Armed Forces in Europe and in the United States. *IRSEM, Notes*, 107, 18.

Desson, Z., Weller, E., McMeekin, P., & Ammi, M. (2020). An analysis of the policy responses to the COVID-19 pandemic in France, Belgium, and Canada. *Health Policy and Technology*, 9(4), 430–446. https://doi.org/10.1016/j.hlpt.2020.09.002

Le Chatelier, G. (2020). Les pouvoirs de police du maire aux temps du covid-19 / The Mayor's power of police in time of covid-19. *Actualité Juridique des collectivités territoriales*, 250, 328–330.

Opillard, F., Palle, A., & Michelis, L. (2020). Discourse and strategic use of the military in France and Europe in the COVID-19 crisis. *Tijdschrift Voor Economische En Sociale Geografie*, 111(3), 239–259. https://doi.org/10.1111/tesg.12451

Opinionway. (2021). *Perception par la population française de la crise sanitaire et du rôle des forces armées dans la gestion de cette crise / French population's perception of the health crisis and the role of the armed forces in managing this crisis* (ANR Army, Éd.).

Section 3

Countries Focused on Population Monitoring and Restrictions

10

Policy Measures, Information Technology, and People's Collective Behavior in Taiwan's COVID-19 Response

Cheryl Lin[1], Pikuei Tu[1], Wendy E. Braund[2], Jewel Mullen[3], and Georges C. Benjamin[4]

[1] Policy and Organizational Management Program, Duke University, Durham, NC, USA
[2] Pennsylvania Department of Health, Harrisburg, PA, USA
[3] Dell Medical School, University of Texas at Austin, Austin, TX, USA
[4] American Public Health Association, Washington, DC, USA

10.1 Introduction

COVID-19 has rampaged globally with devastating consequences on human lives and livelihoods. Two summers into the pandemic, the world continued to battle many uncertainties. By July 2021, total reported cases globally approached 200 million, with over four million deaths. Only a handful of countries had vaccinated more than half of their populations thus far,[1] which was seven months after the vaccine became available. Initial confidence in the success of the vaccine resulted in daily cases plummeting and was followed by widely celebrated reopenings. However, numerous new viral variants and waning vaccine effectiveness led to new surges of infections in most countries.

Taiwan, a democratic island-country with 23.5 million population, was predicted to have the second highest risk of imported cases at the outset[2] and instead registered among the lowest COVID-19 prevalence and mortality rates during year one (33.6 and 0.3 per million, respectively).[3] Using aggressive border controls, extensive contact tracing, strict quarantine polices, and its accessible universal healthcare system, Taiwan went 253 consecutive days (April–December 2020) without local transmission. Citizens heeded public health messaging and embraced masking, handwashing, and physical distancing, all of which limited the tally to 1,000 COVID-19 cases over the first 14 months of the pandemic. It was the calm before the storm: the next 10,000 cases took only 11 weeks.

Relaxed measures, almost nonexistent natural immunity, a global shortage and delayed arrival of vaccines, political complications, and limited testing hindered the country's defenses against new, more transmissible variants that have continued to emerge. In mid-May 2021, the Taiwanese government raised its COVID-19 alert to level III, the second highest, as the country experienced daily cases in the hundreds and deaths in double digits for the first time. Some of the policies and practices that worked well earlier had to be adapted or reinstated quickly. Citizens refrained from going out even in the absence of a "stay at home" order and, further, requested extension of restaurant and business restrictions for caution. In less than three months, daily local cases receded to single digits.

This chapter describes Taiwan's emergency response policies, including the Communicable Disease Control Act (CDCA), pandemic measures in different segments of the population, the role of national health insurance (NHI) and accessible healthcare, innovative integrations of information technology (IT), and amendments to laws and regulations adapted to the evolving situation.

10.2   A Snapshot of Taiwan

Taiwan, formally the Republic of China, is a Democracy with a semi-presidential, multiparty system in which the President is the head of state and elected by the people. Rated 11th on the Democracy Index,[4] the country has a five-branch government (known as Yuans): a unicameral Legislative Yuan which can pass laws without presidential approval (nor can the President veto); an Executive Yuan led by the Premier appointed by the President; an independent Judicial Yuan; a Control Yuan monitoring and auditing government performance; and an Examination Yuan responsible for national examinations including civil service employment.

As a modern, egalitarian society, Taiwan has largely retained much traditional, family oriented, and collectivist culture that places strong emphasis on education and harmony. Located in East Asia, 112 miles from the southeastern coast of China and a three-hour flight from its northern neighbor, Japan, Taiwan has a vibrant, free market economy. It is the 10th largest trading partner of the United States,[5] known for its consumer electronics and machinery products, high-tech industry, hospitable people, and tantalizing foods and teas.

10.2.1   The Legal Framework Pertaining to Pandemic Response

10.2.1.1   Epidemic Control and Public Health Emergency

Taiwan's CDCA was introduced in 1944. Intended to halt the occurrence and spread of communicable diseases, it identified 10 legally defined, severe infectious diseases that required prompt reporting and containment, such as smallpox, plague, and diphtheria, and allowed inclusion of new emerging diseases. The Act has been amended multiple times, most significantly in 1999, the year the Taiwan Centers for Disease Control (CDC) was established,[6] to more explicitly secure people's rights, update border control regulations, and clarify the respective authorities and responsibilities of the central and local governments while increasing the government's power in stipulating and executing disease control measures during an emergency.[7, 8] Also noteworthy was a 2004 amendment after the Severe Acute Respiratory Syndrome (SARS) pandemic to strengthen the country's epidemic control capacity by modernizing the surveillance system, including the creation of the National Health Command Center to centralize ongoing disease monitoring in real time.[9]

In 2011, the Constitutional Court ruled CDCA Article (§48), which mandates detention or quarantine of persons suspected to be infected with a severe communicable disease, to be constitutional and, while limiting personal liberty, not in conflict with the principle of proportionality (Constitution §23) for its purpose of preventing transmission and safeguarding citizens' health and lives.[10] The ruling further prompted CDCA to more clearly specify and inform affected individuals of the isolation parameters and duration (§44).[10, 11] The Act was further updated in June 2019, pre-COVID-19, to stipulate penalties for spreading rumors or misinformation (§63), among other violations.

When CDC detects an imminent outbreak, the Ministry of Health and Welfare (MOHW) can request the Executive Yuan to review and approve the activation of the Central Epidemic Command Center (CECC) and to appoint a commander (§17). Selection of the individual who serves as commander, which may be the CDC director, the Minister of Health and Welfare, or the Premier, usually depends on the level (Three, Two, One [highest]) of the CECC's operation. The change of level status and eventual reclosure of the CECC after the threat is neutralized are determined by the head of MOHW (§8) and/or the CECC's commander.[12] During the COVID-19 pandemic, except for the initial week of January 2020 in which the CDC director was commander while at Level Three, the Minister has served as commander even when the Level was raised to One on 27 February 2020.

Table 10.1 Legal authorities and responsibilities concerning high-risk emerging infectious diseases.

Entity	Rights and authority	Responsibilities
Central government – competent authority being the MOHW (§2)	Classify disease, determine alert level and restrictions (§8), activate CECC (§17); during CECC operation, can mobilize and coordinate other government agencies including military and reserve (§6 & 17), use media with priority (§52), expropriate facilities or commandeer resources for disease control purposes (§53); temporarily shut down potentially contaminated water supplies (§21). Head of MOHW, or commander during CECC operation, has ultimate decision-making authority (SA §7)	Formulate policies and stipulate disease prevention/control measures including: • Immunization, surveillance, case investigation and reporting, testing, quarantine (§5-1.1 & 26), isolate confirmed cases (§44 & 48) • Personal protective equipment (PPE) and related material, device stockpiling, training (§5-1.1 & 20) • Supervises, assesses, and assists the operations of local governments and healthcare institutions (§5-1.2 & 16-2) • Formulate vaccine policy and purchase (§27), promote and implement vaccination (§28); sets up relief funds for vaccine-related injuries (§5-1.3 & 30) • Performs border control and quarantine (§5-1.4), screening and health declaration (§58) • Disseminates international and domestic outbreak information and related measures via mass media (§8-2), correct and fine misinformation (§9 & 63) • Establish Disease Control Medical Network, designate isolation wards, mobilize healthcare resources (§14-1 & 14-2), form mobile squads as needed (§15) • Compensate for expropriation and requisition (§14-3)
Local government – City/County governments and local health departments	Classify disease and determine alert level at the locality and inform central government (§8), form local command center (§16-2)	Develop implementation plans and execute communicable disease control measures, report to central government and may request support (§5-2). Compensate for destroyed disease transmissible foods or animals (§24)
Healthcare institutions	Subsidy for isolation wards (§14); compensation for expropriated facilities, required closures, or requisite resources (§53 & 54; SA §8 & 9); rewards for excellent performance (§73; SA §2)	Secure patient privacy (§10); establish isolation wards; perform disease prevention/control training and drill; stockpile PPE and pharmaceutical supplies; support vaccination policy (§29); execute infection control measures and prevent nosocomial transmission (§32) Subject to fine if institution or its employees were incompliant, refused or interfered with government supervision or inspection (§64 & 65)
Medical professionals	Supplements for extra duties (SA §2), compensation for injury or death from performing disease control-related tasks (§74; SA §2)	Check TOCC (§31), perform test, report confirmed or suspected cases (§39 & 46; PA §15); evaluate and retest patients in isolation to determine further treatment or isolation needs (§45-2); vaccinate; maintain patient privacy (§10), ensure patients' legal rights without discriminate (§11)
"Patients" – including individuals confirmed with or suspected of infection, along with the likely exposed (§13)	Compensation for lost wages during quarantine or due to taking care of family under quarantine (SA §3); subsidy for funeral cost if remains must be examined by autopsy (§50)	Comply with orders for testing, treatment, vaccination, quarantine, or isolation (§36, 43, 45); provide truthful information on TOCC and during case investigation (§31); may be fined and/or prosecuted/imprisoned if refusal or violation caused transmission (§62 & 67; SA §13 & 15)

Sources: Communicable Disease Control Act (updated 19 June, 2019), the Special Act (SA, updated 31 May, 2021), Physicians Act (PA).

The law grants the head of MOHW or the commander when the CECC is in operation, the authority to execute pandemic control-related laws (§17), stipulate and amend policies (§5), and mobilize cross-departmental resources (§6 & 18) – including soliciting assistance from the military and private organizations if necessary (§17, 53 & 54). Emergency rules decree mandatory testing of people at risk of infection (§48), reporting of confirmed cases to the Taiwan CDC (§46), quarantine of suspected individuals, and isolation of confirmed cases (§48), while protecting people's rights and patient privacy (§10-12).[13]

In response to the novel coronavirus, a companion *Special Act for Prevention, Relief and Revitalization Measures for Severe Pneumonia with Novel Pathogens* (hereinafter called the Special Act) was passed in February 2020. It was established to provide subsidies for the mitigation of COVID-19's impact on the economy and society – including compensation and incentives for medical personnel and institutions as well as agencies, organizations, and private citizens involved in or affected by preventive measures such as quarantine or expropriation (§1~5). It also set penalties for price gouging of medical or essential supplies (§12), violation of disease control regulations (§13 & 16) such as quarantine (§15) and disseminating misinformation (§14). Finally, the Special Act authorized the government to increase expenditures to provide an economic stimulus, funded by surplus of the previous fiscal year or debt raising, and subject to the Legislature's review and approval (§11).[14]

Table 10.1 summarizes the rights and responsibilities of various entities based on laws relevant to pandemic response.

10.2.1.2   Personal Information

In Taiwan, privacy is considered one of the basic human rights covered under the Constitution.[15] As individuals may be requested to provide personal data during public health emergencies, the balance of privacy rights versus the population's safety and wellbeing has been regularly debated. The *Personal Data Protection Act* (PDPA),[16] similar to the European Union's privacy legislation and augmented with the *Enforcement Rules of the Personal Data Protection Act*,[17] was promulgated in 1995. People's rights to privacy and secrecy of communications are also safeguarded by the *Communication Protection and Surveillance Act*[18] and the Constitution (§13).[19] These laws are executed and interpreted by Ministry of Justice and National Development Council. Both the central and local governments have the authority to enforce these laws and impose penalties for infringements. The PDPA allows exceptions for a government agency to acquire sensitive personal information when it is necessary to perform its statutory duties (§6) (e.g. contact tracing or medical records as required by the CDCA during an epi/pandemic) and decrees the data can only be used for the specified purpose while considering proportionality (§5). The law also provides individuals the right to request deletion or termination of processing of their personal data (§3).[16]

10.3   The Ominous Beginning of the Pandemic

Given the lessons of SARS in 2003 and proximity to China, the Taiwan CDC was on high alert when online forum chats from China about a mysterious infection in Wuhan began to circulate near the end of 2019. On 31 December, as China reported the unknown pneumonia outbreak to the World Health Organization (WHO), Taiwan CDC started onboard health screening of flights arriving from Wuhan,[20] in what may have been the first response to the novel coronavirus outside of China.

The government activated its CECC on 20 January, 2020, the same day the U.S. Centers for Disease Control and Prevention (US CDC) activated its Emergency Operations Center and prior to COVID-19's entry into the news and public awareness. Within a day, each country confirmed its first imported case, both travelers from Wuhan, when there were only three other reported cases outside of China. Two days later, Wuhan, with its 11 million population, went under lockdown.

On 11 March, the WHO declared COVID-19 a pandemic which had spread to 114 countries, infecting almost 120,000 people and killing more than 4,200 people.[21] Reported cases in the United States topped 15,000 with nearly 200 deaths and on 19 March, the governors of California and New York implemented unprecedented shelter-in-place orders.[22, 23] The U.S. State Department issued its highest global advisory against traveling overseas as Italy's death toll of 3,405 surpassed China's. Over the following month, 42 other states in America issued stay-at-home directives; similar orders promulgated globally, affecting two-third of the world's population,[24] as reported cases exploded to over half a million.

Taiwan thus far had effectively controlled the spread of COVID-19,[25] responding to the outbreak immediately and aggressively with an array of policies and conventional containment measures augmented by technology.[26, 27] While only 18% of the workforce converted to working-from-home and as one of a few countries where schools remained open,[28, 29] the country managed to get through the first global wave by mid-April with fewer than 400 confirmed cases (of which over 85% were imported),[30] followed by a long streak of zero domestic transmission.

10.3.1 Swift Responses Early On

Taiwan's experience with another severe coronavirus outbreak – SARS CoV-1 in 2003, also novel at the time – provided valuable lessons and prompted updated disease control strategies and emergency readiness, including the 2004 amendment to the CDCA and establishment of the Infectious Disease Control Medical Network. Within the first week of 2020, the Taiwan government assembled a cross-departmental taskforce and an expert advisory committee. The healthcare community was notified to screen patients with travel history from Hubei Province (where Wuhan is the capital) and manifesting respiratory symptoms or fever.[27] Contactless infrared temperature checkpoints had been installed at airports and seaports; hospitals swiftly instituted screening stations to monitor entrance traffic, requiring masks and hand sanitizing, and separating individuals with fever or related conditions.

Simultaneously, the Taiwan CDC epidemiology laboratory started developing and producing test kits which leveraged existing diagnostic modalities for pneumonia of unknown etiology. On 12 January, immediately after the viral genome was released to the global scientific community, Taiwan CDC introduced a high sensitivity real-time reverse transcription–polymerase-chain-reaction (RT-PCR) test that yielded results in four hours,[31] increasing domestic testing capacity and case detection amidst a severe shortage and underdevelopment of COVID-19 tests worldwide.

On 15 January, the Taiwan CDC specified the severe pneumonia caused by novel coronavirus as a Category-V Communicable Disease – an emergent infectious disease posing a serious risk to the population's health, as defined by CDCA (§3).[13] On 20 January, the CECC was activated. Medical professionals and laboratories were required to report positive cases to the CDC within 24 hours. Persons testing positive were hospitalized in negative-pressure rooms for treatment and observation and to prevent spread. The central government increased national PPE stockpiles and distributed additional supplies to healthcare facilities, mapped designated isolation wings of responding hospitals in preparation for a surge in patients, and created a nationwide inventory of ventilators and daily available ICU and isolation beds.[32]

Concurrently, numerous regulations and policies as well as personal hygienic practices were put in place and communicated to the public via daily press conferences and hourly public service announcements on TV, radio, the internet, and social media for timely information dissemination (§6-12 & 9).[33, 34] These early measures were effective: when the WHO declared a public health emergency of international concern on 30 January, Taiwan had only 9 reported cases and no deaths.[1]

10.4   Blocking Infection Importation and Local Transmission

10.4.1   Tightened Border Control

In addition to posting travel advisories, the Taiwan CDC enhanced border control, as required by the CDCA (§58). Taiwan CDC officers stationed at airports implemented health screening of passengers and provided healthcare advice. These procedures detected the first COVID-19 case arriving from overseas, who was directly transported to the hospital.[35] Before the end of January 2020, CECC suspended tour groups to and from China and limited visitor entries. Reporting and testing criteria were expanded from China travel history to include persons who had symptoms or close contact with probable exposure. Upon arrival, all travelers were required to undergo entry screening and complete a Health Declaration detailing their symptoms plus travel and contact history in the past 14 days. If completed digitally prior to departure, they received a text confirmation upon arrival to facilitate and expedite the entry and customs process (the utilization rate reached 90% by June 2020).[36] All incoming individuals' cell phone numbers were recorded in the Taiwan CDC's quarantine database; phones were required to be on and with the owner 24 hours a day during the mandated 14-day status monitoring period.[2]

Suspected cases self-reported or detected were tested onsite and taken (by dedicated, government-subsidized "disease prevention taxis") either to designated responding hospitals or a centralized quarantine center to await their test results, based on the border control clinician's evaluation. If positive, passengers sitting two rows ahead and behind the confirmed case along with airline crew who had prolonged interactions were tested as well. Individuals with possible exposure or who showed symptoms, even if they tested negative, were reported to the central database for follow-up or referral to care. Passengers arriving from overseas were required to complete a 14-day quarantine (at home if they have a separate bathroom or at a "disease prevention hotel"), checked by district administrative staff daily via their registered cell phone. Non-responding or incompliant individuals could be fined, tracked down by the police, and/or sent to a centralized quarantine center.

As the global situation continued to intensify, the application of emergency response stipulations widened. An additional week of self-monitoring (i.e. recording temperature and symptoms twice daily, avoiding going out or visiting with others, and wearing a mask and foregoing public transportation if leaving home) was added to the two-week quarantine. After the local case surge in the spring of 2021, all travelers were required to be tested upon arrival, conduct self-testing during quarantine, and take another PCR test before being released from quarantine. If a person tested positive, the individual was picked up by special transportation to be treated at the nearest hospital. The immigration office also restricted confirmed cases from leaving the country to prevent international transmission; such restrictions ceased once the person was no longer contagious based on a negative PCR test result (§58-5 & 58-6).

---

1 For more details on Taiwan's early response measures, including specific policy decisions during the first 50 days of the pandemic, please see Lin et al.[27]. A companion podcast is available at https://tools.cdc.gov/medialibrary/index.aspx#/media/id/406900.
2 Visitors without a workable cell phone could obtain a free phone loan and/or purchase a SIM card for local network connection at the airport.

10.4.2 Rigorous Contact Tracing

Contact tracing is a critical public health tool used in an outbreak to identify and notify people who may be unaware of being exposed to self-monitor their health or seek medical attention, thus preventing further spreading. Taiwan began the earliest comprehensive contact tracing outside of China in late January 2020.[37] Central and regional Taiwan CDC epidemiologists led local health department teams in conducting patient interviews and compiling a list of locations where the infected person had been 2–7 days prior to estimated disease onset together with all identifiable contacts. If a confirmed individual was unable or unwilling to provide certain details (e.g. the exact time, location, or companion), the contact tracing team might work with local law enforcement and use multiple data sources, including medical appointments, business or community security videos, and telecommunication companies' aggregated traffic patterns.[38] As necessary, individual cell phone GPS records and social media posts were utilized (with oral consent) to assist recall, while maintaining confidentiality in accordance with the *Physician Act* ensuring patient privacy and the CDCA's stipulation against revealing patients' identity or medical information (§10).

Detailed information was obtained from individuals who tested positive to help triangulate the source of infection and determine the risk to contacts. It is a violation of the CDCA to refuse interviews or provide false or incomplete information that interferes with the case investigation (§43); guilty parties can be fined US$2,000–10,000.[3] Individuals who are aware of having contracted an infectious disease but transmitted it to others due to their failure to follow regulations are subject to a fine up to US$17,500 or up to three years of imprisonment (§62).[13]

Every close contact is interviewed and scheduled for COVID-19 testing. Those who test positive are transported to treatment hospitals via designated vehicles or ambulance. If negative, they undergo home-quarantine for 14 days. All other contacts are called or texted and asked to self-monitor for the same period. Local environmental departments disinfect identified locations and surrounding areas, if necessary. When there is a potential exposure to the larger public, CECC publicizes the site and date (avoiding naming specific businesses, if possible, to minimize stigma) to alert affected individuals to self-monitor or get tested. When there is a potential cluster of transmission, CECC also seeks assistance from major telecommunication companies to send out cell messages based on mobile GPS signals, without personal identification or breaching confidentiality, to people who were at the same location when or soon after the confirmed and/or suspected individuals were there.[39]

10.4.2.1 Augmentation with Information Technology (IT)

Utilizing IT to augment the labor-intensive investigative operations and increase efficiency, many nations have developed apps to assist in recording and matching individuals' activities for risk notification. Through public–private partnerships, Taiwan developed several platforms. The *Taiwan Social Distance App* is an opt-in self-warning tool, developed by Taiwan CDC and Taiwan AI Labs with built-in security and privacy protections stricter than the European Union's General Data Protection Regulation (the world's toughest law on personal data). The system does not require registration nor track individual users' locations. It randomly generates an irreversible/irretrievable hashed ID (anonymous identifier) for each phone every 15 minutes, allowing the app to chart movements over the previous 14 days. An alert pops up if the phone had come within two meters of a confirmed case for more than two minutes.[40] Participants, if they test positive, are asked to upload their current random ID for the system to alert users at risk of exposure. The information is stored only on the phones and automatically deleted after 10 days.[41]

---

3 For reference, the entry-level hourly wage at McDonald's is approximately US$6 in Taiwan compared to US$8-10 in the United States.

No personal data are collected by any government agency or business. Users can opt out anytime. The record showed that over seven million people have downloaded the app, nearly one-third of the population, but the actual usage or effectiveness is unclear due to the relatively low number of confirmed cases in Taiwan and small proportion of that number who notified the system when they tested positive. Additional promotion as well as education about the purpose and mechanism of the app could likely increase its utility.

An integrated *Contact Tracing Support Platform* was also launched to improve the precision of contact tracing, data-sharing, and decision-making. By creating a dynamic "hot zone map" with trails of infected individuals and voluntary self-surveillance data, the interactive system allowed central and local governments to better monitor cross-region spread, analyze outbreak sources and development, predict imminent clusters, and loop back to identify or update hot zones where cases are increasing quickly. It also enables governments to promptly send cell messages to people who may have been exposed to begin self-quarantine or get tested. The system has stringent privacy oversight, and its use is restricted to government employees involved in contact tracing and pandemic response for that sole purpose.[42]

These laws and measures may be deemed unfeasible or a potential privacy violation in some countries but have been mostly accepted by the Taiwanese. The SARS experience played an important role in shaping people's adaptation to strict rules and inconvenience during emergencies to protect their health and the public's.[34] According to the CDCA, during an outbreak, the public shall cooperate with health authorities' disease prevention measures (§36). Living in a collectivist culture, people are more willing to oblige and expect others to do so in order to avert disease spread. Precautions taken by the government to secure information and promotion of the PDPA in recent years have strengthened people's awareness of their rights.[17] Also, daily press conferences held by CECC and CDC leadership delineating case investigation results have educated the public about transmission routes and underscored the importance of vigilance and cooperation with response regulations.

10.4.3   Enforcing Quarantine – Operations and Mechanism

Although quarantine is a common isolation method for infection prevention, its definition and procedures vary by country.[43] As the CDCA prescribes, the MOHW sets the operation policies and parameters for central and local authorities to test, vaccinate or treat, and quarantine people who had contact with confirmed cases or possible infection (§48). More specifically, "patients" are defined as persons who contracted the disease, had close contact with confirmed individuals, or are likely infected and therefore at risk of transmitting the virus (§13). Confirmed and probable cases cannot refuse testing, investigation, treatment, or confinement (§43). Other than being hospitalized if confirmed or symptomatic, patients are mandated to quarantine for 14 days either at their residence or a designated quarantine hotel or centralized center. At the same time, the rights and privacy of patients, persons under quarantine, their families, and medical professionals must be protected, without discrimination (§11).[13]

10.4.3.1   Provisions, Compensation, and Penalties During Quarantine

To minimize obstacles and promote compliance, the Taiwan legislature enacted new laws containing both incentives and deterrents to manage quarantine with wraparound services. Upon receiving information from CECC's centralized database, staff at local civil offices or health departments call or text people under mandated quarantine to establish communication, set smart phone GPS homebound parameters, and provide instructions and sometimes a care package.[44] [4]

Monitoring consists of electronic location confirmation and one–two phone calls/texts daily to check health status and offer support. A 24-hour hotline provides counseling and information. Individuals are required to call to arrange transportation and appointments if they have symptoms or need medical care. If symptoms are deemed mild or unrelated by either phone or in-person counseling and the individual not admitted to a hospital, a healthcare provider follows up by phone to evaluate throughout the quarantine or the additional seven-day self-monitoring. Further, local environmental protection departments collect garbage weekly separately from the general public to minimize contamination. Staff or volunteers from local Quarantine Care Centers pay home visits to provide assistance such as arranging grocery and meal delivery or childcare, if needed.

To compensate for financial losses or other damages stemming from disease prevention measures stipulated by CECC, the government passed the *Special Act,* and the Legislature created an emergency fund. To help cover wages lost while under quarantine, the Act provides a supplement of NT$1,000/day for 14 days (US$500 total)[5] for those without paid sick leave or caregiver days who are supporting an ill or quarantined child or elderly family member (§3).[46] Employers are required to allow exemption leave, rather than personal leave, and not use employees' absences as the basis for bonuses or dismissal.[14] Employers are encouraged to pay employees their regular salary; they may receive tax credit double the amount paid (§4). Individuals whose livelihood is adversely affected due to mandated isolation can seek help through the *Public Assistance Act.*

Determined to minimize community spread, the CECC established tight control and increased penalties. Violators of quarantine could be fined US$3,500–35,000, depending on the length of time violating confinement or potential for exposing others (e.g. taking public transportation or holding/attending parties) and required to forfeit financial compensation.[47] Police are dispatched to track down violators within hours of notification. Repeat offenders are taken to centralized quarantine facilities for the remainder of their 14-day period. Smaller misdemeanors, such as not responding to quarantine spot checks, putting down false information on a Health Declaration, or not reporting related symptoms are subject to a US$300–5,000 fine. As the number of quarantined persons grew, a supplementary two-way monitoring chatbot was implemented. The application of this digital fence reduced quarantine violations from 30 to 0.3%.[36] These extraordinary efforts helped contribute to the low case rate in Taiwan, limited community spread to predominantly small, isolated clusters.[48, 49]

As case counts rise again, more countries including Canada, New Zealand, and Australia have employed comparably strict quarantine mandates.[50-52] Some of the aggressive preventive measures, including innovative use of big data and technology similarly implemented in South Korea and Iceland as in Taiwan, have raised concerns elsewhere.[53-55] Taiwan ranks second highest in freedom in Asia[56] [6]; the government has attended to upholding people's rights and

---

4 Items commonly include masks, thermometer, health education materials, free passwords for on-demand movies or e-books/learning channels, snacks and instant noodles, or canned food, hand sanitizer or alcohol-based cleanser; some cities also sent a note from the mayor and online shopping vouchers.[45]

5 The average monthly earnings in Taiwan is approximately US$1,800 in 2020. Most people used the daily supplement to help cover part of the quarantine hotel charges, which generally cost NT$1,500–5,000 per night depending on the location and amenity.

6 In[56] global report, Taiwan scored 94/100 total on freedom, with 38/40 on political rights and 56/60 on civil liberties. For reference, the United States scored 83, 32, and 51 and Japan – the highest in Asia – scored 96, 40, and 56, respectively.

considers possible reactions or protest to new policies. During a public health emergency, the Taiwanese people prefer to opt for temporary restraints to preserve long-term freedom and the larger populations' well-being; they have embraced these "sacrifices" and are grateful for the resulting COVID-19 containment in the country.

10.5 Active Participatory Role of the Public – Awareness and Preventive Behavior

While laws and regulations are intended to protect individuals' well-being and the greater societal good, the public's behavior and level of compliance determine their impact and success. Memories of SARS lingered in Taiwan, and the initial COVID-19 epidemic heightened adherence to protective, proactive behaviors. The temperature monitoring instituted in airports and seaports in 2003 were speedily added to hospitals, restaurants, offices, businesses, congregate living, and public events. Hand sanitizers and surface disinfectants were widely placed in public spaces to ensure access and encourage routine usage. When schools returned to session after the first winter break, all students had their temperature checked and hands sanitized every morning entering campuses.[57, 58] A March 2020 poll on the cusp of the pandemic's explosion indicated 90% of Taiwanese wore a mask in public because of the outbreak,[29] in sharp contrast with the attitude of citizens in the West.[59, 60]

10.5.1 Common Use of Masks and Response to Shortage

Taiwanese are familiar with mask-wearing during flu seasons, on high air particulate matter days or crowded subway rides, and by those who are sick or high risk. Despite Taiwan CDC's initial guideline that healthy individuals need not wear a mask except in hospitals or crowded, enclosed areas, they were immediately in high demand. Anticipating an international shortage of masks, the Taiwanese government acted early. It suspended mask exports in late January 2020, requisitioned domestic supplies, accelerated production in partnership with local companies,[7] and instituted a rationing system in early February to improve distribution and prevent price hikes. Residents can obtain masks locally by swiping their NHI card, already linked to pharmacies and local health centers nationwide. In addition, a government-funded mobile app helped citizens locate distribution points and showed updates on availability. Responding to the 2021 spring surge, CECC raised the alert level to III and mandated mask wearing in public. With a low vaccination rate at the time, the public's diligent compliance with this policy likely contributed to bending the curve of community transmission.

The requisition and mobilization were supported by the CDCA, which grants CECC the power during emergencies to expropriate products and properties and compensate affected parties accordingly (§53 & 54) as well as set prices (§55).[13] Other laws prohibit price gouging and hoarding with fines and jail sentences as deterrents.[14]

10.5.2 Promoting and Self-Adhering to Social Distancing

After COVID-19 spread exponentially from Asia to Western Europe and then to the United States in the spring of 2020, movement restriction and physical distancing policies were adopted.

---

7 Dozens of engineers from private industries voluntarily formed a "national team" to help factories refit and build production lines to hasten manufacturing. In less than a month, Taiwan became the second largest mask-producing country in the world.[61] The increased supply eased the public anxiety of shortage and later enabled Taiwan to donate to the urgent needs of other countries, including hundreds of millions sent to Europe and the United States.[62, 63]

In April 2020, approximately 95% of Americans and half of the world's population were under some type of shelter-in-place orders.[64, 65] Rather than closing schools and businesses or prohibiting all public events, CECC provided guidelines on physical distancing for crowd control and event operations; citizens were encouraged to stay home on weekends. Elementary schools used plexiglass dividers on desks to reduce respiratory droplet spread.[57] Similar transparent devices were installed at food courts, banks, and other public-facing services and later became a requirement (in addition to masking) for operation during periods of increasing cases.

Although physical gestures of affection are less customary in Taiwan than in other countries, close social interactions and eating out with friends are common, so the feasibility of social distancing without a formal stay-at-home policy was initially questioned. The distinctive culture of collectivism and perseverance was evident when Taiwan observed daily cases in the hundreds in May 2021 and the alert level was raised from II to III (second highest). Campuses were closed for the first time and restaurants could only offer take-out. Entertainment venues and most tourist sites were shut down. Without a "hunker down" mandate, streets were almost empty the next day and public transportation ridership dropped by over 80%. The citizens' self-regulation coupled with modified testing criteria and assertive measures brought down the case numbers. Despite the desire to return to normal life and resume business after more than two months of intense alert, when the CECC announced the relaxing parameters, the people demanded an extension of certain restrictions.[66] Even with occasional disagreements between the government and the people in executing and disputing laws or policies, the social norms of caution, self-protection, and conformity in Taiwan reinforced the effect of many disease control measures.

10.6 Healthcare System and Capacity

10.6.1 National Health Insurance (NHI) and Data Integration

Taiwan has a single payer universal healthcare system that provides affordable, quality care,[67] of which approximately 70% are private medical facilities and 30% public in a free, competitive market. Key to this system is Taiwan's NHI, with its provision written in the Constitution Amendment (§10-5),[68] covering 99.9% of the population with comprehensive services supported by cutting-edge IT.[69, 70] Established in 1994, it has been consistently ranked among the best worldwide and reported public satisfaction exceeding 85%.[67, 71, 72] The universal model enhances the country's healthcare capacity and mobilization. Taiwanese (as well as foreign residents and students) can seek medical attention for any issue without referral, minimum wait time, and little fear of financial burden; premiums and co-pays are subsidized or waived for low-income families.[8]

The centralized, secure cloud-based electronic health records have played an instrumental role in risk identification and case investigation throughout the pandemic, as for other outbreaks and communicable diseases such as dengue fever and norovirus. Because providers are required to submit claims to the single-payer platform within 24 hours, the NHI database has near real-time information that allows clinicians and Taiwan CDC to track medical visits and disease trends. The NHI patient records contain complete health history, underlying health conditions, and recent progression of symptoms, treatments or prescriptions, and hospitalization. During COVID-19, although

---

8 The NHI comprehensive coverage includes preventive, specialist, dental, vision, and mental healthcare as well as prescription drugs and traditional Chinese medicine. The funding is primarily payroll-based, with the government, employer, and individual each responsible for approximately one-third of the premium (varies by occupation). The healthcare is not tied to employment so people stay insured even when they change or lose their jobs. Patients with certain rare or severe diseases are offered reduced co-pays.[69]

CDCA requires healthcare providers to ask patients' TOCC during a visit (§31), some patients may not disclose full information. At the CECC's request, the NHI integrated with the Customs and Immigration database to flag those recently visited highly impacted countries, so providers would be aware of patients' potential exposure.[27] Records of all confirmed and suspected case contacts reported to Taiwan CDC as well as quarantine or self-monitoring timeframe and COVID-19 test results were also added to the NHI database for follow up until the individuals were released from hospital, asymptomatic, or tested negative twice.[73]

Combining these data and CDC's communicable disease surveillance helped pinpoint high-risk patients and persons likely to have had contact with infected cases. In addition, the NHI database assisted Taiwan CDC to quickly identify new patterns of symptoms or case clusters and the source or path of infection. The high security and privacy policy of the NHI IT system, protected by multi-keyed de-identification algorithm, has stringent rules on data-sharing accessibility and expiration stipulated and enforced for pandemic response only.[74] Any integration of data systems was restricted to one-way transmission of specific information from other departments to the NHI database, and no health records or personal information were available to anyone outside the health system.

The advanced IT and single-payer model further contribute to the exceptional efficiency in keeping administrative costs at about 1% of the national healthcare expenditure and out-of-pocket costs low.[70, 75] The accessibility of the universal healthcare system has helped deter community spread by casting a wider net to identify suspected cases, including those with minor or originally seemingly unrelated symptoms.

10.6.2 Infectious Disease Control Medical Network

As a Category-V severe communicable disease, required testing and treatment for COVID-19 are covered by the government. The MOHW commands an extensive Infectious Disease Control Medical Network connecting selected public hospitals and medical centers across the country, divided into six regions. As prescribed by the CDCA, the network is poised to mount a coordinated response with predefined responsibilities during emergencies and medical surges, including designating responding and treatment hospitals (§6), establishing isolation wards (§12), and separating and admitting patients. Every region is supervised by a commander, appointed by the minister, and one or two deputies (§3). These leadership roles are generally served by an expert from a medical center, CDC regional director, or senior staff from the local health department's disease control division to ensure familiarity with the local environment and needs; they have the power to direct and audit all local governments and healthcare facilities in the region in disease control efforts (§4.1 & 4.2). The Network Regulations dictate regional commanders' authority and duty to assess and control pandemic situations in their jurisdictions, mobilize healthcare facilities and human resources, including expropriation or cross-region support as needed, and activate isolation hospitals (§4 & 5).[76]

Isolation hospitals hold three-year designations and must employ infectious disease specialists (§9 & 7). Their responsibility to treat confirmed patients ends when the CECC is closed. Hospitals' loss of income due to reserved, unused isolation wards during an outbreak is repaid by the government (§12). Such designation releases private clinics and medical centers to continue to treat and hospitalize non-COVID patients and helps prevent nosocomial infection.

In early 2020, CECC enacted additional infection prevention guidelines for hospitals, including separation of wards, patients and their visitors, healthcare professionals, housekeeping, and administrative staff. Potentially infected individuals identified at screening stations were put in protective gear and escorted to isolation rooms for testing. Confirmed cases were maintained in isolation rooms for observation and treatment or transferred to designated treatment hospitals and discharged only after testing negative two or three times.

The structure of the nation's universal healthcare system and relatively small number of cases allowed Taiwan to adhere to these comprehensive policies consistently for the large part of the pandemic, including admitting patients with minor or no symptoms, thus minimizing community transmission and avoiding unanticipated death due to lack of care or sudden disease progression. Until 16 March 2020, Taiwan had experienced single-digit daily new cases. In the following weeks, even with study-abroad students and travelers rushing home because of university campus closures and the first wave hitting the United States and Europe, the daily new case number was contained to under 30 with enhanced border control and vigilant quarantine and surveillance measures. By the end of 2020, there were seven deaths from COVID-19 in Taiwan, six of whom had preexisting chronic diseases.[3] However, as encountered by many countries earlier, the healthcare system and capacity were challenged when a larger surge occurred with the Alpha variant in May 2021; some of the stringent practices had to be more flexible when adapting to the evolving situation, such as directing asymptomatic confirmed cases to stay home for self-isolation and monitoring, converting regular wards into isolation rooms and placing patients with marginal symptoms in double-rooms for observation, and releasing patients when tested negative once.

10.6.3 Assuring Care and Support for the Providers

Taiwan took steps intended to protect healthcare personnel from the start of the pandemic. CECC increased hospital reserves of essential medical supplies and PPE and reevaluated PPE standards and procedures for high-risk workers (e.g. frontline infection control staff, police, and airline crews) as the pandemic evolved. Policy stipulated that healthcare workers with a fever above 38 °C (100.4 °F) or related symptoms were to be isolated, screened for COVID-19, placed off-duty while awaiting results or under treatment, and allowed to resume working only after two negative test results 24 hours apart. If they tested positive, all patients and personnel in close contact for the past 14 days were also tested, and impacted wards were cleared for decontamination. Others who were potentially exposed were asked to undergo two weeks of self-monitoring. Providers caring for confirmed patients could receive supplements for additional duties or extra hours and increased risks.

Direct care and other hospital workers and members of the greater disease prevention network, such as those monitoring quarantine, who were infected from conducting COVID-19 related duties, could apply for a one-time government compensation up to U.S.$12,000 in addition to paid sick leave.[77] If they died, their families became eligible for a U.S.$330,000 payment, as well as subsidies for education expenses of the children of the deceased.[78] Incentives and awards for organizations (i.e. public agencies, medical facilities, schools, and private groups) with outstanding performance in disease prevention or pandemic response efforts were also enacted into law (§2). Healthcare institutions that temporarily closed in cooperation with CECC's orders were compensated (§9).

10.7 The Heights of Cases, Anxiety, and Dilemmas

For the first year of the pandemic, Taiwan reported an average 0.6% test positivity rate, experienced a total of seven deaths in its 799 confirmed cases, and tabulated 253 consecutive days averting local transmission from April through December. These statistics put Taiwan among the top echelon of nations, including New Zealand, Australia, Singapore, South Korea, and Vietnam, in terms of having handled the pandemic effectively.[25, 26, 48] Compared to most other nations, Taiwan's economy was well sustained,[9] reporting 3.11% growth in 2020,[79] though many hourly labors and small businesses suffered.

Over the early part of 2021, except for a nosocomial cluster at a large ministerial hospital that stemmed from a physician infected when treating an imported case,[80] the country charted another 72 consecutive days without domestic cases. Yet, the relatively calm environment amidst the devastating global situation rendered the Taiwanese population almost no natural immunity and at low defense against the more transmissible virus mutations.[81]

10.7.1 The Surge of Spring/Summer 2021

On 15 May, 2021, the daily case count exceeded 100 for the first time. The CECC raised the Alert Level to III (the second highest) with added restrictions. Streets were nearly empty due to voluntary lockdowns. Even for the traditional dragon boat festival holiday, sales of train tickets dropped to less than a quarter of the normal volume. Schools reluctantly closed campuses.[10] Masks were required both indoors and outdoors, including in private vehicles carrying multiple passengers.[82]

Taiwan had only received 433,000 doses of vaccines, or 2% of the nearly 20 million international orders placed, by that time. The CECC, at local governments' requests, allocated additional PPE and essential supplies to increase hospital stockpiles.[83] As the surge continued, it included a handful of hospital and institutional outbreaks. When the daily inventory of available ICU and isolation beds indicated near capacity in a particular city, patients were transferred to other responding hospitals within the region as designated by the Infectious Disease Control Medical Network. Some regular wards were cleared to be used as isolation rooms. Several hotels were also refitted to house confirmed patients with minor or no symptoms for observation by healthcare teams; asymptomatic suspected cases were advised to stay home.[84]

In response to the first, small cluster of Delta variant infections found in the southern part of the country, measures were heightened both domestically and at the border. Arriving passengers reporting any symptoms in the previous 14 days had to take a PCR test at the airport and wait at a government quarantine center for results; passengers arriving from high-risk countries were required to stay at the center for two weeks. All other travelers were to check-in to quarantine hotels and take a PCR test twice – upon arrival and at the end of quarantine period – plus another rapid self-test in between.

The ongoing measures of prompt communication, testing, contact tracing, isolation/quarantine, and treatment that had been key to Taiwan's success at controlling COVID-19 proved to be challenging when cases suddenly soared, and the healthcare system became strained. At the same time, it was difficult for the whole country, especially cities experiencing zero or single-digit cases, to sustain high restrictions. Both the government and citizenry were apprehensive about the country's reopening – a daunting dilemma that all nations faced. In due course, the more aggressive testing and largely self-imposed movement restrictions suppressed community spread relatively quickly; daily confirmed cases receded from 500-700 at the peak to less than 50 in seven weeks.

The CECC set its criteria to release from Level III: no more than three clusters per week or 10 local cases with unknown source per day.[85] By early July, daily cases were down to fewer than 30. In preparation for lowering alert level, the CECC announced a few relaxed policies, including resuming the operations of childcare, museums, movie theaters, and dine-in at restaurants with

---

9 For context, the 2020 US GDP growth was negative 3.5%, German economy shrank by 5%, Japan decreased by 4.83%, and the world fell 3.8%.

10 By April 2020, over 160 countries had moved classes remotely with nearly 90% of the students worldwide affected due to the first wave of COVID-19; Taiwan was one of few countries where schools stayed open during the first year of the pandemic.[28]

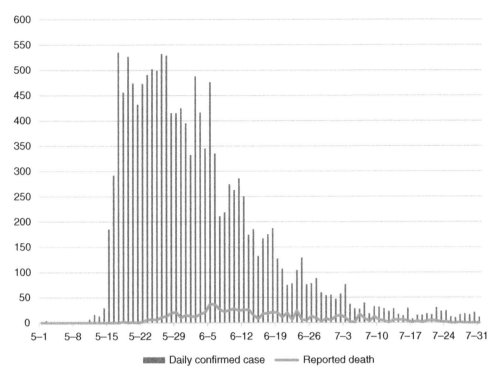

Figure 10.1   Taiwan local COVID-19 infections during 2021 spring/summer surge. Source: Taiwan CDC.

limited capacity.[86] Although the nation was eager to reopen, the people demanded an extension of the dine-in restriction, preferring caution. The public's voice induced the majority of mayors and county commissioners to uphold tighter measures than the CECC's updated national policies.[66] Though local governments have the authority to stipulate discrete public health measures and enforce policies in their jurisdictions when an emergency is at a regional level, such discrepancy or opposition was uncommon.[87] Level III eventually concluded on 26 July. Even then, some cities waited several more weeks before reopening dine-in restaurants and other venues such as swimming pools. Figure 10.1 presents the trends and numbers in confirmed cases and deaths during the largest surge in Taiwan thus far.

10.7.2   Amended Policies and Reflections of the Surge

Although Taiwan sustained more than a year of minimal community transmission, border control with temperature monitoring and symptom reporting were later proven insufficient as scientific evidence indicated that asymptomatic and presymptomatic individuals infected with COVID-19 could spread the virus. While Taiwan has a strict 14-day quarantine mandate for incoming passengers, the CECC permitted reduced time for airline crews considering the nature of their work. Crews from long-haul flights were required to quarantine for seven days plus seven days of self-monitoring since January 2021.[11] The rule was relaxed to five-day quarantine plus nine-day self-monitoring in March and further lowered to three plus eleven on 15 April.[88] A large cluster of infections involving crew, staff at an airline-commissioned quarantine hotel, and their families occurred two weeks later.[89] After two more weeks, local cases exploded[90, 91]; contact tracing did

---

11 Crews from short flights need to only self-monitor for two weeks if they did not deplane in a foreign country.

not identify a direct link other than confirming many were infected with the same viral strain.[92] The policy was reversed a month later.[93]

Some experts and politicians also questioned CECC's resistance to performing mass or random testing and the rigid criteria for free testing which missed an unknown number of asymptomatic cases that could have been causing community spread.[80, 90, 94] The mayors of the two most impacted cities made timely executive decisions to establish rapid testing stations. As both testing numbers and confirmed cases jumped to new highs with the positive rate ranging from 5 to 11% in some pockets of the capital, more pop-up testing stations were installed around the country.[95, 96]

The CECC overhauled its testing policy, including provision of subsidies for setting up testing stations and supplements for technicians and staff[97] as well as enabling local governments and private organizations to purchase additional rapid PCR test machinery to quickly increase community testing capacity.[98] Participating corporations were required to have medical staff conducting the tests, provide isolation accommodation for employees who were positive from rapid test and waiting for PCR results, and report confirmed cases to Taiwan CDC.[99] At the border, in addition to the requirement of a negative test report within three days prior to departure that was in place since December 2020, a PCR test upon arrival was added for all incoming passengers in June 2021. Testing booths were also installed at domestic airports to keep symptomatic and positive individuals from boarding a plane to prevent cross-region transmission.[100] Further, under the CDCA, CECC offered awards for primary care physicians who identified and referred suspected cases that subsequently tested positive and for medical facilities that reported back referral follow-up (§5). To preserve healthcare capacity and prevent nosocomial transmission, hospitals reduced out-patient and elective services, and required all patients to have a PCR test before hospitalization or surgery as well as all caregivers staying with patients at wards.[101] Several outbreaks were reported at traditional markets and private companies. When a cluster seemed to grow uncontrollably, CECC set up a mobile command center onsite to assist local governments with testing, containment, and even vaccination. These and other measures brought down positivity rates to below 1% again by July 2021.

Comparing to seven deaths in Taiwan in 2020, the sharp surge claimed over 770 lives in two months, with approximately 90% aged 60 or older. A CECC spokesperson acknowledged that the response did not pivot quickly enough, attributed to the higher-than-normal case fatality rate and the delay in ramping up the containment plan.[102]

10.8   Vaccine Supply, Hesitancy, and Distribution

10.8.1   Slow Delivery and Shortage of Supply

With a worldwide shortage of vaccine supplies and manufacturing behind schedule, small shipments started to reach Taiwan in March 2021, with a meager 117,000 doses of AstraZeneca in the first allotment. Supply chain unpredictability challenged mass vaccination planning. Because of the low number of cases and deaths in the country for the first 14 months of the pandemic, initial public interest in vaccination was low.[92] By June, demand soared as the country experienced its worst surge of infections and cases approached 9,000, but Taiwan received just 876,600 doses of the nearly 20 million purchased; only 3% of the population were vaccinated, almost all of them medical professionals. The annual national college admission examination was postponed to allow time for all proctors to get vaccinated before the huge gathering (and hoping for the surge to pass).

Several vaccine manufacturers in countries combating new surges suspended or delayed exports, exacerbating problems in Taiwan.[103] On 4 June, Japan donated and flew 1.24 million doses of

AstraZeneca vaccines, the first of multiple shipments, to Taiwan. This timely expression of friendship was prompted by suggestions from the Japanese people and parliament as a reciprocal gift for the supplies and monetary assistance the Taiwanese provided Japan in 2011 for the magnitude 9.0 Fukushima earthquake.[104] [12] Then, the United States provided 2.5 million doses of Moderna to Taiwan, which arrived on 20 June. Soon the preliminary goal of 25% coverage (at least one dose) was achieved ahead of schedule on 24 July, though fewer than 1% of the population was fully vaccinated.

10.8.2 Vaccine Hesitancy and Demand

The evolving science about the virus and the newness of the vaccine prompted global skepticism and reservations about the COVID-19 vaccines,[106] including in Taiwan. *Vaccine hesitancy* is defined as context- and vaccine-specific "delay in acceptance or refusal of vaccines despite availability and quality of vaccine service.[107]" On 22 March, as the nationwide vaccination program was initiated, Taiwan recorded another 41 days without local transmission and over two weeks without any deaths, which dampened any sense of urgency.[92] The Taiwanese also had concerns about the AstraZeneca vaccine due to blood clots and other internationally reported adverse effects.[108]

After providing high-risk healthcare professionals and frontline pandemic response workers a first dose, the government turned to vaccinating senior citizens. The first cohort of ages 85 and older included a large majority with comorbidities and restricted physical functions, and in the initial days of the program, dozens of sudden deaths occurred within 72 hours of vaccination.[109] This further increased vaccine hesitancy, even though many experts believed these deaths were due to conditions unrelated to the vaccine itself, such as long commutes, waiting in long lines in a summer heat wave, and comorbidities. Families and physicians were also reticent to suggest vaccination to seniors, despite the fact that they were most at risk.[110] Some cities experienced no-shows at half of their appointments. Although the CDCA provides compensation and assistance for people injured from taking vaccines (§30-1), a direct link was tenuous. Because the CECC had discretion to determine compensation (§30-3 & 50-4), it offered US$10,000 for funeral assistance if the family agreed to an autopsy. However, the policy was not well received due to the cultural preference for burial of the body intact and the possible perception that families foregoing tradition were doing so for monetary incentives.

Despite vaccine demand abruptly escalating with the COVID-19 surge in mid-May 2021, continuing doubts about the AstraZeneca vaccine fueled preference for the mRNA vaccines; but before the donation from the United States, only 390,000 of the 5.05 million Moderna doses purchased had been delivered. To help fulfill the urgent demand for vaccines, two Taiwanese high-tech companies, Hon Hai together with its Young Lin Foundation and TSMC,[13] each announced plans to purchase 5 million doses of the Pfizer-BioNTech vaccine.[111] Soon thereafter, TzuChi Foundation, a Taiwanese international humanitarian organization heavily involved in long-term global medical aid and disaster relief, secured a deal on 22 July for another five million vaccines to be donated to the government for distribution.[112] These efforts on top of previously government-purchased supplies would enable 75% of the population to be fully vaccinated.

---

12 The 11 March 2011 earthquake in Fukushima was the strongest in Japan's recorded history, measuring a magnitude of 9.0. It triggered a tsunami up to 40 m (132 ft) high, left over 450,000 people homeless and killed more than 15,500 people. The donations from the Taiwanese governments, charities and private organizations, and the general public totaled ¥20 billion Japanese Yen (approximately US$182 million) – the largest donation of all countries for this natural disaster ([105]).

13 Hon Hai (perhaps better known as Foxconn) is the largest electronic manufacturer worldwide with 1.3 million employees. TSMC (Taiwan Semiconductor Manufacturing Company) is the largest global producer of processor chips for smartphones, computers, and automobiles.

10.8.3 Vaccine Prioritization and Administration

Taiwan's COVID-19 vaccination group classification is a mix of occupation, age, and risk of infection and transmission.[113] In addition to the public and media's questions and disputes about the vaccine purchasing decisions and undisclosed contract details,[80, 89, 114] the prioritization list's rationale and multiple revisions have faced criticism, including reshuffling of subgroups and nebulous definitions of certain categories.[92, 115] However, some re-prioritizations were widely accepted, such as cohabitating family members of healthcare professionals treating suspected or infected patients. Furthermore, after an outbreak in an airport quarantine hotel housing airline crews, domestic crews were added to group 3 as a newly created category: high-contact frontline workers.[14]

The CECC is in charge of allocating and distributing the national vaccine supply to local health departments, generally based on population, inoculation capacity, and recent case incidence. As demand heightened and delivery lagged, several dilemmas emerged, such as whether to adopt mixing different vaccine brands, increase the interval between shots to stretch supply, and use limited inventory to fully vaccinate at-risk populations or give more people a first dose to broaden basic coverage. These questions involving logistical feasibility, evolving scientific evidence, and equity have continued to be debated.

10.9 Reflections and Conclusions

The complexity and anxiety of everything surrounding COVID-19, including unknown risks, the initial mask and vaccine shortages, social isolation, and the disruption of normal routines have affected the lives of Taiwanese, as well as billions of people worldwide.

Taiwan's comparatively small case numbers may be attributed to a strict disease control model in an island nation which can more easily secure its borders, along with public acceptance of public health measures. These actions included preemptive health screening by airport and maritime border controls, expansive contact tracing, and daily electronic check-ins by people under mandated quarantine. The legislature formulates and enacts the laws and the CECC stipulates the pandemic policies. Still, it is a collective decision of the government and the people to deliberate (or determine) the acceptable balance between public health and civil liberty. Even the best implementation of public health measures, medicine, and the most-advanced digital tracing or surveillance tools could not contain the spread if few people voluntarily participate in the system or comply with the guidelines. The citizens' proactive, cautionary behavior – from the high prevalence of mask-wearing since January 2020 to self-imposed sheltering at home when the case number jumped – reinforced the effects of the measures; the tangible results of an attenuated condition then made the restrictions more endurable.

For much longer than anyone had anticipated or ever imagined, people the world over have lived in a series of paradoxes during this pandemic: feeling despair and hopefulness; isolated yet connected; relinquishing freedom and making uncomfortable choices; rethinking the meaning of life and longing for a return to "normal"; losing track of time and counting the days. Likewise, governments face the intricate dilemma of reopening the economy or prioritizing population health through continued restrictions. It poses a particular challenge for Taiwan, once a lauded model in combating the pandemic,[116] to forgo the COVID-zero approach and lift its stringent border control.[51, 91] While the shock of the sudden surge in May 2021 lingers, Taiwan recognizes the need to reconnect with the world in order to fully recover the economy and people's livelihood. With the

---

14 Subsequently, seaport personnel, taxi drivers who transport suspected cases or people under quarantine, and staff working at quarantine hotels were added to the high-contact frontline workers category.

public's demand and global trend of moving toward the new normal of living with COVID-19, the CECC plans gradual stepwise removal of most domestic constraints once 60% of the population is fully vaccinated by the end of 2021[15] and will eventually reduce quarantine requirements for incoming passengers later in 2022. The nation continues to learn from these experiences and fine-tune its response. The lessons obtained from the previous experience with SARS Cov-1 resulted in an elevated emergency alert system and strengthened public health preparedness and response capacity. The national experience from the COVID-19 pandemic and the new lessons learned shall also enable Taiwan to improve its readiness and operations to defend against future public health crises.

References

1 Our World in Data. Coronavirus Pandemic (COVID-19) – Statistics and Research. Our World in Data. Published updated daily 2021. Accessed October 1, 2021. https://ourworldindata.org/coronavirus#coronavirus-country-profiles

2 Gardner L. Modeling the Spreading Risk of 2019-nCoV. JHU-Center for Systems Science and Engineering. Published January 31, 2020. Accessed May 1, 2020. https://systems.jhu.edu/research/public-health/ncov-model-2/

3 Taiwan CDC. Taiwan CDC Press Release 2020-12-31. Taiwan CDC. Published December 31, 2020. Accessed November 7, 2021. https://www.cdc.gov.tw/Bulletin/Detail/81weVaSfZeMRFpFRWhaNqg?typeid=9

4 The Economist Intelligence Unit. Democracy Index 2020. Economist Intelligence Unit. Published 2020. Accessed September 8, 2021. https://www.eiu.com/n/campaigns/democracy-index-2020/

5 Taiwan | United States Trade Representative. Office of the United States Trade Representative. Published 2020. Accessed September 8, 2021. https://ustr.gov/countries-regions/china/taiwan

6 Taiwan CDC. History and achievements of Taiwan Centers for Disease Control. Taiwan Centers for Disease Control. Published April 30, 2014. Accessed September 3, 2021. https://www.cdc.gov.tw/Category/Page/MTqnNaOG-jHJxOJ-HsxYyg

7 Yang S. Introduction of the Communicable Disease Control Act. *Taiwan Epidemiol Bull.* 2000;16(5):145–150. Accessed September 3, 2021. https://www.cdc.gov.tw/EpidemicTheme/Detail/zKNFqsVWxUoUqE6fyhmBNA?archiveId=8khq0Ve_-PEB4OD3i9BB-Q

8 Yang S. Understanding and application of Communicable Disease Control Act. *Taiwan Epidemiol Bull.* 2003;19(3):125–142. https://www.cdc.gov.tw/File/Get/Lt18vGCeP_7gSjUKlODLzg

9 Taiwan CDC. Establishment of National Health Command Center (NHCC). Taiwan Centers for Disease Control. Published December 17, 2018. Accessed September 3, 2021. https://www.cdc.gov.tw/Category/MPage/6CJ7RCriP1wF4BmtgAhKuA

10 Judicial Yuan. Constitutional Court Ruling and Interpretation #690. Constitutional Court, ROC. Published September 30, 2011. Accessed September 2, 2021. http://cons.judicial.gov.tw/jcc/zh-tw/jep03/show?expno=690

11 Yeh MJ, Cheng Y. Policies Tackling the COVID-19 Pandemic: A Sociopolitical Perspective from Taiwan. *Health Secur.* 2020;18(6):427–434. https://doi.org/10.1089/hs.2020.0095

12 Taiwan Ministry of Health and Welfare. Enforcement Regulations Governing the Central Epidemics Command Center. Laws & Regulations Database of The Republic of China. Published January 28, 2008. Accessed September 14, 2021. https://law.moj.gov.tw/ENG/LawClass/LawAll.aspx?pcode=L0050025

---

15 (Update after initial writing) By 6 December 2021, 76.8% of the Taiwan population received at least one dose and 60.2% were fully vaccinated. As of May 2022, 78.8% were fully vaccinated and 62.5% also had a booster.

13 Taiwan Ministry of Health and Welfare. Communicable Disease Control Act. Laws & Regulations Database of The Republic of China. Published June 19, 2019. Accessed July 25, 2021. https://law.moj.gov.tw/ENG/LawClass/LawAll.aspx?pcode=L0050001

14 Taiwan Ministry of Health and Welfare. Special Act for Prevention, Relief and Revitalization Measures for Severe Pneumonia with Novel Pathogens. Laws & Regulations Database of The Republic of China. Published May 31, 2021. Accessed July 25, 2021. https://law.moj.gov.tw/ENG/LawClass/LawAll.aspx?pcode=L0050039

15 Ho C. Configuration of the Notion of Privacy as a Fundamental Right in Taiwan – A Comparative Study of International Treaties and EU Rules. In: Cohen JA, Alford WP, Lo C-fa, eds. *Taiwan and International Human Rights: A Story of Transformation*. Economics, Law, and Institutions in Asia Pacific. Springer; 2019:423–436. https://doi.org/10.1007/978-981-13-0350-0_24

16 Taiwan National Development Council. Personal Data Protection Act. Laws & Regulations Database of The Republic of China. Published December 30, 2015. Accessed August 27, 2021. https://law.moj.gov.tw/ENG/LawClass/LawAll.aspx?pcode=I0050021

17 National Development Council. Enforcement Rules of the Personal Data Protection Act. Laws & Regulations Database of The Republic of China. Published March 2, 2016. Accessed September 14, 2021. https://law.moj.gov.tw/ENG/LawClass/LawAll.aspx?pcode=I0050022

18 Ministry of Justice. The Communication Security and Surveillance Act. Laws & Regulations Database of The Republic of China. Published May 23, 2018. Accessed September 14, 2021. https://law.moj.gov.tw/ENG/LawClass/LawAll.aspx?pcode=K0060044

19 Office of the President. Constitution of the Republic of China (Taiwan). Laws & Regulations Database of The Republic of China. Published January 1, 1947. Accessed September 14, 2021. https://law.moj.gov.tw/ENG/LawClass/LawAll.aspx?pcode=A0000001

20 Taiwan CDC. CDC continues border control with on-board health screening of flights from Wuhan due to pneumonia outbreak in China. Taiwan CDC Press Release. Published December 31, 2019. Accessed October 17, 2021. https://www.cdc.gov.tw/Bulletin/Detail/zicpvVlBKj-UVeZ5yWBrLQ?typeid=9

21 WHO Director-General. WHO Director-General's opening remarks at the media briefing on COVID-19 – 11 March 2020. World Health Organization. Published March 11, 2020. Accessed April 2, 2020. https://www.who.int/dg/speeches/detail/who-director-general-s-opening-remarks-at-the-media-briefing-on-covid-19---11-march-2020

22 Andrew M. Cuomo. No. 202.6: Continuing Temporary Suspension and Modification of Laws Relating to the Disaster Emergency. New York State Governor Executive Order. Published March 18, 2020. Accessed May 2, 2020. https://www.governor.ny.gov/news/no-2026-continuing-temporary-suspension-and-modification-laws-relating-disaster-emergency

23 Office of Governor. Governor Gavin Newsom Issues Stay at Home Order. California Governor. Published March 19, 2020. Accessed May 2, 2020. https://www.gov.ca.gov/2020/03/19/governor-gavin-newsom-issues-stay-at-home-order/

24 Mervosh S, Lu D, Swales V. See Which States and Cities Have Told Residents to Stay at Home. *The New York Times*. Published March 31, 2020. Accessed April 2, 2020. https://www.nytimes.com/interactive/2020/us/coronavirus-stay-at-home-order.html

25 Frieden T. Which Countries Have Responded Best to Covid-19? *Wall Street Journal*. Published January 1, 2021. Accessed October 18, 2021. https://www.wsj.com/articles/which-countries-have-responded-best-to-covid-19-11609516800

26 Dewan A, Pettersson H, Croker N. As governments fumbled their coronavirus response, these four got it right. Here's how. CNN. Published April 16, 2020. Accessed April 25, 2020. https://www.cnn.com/2020/04/16/world/coronavirus-response-lessons-learned-intl/index.html

27 Lin C, Braund WE, Auerbach J, et al. Policy Decisions and Use of Information Technology to Fight COVID-19, Taiwan – Volume 26, Number 7 – July 2020 – Emerging Infectious Diseases journal – CDC. *Emerg Infect Dis.* 2020;26(7). https://doi.org/10.3201/eid2607.200574

28 Mokhtar F, Gross S. Should Schools Close to Fight Virus? These Places Say No. *Bloomberg.com.* Published March 27, 2020. Accessed April 25, 2020. https://www.bloomberg.com/news/articles/2020-03-27/should-schools-close-to-fight-virus-these-countries-say-no

29 TVBS Poll Center. Satisfaction and impact survey of president and COVID-19. TVBS. Published March 26, 2020. Accessed April 26, 2020. https://cc.tvbs.com.tw/portal/file/poll_center/2020/20200326/d1c2bea9ec4cc133b96a8369f5115382.pdf

30 Taiwan CDC. Total confirmed cases 398 and 178 released from isolation. Taiwan CDC. Published April 18, 2020. Accessed November 7, 2021. https://www.cdc.gov.tw/Bulletin/Detail/VNT5yumlWAFQo1i4digYdg?typeid=9

31 Taiwan CDC. First death from Wuhan outbreak, Taiwan CDC has instituted response plan. Taiwan CDC Press Release. Published January 11, 2020. Accessed August 17, 2021. https://www.cdc.gov.tw/Bulletin/Detail/YsgfiNEJSbxUqOBP4YgYsQ?typeid=9

32 Taiwan CDC. CDC activated Central Epidemic Control Center to prevent novel coronavirus spread. Taiwan CDC. Published January 20, 2020. Accessed November 7, 2021. https://www.cdc.gov.tw/Bulletin/Detail/32NPG1QXFhAmaOLjDOpNmg?typeid=9

33 Griffiths J. Taiwan's coronavirus response is among the best globally. CNN. Published April 5, 2020. Accessed April 10, 2020. https://www.cnn.com/2020/04/04/asia/taiwan-coronavirus-response-who-intl-hnk/index.html

34 Williams H. How Taiwan was coronavirus-ready while the U.S. got caught with its "pants down". *CBS News.* Published May 26, 2020. Accessed November 7, 2021. https://www.cbsnews.com/news/coronavirus-in-taiwan-how-taipei-was-ready-while-us-got-caught-with-pants-down-expert-says/

35 Taiwan Centers for Disease Control. Taiwan timely identifies first imported case of 2019 novel coronavirus infection returning from Wuhan, China through onboard quarantine. Taiwan Centers for Disease Control. Published January 21, 2020. Accessed May 1, 2021. https://www.cdc.gov.tw/En/Bulletin/Detail/pVg_jRVvtHhp94C6GShRkQ?typeid=158

36 Taiwan Centers for Disease Control. Establishing health safety net, advancing intelligent disease control with technology. Published June 1, 2020. Accessed August 21, 2021. https://www.cdc.gov.tw/Bulletin/Detail/Mtrg60_RrPSBQP4kuO_snQ?typeid=9

37 Ritchie H, Ortiz-Ospina E, Beltekian D, et al. Coronavirus Pandemic (COVID-19): Testing and Contract Tracing. *Our World Data.* Published 2020. Accessed August 3, 2021. https://ourworldindata.org/covid-testing-contact-tracing

38 Huang YY. Ceasing the golden 10-hours: Keys to Taiwan blocking virus transmission (in Chinese). Mirror Media. Published March 31, 2020. Accessed April 26, 2020. https://www.mirrormedia.mg/story/20200331inv001/

39 Huang YY. Setting three technology blocks in contact tracing. *Mirror Media.* Published March 31, 2020. Accessed November 7, 2021. https://www.mirrormedia.mg/story/20200331inv005/

40 Taiwan CDC. Taiwan Social Distancing App. Taiwan Centers for Disease Control. Published 2021. Accessed July 27, 2021. https://www.cdc.gov.tw/Category/Page/R8bAd_yiVi22CIr73qM2yw

41 Liu N. Must download, social distance app will alert you if contacted with confirm case. FETnet. Published 2021. Accessed July 19, 2021. http://www.fetnet.net:80/content/cbu/tw/lifecircle/tech/taiwan-social-distance-app.html

42 Taiwan Centers for Disease Control. Contact tracing support platform. Taiwan Centers for Disease Control. Published July 24, 2021. Accessed July 28, 2021. https://www.cdc.gov.tw/Bulletin/Detail/rVZ1dkbtACeqf4cypmsrkg?typeid=9

43 Collins F. The Challenge of Tracking COVID-19's Stealthy Spread. NIH Director's Blog. Published April 23, 2020. Accessed April 25, 2020. https://directorsblog.nih.gov/tag/contact-tracing/

44 Schifrin N. Taiwan's aggressive efforts are paying off in fight against COVID-19. PBS NewsHour. Published April 1, 2020. Accessed April 2, 2020. https://www.pbs.org/newshour/show/taiwans-aggressive-efforts-are-paying-off-in-fight-against-covid-19

45 Global View Monthly. Unboxing the varieties of local governments' quarantine care packages. Global View. Published March 8, 2020. Accessed April 2, 2021. https://www.gvm.com.tw/article/71464

46 Taiwan Centers for Disease Control. Quarantine Compensation Policies during COVID-19 Pandemic (Amendment). Taiwan Centers for Disease Control. Published June 17, 2020. Accessed August 1, 2021. https://www.cdc.gov.tw/File/Get?q=66HT6AZdVjKmPmyJ9OclbL2OM3Z7s5d_tNSgsa7dr8LvZCDnVz3qFD6gbW8izKVfqknFLsmUqeTntncPA7AO75brZevhYNO0VKFbf8_fr-V8Q6PRuWixmNBfckpntu_9i1DGotxmOk76G1SMKpRVVxuaSrC74_xIvPOyFsh2W9JrW0hQUCa6KQkZpSMY9_pQnDSJCryGYl9mAUv2oxDqSQ

47 Taiwan Centers for Disease Control. Penalties for Violating Quarantine Mandate. Published April 17, 2020. Accessed August 1, 2021. https://www.cdc.gov.tw/File/Get?q=66HT6AZdVjKmPmyJ9OclbPftHQmDIEe9W-zuEasTmGaEBtuXEmU2Og94RTn6wuHIIC9wK7yBliOgFOrqJFgqTUkbBcGdFfMFjqSHSO4WHTv7sCycgkclxjbW5TUXrGuhfgXVYSQg34WKXcUFigTTBiODC4ATZhupYo4jSI089CObEu3em9nuE7k3UQOBiz9-59IOC1Nts3cHqXilo_lmxwEyFq7vUlyxnV-b2cQtmr7LayYdroqLM4Btp_vJ5cUv8lqHzF94ermqORLHxgzSAuS1ghiA3xyRV5MxndDKJVyArQ_id3rS_A8oH9Yd48tMOVnvEj9OWUBEp4ggrw9_p6iVLuqqqV__NdwidxyQEm4

48 Farr C, Gao M. How Taiwan beat the coronavirus. CNBC. Published July 15, 2020. Accessed October 18, 2021. https://www.cnbc.com/2020/07/15/how-taiwan-beat-the-coronavirus.html

49 Lin C, Mullen J, Braund WE, Tu P, Auerbach J. Reopening safely – Lessons from Taiwan's COVID-19 response. *J Glob Health.* 2020;10(2):020318. doi:https://doi.org/10.7189/jogh.10.020318

50 Cave D. Australia Is Betting on Remote Quarantine. Here's What I Learned on the Inside. *The New York Times.* Published August 20, 2021. Accessed November 14, 2021. https://www.nytimes.com/2021/08/20/world/australia/howard-springs-quarantine.html

51 Cortez MF, Hong J, Bloomberg. For 'COVID Zero' success stories, opening up is hard to do. Fortune. Published May 14, 2021. Accessed November 14, 2021. https://fortune.com/2021/05/14/covid-zero-reopen-hong-kong-singapore/

52 O'Grady S. To keep coronavirus out, Canada's smallest province kept the rest of the country away. Now outsiders are returning. *Washington Post.* Published July 6, 2020. Accessed November 14, 2021. https://www.washingtonpost.com/world/2020/07/06/prince-edward-island-canada-coronavirus-atlantic-bubble-reopening-travel/

53 Ferretti L, Wymant C, Kendall M, et al. Quantifying SARS-CoV-2 transmission suggests epidemic control with digital contact tracing. *Science.* Published March 31, 2020. https://doi.org/10.1126/science.abb6936

54 Radio New Zealand. App being developed to improve Covid-19 contact tracing. RNZ. Published April 9, 2020. Accessed April 25, 2020. https://www.rnz.co.nz/news/national/413892/app-being-developed-to-improve-covid-19-contact-tracing

55 Wetsman N. What is contact tracing? The Verge. Published April 10, 2020. Accessed November 7, 2021. https://www.theverge.com/2020/4/10/21216550/contact-tracing-coronavirus-what-is-tracking-spread-how-it-works

56 Freedom House. Freedom in the World 2021-Countries and Territories Scores. Freedom House. Published 2021. Accessed October 17, 2021. https://freedomhouse.org/countries/freedom-world/scores

57 Taylor C, Kampf S, Grundig T, Common D. Taiwan is beating COVID-19 without closing schools or workplaces. Can Canada do the same? CBC. Published March 21, 2020. Accessed April 2, 2020. https://www.cbc.ca/news/business/taiwan-covid-19-lessons-1.5505031

58 Will M. How Schools in Other Countries Have Reopened. *Education Week*. https://www.edweek.org/policy-politics/how-schools-in-other-countries-have-reopened/2020/06. Published June 11, 2020. Accessed October 18, 2021

59 Griffiths J. Asia may have been right about coronavirus and face masks, and the rest of the world is coming around. CNN. Published April 1, 2020. Accessed April 25, 2020. https://www.cnn.com/2020/04/01/asia/coronavirus-mask-messaging-intl-hnk/index.html

60 Onishi N, Méheut C. Mask-Wearing Is a Very New Fashion in Paris (and a Lot of Other Places). *The New York Times*. Published April 9, 2020. Accessed April 16, 2020. https://www.nytimes.com/2020/04/09/world/europe/virus-mask-wearing.html

61 Huang T-H. Taiwan emerges as 2nd largest face mask producer to fight epidemic. Taiwan News. Published February 14, 2020. Accessed April 26, 2020. https://www.taiwannews.com.tw/en/news/3876286

62 Chen Y, Chang CC, Yeh J. 10 million masks to be donated to U.S., 11 European countries, allies. Focus Taiwan. Published April 1, 2020. Accessed April 16, 2020. https://focustaiwan.tw/politics/202004010014

63 Liberty Times. President of the European Commission publicly thanked Taiwan for donating 5.6 million masks. *Liberty Times*. Published April 2, 2020. Accessed November 7, 2021. https://news.ltn.com.tw/news/politics/breakingnews/3120736

64 Buchholz K. Infographic: What Share of the World Population Is Already on COVID-19 Lockdown? Statista Infographics. Published April 7, 2020. Accessed April 10, 2020. https://www.statista.com/chart/21240/enforced-covid-19-lockdowns-by-people-affected-per-country/

65 Dunford D, Dale B, Stylianou N, Lowther E, Ahmed M, Torre Arenas I de la. The world in lockdown in maps and charts. *BBC News*. Published April 7, 2020. Accessed April 10, 2020. https://www.bbc.com/news/world-52103747

66 Cheng WC. The whole island "counter-clocked" to prohibit dine-in at restaurants. *United Daily News*. Published July 11, 2021. Accessed August 19, 2021. https://udn.com/news/story/122173/5593008

67 Ireland S. Revealed: Countries With The Best Health Care Systems, 2019. CEOWORLD magazine. Published August 5, 2019. Accessed April 25, 2020. https://ceoworld.biz/2019/08/05/revealed-countries-with-the-best-health-care-systems-2019/

68 Office of the President. Additional Articles of the Constitution of the Republic of China. Laws & Regulations Database of The Republic of China. Published June 10, 2005. Accessed September 14, 2021. https://law.moj.gov.tw/ENG/LawClass/LawAll.aspx?pcode=A0000002

69 National Health Insurance Administration. 2020-2021 National Health Insurance in Taiwan Annual Report. National Health Insurance Administration. Published October 4, 2021. Accessed October 18, 2021. https://www.nhi.gov.tw/English/Content_List.aspx?n=2BDB331B84E5BC43&topn=ED4A30E51A609E49&Create=1

70 Scott D. Taiwan's single-payer success story – and its lessons for America. Vox. Published January 13, 2020. Accessed April 16, 2020. https://www.vox.com/health-care/2020/1/13/21028702/medicare-for-all-taiwan-health-insurance

71 BioSpectrum. Taiwan emerges as pioneer in strengthening global healthcare. BioSpectrum. Published December 21, 2019. Accessed April 25, 2021. https://www.biospectrumasia.com/news/55/15136/taiwan-emerges-as-pioneer-in-strengthening-global-healthcare.html

72 National Health Insurance Administration. Public Satisfaction with National Health Insurance System Hits Historical High of 89.7%. National Health Insurance Administration, Ministry of Health and Welfare. Published November 26, 2019. Accessed October 17, 2021. https://www.nhi.gov.tw/English/News_Content.aspx?n=996D1B4B5DC48343&sms=F0EAFEB716DE7FFA&s=B8D5EE50036E8B4D&Create=1

73 Taiwan CDC. NHI cloud record to note negative and self-monitoring cases. Published May 17, 2021. Accessed September 3, 2021. https://www.cdc.gov.tw/Bulletin/Detail/FPFUTJ_xdE8deRN7mtAgtQ?typeid=9

74 Tsai M, Hwang A. Taiwan using national health insurance data to enable AI-based smart medical care development. DIGITIMES. Published March 6, 2020. Accessed April 16, 2020. https://www.digitimes.com/news/a20200305PD210.html

75 NHI Profile. National Health Insurance in Taiwan Annual Report 2017-2018. National Health Insurance Administration. Published October 1, 2019. Accessed May 2, 2020. https://www.nhi.gov.tw/ENGLISH/Content_List.aspx?n=8FC0974BBFEFA56D&topn=ED4A30E51A609E49&Create=1

76 Ministry of Health and Welfare. Regulations Governing Operation of the Communicable Disease. Published December 18, 2015. Accessed May 1, 2021. 118b9c01-7d92-4c2b-bc15-d0b02cee1b3d.pdf

77 Wu Y. Healthcare providers infected while treating patients could receive NT$350,000 in compensation. *Mirror Media*. Published January 12, 2021. Accessed December 18, 2021. https://www.mirrormedia.mg/story/20210112edi042/

78 Taiwan Ministry of Health and Welfare. Regulations Governing Subsidies for Injuries, Illnesses or Deaths due to Performing Control Measures against Category V Communicable Diseases. Laws & Regulations Database of The Republic of China (Taiwan). Published September 3, 2021. Accessed May 18, 2022. https://law.moj.gov.tw/ENG/LawClass/LawAll.aspx?pcode=L0050027

79 The Economist Intelligence Unit. Taiwan Economy, Politics and GDP Growth Summary. Published 2021. Accessed July 30, 2021. https://country.eiu.com/taiwan

80 BBC News. Taiwan faces the worst crisis: TaoYuan Hospital cluster tests response measures. BBC News Chinese. Published January 26, 2021. Accessed October 19, 2021. https://www.bbc.com/zhongwen/trad/chinese-news-55808601

81 Strong M. Complacency, sluggish vaccination behind Taiwan's COVID surge: Bloomberg. *Taiwan News*. Published May 20, 2021. Accessed October 18, 2021. https://www.taiwannews.com.tw/en/news/4207160

82 Taiwan CDC. CECC raises alter level to III in two northern cities, tightening restrictions in communities. Taiwan CDC. Published May 15, 2021. Accessed August 19, 2021. https://www.cdc.gov.tw/Category/ListContent/EmXemht4IT-IRAPrAnyG9A?uaid=E7bi2j8UYj1Rmz73OPE7Yg

83 Taiwan Centers for Disease Control. June 1 National Pandemic Response Meeting Report. Taiwan CDC Press Release. Published June 1, 2021. Accessed July 24, 2021. https://www.cdc.gov.tw/Bulletin/Detail/K36ktrFXahLqSBuiwMYlJw?typeid=9

84 Chen YT. Taipei set up makeshift hospitals at quarantine hotels for patients with no or minor symptoms. CNA. Published May 21, 2021. Accessed June 19, 2021. https://www.cna.com.tw/news/firstnews/202105210233.aspx

85 United Daily News. COVID-19 guidelines – Criteria and measures of four levels of alert. *United Daily News.* https://health.udn.com/health/story/121019/5448646. Published May 11, 2021. Accessed August 19, 2021

86 Chen YT. Level II extended through 8/23 with relaxed restrictions, dine-in allowed for restaurants. *Liberty Times Net.* https://news.ltn.com.tw/news/life/breakingnews/3613704. Published July 23, 2021. Accessed May 19, 2022

87 Mandarin Daily News. Slight relaxation from Level III, many cities still prohibit dine-in at restaurants. *Mandarin Daily News.* Published July 10, 2021. Accessed August 19, 2021. https://www.mdnkids.com/content.asp?sub=1&sn=2925

88 Central Epidemic Control Center. Central Epidemic Control Center press conference. Presented at: August 13, 2021.

89 BBC News. Model of anti-pandemic Taiwan in doubt: Pilots infected and community cases rising. BBC News Chinese. Published May 12, 2021. Accessed October 19, 2021. https://www.bbc.com/zhongwen/trad/chinese-news-57086046

90 Ellis S, Wang C, Cortez MF. Complacency Let Covid Erode Taiwan's Only Line of Defense. *Bloomberg.* Published May 18, 2021. Accessed October 18, 2021. https://www.bloomberg.com/news/articles/2021-05-18/complacency-let-covid-break-down-taiwan-s-only-line-of-defense

91 Inocencio R. Why Taiwan, long a COVID success story, is seeing a record surge in cases. *CBS News.* https://www.cbsnews.com/news/taiwan-covid-cases-previous-success-story-now-record-coronavirus-surge/

92 BBC News. Global pandemic myth shattered: How did Taiwan get here. *BBC News.* Published May 25, 2021. Accessed October 18, 2021. Published May 20, 2021. Accessed November 7, 2021. https://www.bbc.com/zhongwen/trad/57187804

93 Taiwan CDC. Modifying quarantine measure for domestic airline crews. Taiwan CDC. Published June 14, 2021. Accessed September 3, 2021. https://www.cdc.gov.tw/Bulletin/Detail/Aaw09pr_bNORqPc8F1fUSA?typeid=9

94 Pon ZC. Taipei mayor confronting CECC commander: Rapid tests found large number of cases. Global Views. Published May 20, 2021. Accessed October 18, 2021. https://www.gvm.com.tw/article/79652

95 Chen YC. Taipei testing center positivity rate decreasing from 11 to 4.7% in 5 days. *CNA-Focus Taiwan.* Published May 18, 2021. Accessed August 19, 2021. https://www.cna.com.tw/news/firstnews/202105180256.aspx

96 Chen YT, Lin CS. Taipei city added 20 rapid testing centers: Come if you have symptoms or contact. CNA. Published May 23, 2021. Accessed June 19, 2021. https://www.cna.com.tw/news/firstnews/202105230135.aspx

97 Taiwan CDC. Subsidy for community testing centers. Taiwan CDC. Published May 30, 2021. Accessed September 3, 2021. https://www.cdc.gov.tw/Bulletin/Detail/1Q_whSnJYilR4qZB9zso7w?typeid=9

98 Taiwan CDC. Subsidy for purchasing rapid PCR test machinery to accelerate community testing capacity. Taiwan Centers for Disease Control. Published June 15, 2021. Accessed September 3, 2021. https://www.cdc.gov.tw/Bulletin/Detail/84kDjSBTHU75sIoWKAdKcg?typeid=9

99 Taiwan CDC. National Disease Control Committee post-meeting press conference report. Taiwan CDC. Published June 1, 2021. Accessed September 3, 2021. https://www.cdc.gov.tw/Bulletin/Detail/K36ktrFXahLqSBuiwMYlJw?typeid=9

100 Taiwan CDC. Department of Transportation set up testing booths at 5 airports. Taiwan CDC. Published May 31, 2021. Accessed September 3, 2021. https://www.cdc.gov.tw/Bulletin/Detail/XA0ksHRpXczO_NWgNKC8iQ?typeid=9

101 Taiwan CDC. CECC announced 4 response strategies to conserve medial capacity. Taiwan CDC. Published May 16, 2021. Accessed September 3, 2021. https://www.cdc.gov.tw/Bulletin/Detail/_czNqXB2n2A3JZrciBnMhQ?typeid=9

102 Yang CL. Bloomberg accounted complacency as cause for Taiwan breaching COVID defense, CDC spokesperson responded. Newtalk. Published July 26, 2021. Accessed July 28, 2021. https://newtalk.tw/news/view/2021-07-26/610624

103 Yasir S. A vaccine maker in India signals it won't export doses before year's end, slowing aid to the world's poorest. *The New York Times*. Published May 19, 2021. Accessed July 24, 2021. https://www.nytimes.com/2021/05/19/world/india-serum-institute-vaccines.html

104 Lian UY. 1.24 million AZ vaccines arriving Taiwan! Why is Japan donating and why AZ? *Common Health*. Published June 4, 2021. Accessed August 19, 2021. https://www.commonhealth.com.tw/article/84380

105 Chaou K, Wen Y. Stories behind the number: 6.8 billion donations from Taiwan for the Eastern Japan earthquake. nippon.com. Published April 6, 2018. Accessed July 22, 2021. https://www.nippon.com/hk/features/c04918/

106 Lin C, Tu P, Beitsch LM. Confidence and Receptivity for COVID-19 Vaccines: A Rapid Systematic Review. *Vaccines*. 2020;9(1), 16. https://doi.org/10.3390/vaccines9010016

107 MacDonald NE, SAGE Working Group on Vaccine Hesitancy. Vaccine hesitancy: Definition, scope and determinants. *Vaccine* 2015;33(34):4161–4164. https://doi.org/10.1016/j.vaccine.2015.04.036

108 BBC News. Taiwan accepted 400 thousand doses of AstraZeneca in emergency, but some citizens refused. BBC News. Published May 20, 2021. Accessed October 19, 2021. https://www.bbc.com/zhongwen/trad/world-57186822

109 Chou CR. 43 deaths after vaccination: Comparing international data. *TVBS*. Published June 18, 2021. Accessed August 19, 2021. https://news.tvbs.com.tw/life/1530488

110 Lian UY. Identifying risk factors is more important than post-vaccination death rate. *Common Health*. Published July 3, 2021. Accessed August 19, 2021. https://www.commonhealth.com.tw/article/84586

111 Foxconn. TSMC and Hon Hai/YongLin Foundation Donate 10 Million Doses of BNT Vaccine to Taiwan CDC. Foxconn Technology Group. Published July 12, 2021. Accessed November 6, 2021. https://www.honhai.com/en-us/press-center/events/csr-events/646

112 Reuters. Taiwan bumps BioNTech vaccine order to 15 mln with Buddhist donation. *Reuters*. Published July 21, 2021. Accessed August 19, 2021. https://www.reuters.com/world/asia-pacific/taiwan-buddhist-group-buy-5-mln-biontech-vaccines-2021-07-21/

113 Wang CL. CDC announces the latest top 10 priorities for COVID-19 vaccination. Heho. Published February 26, 2021. Accessed July 24, 2021. https://heho.com.tw/archives/163903

114 BBC News. Local cases continue to exceed 100, why Taiwan's vaccination program struggling. BBC News. Published May 19, 2021. Accessed October 19, 2021. https://www.bbc.com/zhongwen/trad/chinese-news-57156901

115 Shieh WZ. 410,000 AZ vaccines starting today, policemen upgraded to priority category 5. Mirror Media. Published May 28, 2021. Accessed July 24, 2021. https://www.mirrormedia.mg/story/20210528edi011/

116 Bourke L. Zero-COVID countries face 'genuine dilemma' about how to reopen: WHO. The Sydney Morning Herald. Published June 7, 2021. Accessed November 14, 2021. https://www.smh.com.au/world/europe/zero-covid-countries-face-genuine-dilemma-about-how-to-open-up-who-20210608-p57yyg.html

11

The Legislative and Political Responses of Viet Nam to the Covid-19 Pandemic: The Balancing of Public Health and Collective Civil Liberties

Nguyen T. Trung[1] and Nguyen Q. Duong[2]

[1]*Research fellow, Max Planck Institute Luxembourg for International, European and Regulatory Procedural Law, Luxembourg*
[2]*Ministry of Foreign Affairs, Vietnam*

Disclaimer

The authors would like to thank Mrs. Le Duc Hanh for her insightful ideas on certain parts of the manuscript. This chapter represents the opinions of the authors and is the product of professional research. It is not meant to represent the position or opinions of the Vietnamese government on the topic. Any errors are the fault of the authors.

11.1 Introduction

31 December of 2020 was quite a particular New Year's Eve. Contrary to the many previous years, most, if not all, New Year events were canceled as citizens worldwide were being placed under strict lockdown to curb the spread of the Covid-19 pandemic. Yet, in South East Asia, the people of Viet Nam were celebrating the New Year as if the pandemic did not exist. This was made possible by the country's remarkable handling of this public health crisis, despite being one of the first countries with a confirmed case of Covid-19 outside of China (Coleman 2020).

Viet Nam's success story has attracted attention from commentators as it has remained one of the few countries that were not forced to undergo a prolonged lockdown and restriction of all its social and economic activities during the Covid-19 pandemic. These studies focus primarily on the effective response of the Vietnamese government to the pandemic, the measures that were put into place to curb the spread of this novel virus, and the contribution of the general public and other non-state actors in Viet Nam in the process of coping with the pandemic. In the context of analyzing the law and policy contexts of Covid-19 in Asian countries, Nguyen and Phan explained Viet Nam's success in terms of its past experiences with other contagious diseases, such as the Severe Acute Respiratory Syndrome (SARS) in 2003, its centralized and unified decision-making process to combat the spread of the virus and the flexible response of the Vietnamese government by combing "coercive means with deliberate action, public education, effective governance, and effective coordination with the community and the private sector" (Nguyen and Phan 2020, p. 58). The authors argued that the country is on the right track in the "Covid-19 campaign" as it gathered support from the general public by prioritizing public health over economic growth. In a more

Impacts of the Covid-19 Pandemic: International Laws, Policies, and Civil Liberties, First Edition. Edited by Nadav Morag.
© 2023 John Wiley & Sons, Inc. Published 2023 by John Wiley & Sons, Inc.

recent study, Le et al. analyzed the "policy documents" issued by the Vietnamese authorities in the first two waves of the Covid-19 virus in Viet Nam (from January 2020 to July 2020) (Le et al. 2021). Based on the assessment of close-to-1000 policy documents issued by 33 government agencies in Viet Nam since the virus first appeared, the authors demonstrated the multidimensional approaches taken by the Vietnamese authorities, which put in place several key measures to contain the spread of the virus, including outbreak announcements, medical treatments, school closure, border control, tracing and tracking of confirmed and suspicious cases, and quarantine measures. In their findings, the authors found that special policies were put in place that did not previously exist before the pandemic, such as nationwide school closure, financial support for quarantined people at home or in centralized centers, and inbound flight restrictions with "quarantine" and "isolation" being the most mentioned keywords in these policy documents. Ultimately, these studies, as well as others (Black 2020; Reguly 2020; Pollack et al. 2021), converged on the point that the responses of the Vietnamese government have been effective in identifying infection's strings, preventing the spread of the virus and suppressing the social effects of the pandemic in the public.

While concurring, in principle, with the ultimate findings of the abovementioned studies, this chapter seeks to take matters a step further in addressing two issues: first, whether there has been a paradigm shift in the legal and political responses of the Vietnamese government during the different waves of the Covid-19 pandemic; and, second, whether the enjoyment of civil liberties in Viet Nam have been adversely affected as a the result of the measures put into place by the Vietnamese authorities to combat the Covid-19 virus. The first research question is important because as Covid-19 is an infectious virus that constantly changes through mutation (CDC 2022), it is expected that government responses and tactics should be adopted accordingly to curb the appearance of new variants. The aforementioned studies were all concluded when Viet Nam successfully contained the first (23 January– 9 April 2020) and second waves (25 July–2 September 2020) of Covid-19 infections. Since then, Viet Nam has witnessed two more waves of infections (from 28 January to 13 March 2021 and from 27 April to the time of writing this chapter). As such, this is a good time to re-evaluate what has changed (if anything) in the legal framework and the Vietnamese government's current strategy to combat the Covid-19 virus. The second question is significant because, in times of pandemic emergency, it is expected that individual human rights and civil liberties will be limited in the public interest. Nevertheless, there have been concerns that such limitations would adversely affect basic civil liberties by means of intrusion into an individual's privacy rights through tracking and surveillance, preventing free speech and coercing in quarantine and isolation (Orzechowski et al. 2021, p. 146). An assessment of whether the measures implemented by the Vietnamese government are proportionate to the risks caused by the Covid-19 will shed light on the country's balancing of public health and civil liberties in times of pandemic.

The remainder of this chapter will be divided into the following sections: Section 11.2 begins by providing a descriptive background of the four waves of Covid-19 in Viet Nam. Section 11.3 delivers an overview of the legal framework in combating infectious diseases in Viet Nam, including the 2013 Constitution, the 2007 Law on prevention and control of infectious diseases, the Criminal Code 2015, related governmental decrees, and administrative documents. Section 11.4 will focus on the measures implemented by the Vietnamese government to address the Covid-19 pandemic, such as the tracking and tracing system and the rules on mandatory quarantine and social distancing measures. Section 11.5 will address the abovementioned research questions in this contribution, namely the paradigm shift in the legal and political responses of the Vietnamese government to address Covid-19 and its balancing of public health and civil liberties in times of pandemic. Section 11.6 will provide conclusions on Viet Nam's approach.

11.2 Background: The Four Waves of Covid-19 in Viet Nam

23 January 2020 marked the first day the virus appeared in Viet Nam with two cases imported from Wuhan, China. From that day until 17 May 2021, there are four waves that the virus was domestically spread: (i) 23 January–19 April 2020, (ii) 25 July–2 September 2020, (iii) 28 January–13 March 2021, and (iv) 27 April–15 July 2021.

We gathered and calculated the data of domestically infected cases and Covid-19-related deaths through the daily tallies from notices of the Ministry of Health of Viet Nam, official Vietnamese newspapers, such as Vnexpress and Tuoitrenews, and reports of the Vietnamese government to the World Health Organization. The reason for the reference from multiple sources is that the daily tallies of infected cases in the official government portal include both domestic and imported cases. We excluded the tallies of imported cases from our graphic, making our data collection method different from sources such as https://www.worldometers.info. The rationale for this approach is that the Vietnamese government had restricted commercial flights coming into Viet Nam when the virus first emerged. Instead, passenger flights into Viet Nam were for the humanitarian purpose of rescuing tourists, students and workers aboard whose visas have expired in the infected region (Doan 2020). Moreover, all incoming passengers, either by air, sea, or ground routes, were immediately quarantined as soon as they arrived in the Vietnamese territory. Consequently, it is likely to assume that all imported positive cases were infected while abroad or during the flights. As such, these imported cases are extraordinary and do not reflect the assessment of the effectiveness of Covid-19-related measures in preventing the spread of the virus within the jurisdiction of the state. Our data collection cut-off date is 15 July 2021.

11.2.1 The First Wave (23 January–19 April 2020)

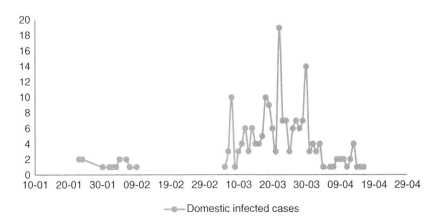

The first wave started from 23 January to 19 April 2020. During this period, there was approximately 1–2 case(s) daily, which were all related to people arriving from Wuhan (Bach Mai 2020). One week after identifying the first case in Viet Nam, Prime Minister Nguyen Xuan Phuc established the Covid-19 National Steering Committee, composing representatives of all relevant agencies, such as Ministries of Health, Communication, Foreign Affairs, Transportation, and Defense (Decision 170/QĐ-TTg dated 30 January 2020). The Committee coordinated all activities related to prevention and combating the pandemic and provided daily reports to the prime minister (Article 2 of the Decision). On 1 February, the prime minister issued Decision 173/QĐ-TTg, officially declaring Covid-19 as a pandemic in Viet Nam. Acknowledging that most cases at that time were related to people arriving from Wuhan, on 7 February, the Health Ministry issued Decision 344/QĐ-BYT requiring all arrivals from Wuhan to stay in quarantine camps for at least 14 days.

After new arrivals from the United States, the EU, and South Korea tested positive for Covid-19, on 18 March, the Vietnamese government decided to pause issuing visas for Viet Nam and decided to restrict flights from abroad (Notice 102/TB-VPCP dated 18 March 2020). Furthermore, all people arriving in Viet Nam were required to stay in quarantine camps run by soldiers and medical staff for at least 14 days. Contact tracing and testing procedures were quickly implemented during this period, and this contact tracing identified 46 relevant cases in Hà Nội and 18 relevant cases in Hồ Chí Minh City (Bach Mai 2020). From March until April 2020, the prime minister issued three important directives (Directive 15/CT-TTg on 27 March, Directive 16/CT-TTg on 31 March and Directive 19/CT-TTg on 24 April) to temporarily implement social distancing measures, including the prohibition of public gatherings, restriction of transportation, and the closure of nonessential businesses. After implementing the three directives, daily new cases decreased significantly, with only 13 cases identified from 6 to 15 April.

During the 86 days of the first wave, around 200 positive cases were domestically infected throughout Viet Nam compared to more than 2 million cases recorded worldwide. The government of Viet Nam quickly responded to the emergence of the novel virus by implementing several administrative and executive measures, including the establishment of the National Steering Committee, the approval of Directives 15, 16, and 19, all of which will be effective tools for Viet Nam to prevent and combat the pandemic in later waves.

11.2.2 The Second Wave (25 July–2 September 2020)

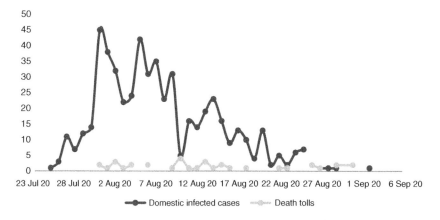

The second wave started on 25 July 2020 with a patient zero in Đà Nẵng, a tourist city in the middle part of the country. Immediately after the patient tested positive for Covid-19, contact tracing and testing in Đà Nẵng's hospitals for suspected cases were implemented (Tuan 2020). Recognizing the potential seriousness of this wave, the prime minister required Đà Nẵng city to undertake quarantine measures and allowed the local head of the governing administrative unit (Chairpersons of the People's Committee) to decide the application of either Directive 16 (more restrictive) or Directive 19 (less restrictive), whichever is appropriate in the current situation (Notice 262/TB-VPCP dated 29 July 2020). The Chairperson of Đà Nẵng decided to apply Directive 16 to six central districts and Directive 19 to two suburban districts (Binh 2020). Similarly, the provincial leaders of other provinces and cities, such as Hà Nội, decided to apply Directive 19 to the whole city and test all people returning from Đà Nẵng (Chinh 2020). The infection expanded to some northern Vietnamese provinces, such as Hà Nội, Lạng Sơn, and Hải Dương, but most cases were in Đà Nẵng City and its neighboring provinces. Together with contact tracing, the Covid-19 National Steering Committee and the Ministry of Health adopted several guidelines to tighten social distancing in hospitals, which was not covered by previous Directives (Telegram 1158/CĐ-BCĐQG dated 27 July 2020 and Telegram 1212/CĐ-BYT dated 3 August 2020). On 18 August, the Health Ministry required all hospitals and healthcare facilities to suspend unauthorized people from visiting resident patients (Document 4393/BYT-KCB dated 18 August 2020, para. 7).

The date of 31 July recorded the highest number of daily new cases in Viet Nam in the first two waves, at 45 patients and the first death, a patient who had previously suffered chronic kidney failure for over 10 years (N. Le 2020). In one month from 31 July to 31 August 2020, Viet Nam recorded 34 deaths in total, most of who are elders in Đà Nẵng hospital with serious comorbidity.

The second wave in Viet Nam recorded more than 500 cases in more than one month, which means 17 daily cases on average compared to more than 400,000 cases daily on average worldwide. Many of the administrative frameworks approved by the first wave were used, such as Directives 16 and 19. On the other hand, some new steps include authorizing the chairpersons to decide the appropriate social distancing and quarantine measures in their province.

11.2.3 The Third Wave (28 January–13 March 2021)

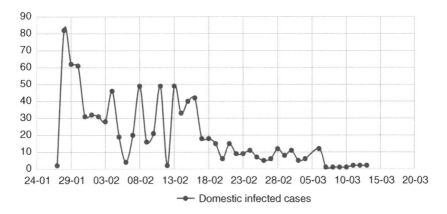

The third wave of Covid-19 spread in Viet Nam started on 27 January 2021, with two patients in Quảng Ninh and Hải Dương in northern Viet Nam. One patient was a worker in an industrial zone in Hải Dương, who came in close proximity with the patient zero tested positive for Covid-19 after arriving in Japan from Viet Nam, and the other served as a staff of Vân Đồn Airport of Quảng Ninh (Dinh 2021). During the Covid-19 National Steering Committee meeting, the Vietnamese authorities decided to mobilize experts from central hospitals to support Hải Dương with mass testing and establishing field hospitals on the next day (Dinh 2021). With mass testing, 28 January 2021 witnessed the highest number of daily new cases in Viet Nam in the first three waves, reaching 82 patients, including 77 patients in Hai Duong and 11 others in Quảng Ninh (Thuong 2021b). On the same day, the prime minister adopted Directive 5/CT-TTg, requiring a city in Hải Dương province to quarantine under Directive 16 and all other provinces to implement social distancing measures. The directive also suspended all activities of Van Don Airport and authorized the Chairpersons of Hải Dương and Quảng Ninh province to decide on Covid-19-related measures based on either Directive 15 or 16. The Chairperson of Quảng Ninh immediately decided to apply Directive 16 to some high-risk areas on 29 January for 21 days (Tuan 2021). Meanwhile, the Hải Dương People Committee decided to establish containment zones in several villages and hamlets for 21 days in accordance with the spirit of Directive 19 (Decision 383/QĐ-BCĐ dated 2 February 2021) and, later, to quarantine the entire province on 15 February based on Directive 16 for 14 days.

The third wave recorded more than 900 patients with no deaths in 45 days. A new measure was the establishment of three field hospitals in Hải Dương province, which may have been due to the main characteristics of patients in Hải Dương, almost all of whom were workers in industrial zones, in contrast to elderly patients admitted to hospitals during the second wave.

11.2.4 The Fourth Wave (27 April–15 July 2021)

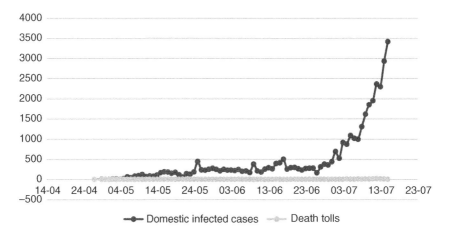

A patient infected from a quarantine zone in Yen Bai was officially recorded on 27 April 2021, ended a one-month period without a positive case in Viet Nam, and marked the beginning of the fourth wave (Hoang 2021b). As a holiday in Viet Nam was coming on 30 April, many large cities throughout the country immediately suspended annual public-gathering events, such as firework performances and festivals, to prevent a new wave of infections. On 29 April, six more patients were tested positive for Covid-19, including one patient who tested positive after more than 14 days of staying in quarantine camps (Xuan 2021). The number of cases climbed up significantly daily, reaching nearly 3,500 cases on 15 July 2021, and spread widely, affecting 58/63 provinces of Viet Nam (WHO Report 50 2021c). The outbreak primarily affected northern provinces, including Bắc Giang and Bắc Ninh, but then new clusters emerged and quickly transmitted in Hồ Chí Minh city and other southern provinces (WHO Report 46 2021b). There were various cases in different provinces with unknown sources of transmission (WHO Report 50 2021c). The need to implement the "dual objectives" of pandemic prevention and control and economic and social development was reaffirmed by Telegram dated 27 April of the Permanent Secretariat and Telegrams 789/CĐ-TTg dated 5/6/2021 of the Prime Minister. Under these directives, each province adopted measures to prevent and control the pandemic at the local level. For example, after recorded 133 cases from 26 to 30 May 2021, the Chairperson of Hồ Chí Minh City decided to apply Directive 15 to the whole city and Directive 16 to some local clusters as of 31 May. Directive 16 has been applied to the whole Hồ Chí Minh City since 9 July, after recording 13,012 cases since 27 April (WHO Report 50 2021c). During this wave, the number of deaths also increased; the highest record was 18 deaths on 12 July 2021, bringing about the total deaths in this wave to 172.

In summary, a number of conclusions can be drawn from the four waves of Covid-19 in Viet Nam. First, the number of daily new cases increased through the four waves. The latest wave has lasted the longest and recorded nearly 3,500 infections a day at the most, in comparison to only 80 infections a day during the third wave. However, the mortality rate and the proportion of the number of patients to the population as a whole are relatively low. Second, all waves have involved cluster transmissions, focused in particular provinces instead of being characterized by uncontrollable spread throughout the country. Finally, the Vietnamese government has responded immediately to new outbreaks with containment measures, such as quarantine, social distancing, and mass testing, to prevent the Covid-19 virus from spreading in public.

11.3 The Legislative Framework in Combating Infectious Disease

This section will analyze Vietnamese legal and administrative instruments on which the framework for preventing and combating infectious disease is based, particularly with respect to the Covid-19 pandemic. Going further than previous work (Nguyen and Phan 2020), we will not only look at primary law, namely the 2013 Constitution, the 2007 Law on Prevention and Control of Infectious Diseases, and the 2015 Criminal Code but also include secondary law, such as governmental decrees and the interpretative document issued by the People's Supreme Court that interprets these laws. Moreover, given their central role in providing guidelines to the implementation of Covid-19-related measures, we will analyze other administrative documents, such as directives and telegrams.

11.3.1 Legislative and Administrative Documents in Vietnam

Under the 2015 Law on Promulgation of Legislative Documents, legislative documents are defined as documents that contain normative regulations, which are general rules of conduct, legally binding, and enforceable on agencies, organizations, and individuals (Article 2(1) and 3(1)). The system of legislative documents includes (i) the Constitution, (ii) codes, laws, and resolutions of the National Assembly, (iii) Ordinances, Resolutions of the Standing Committee of the National Assembly, (iv) Decrees of the government, (v) Decisions of Prime Minister, (vi) Circulars of ministerial agencies, and (vii) Decisions of local authorities (Article 4 of the 2015 Law).

Apart from legislative documents, administrative documents also contribute to the regulation of the conduct of agencies, organizations, and individuals in Viet Nam. Administrative documents are formed when a government authority performs its management, governance, and other core business functions (Article 3(3), Article 7 of the Decree 30/2020/NĐ-CP dated 5 March 2020 on Records Management). Administrative documents are not legislative documents and, thus, they do not contain normative regulations. Nevertheless, certain types of administrative documents, such as directives of the prime minister and telegrams of the government and ministries, play an important role in providing guidelines for the implementation of legislative documents and prescribing executive measures for specific issues. Additionally, since administrative documents do not need to undergo the legislative process at the National Assembly, they can be adopted in a timely manner to address changing circumstances.

11.3.2 The Constitution

The 2013 Constitution is the supreme law in Viet Nam and supersedes all other laws. Relating to combating infectious diseases, the 2013 Constitution provides for a framework for the protection of human rights, the hierarchy of powers of national agencies, and the authority to declare a state of emergency.

While Article 61 of the 1992 Constitution provided for a general entitlement to a regime of health protection, Article 38 of the 2013 Constitution stipulates more specific rights of every citizen relating to health protection, including equal access to healthcare and medical services. These rights come with the duty to comply with disease-control regulations, such as prophylactics, medical examination, and treatment. Moreover, this provision also prohibits any acts of threatening the life and health of other people.

Regarding the hierarchy of powers, the National Assembly is the highest legislative organ in Viet Nam, responsible for making and amending legislation (Article 69, 70(1) of the Constitution). The government is the highest administrative body, comprising of the prime minister, deputy prime ministers, and heads of ministerial-level agencies (Article 94(1), 95(1) of the Constitution). The government shall organize the implementation of the Constitution, laws and resolutions of the National Assembly (Article 96(1) of the Constitution). The prime minister, as the head of the government, shall be responsible for leading the work of the government, formulation of policies, and organize the implementation of laws as well as the work of the state administration system from the central to the local level (Article 98 of the Constitution). Ministers and heads of ministerial-level agencies, as members of the government, shall lead the work of their respective ministries and perform the management of the sectors and fields under their charge as well as monitor nationwide the implementation of relevant laws (Article 99 of the Constitution). The implementation of the Constitution and laws in their locality is the responsibility of local administrative authorities, which are the People's Committees of provinces, districts, and communes (Article 110 of the Constitution). As such, local authorities are given the autonomy to choose the most appropriate way to implement the law in their respective jurisdiction. Nevertheless, under the 2015 Law on the organization of the local government, this autonomy is subjected to the inspection and guidance of the central government and the ministerial-level agencies within the relevant sectors (Article 36).

The Constitution provides the National Assembly the power to proclaim the state of emergency in times of war and other national crises (Article 70(13) of the Constitution). Such a state of emergency, which can be national or limited to a particular locality, can be declared (or canceled) by the Standing Committee of National Assembly or by the president either based on the resolutions of the Standing Committee or when the Standing Committee cannot meet (Article 74(10), Article 88(5) of the Constitution). The Government shall be responsible for carrying out the orders to proclaim a State of Emergency (Article 96(3) of the Constitution). The specific procedures to declare the state of emergency in cases of dangerous epidemics are stipulated in the 2007 Law on Prevention and Control of Infectious Diseases ("the 2007 Law") (Report 297/BTP-PLHSHC of the Ministry of Justice to the Prime Minister; Thu 2020). Nevertheless, at the time of writing this chapter, the state of emergency has not been declared by the Vietnamese government.

11.3.3 The 2007 Law on Prevention and Control of Infectious Diseases

The 2007 Law categorizes three classes of infectious diseases, among which Class-A disease is defined as "extremely dangerous infectious diseases that can transmit very rapidly and spread widely with high mortality rates or with unknown agents" (Article 3). Subsequently, the Covid-19 virus is classified as a Class-A disease by Decision 07/2020/QĐ-TTg dated 26 February 2020 of the Prime Minister.

The 2007 Law, which was implemented by Decree 101/2010/NĐ-CP dated 30 September 2010 and Decree 117/2020/NĐ-CP dated 28 September 2020, provides for (i) prevention measures, (ii) combating measures, and (iii) prohibited acts relating to the prevention and control of diseases.

11.3.3.1 Prevention Measures

Prevention measures include information, education, and communication; infectious disease surveillance; use of vaccines and measures against transmission within the medical examination establishment. Accordingly, information, education, and communication on prevention and control of infectious diseases should be accurate, clear, easily understandable, timely, practical, and readily available to all citizens (Article 11). The content and direction of information, education, and communication are the responsibility of the Ministry of Health, Information and Communication, Education and Training, and local authorities (Article 1).

The surveillance of infectious diseases shall be applied to both patients and suspected cases. When there is a Class-A epidemic, patients and suspected cases should make health declarations, and health establishments should report promptly to competent health agencies; local authorities are responsible for surveillance in localities (Articles 20, 22, and 23). The information to be collected relates to "places, time and causes of morbidity and mortality; status of disease; status of immunology; major demographic characteristics and other necessary information" (Article 21). Surveillance reports should be made weekly or monthly, or yearly; quick and irregular reports, including case and cluster reports, may also be made if necessary (Article 22). Specific form for each type of report is provided in Circular 54/2015/TT-BYT dated 28 December 2015 issued by the Ministry of Health.

Regarding the use of vaccines, Article 8 of the 2007 Law provides that "everyone has the right to use vaccines and medical-biological products to protect their health and that of their community." On 8 March 2021, Viet Nam launched Phase 1 of the Covid-19 vaccination campaign, during which healthcare workers at healthcare facilities, frontline workers working on outbreak prevention and response in 19 provinces were prioritized for access (WHO Report 42 2021a). As of 16 May, there have been 979,238 doses of vaccines administered cumulatively, and the target of securing 150 million doses for 70% of the population was set for the next year (WHO Report 42 2021a).

The 2007 Law also provides measures to prevent transmission within health establishments, including isolation of patients, disinfection and sterilization of the environment, waste treatment, and personal hygiene (Article 31). It is also the responsibility of the patient's relatives to "follow instructions of medical practitioners and health workers and rules of medical examination and treatment establishments" (Article 34). On this basis, the number of relatives allowed to take care of a patient in hospitals was limited, and patients' relatives were not allowed to make unnecessary visits to the patient during the pandemic.

11.3.3.2 Combating Measures

The 2007 Law provides for combating measures against a pandemic, including the announcement of an epidemic, the establishment of a national steering committee, the restriction on activities and the mobilization of other medical services. Article 3 of the Law classified three types of epidemics based on their level of fatality and transmittal: Class-A is comprised of extremely dangerous infectious diseases that can transmit very rapidly and spread widely with high mortality rates or with unknown agents, such as A-H5N1, SARS, or Ebola virus; Class-B epidemic includes dangerous infectious disease that can rapidly transmit and be fatal; and Class-C epidemic consisting of less dangerous infectious diseases that are not rapidly transmittable (Article 3 of the 2007 Law). The Law stipulates that the announcement of Class-A epidemic will be made by the prime minister based on the recommendation by the Minister of Health (Article 38 of the 2007 Law, Article 3 of Decision 02/2016/QĐ-TTg). On this basis, former Prime Minister Nguyen Xuan Phuc has made the announcement of the Covid-19 pandemic in Decision 447/QĐ-TTg dated 1 April 2020. This event marked a turning point in the country's campaign against the Covid-19 virus since it has provided the basis for the government authorities to adopt further action to combat the spread of the virus in public.

Establishing a national steering committee is a strategic measure to combat the pandemic. Article 46 of the 2007 Law stipulates that the committee be composed of "representatives of health, finance, information-communication, foreign affairs, defense, public security and other related agencies," led by either the prime minister or a designated deputy prime minister or Minister of Health. Moreover, the prime minister is authorized to issue specific regulations on the setting up of anti-epidemic steering committees at all levels. On this basis, the Covid-19 National Steering Committee was established only one week after the first Covid-19 case was discovered in Viet Nam with representatives of all agencies to ensure a coherent approach toward combating the pandemic.

Controlling transportation and public gathering activities are also listed in the 2007 Law as measures to combat infectious diseases. Accordingly, persons and means of transport are restricted from entering or leaving epidemic zones (Article 53). Based on this provision, transportation from and to clusters such as Đà Nẵng in the second wave or Hải Dương in the third wave was restricted. The 2007 Law also authorizes competent national agencies to suspend the operation of service providers, such as those selling food and beverages, and to prohibit public gatherings, activities, and services in public places in epidemic zones (Article 52). The procedure for such suspension in the case of a Class-A epidemic is detailed in Decree 101/2010/NĐ-CP, where the suspension of public services and prohibition of public gatherings, activities, and services in public places shall be approved by either chairperson of the related district, chairperson of the province, or the Minister of Health, depending on the scope of the closure (Articles 15(3) and 17(3) of Decree 101). These approved measures shall be published in the appropriate public media no later than six hours from the time of issuance (Article 18 of Decree 101).

Other anti-epidemic measures include the organization of first aid, medical examination, treatment, and medical isolation. Article 48 of the 2007 Law opens the possibility to establish medical treatment and send mobile teams to epidemic zones, which provided the basis for field hospitals in the third and fourth waves. The 2007 Law also reaffirmed the obligation for patients and suspected cases to quarantine or isolate at home, in medical facilities, or in other establishments (Article 49).

11.3.3.3 Prohibited Activities and Fines for Failures to Implement Prevention and Combating Measures

Article 8 of the 2007 Law provides for several prohibited acts relating to prevention and controlling infectious diseases, including, *inter alia*, intentionally transmitting agents of infectious disease, concealing and failing to report cases of contracting infectious diseases, declaring or reporting false information, and failing to comply with measures for preventing and controlling infectious diseases at the request of the competent authorities.

Violations of prevention and controlling of infectious diseases, including prohibited acts, are fined under Decree 117/2020/NĐ-CP prescribing penalties for administrative violations in the medical sector ("Decree 117"), which replaces the Decree 176/2013/NĐ-CP dated 14 November 2013. The Decree 117 was promulgated in response to the Covid-19 pandemic since it has raised the bar for fines of Class-A infectious diseases, including the Covid-19 virus, to the highest. Local authorities may impose such fines at the district level. Regarding measures for prevention, Decree 117 stipulates that, in cases of attempts to block the dissemination of information and education, penalties shall be imposed if there are failures to organize such dissemination for employees or to (properly) implement regulations on broadcasting or to provide accurate and timely information on an epidemic according to disseminate content provided by competent agencies; or if there is an attempt to charge for the provision of information and education through mass media (Article 5 of the Decree). Those failing to provide accurate and timely information may be fined 10 million to 15 million VND (500–750 USD), which is the highest penalty for individuals. For surveillance purposes, failure to perform tests at the request of a competent health agency may be fined up to 3 million VND (Article 7). Meanwhile, serious penalties from 10 to 20 million VND shall be imposed if there is an attempt to conceal, fail to report, or delay the reporting on the status of infection, or deliberately providing false reports on Class-A infectious diseases (Article 7 of the Decree 117).

Regarding measures to combat the epidemic, fines shall be imposed for failures to implement medical isolation and epidemic management measures. People infected with Class-A infectious diseases who refuse to quarantine or isolate may be fined from 15 to 20 million VND (Article 11 of the Decree 117). Meanwhile, violations against regulations on personal protective measures, including wearing face masks, shall be fined 1–3 million VND, a sum that was increased 10 times in comparison to the previous fine under Decree 176/2013/NĐ-CP. Those concealing the status of infection or failures to implement cleaning, disinfection, and sterilization measures in an epidemic zone shall also be fined up to 10 million VND (Article 12(2) of the Decree 117). Restaurants shall be fined up to 20 million VND if they fail to fully comply with the lockdown decisions of competent authorities (Article 12(3) of the Decree). Individuals can be fined, up to 30 million VND, if they fail to comply with decisions on health inspection, surveillance, and control prior to entering or leaving epidemic areas (Article 12(4) of the Decree).

These fines are financially significant, taking into account Viet Nam's minimum salary of employees is set between 3 and 4.4 million VND per month (135–195 USD) (Article 3 of Decree 90/2019/NĐ-CP dated 15 November 2019 stipulating region-based minimum wages applied to employees working under labor contracts). As such, they have been an effective means to prevent violations of Covid-19 measures.

11.3.4 The Criminal Code

Violations of laws and regulations relating to preventing and combating the Covid-19 pandemic may constitute criminal offenses under the 2015 Criminal Code ("2015 Code"), as interpreted by the People's Supreme Court in Document 45/TANDTC dated 30 March 2020 ("Document 45"). In particular, Document 45, a guideline for lower levels of People's Court in application and adjudication, lists relevant offenses for Covid-19-related measures, including, *inter alia*, (i) violations of prevention and combating measures, (ii) inappropriate dissemination of information and communication on the pandemic, and (iii) abuse of the pandemic for illegal profits.

Regarding violations of measures to prevent and combat the Covid-19 pandemic, the Code criminalizes the acts of spreading dangerous diseases to humans (Article 240 of the 2015 Code). In particular, a confirmed patient with Covid-19 or a suspected person returning from an infected area may be punished up to 12 years of imprisonment if that person (i) escapes from quarantine camps, (ii) disobeys rules on quarantine, (iii) refuses or evades the application of medical isolation and enforced medical isolation, or (iv) refuses to make health declaration or declare inaccurate or insufficient information. Recently, several individuals have been prosecuted for failing to obey mandatory quarantine after arriving from high-risk areas and transmitting Covid-19 to others (Thang 2020; Thuong 2021a).

Article 295 of the 2015 Code also provides for offenses relating to public safety in a crowded area with a penalty of 1–12 years of imprisonment. Document 45 has stipulated that this provision and penalty are applicable in cases where an owner or manager of a service-providing establishment (bar, karaoke, massage, or spa) does not comply with requests on suspending all activities to prevent and combat the Covid-19 and causes a loss of over 100 million for correction. In June 2021, the director of a spa in Đà Nẵng was prosecuted for requesting 30 staff not to wear facemasks during a meeting, resulting in 65 patients of Covid-19 and a loss of 7 billion VND for treatment (Phong 2021).

Furthermore, Document 45 stipulates that any person using violence, the threat of violence, or otherwise obstructs a law enforcement officer from performing their official duties of prevention and combating the pandemic may constitute an offense carrying a penalty of 6 months–7 years of imprisonment under Article 330 of the 2015 Code. Moreover, an offense of negligence can occur when a person who is responsible for prevention and combating the Covid-19 pandemic does not implement the required measures or fails to implement them in a timely and/or sufficient manner, as provided by law and this results in serious consequences. Offenders may face a penalty of up to 12 years of imprisonment under Article 360 of the Code. From April 2020 to 21 June 2021, 45 criminal cases were successfully prosecuted that entailed a penalty of 9–15 months of imprisonment due to these types of offenses (Phap 2021).

Regarding inappropriate dissemination of information and communication relating to the pandemic, Article 288 of the 2015 Code criminalizes the act of uploading fake or distorted information on the state of Covid-19 pandemic to telecommunication networks and imposes penalties of up to 1 billion VND and seven years of imprisonment (Document 45). In May 2020, a person was sentenced to nine months of probation for uploading fake news on deaths due to Covid-19 in Viet Nam on the basis of Article 288 (Thanh 2020).

Concerning the abuse of the pandemic for illegal profits, including fraud, smuggling, and hoarding, Document 45 stipulates that the 2015 Code prohibits the act of fraud involving the dissemination of fake news on the effectiveness of medicine and medical equipment relating to the disease in order to obtain others' property. On 28 April 2021, a person who resided in Ha Noi was sentenced to 15 years of imprisonment for conducting fraudulent deals on digital thermometers and medical facemasks in 2020 and illegally obtained 1.4 billion VND (Truong 2021). Meanwhile, a charge of smuggling may also be brought against a person who exports Covid-19-related medicine and medical equipment to gain illegal profits. The act of "hoarding" has also been defined in Document 45 and includes acts that involve taking advantage of scarce items or the creation of an erroneous sense of scarcity during the Covid-19 pandemic in order to buy in large quantities of items from price stabilization programs issued by the state.

11.3.5 Three Directives of the Prime Minister

In the campaign to prevent and combat Covid-19, the Vietnamese government has implemented several administrative documents, most notably the Directive 15/CT-TTg dated 27 March 2020 ("Directive 15"), Directive 16/CT-TTg dated 31 March 2020 ("Directive 16"), and Directive 19 dated 24 April 2020 ("Directive 19"). As previously mentioned, these directives are not legislative documents within the meaning of the 2015 Law since they do not contain normative regulations and are not adopted via the legislative procedures. They, indeed, are administrative documents specifically adopted to manage the work of ministerial-level agencies and local administration authorities to combat the Covid-19 epidemic during the first wave in 2020. Their repeated application in case of outbreaks is not unconditional as legislative documents but requires further implementation by local authorities.

In general, these directives are issued by the prime minister and set out regulations regarding the public gathering, social distancing, business operations, and transportation and mobility under different scenarios for governmental agencies and local authorities to perform.

The differences between Directives 15, 16, and 19 (HCDC 2021)

	Directive 15	Directive 16	Directive 19
Public gatherings	Postponement of cultural, sport, and entertainment activities. Prohibition on gatherings of more than 20 people indoors and more than 10 people in public venues.	Prohibition on gatherings of more than 2 people.	Postponement of cultural, sport, religious and entertainment activities. Prohibition on a gathering of more than 20 people (for metropolitan areas) or 30 people (in other cities).
Minimum physical distancing	2 m	2 m	1 m
Operation of businesses	Closure of all nonessential businesses.	Closure of all nonessential businesses.	Closure of karaoke, bars, massage parlors and spas, beauty parlors, discos. Opening of restaurants, gyms, retail stores, and tourism sites.
Transportation and mobility	Restriction of transportation in metropolitans.	Restriction of all interprovincial transportation.	No restrictions.

Accordingly, Directive 16 is the most restrictive as it involves close to a full lockdown of all social and economic activities. Whereas, Directives 15 and 19 are more lenient and are based on maintaining sanitary practices and social distancing while keeping the economy open to a certain extent.

In summary, the 2013 Constitution and the 2007 Law on Prevention and Control of Infectious Disease provide a framework to prevent and combat infectious diseases outbreak, such as the Covid-19 pandemic. Regarding enforcement, the violators of measures aimed at preventing the spread of infectious diseases may face administrative fines under Decree 17/2020/ND-CP and criminal punishments under the 2015 Criminal Code, in which several penalties have been clarified by the People's Supreme Court in Document 45/TANDTC in the case of Covid-19-related measures. There have been two new legislative documents adopted in response to Covid-19, namely the Decree 117/2020/NĐ-CP on administrative fines and the Decision 07/2020/QĐ-TTg of the Prime Minister categorizing the Covid-19 pandemic as a Class-A infectious disease, which facilitate the application of all previous frameworks to combating the pandemic. The specific instructions and Covid-19-related measures are found in administrative documents, such as Directives 15, 16, and 19, which are to be applied by the local administrative authorities depending on the particular circumstances of each region, taking into account recommendations of the central government and related ministries.

11.4 The Policy Responses of the Vietnamese Government During the Pandemic

This section will examine three measures that were implemented by the Vietnamese government to curb the spread of the virus in all four waves of the pandemic, namely (i) the contact tracing system, (ii) quarantine regulation for confirmed and suspected cases, and (iii) the social distancing measures, which included rules on public gathering, closure of nonessential businesses, and school closures. These are not the only measures implemented by the Vietnamese government in the fight against the Covid-19 pandemic (Le et al. identified 13 large-scheme measures implemented by the Vietnamese government specifically in response to the Covid-19 context. See Le et al. 2021, p. 11). However, the authors choose to focus on analyzing these measures because they affect the basic civil liberties of the citizens (WHO Document 2007, pp. 9–11) and, as such, this assessment will help shed light on the impact to these liberties during a pandemic. The purpose of this section is also to help determine whether there has been a paradigm shift in the strategy of the government's approach to combating Covid-19 from when the virus first appeared to the present (which will be dealt with in the later part of this chapter).

11.4.1 The Contact Tracing System

The contact tracing system is described in the Handbook of guidelines for tracking persons that come into contact with SAR-COV-2 (Covid-19) positive patients ("Handbook") (attached to Decision 5053/QĐ-BYT dated 03 December 2020 of the Ministry of Health). The contact tracing system aims to identify the confirmed and suspected cases of the virus and methodically track all those who have come in close contact with the patients to effectively prevent the spread of the virus in public (Preamble of the Handbook). This system comprises several components, namely (i) the identification system and (ii) the tracking and tracing system that aims at "detecting the string of infections in public to promptly prevent the spread of the virus" (Article I of the Handbook).

Regarding the identification system, though only formally defined in the Handbook, it has been used by the Vietnamese authorities to classify confirmed and suspected cases since the beginning of the campaign, even prior to the Covid-19 virus being classified as a global pandemic by the WHO. Accordingly, confirmed cases are classified as an F0 with a number affixed to identify the travel record, health condition, and other statuses of the patient (e.g. patient 1); F1 are those that have come in close proximity (within 2m) with F0 within three days of the latter's showing of symptoms and F2 are those that come in close contact with F1 (Article IV of the Handbook). This identification system has a dynamic character in the sense that the "F-status" of an individual can change over time depending on the status of the person they originally came in contact with (Hardy et al. 2021; Mai 2021b). Consequently, if an F1 becomes a confirmed case (F0), the F-status of all their contacts will be "upgraded," and an F2 will become F1, and so on.

After having identified the F0, Article V of the Handbook lays down the procedures for the Vietnamese authorities to track and trace suspected cases. Accordingly, the F0s must provide their "epidemiological points," including their travel records and destinations that the patients have visited and the people they have come in close proximity with for the past 72 hours since showing symptoms (Article V of the Handbook). Such "epidemiological points" are then disclosed to the public via mainstream media, social network messaging, and tracking applications (Hutt 2020; Nguyen 2021). Then, the suspected cases, namely F1, are traced based on information obtained from the F0 patient, the patient's habitat area, and the people that were likely to be presented at the epidemiological points. The same procedure applies to F2 and so on. This process is conducted by a network of healthcare and social workers from the central disease control agency to the provincial and communal level, depending on the epidemiological points.

Recently, with the spread of new and more contagious variants in public, there have been some changes to the contact tracing system. Specifically, the identification system has extended the status of suspected cases to F5 in provinces where there are many positive patients, such as Quảng Ninh and Thái Bình (Minh 2021; Mai 2021a; Hutt 2020), which led to an increasing number of suspected cases that need to be contacted and monitored by the local authorities. Moreover, there has been an increased use of technology to track and trace suspected cases. Apart from the Blue-zone application, which was used at the early stage of the campaign, the Ministry of Information and Communication has introduced the Guideline on Information technology solutions to prevent and combat Covid-19 ("IT Guideline"), which provides other solutions to effectively track and trace suspected cases, namely the voluntary health declaration system for the residents (NCOVI), the Vietnam Health Declaration for foreigners, the QR code system to monitor visitors in public places, such as restaurants, schools, and supermarkets, and a real-time Covid-19 map (https:// antoancovid.vn/) that marks the epidemiological points of confirmed and suspected cases.

Regarding the patient's identity, initially, the information regarding their whereabouts and travel record was disclosed to the public via mainstream media. Though the names of these patients are often redacted, it was often possible for the public to have knowledge of the identity of the patient, thus leading to an intrusion into the privacy rights of that patient (S. Nguyen 2020; T. Nguyen 2020). Accordingly, the Ministry of Health subsequently instructed the relevant authorities, including the Vietnamese news media, not to disclose personal information, travel records and lists of contacts of Covid-19 patients; rather, only the epidemiological points that the person visited is made publicly available (Decision 4191/BYT-TT-KT dated 21 May 2021, para. 2).

11.4.2 Quarantine Regulation

Quarantine regulation in Viet Nam can be divided into three main scenarios, depending on the level of exposure to the Covid-19 virus (Decision 878/QĐ-BYT dated 12 March 2020 of the Ministry of Health):

(i) Hospital quarantine: Confirmed cases or F0 are quarantined and treated in specialized sections of central or provincial hospitals.
(ii) Medical facility quarantine: Suspected cases or F1 are required to quarantine in state-run medical facilities or camps established throughout the country. This rule also applies to foreigners or returning Vietnamese citizens who enter Viet Nam from abroad.
(iii) At-home quarantine: F2s are required to self-quarantine at home. During that time, if the F1, whom that person contacts with, turns out to be positive, F2 will become F1 and needs to be quarantined in a medical facility.

Initially, the quarantine time for suspected cases was at least 14 days at the medical facility and another 14 days at home after exiting the facilities. However, with the presence of the new variants in the latest wave, which may have a longer incubation period, the in-camp quarantine time has been extended to 21 days, and the additional at-home quarantine time has been adjusted to seven days for suspected cases (Telegram 600/CĐ-BCĐ dated 5 May 2021 of the Covid-19 National Steering Committee). During this time, the suspected cases are subjected to at least three polymerase chain reaction ("PCR") tests, and their health conditions are monitored regularly by healthcare staff at the medical facility. Moreover, with confirmed cases spotted in crowded places, such as industrial areas in Bắc Ninh and Bắc Giang, the Head of the Covid-19 National Steering Committee has suggested that local authorities should consider implementing a pilot system to quarantine F1 at home where they would be subjected to surveillance by technology means (camera, GPS bands) and their neighbors (Viet 2021).

Regarding costs for quarantine, before September 2020, quarantine in state-run facilities and medical treatment is provided free of charge for suspected cases. Subsequently, to provide relief for the government budget as tens of thousands of people are required to be quarantined in camps, people coming from aboard are charged a daily quarantine fee, which includes transportation service, Covid-19 test, and other accommodation expenses (Notice 313/TB-VPCP dated 29 August 2020, para. 11. See also Article 1 of Resolution 16/NQ-CP dated 8 February 2021).

11.4.3 Social Distancing Measures

Social distancing measures were implemented by the Vietnamese government throughout the pandemic. The first social distancing measure, taken under Telegram 156/CĐ-TTg dated 2 February 2020 of the Prime Minister, was the cancellation of all public events (festivals, religious, and tourism activities) in provinces that announced that they had a confirmed case (N. Nguyen, 2020). Subsequently, in response to a rise in confirmed cases across the country, a national lockdown was put into place by Directive 16. Accordingly, for 15 days as of 1 April 2020, nonessential workers were required to stay indoors, and all citizens were obligated to wear facemasks when going out for valid reasons. In addition, nonessential businesses were closed, and a ban on the gathering of more than two persons was put in place. Later, it was elaborated that the nationwide quarantine was designed not to isolate but rather to ensure that social distancing rules were respected while ensuring that the production of essential goods, such as food and medical supplies, be uninterrupted (Viet 2020). To date, this has remained the sole instance in which a lockdown was imposed at the national level.

Notably, the social distancing regulation does not apply to each suspected case individually but can extend to the locale where a person lives or visits. Specifically, when there are confirmed and suspected cases, the entire building or town is placed under in-home isolation to prevent the potential spread of the virus outside the epidemiological points. For example, the entire commune of Đồng Văn in the Lạng Sơn province, consisting of 7,623 people, were placed under isolation following the discovery of a single case in the area (patient 268) (Thai 2020). Similarly, an apartment complex of more than 1,500 residents in Ha Noi was placed under lockdown due to a single confirmed case of a resident living on the 24th floor of the building (Vietnamnews 2021).

Another aggressive social distancing measure is the closure of public and private schools. After the announcement of the virus on 1 February 2020 by the prime minister (Decision 173/QĐ-TTg), all 63 provincial chairpersons of Viet Nam decided to close all education centers in the country, from kindergarten to university level, to prevent the spread of the virus (Center of Media Education 2021). This closure took place immediately after the Lunar New Year's vacation, which ended on 30 January 2020, and stayed effective until the end of April when the country did not report any new confirmed case for a few weeks (Vu 2020). In the current wave, nationwide school closures were not implemented; rather, each provincial authority was allowed to develop its own criteria for school closure based on the specific circumstances and context of the province. For example, while all students in Hà Nội and Bắc Giang are required to stay at home due to the increase in confirmed cases, those in the 9th and 12th grade in Hải Phòng are allowed to continue their study to prepare for the examinations (Hoang 2021a).

11.5 The Paradigm Shift in the Legal and Political Responses and the Balancing of Public Health and Civil Liberties

This section will address the research questions posited at the beginning of this chapter: (i) whether there has been a paradigm shift of the legal and political responses of the Vietnamese government in the different waves of the Covid-19 pandemic and (ii) whether the enjoyment of civil liberties in Viet Nam are adversely affected as a result of the measures put into place by the Vietnamese authorities to combat the Covid-19 virus.

11.5.1 The Paradigm Shift in the Legal and Political Responses

Concerning the first question, our analysis in Section 11.3 and 11.4 of this chapter has identified several conclusions with respect to the actions of the Vietnamese government in the campaign against the Covid-19 virus from the first wave to the current wave:

First, contrary to the approach taken by other countries, the Vietnamese government did not officially declare a state of emergency during the Covid-19 pandemic. Moreover, it has not engaged in any major legislative act to promulgate new laws to implement its Covid-19-related measure (with the exception of Decree 117/2020/NĐ-CP, a secondary law that raises administrative fines for public health violations). The rationale for this approach could be that the current legislative framework has provided the executive branch with enough power to undertake appropriate measures, including quarantine, lockdown, and closure of business to prevent and combat highly transmissible diseases. This is likely to be the case considering that these laws and regulations were adopted after the experience of combating the SARS outbreak in Viet Nam in 2003. Instead, the Vietnamese government has augmented existing laws with a system of "soft laws," such as directives of the prime minister and decisions of the Covid-19 National Steering Committee to react malleably to the situations.

Second, there has been a trend toward decentralization of the decision-making process from the central government to the provincial governments. In contrast with the legislative approach taken by other countries in the region (Ramraj 2021, pp. 18–19), as an alternative to imposing a nationwide measure, the latest directive of the prime minister (Directive 05/CT-TTg dated 28 January 2021) has delegated decision-making power to the provincial chairpersons to decide on containment measures, such as the closure of businesses, school closures, and other social distancing measures, in their province (paras. 1–2). Consequently, provincial governments have issued their policy documents based on these guidelines and the particular circumstances of each province. In this way, Vietnamese provincial governments can respond malleably to new developments that have taken place since the virus first appeared in the country.

Third, the measures implemented by the Vietnamese government have become more proportionate to the risk of the transmissibly of the virus. At the early stage, the Vietnamese government took drastic actions, such as border control, quarantine, and contact tracing, to curb the spread of the virus even when there has not been widespread community transmission of the virus (Navarro 2021, p. 263). For example, the national lockdown of 63 cities and provinces was imposed on 31 March 2020 for 15 days when there were less than 200 cases in 5 cities of the country (Yen 2020). Accordingly, social distancing measures, such as the shutdown of schools and closure of nonessential businesses, took place in cities or provinces where there were no Covid-19 patients or suspected cases at the time. Moreover, the in-camp quarantine regulation was applied to all persons coming from abroad or who have come in close contact with the patient, which, at times, has increased the number of suspected cases in medical facilities to more than 42,000 (Ministry of Health 2021).

Recently, with the increased understanding of the virus and the progress of the vaccination campaign, the Vietnamese government has taken a more lenient approach. In contrary to the policy responses in the previous waves, which had the sole objective of bringing Covid-19 positive cases to zero, the Vietnamese government has opted for the "dual objectives" of preventing the spread of the virus as well as maintaining socioeconomic growth in the fourth wave (Nhat 2021). As such, the central government had not declared another national lockdown despite having 60 times more infected cases compared to the period when the first national lockdown was put into place. Instead, the Vietnamese authorities have recourse to imposing partial lockdowns in specific communes or cities where a Covid-19 patient was discovered. This measure is less drastic and more similar to the approach taken by other countries in the region that seeks to minimize the effect of the pandemic on the public health system while maintaining economic growth (Ramraj 2021). Moreover, while the quarantine duration has remained the same (28 days in total), there have been increasing calls from government officials and health experts to allow suspected cases, especially young children, to be quarantined at home to relieve depression and the pressure on patients and medical workers (Chau and Han 2021; Long and Mai 2021).

11.5.2 The Balancing of Public Health and Civil Liberties

With respect to the impact of public health measures on civil liberties in Viet Nam, since the start of the pandemic, there has been concern about the so-called "pandemic backsliding" problem, whereby governments, under the guise of responding to the virus, would exercise excessive emergency powers for political gains and undermine liberal-democratic standards, such as the freedom of expression and mobility (Flood et al. 2020; Daly 2021). Comparative studies of the effects of Covid-19-related measures on democratic standards in numerous countries around the world had identified a variety of pressing problems when countries undertook public health measures to respond to the spread of the virus, including abuse of emergency powers by the executive branch, parliaments being sidelined, or a failure of courts to safeguard constitutional rights (Alizada et al. 2021; Grogan 2021).

Measures taken in response to curbing the spread of a global epidemic entail trade-offs between the collective goals of protecting public health and citizens' rights and liberties (Gostin et al. 2020, p. 10; Gostin and Wiley 2020). However, such measures also need to be necessary, reasonable, and proportionate to the risks being dealt with (WHO Document 2007, pp. 3–4; *Van Hulst v. Netherland* 2004, para. 7.6) Put differently, in the case of the Covid-19 pandemic, national authorities need to conduct a balancing exercise wherein they have to weigh the contribution of their measures to preventing new infections in public against the enjoyment of civil liberties. Accordingly, to analyze how the Vietnamese government's measures have struck a balance between the goal of protecting public health and the safeguard of civil liberties, we will examine (i) the objective or goal that the measures aim to pursue, (ii) the contribution of the measure to the said objective or goal, and (iii) the impact of the measure on the citizens' enjoyment of civil liberties.

First, it is undoubtedly true that, amid a pandemic, the protection of public health is the utmost important goal in the policy planning of any country. However, the degree of such protection can differ depending on the national Covid-19 strategy of each country. For example, from the onset of the pandemic, countries such as Sweden embarked on a *de facto* "herd immunity approach," which accepted a certain level of community transmission and aimed to protect the most vulnerable from the virus (Claeson and Hanson 2020). On the contrary, the Vietnamese government has opted for a low-risk tolerance of the virus, which aims at eliminating any presence of the virus in the community. In general, governments have the discretion to set their appropriate level of protection, and it is not uncommon for countries to accept low risks when it comes to the protection of public health. In the *Bellio* case, the European Court of Justice upheld the right of European countries to pursue the policy of "zero tolerance" with regard to the contamination of animal feed that possibly contained agent that causes the bovine spongiform encephalopathy (or "Mad cow") disease, even in the face of scientific uncertainty (Bellio F.lli Srl v Prefettura di Treviso 2004, paras. 39, 53, 58). The low-risk tolerance exhibited by the Vietnamese policy-makers can be discerned from their statements and actions to isolate and quarantine patients and suspected cases, even amid conflicting theories concerning the transmissibility of the new virus (S.M. Le 2020; T.H. Le 2020). As early as January 2020, when the Covid-19 virus has only appeared in eight countries and territories, the Vietnamese government has promptly imposed strict border control, including mandatory medical declaration at all ports of entry (Trang 2020). Subsequently, the Vietnamese government issued an unequivocal message that the Covid-19 virus is an "aggressor" and that it is a national duty for every citizen to unite and eradicate the virus in the community. As noted by the former Prime Minister Nguyen Xuan Phuc: "Every business, every citizen, every residential area must be a fortress to prevent the epidemic" (Pham 2020). Additionally, the objective of pursuing a low-risk tolerance is evident in the manner in which the Vietnamese authorities maintained a strict intolerance for community infection and, thus, only lifted lockdown measures when there were no new cases in the community for at least several days (Smith 2020).

Second, in pursuing such a high level of protection of public health, the Vietnamese government took a set of early and decisive measures to combat and prevent the spread of the Covid-19 virus in public. The question remains: whether these measures were solely aimed at the said objective or served as a disguise to fulfill another purpose. Studies have shown that countries can use Covid-19 measures to further political aims, such as attracting constituencies in an election, consolidating power, or suppressing freedom of speech (Alizada et al. 2021; Daly 2021; Grogan 2021). Jasanoff and Hilgartner argued that the "stress test" to distinguish a "control" or a "chaos" governance can be discerned in whether a government has maintained a coherent response or entailed conflict and contradiction over its Covid-19 policy (Jasanoff and Hilgartner 2021).

Within this paradigm, it can be argued that the Vietnamese government's measures to combat and prevent the Covid-19 virus aim to address the health crisis instead of pursuing political objectives. By establishing the Covid-19 National Steering Committee, an interministerial body that includes ministries in health, public security, commerce, and communication, the Vietnamese government aimed at maintaining a holistic and coherent approach in combating and preventing the Covid-19 virus over the key and interrelated areas of public health, politics, and the economy. There have been certain criticisms that the Vietnamese government, when implementing Covid-19 measures, has suppressed the freedom of speech (Edgell et al. 2020, pp. 4–5). However, the measures taken by the Vietnamese authorities on social media are targeted at censoring pseudo-science statements and "hoax spreaders" that spread fake news and downplayed the importance of vaccines and social distancing (Nguyen and Pearson 2020). As such, these measures are aimed at preventing misinformation, which can hinder the collective efforts of combating the spread of the virus and causes confusion in public, rather than to be considered suppression of the freedom of expression on social media.

By taking into account past experiences when dealing with other respiratory diseases (e.g. the SARS virus), the Vietnamese health law has granted the executive branch ample power in enacting measures that may affect the normal livelihood of the citizens (see Section 11.3). Thus, it is highly improbable that there would be a need for the Vietnamese government to bypass the legislative process in issuing measures to protect public health.

Finally, it is obvious that Covid-19-related measures can have a negative impact on the enjoyment of civil liberties, such as the right to mobility, education, work, and the safeguarding of personal information. The mandatory quarantine regulations imposed by the Vietnamese government effectively isolated tens of thousands of people in medical facilities. The lockdown and related measures adversely affected the country's economy in terms of reducing the GDP growth rate and increasing the unemployment rate (Nguyen and Phan 2020, p. 69). Moreover, at times, the contract-tracing and surveillance system, which required disclosing one's whereabouts and travel record, accidentally disclosed the patient's identity (Max 2020). Together with the propaganda system that emphasizes the danger and transmissibility of the virus, the measure has caused a backlash that has facilitated the public stigmatization of Covid-19 patients (S. Nguyen 2020).

Despite these setbacks, the Vietnamese government has implemented several "balancing" measures to reduce the impacts of Covid-19-related measures on the enjoyment of civil liberties by its citizens. At the outset, the concept of civil liberties in the Vietnamese context needs to be understood in the collective instead of the individual sense. As posited by Brems, Asians, "especially those influenced by Confucianism, are said to value the community over the individual, to strive for consensus and to respect an authority that takes care of its citizens" (Brems 2001, p. 86). As such, in the context of Viet Nam – an Asian country whose society strongly reflects the core values of Confucianism, the enjoyment of civil liberties amid a pandemic is to be understood on the basis of solidarity, which emphasizes the preservation of community rights, the respect for authority and social harmony (Ivic 2020, pp. 345–346). As such, the mandatory quarantine regulation, while is perceived by some as "ruthlessly efficient" (Strangio 2021), has played a key role in safeguarding the collective civil liberties of the community through the protection of public health and the maintenance of public order. Moreover, it should be noted that Viet Nam's healthcare facilities are relatively undeveloped compared to other countries in the region (placing 66/89 countries, see Ireland, 2021). With a large and crowded population of tens of millions in large metropolitans, such as Hà Nội and Hồ Chí Minh City, the impacts on civil liberties, including the right to healthcare and life, would be disastrous if the virus were to remain uncontrolled.

Moreover, although the Vietnamese government has prioritized the collective over individual interests, it has put forward measures to ease the impact on the public. Economically, the government has provided financial support in terms of tax breaks, fee waivers, and direct payments to the employee, laid-off workers, and poor households who have been negatively affected by lockdown measures (Directive 11/CT-TTg dated 4 March 2020 of the Prime Minister, Resolution 42/NQ-CP dated 9 April 2020 of the Government). In addition, after a few incidents where the patient's identity was accidentally disclosed, the government has taken steps to direct the Vietnamese news media not to reveal personal information of the patients or suspected cases to the public.

In sum, the Vietnamese government has maintained a coherent policy to combat and prevent the pandemic. Despite conflicting theories when the virus first emerged, the Vietnamese authorities have taken the precautionary approach in treating the Covid-19 virus as a highly transmissible and deathly disease and, as such, conveying a clear and transparent message to the public on the danger of the virus and the importance of social distancing. While the legal framework has not fundamentally changed, the central government has adapted its response by delegating more decision-making power to provincial governments and tailoring measures to new developments in the virus' behavior. These responses allowed the Vietnamese authorities to react malleably to the situations on the ground and to strike a balance between the pursuit of low-risk tolerance in protecting public health and the enjoyment of civil liberties by the citizens. A strategy based on the community's solidarity has allowed the Vietnamese government to lift Covid-19 measures after a few weeks instead of forcing its citizens to go through a prolonged lockdown like many other countries.

11.6 Conclusion

This chapter analyzes the approach of Viet Nam, a country that was among the first to encounter the virus outside of China, in balancing the protection of public health and civil liberties from the legal and political perspective. The unpredictability of the novel virus and its variants has put a burden on governments to adopt an appropriate approach to protect public health and maintain the enjoyment of civil liberties by its citizens. Apart from the public health and economic consequences, there is another fear that the virus will have a negative effect on democracy and human rights standards, something that has already been the case in some countries.

Our research shows that, contrary to other countries, the Vietnamese government has not implemented any legislative changes to its Covid-19 laws nor invoked the national emergency clause to give the executive branch more power. One of the reasons can be that, given the country's experience in dealing with the SARS virus outbreak in 2003, Vietnamese legislators decided to give authorities broad discretion to swiftly deal with the outbreak of a pandemic, which is evident in the 2007 Law of prevention and control of infectious disease and other health legislation. Instead of promulgating new legislative acts, the Vietnamese authorities have relied on administrative documents, such as directives of the prime minister, which have played a major role in addressing new developments and clarifying the government's measures. Moreover, there has also been a trend of decentralization, in which the central government has delegated decision-making authority to the provincial leaders to react flexibly to the situations on the ground. Consequently, the fear of parliamentary bypass is not present in the case of Viet Nam.

Moreover, in limiting the negative effects of Covid-19-related measures, the Vietnamese government has adapted its response to new developments in the country's situation. The overarching policy of the Vietnamese authorities concerning the campaign to combat and prevent the virus has remained consistent from the beginning – that is, to emphasize containment measures, such as quarantine and track and tracing to limit and eradicate the presence of the virus in public. However, recently, the Vietnamese government has taken a more lenient approach in dealing with the virus, which results in partial lockdowns of infected areas, instead of a comprehensive national lockdown; in-house quarantine, instead of in-camp isolation for suspected cases; and nondisclosure of the identity of patients to protect private information. This approach reflects the "dual objectives" of minimizing the effect of the pandemic on public health and maintaining socioeconomic growth in the country.

At the time of writing, Viet Nam is experiencing its worst Covid-19 virus spike to date, with thousands of positive cases daily and hundreds of deaths. As such, the low-risk tolerance and the "dual objectives" that the Vietnamese government has been pursuing are being challenged by the emergence of more contagious variants of the virus. Its stringent quarantine and lockdown measures have faced a backlash because they negatively affected the lives of millions of people and put a toll on economic growth, and negatively impacted the employment rate. Moreover, the mandatory quarantine for all non-symptoms patients and suspected cases has stretched the public healthcare's capacity in treating Covid-19-related and non-related patients. Nevertheless, these restrictions must be assessed from the perspective of safeguarding the collective civil liberties of the community through the protection of public health and the maintenance of public order. Given Viet Nam's overcrowded metropolitan areas and relatively poor healthcare facilities, had the government not adopted drastic measures to curb the spread of the virus, the toll on human health would have been devastating.

In the years ahead, we might have to adapt to the "new normal" as it remains to be seen how this global pandemic will unfold. The shift to a less drastic approach of the Vietnamese government in preventing and combating the Covid-19 virus has signaled that the country is prepared for a marathon war against the pandemic with the unity of the government and people. The balancing exercise between the goal of protecting public health and the citizens' enjoyment of civil liberties remains at the heart of the campaign.

References

1. Cited Cases
Case C-286/02 *Bellio F.lli Srl v Prefettura di Treviso*, ECLI:EU:C:2004:212, 1st April 2004, Court of Justice of the European Union [CJEU].
Van Hulst v. Netherlands, Comm. 903/1999, U.N. Doc. A/60/40, Vol. II, at 29 (HRC 2004).

2. Books/Book Chapters
Brems, E. (2001) *Human Rights: Universality and Diversity*, Kluwer Law International, The Hague.
Nguyen, C., and Phan, T. (2020) Vietnam: marshalling state and non- state actors, in *COVID-19 in Asia: Law and Policy Contexts* (eds. Ramraj, V.V.), Oxford University Press, New York, NY.
Ramraj, V.V. (ed.) (2021) *Covid-19 in Asia: Law and Policy Contexts*, Oxford University Press.

3. Journal Articles
Claeson, M., and Hanson, S. (2020) COVID-19 and the Swedish Enigma. *The Lancet*, 397, 259–261.
Daly, T.G. (2021) Democracy and the global pandemic. https://intr2dok.vifa-recht.de/receive/mir_mods_00010528 (accessed 24 June 2021).
Flood, C.M., MacDonnell, V., Thomas, B., and Wilson, K. (2020) Reconciling civil liberties and public health in the response to COVID-19. *FACETS*, 5 (1), 887–898.
Gostin, L., and Wiley, L. (2020) Governmental public health powers during the COVID-19 pandemic: stay-at-home orders, business closures, and travel restrictions. *JAMA*, 323 (21), 2137–2138.
Gostin, L., Friedman, E., and Wetter, S. (2020) Responding to Covid-19: how to navigate a public health emergency legally and ethically. *The Hastings Center Report*, 50 (2), 8–12.
Grogan, J. (2021) Power, law and the COVID-19 pandemic – Part I: the year of pandemic. *VerfBlog*. https://intr2dok.vifa-recht.de/receive/mir_mods_00010624 (accessed 24 June 2021).
Ivic, S. (2020) Vietnam's response to the COVID-19 outbreak. *Asian Bioethics Review*, 12, 341–47.
Jasanoff, S., and Hilgartner, S. (2021) A stress test for politics: insights from the comparative Covid response project (CompCoRe). *VerfBlog*. https://verfassungsblog.de/a-stress-test-for-politics-insights-from-the-comparative-covid-response-project-compcore-2020/ (accessed 24 June 2021)
Le, T.-A.T., Vodden, K., Wu, J., and Atiwesh, G. (2021) Policy responses to the COVID-19 pandemic in Vietnam. *IJERPH*, 18 (2), 559.
Navarro, V. (2021) Why Asian countries are controlling the pandemic better than the United States and Western Europe. *International Journal of Health Services*, 51 (2), 261–264.
Orzechowski, M., Schochow, M., and Steger, F. (2021) Balancing public health and civil liberties in times of pandemic. *Journal of Public Health Policy*, 42 (1), 145–153.

4. Blog Posts
Le, S.M. (2020). Containing the Coronavirus (Covid-19): Lessons from Vietnam. *World Bank Blogs*.
Le, T.H. (2020). Vietnam's Successful Battle against Covid-19. *Council of Foreign Relations*.
Nguyen, T. (2020). Patient 17: A Turning Point for Vietnam's 'Wartime Spirit' during COVID-19. *National University of Singapore Faculty of Law*.
Pham, P. (2020). Can Vietnam's COVID-19 Response be Replicated? *Asia & the Pacific Policy Society*.

5. Newspapers Articles and other documents
Alizada, N., Cole, R., Gastaldi, L., and Grahn, S. (2021). Autocratization Turns Viral: Democracy Report 2021. University of Gothenburg: V-Dem Institute (March).
Bach Mai (2020). "Cuộc Chiến" Chống Dịch COVID-19 Tại Việt Nam: 100 Ngày Nhìn Lại. *Bach Mai Hospital* (4 May). http://www.bachmai.gov.vn/en/tin-tuc-va-su-kien/tin-trong-nganh-menuleft-34/

6232-cuoc-chien-chong-dich-covid-19-tai-viet-nam-100-ngay-nhin-lai.html (accessed 15 July 2021).

Binh, T. (2020). Từ 0 Giờ Ngày 28-7-2020: Thực Hiện Cách Ly Xã Hội Theo Chỉ Thị Số 16/CT-TTg Tại 6 Quận Trong Vòng 15 Ngày. *Da Nang City Portal* (27 July). https://danang.gov.vn/chinh-quyen/chi-tiet?id=40207&_c=3 (accessed 15 July 2021).

Black, G. (2020). Vietnam May Have the Most Effective Response to Covid-19. *The Nation* (24 April). https://www.thenation.com/article/world/coronavirus-vietnam-quarantine-mobilization/ (accessed 15 July 2021)

CDC (2022). Centers for Disease Control and Prevention of the United States of America, About Variants (26 April 2022). https://www.cdc.gov/coronavirus/2019-ncov/variants/about-variants .html?CDC_AA_refVal=https%3A%2F%2Fwww.cdc.gov%2Fcoronavirus%2F2019-ncov%2Fvariants %2Fvariant.html (accessed 15 July 2021)

Center of Media Education (2021). 63/63 tỉnh, thành cho học sinh nghỉ học để phòng dịch nCoV. *Ministry of Education and Training*.

Chau, L. and Han, V. (2021). Cách Ly F1 Tại Nhà, Đừng Ngại! *Thanhniennews* (17 June). https:// thanhnien.vn/thoi-su/cach-ly-f1-tai-nha-dung-ngai-1400052.html (accessed 15 July 2021).

Chinh, P. (2020). Hà Nội Áp Dụng Các Biện Pháp Phòng, Chống Dịch Theo Tinh Thần Chỉ Thị 19. *Viet Nam Government Press* (30 July). http://baochinhphu.vn/Hoat-dong-dia-phuong/Ha-Noi-ap-dung-cac-bien-phap-phong-chong-dich-theo-tinh-than-Chi-thi-19/402430.vgp (accessed 15 July 2021).

Coleman, J. (2020). Vietnam reports first coronavirus cases. *The Hill* (23 January). https://thehill.com/ policy/healthcare/public-global-health/479542-vietnam-reports-first-coronavirus-cases/ (accessed 15 July 2021).

Dinh, N. (2021). Phát Hiện 2 ca Lây Nhiễm COVID-19 Trong Cộng Đồng ở Hải Dương, Quảng Ninh. *Ministry of Health Portal* (28 January). https://moh.gov.vn/hoat-dong-cua-lanh-dao-bo/-/asset_ publisher/TW6LTp1ZtwaN/content/phat-hien-2-ca-lay-nhiem-covid-19-trong-cong-ong-o-hai-duong-quang-ninh (accessed 15 July 2021).

Doan, L. (2020). Vietnam postpones plan to bring home citizens on commercial flights. *Vnexpress* (2 December). https://e.vnexpress.net/news/news/vietnam-postpones-plan-to-bring-home-citizens-on-commercial-flights-4200187.html (accessed 15 July 2021).

Edgell, A., Grahn, S., Lachapelle, J., and Maerz, S. (2020). An update on pandemic backsliding: democracy four months after the beginning of the Covid-19 pandemic. University of Gothenburg: V-Dem Institute (June). https://www.v-dem.net/media/filer_public/b9/2e/b92e59da-2a06-4d2e-82a1-b0a8dece4af7/v-dem_policybrief-24_update-pandemic-backsliding_200702.pdf (accessed 15 July 2021).

Hardy, A., Shum, M., and Quyen, V. (2021). The "F-System" of targeted isolation: a key method in Vietnam's suppression of Covid-19. *Competing Regional Integrations in Southeast Asia* (2 March). https://halshs.archives-ouvertes.fr/halshs-03151062/document (accessed 15 July 2021).

HCDC (2021). Sự Khác Biệt Giữa Chỉ Thị 15, Chỉ Thị 16 và Chỉ Thị 19 Của Thủ Tướng. *Hanoi Center for Disease Control*. https://hcdc.vn/hoidap/index/chitiet/c885f7ce005a3a83daf6c7281501c8c7 (accessed 15 July 2021).

Hoang, K.A. (2021a). Danh Sách Tỉnh, Thành Cho Học Sinh Nghỉ Học Phòng Covid-19. *LuatVietnam* (9 May). https://luatvietnam.vn/tin-phap-luat/danh-sach-cac-tinh-thanh-cho-hoc-sinh-nghi-hoc-phong-covid-19-230-30096-article.html (accessed 15 July 2021).

Hoang, L. (2021b). Chiều 27-4: Việt Nam Thêm 5 ca COVID-19, 1 ca Lây Nhiễm Tại Nơi Cách Ly. *Tuoitrenews* (27 April). https://tuoitre.vn/chieu-27-4-viet-nam-them-5-ca-covid-19-1-ca-lay-nhiem-tai-noi-cach-ly-20210427173750442.htm (accessed 15 July 2021).

Hutt, D. (2020). The Coronavirus Loosens Lips in Hanoi. *Foreign Policy* (15 April). https://foreignpolicy .com/2020/04/15/coronavirus-vietnam-communist-party-hanoi/ (accessed 15 July 2021).

Ireland, S. (2021). Revealed: countries with the best health care systems, 2021. *CEOWorld Magazine* (27 April). https://ceoworld.biz/2021/04/27/revealed-countries-with-the-best-health-care-systems-2021/ (accessed 15 July 2021).

Le, N. (2020). Vietnam reports first Covid-19 death. *Vnexpress* (31 July). https://e.vnexpress.net/news/news/vietnam-reports-first-covid-19-death-4139149.html (accessed 15 July 2021).

Long, T. and Mai, T. (2021). TP.HCM Nghiên Cứu Cách Ly F1 Tại Nhà. *Tuoitrenews* (14 June). https://tuoitre.vn/tphcm-nghien-cuu-cach-ly-f1-tai-nha-20210614181633717.htm (accessed 15 July 2021).

Mai, T. (2021a). Một Trường Hợp F1 Trở Thành F0 ở Thái Bình. *Nhan Dan* (19 May). https://nhandan.com.vn/tin-tuc-y-te/mot-truong-hop-f1-tro-thanh-f0-o-thai-binh-646755/ (accessed 15 July 2021).

Mai, T. (2021b). Thái Bình Phân Loại, Kiểm Soát Trường Hợp Có Nguy CơMắc Covid-19. *Nhan Dan* (22 March). https://nhandan.com.vn/tin-tuc-y-te/mot-truong-hop-f1-tro-thanh-f0-o-thai-binh-646755/ (accessed 15 July 2021).

Max, D.T. (2020). The public-shaming pandemic. *The New Yorker* (21 September). https://www.newyorker.com/magazine/2020/09/28/the-public-shaming-pandemic (accessed 15 July 2021).

Minh, H. (2021). Quảng Ninh Truy Vết, Khoanh Vùng Dịch Đến Tận F4. *Quang Ninh Portal* (19 May). https://www.quangninh.gov.vn/Trang/ChiTietTinTuc.aspx?nid=96441 (accessed 15 July 2021).

Ministry of Health (2021). Bản tin dịch COVID-19 sáng 21/6: Thêm 47 ca mắc COVID-19, Việt Nam ghi nhận tổng cộng 13.258 bệnh nhân. *Ministry of Health Portal.*

Nguyen, D. (2021). Những người truy vết Covid-19. *Vnexpress* (1 May). https://vnexpress.net/nhung-nguoi-truy-vet-covid-19-4270880.html (accessed 15 July 2021)

Nguyen, N. (2020). Các tỉnh đã công bố dịch dừng tất cả lễ hội, quyết định cho học sinh nghỉ học. *Vnexpress* (2 February). https://moh.gov.vn/chuong-trinh-muc-tieu-quoc-gia/-/asset_publisher/7ng11fEWgASC/content/cac-tinh-a-cong-bo-dich-dung-tat-ca-le-hoi-quyet-inh-cho-hoc-sinh-nghi-hoc (accessed 15 July 2021)

Nguyen, S. (2020). Coronavirus: social media anger in Vietnam at jet-setter linked to new cluster in Hanoi. *South China Morning Post* (10 March). https://www.scmp.com/week-asia/health-environment/article/3074493/coronavirus-social-media-anger-vietnam-jet-setter (accessed 15 July 2021).

Nguyen, P. and Pearson, J. (2020). Vietnam introduces "fake News" fines for coronavirus misinformation. *Reuter* (15 April). https://www.reuters.com/article/us-health-coronavirus-vietnam-security-idUSKCN21X0EB (accessed 15 July 2021).

Nhat, B. (2021). Thực Hiện Mục Tiêu Kép Để Đem Lại Hạnh Phúc, Ấm No Cho Nhân Dân. *Viet Nam Government Press* (3 July). http://baochinhphu.vn/Thoi-su/Thu-tuong-chu-tri-hop-Thuong-truc-Chinh-phu-ve-COVID19/401840.vgp (accessed 15 July 2021).

Phap, L. (2021). Tổng Hợp Thông Tin Các Trường Hợp Bị Xử Lý Hình Sự Liên Quan Covid-19. *Thuvienphapluat* (22 July). https://thuvienphapluat.vn/tintuc/vn/thoi-su-phap-luat/thoi-su/35833/tong-hop-thong-tin-cac-truong-hop-bi-xu-ly-hinh-su-lien-quan-covid-19 (accessed 15 July 2021).

Phong, T. (2021). Khởi Tố Giám Đốc AMIDA vi Phạm Quy Định Phòng Chống COVID-19. *Viet Nam Socialist Party Portal* (21 June). http://baochinhphu.vn/Phap-luat/Khoi-to-Giam-doc-AMIDA-vi-pham-quy-dinh-phong-chong-COVID19/435367.vgp (accessed 15 July 2021).

Pollack, T. et al. (2021). Emerging COVID-19 success story: Vietnam's commitment to containment. *OurWorldinData* (5 March). https://ourworldindata.org/covid-exemplar-vietnam (accessed 15 July 2021).

Reguly, E. (2020). With zero pandemic deaths, Vietnam sets the standard for COVID-19 fight. *The Globe and Mail* (27 May). https://www.theglobeandmail.com/world/article-with-zero-pandemic-deaths-vietnam-sets-the-standard-for-covid-1/?fbclid=IwAR3lMET9mhDF2dWWn6nyqA75OTXVIbos8dOjkZvlE3N-iTbygrzXtG1ZQms (accessed 15 July 2021).

Representative Office for Viet Nam (2021a). Viet Nam COVID-19 Situation Report 42 (16 May). https://www.who.int/vietnam/internal-publications-detail/covid-19-in-viet-nam-situation-report-42 (accessed 15 July 2021).

Representative Office for Viet Nam (2021b). COVID-19 in Viet Nam Situation Report 46 (15 June). https://www.who.int/vietnam/internal-publications-detail/covid-19-in-viet-nam-situation-report-46 (accessed 15 July 2021).

Representative Office for Viet Nam (2021c). Viet Nam COVID-19 Situation Report 50 (13 July). https://www.who.int/vietnam/internal-publications-detail/covid-19-in-viet-nam-situation-report-50 (accessed 15 July 2021).

Smith, N. (2020). Vietnam lifts lockdown: how a country of 95m bordering China recorded zero coronavirus deaths. *The Telegraph* (23 April). https://www.telegraph.co.uk/news/2020/04/23/vietnam-lifts-lockdown-country-97-million-bordering-china-recorded/ (accessed 15 July 2021).

Strangio, S. (2021). COVID-19 stages another comeback in Vietnam. *The Diplomat* (4 May). https://thediplomat.com/2021/05/covid-19-stages-another-comeback-in-vietnam/ (accessed 15 July 2021).

Thai, B. (2020). Phong Toả Toàn Bộ Thị Trấn Đồng Văn -Hà Giang Để Phòng Chống Dịch COVID-19. *Sức Khỏe và Đời Sống* (22 April). https://suckhoedoisong.vn/phong-toa-thi-tran-dong-van-ha-giang-de-phong-chong-dich-n172851.html (accessed 15 July 2021).

Thang, Q. (2020). Flight attendant faces criminal charge for flouting quarantine rules, spreading infection. *Vnexpress* (3 December). https://e.vnexpress.net/news/news/flight-attendant-faces-criminal-charge-for-flouting-quarantine-rules-spreading-infection-4200865.html (accessed 15 July 2021).

Thanh, H. (2020). Lĩnh Án vì Tung Tin Một Người Chết Do Nhiễm NCoV. *Vnexpress* (6 May). https://vnexpress.net/linh-an-vi-tung-tin-mot-nguoi-chet-do-nhiem-ncov-4095068.html (accessed 15 July 2021).

Thu, H. (2020). Ban Bố Tình Trạng Khẩn Cấp về Dịch Do Virus Corona: Phải Tuân Thủ Quy Định Pháp Luật. *Viet Nam Socialist Party Portal* (1 February). https://dangcongsan.vn/phong-chong-dich-covid-19/ban-bo-tinh-trang-khan-cap-ve-dich-do-virus-corona-phai-tuan-thu-quy-dinh-phap-luat-547703.html (accessed 15 July 2021).

Thuong, H. (2021a). Khởi Tố vụ Án Liên Quan Hành vi Làm Lây Lan Dịch COVID-19 Rất Lớn ở Mỹ Tho. *Tuoitrenews* (6 July). https://tuoitre.vn/khoi-to-vu-an-lien-quan-hanh-vi-lam-lay-lan-dich-covid-19-rat-lon-o-my-tho-2021070617350305.htm (accessed 15 July 2021).

Thuong, T. (2021b). Thêm 72 ca Mắc Mới ở Hải Dương, 10 ca ở Quảng Ninh. *Bach Mai Hospital.* (28 January). http://bachmai.gov.vn/tin-tuc-va-su-kien/y-hoc-thuong-thuc-menuleft-32/6906-82-ca-duong-tinh-sars-cov-2-tai-hai-duong-va-quang-ninh.html (accessed 15 July 2021).

Trang, T. (2020). Phó Thủ Tướng Vũ Đức Đam: Thực Hiện Ngay Việc Khai Báo y Tế ở Tất Cả Các Cửa Khẩu. *Hanoinews* (20 January). http://www.hanoimoi.com.vn/tin-tuc/Suc-khoe/956398/pho-thu-tuong-vu-duc-dam-thuc-hien-ngay-viec-khai-bao-y-te-o-tat-ca-cac-cua-khau (accessed 15 July 2021).

Truong, N. (2021). 15 Năm Tù Cho Thanh Niên Lừa Bán Khẩu Trang, Nhiệt Kế Điện Tử. *Vnexpress* (28 April). https://vnexpress.net/15-nam-tu-cho-thanh-nien-lua-ban-khau-trang-nhiet-ke-dien-tu-4269969.html (accessed 15 July 2021).

Tuan, D. (2020). Thủ Tướng Chủ Trì Họp Thường Trực Chính Phủ về COVID-19. *Viet Nam Government Press* (25 July). http://baochinhphu.vn/Thoi-su/Thu-tuong-chu-tri-hop-Thuong-truc-Chinh-phu-ve-COVID19/401840.vgp (accessed 15 July 2021).

Tuan, C. (2021). Từ 0h Ngày 29/1, Quảng Ninh Thực Hiện Giãn Cách Xã Hội Một Số Khu Vực Có ca Mắc COVID-19. *Ministry of Health Portal* (28 January). https://ncov.moh.gov.vn/en/-/6847426-845 (accessed 15 July 2021).

Viet, T. (2020). Thủ Tướng Giải Thích về "Cách Ly Toàn Xã Hội". *Vnexpress* (1 April). https://vnexpress .net/thu-tuong-giai-thich-ve-cach-ly-toan-xa-hoi-4077911.html (accessed 15 July 2021).

Viet, T. (2021). Thí Điểm Cách Ly F1 Tại Nhà. *Vnexpress* (20 May). https://vnexpress.net/thi-diem-cach-ly-f1-tai-nha-4281465.html (accessed 15 July 2021).

Vietnamnews (2021). Apartment building in Hà Nội locked down after Indian Expert Tests Positive for COVID-19. *Vietnamnews* (4 May). https://vietnamnews.vn/society/939700/apartment-building-in-ha-noi-locked-down-after-indian-expert-tests-positive-for-covid-19.html (accessed 15 July 2021).

Vu, K. (2020). Vietnam reopens schools after easing coronavirus curbs. *Reuter* (11 May). https://www .reuters.com/article/us-health-coronavirus-vietnam-schools-idUSKBN22N0QB (accessed 15 July 2021).

World Health Organization (2007). Ethical considerations in developing a public health response to pandemic influenza. World Health Organization. (WHO Document)

Xuan, M. (2021). Tối 29-4: Việt Nam Thêm 45 ca COVID-19, Có 6 ca Cộng Đồng Tại Hà Nam và TP.HCM. *Tuoitrenews* (27 April). https://tuoitre.vn/toi-29-4-viet-nam-them-45-ca-covid-19-co-6-ca-cong-dong-tai-ha-nam-va-tp-hcm-20210429193631048.htm (accessed 15 July 2021).

Yen, H. (2020). Bản tin dịch COVID-19 trong 24h qua: Chuẩn bị mọi điều kiện sẵn sàng ứng phó với dịch bệnh trên diện rộng. *Ministry of Education and Training*.

12

Singapore United

Jacinta I-Pei Chen[1], Sharon H.X. Tan[1], Peak Sen Chua[1], Jeremy Lim[1,2], and Jason Chin-Huat Yap[1]

[1] *Saw Swee Hock School of Public Health, National University of Singapore and National University Health System, Singapore*
[2] *HealthServe, Singapore*

12.1 Governing Philosophy and Laws

Singapore is a geographically compact island country with a multiracial population of 5.7 million, most of whom are ethnically Chinese (gov.sg 2019; Department of Statistics, Singapore 2021a). It has traditionally been a popular destination for Chinese tourists (Singapore Tourism Board 2020) and was one of the first countries to report imported cases of COVID-19 in early February 2020. It underwent a suite of island-wide measures (termed the "Circuit Breaker" and similar to a lockdown) from April to June 2020, and then a "Heightened Alert" state from May to June 2021 with the implementation of tighter measures. All in all, Singapore's management of the COVID situation has been cited as a successful model in terms of the control of community spread, mortality rates, and livability (Kuguyo et al. 2020; eca International 2021; Hong 2021; Moss 2021) despite the several instances when the virus broke through in specific subpopulations. This chapter examines the movement control and monitoring orders implemented in the context of legal frameworks, policy approaches, and issues in enforcement and compliance, up until August 2021.

Singapore is a parliamentary democracy with a single-party dominant system and an elected, nonexecutive presidency. Its model of governance is marked by strong political centralization and high levels of social compliance among citizens and residents, founded on a longstanding relationship of sociopolitical trust between the people and the government that is in turn predicated on the latter's historical and continued performance of efficient and effective public administration and strong governance (Huff 1995; Perry et al. 1997; Liow 2012; Woo 2020). Such trust is marked by the populace's general acceptance of government intervention in social and personal spaces, as seen in the country's historical national campaigns that encouraged the speaking of good English, being courteous, and even having smaller or larger families in line with the prevailing population policy (Wong and Yeoh 2003; Kanagaratnam 1968; Chen et al. 2020).

The national emphasis on governmental efficiency stems partially from a historical preoccupation with vulnerability and survival. The "island mentality" of a small nation-state with limited resources and having "to do it on our own" has fostered a psyche of vigilance and competitiveness (Schein 1996; Chew 2000; Chang and Sivam 2004). This underlying mindset has led to survivalist policies such as the accumulation of fiscal reserves, the fostering of multiracial social stability, water recycling efforts, and long-term climate change measures (Tortajada 2006; gov.sg 2019;

Impacts of the Covid-19 Pandemic: International Laws, Policies, and Civil Liberties, First Edition. Edited by Nadav Morag.
© 2023 John Wiley & Sons, Inc. Published 2023 by John Wiley & Sons, Inc.

Bloomberg 2020), and underpins its foreign policy principles of maintaining a deterrent-based military defense and high level of regional engagement alongside an open market economy (Singapore is a highly developed free-market economy which has been ranked as the most open in the world) (Charlton 2019; Ovais 2020; Ministry of Foreign Affairs 2021). The SARS experience, marked by a disproportionate impact from nosocomial outbreaks, was deeply etched in the country's collective consciousness and further sharpened this national vigilance, especially toward threats from infectious diseases (Dan et al. 2009; Vaswani 2020; Lim 2020a). This translated to a culture and practice of readiness for future outbreaks in the healthcare sector prior to the COVID outbreak (Lum et al. 2016; Chen et al. 2020; Chotirmall et al. 2020).

This national survivalist mindset has evolved a populace accustomed to and more accepting of the notion of trade-offs in personal spaces and individual liberties for the sake of societal interests, economic progress, and national peace and order.

Singapore's legal system, inherited from and based on English law, evolved to meet the needs of and reflect the sociopolitical system within which it operates. The principles and framework of the organs of government are laid down by a written constitution, with the Executive (the Cabinet) responsible for the general direction of the government and accountable to Parliament, the Legislature (the Parliament) responsible for enacting legislation, and the Judiciary responsible for administering justice independently, adjudicating conflicts between the different branches of the government, between the government and the people, and between people. The Elected President adds to the overall scheme of system checks through the discretionary power to block certain government actions (Gill et al. 2021; Prime Minister's Office Singapore 2021a).

With the Cabinet formed from members of the ruling party in the Parliament and the Executive possessing delegated power to issue subsidiary legislation, there is a close union between the Legislature and the Executive (The Singapore Government 2020r; Giffard 1999; Lee 2020). The Judiciary has also been characterized as playing a supporting role in promoting good and fair governance through the clear articulation of rules and principles that the Parliament and Executive should uphold internally as trusted leaders and through the political process, rather than playing the adversarial role of "negative" scrutiny of public administration. Unlike the English constitutional model, which is founded on distrust of and separation of powers between the three branches to create checks and balances, the relationship between the branches in Singapore has been less combative and one of "partnership and cooperation within a framework of governance and legality" (Menon n.d.; Thio 2011; Friedrich 1974; Chan 2010; Lee 2020).

With such a cooperative stance between branches of government, and the historically strong emphasis on governmental efficiency and national survival, the conferral of emergency or emergency-like powers on the Executive to deal with threats to national stability is unexceptional in Singapore. Laws such as the Criminal Law (Temporary Provisions) Act and Internal Security Act, originally enacted in 1955 and 1960, respectively, still empower the Executive today to exercise powers of preventive detention in the interests of public order and national security (Internal Security Act 1985; Criminal Law 2000; Lee 2020). Singapore's constitutional culture, expressed especially through criminal law, has been described to reflect a value system that prizes "nation before community and society above self" (White Paper on Shared Values 1991; Lee 2020).

This constitutional culture, backed by a predicated relationship of trust between the government and populace, and the national preoccupation with survival, are important pre-existing conditions that shape and affect Singapore's national COVID response in terms of the choice of legal frameworks, the implementation approach, its swiftness in execution, and the public's reaction.

Other important influencing factors include the nation's wealth, built from years of strong economic performance and accumulated reserves, and the country's geographic location with a regional hub status and reliance on trade and open borders to bring in revenue. The small size of the island nation with its well-defined borders also facilitates ease of border controls without the added complexity of interstate travel and coordination of policy formulation and implementation across states or provinces (Chen et al. 2020; Woo 2020).

12.2 Early Response to Circuit Breaker (February–May 2020)

Singapore reported its first imported case on 23 January 2020 and registered an initial rise in imported cases in the last week of January 2020. Rising locally transmitted cases in February 2020 prompted a series of broad-scale public health measures (Chen et al. 2020; Mahmud and Yong 2020; Goh 2020a). Border control measures, starting as temperature screening, health advisory notices, and travel advisories directed at travellers from/to Hubei, progressively extended to the denial of entry or transit for travellers from Hubei and mainland China by early February 2020. Rapid testing, isolation of cases, contact tracing, and physical distancing orders to suspect cases were initiated and scaled up to identify and separate infected individuals from the larger community (Chen et al. 2020; Ministry of Health, Singapore 2021a). (See Table 12.1 for the timeline of movement control/monitoring orders and legal frameworks used.) These measures were applied pursuant to powers under the Immigration Act and the Infectious Diseases Act, strengthened during the SARS outbreak in 2003 (Lee 2020).

Regular directives from the Ministry of Health to all licensed medical practitioners supported national detection and case management efforts, providing updates to evolving suspect case definitions and patient triage protocols. A network of private primary care clinics, called "Public Health Preparedness Clinics" (PHPCs) and registered and prepared in pre-emergent times to perform roles such as screening, dispensing medications, and supporting acute hospitals during public health emergencies, further enabled swift activation of case management and surveillance capacity in the community (Chen et al. 2020; Chotirmall et al. 2020; Chen et al. 2021a).

The initial rise in cases plateaued toward the end of February. A second and much larger wave of infections, triggered by residents returning from other countries in the evolving pandemic situation, led to a closure of borders followed by a suite of significantly stricter island-wide measures termed the Circuit Breaker on 7 April 2020. (See Figure 12.1 for Singapore's epidemic curve of COVID cases.) This response also involved the closure of most workplaces and to full home-based learning for schools (Mohan and Ang 2020; Channel News Asia 2020a).

As the country shifted into the Circuit Breaker (its term for a nationwide partial lockdown), large clusters emerged in foreign worker dormitories, worsening and complicating the already severe epidemic situation (Chen et al. 2020; Chen et al. 2021a). A dedicated interagency taskforce was set up to tackle the outbreaks in these dormitories (see section on "Migrant Worker Dormitories" for the strategy and measures instituted). With the Circuit Breaker, where extensive movement control measures were enforced nationwide, powers provided under the Infectious Diseases Act and Immigration Act were no longer adequate, and the COVID-19 (Temporary Measures) Bill, containing a host of measures ranging from the Circuit Breaker, provisions for virtual meetings and court hearings, to contracts and insolvency relief, was passed on 7 April 2020. As pointed out in an academic article, the government "evidently had no doubt that the Bill would pass," and a Ministry had already deployed its officers on the day that the Bill was debated in Parliament (Chua and Neo 2021; Lee 2020).

The COVID-19 (Temporary Measures) Act (CMTA) granted wide rule-making powers and discretion to the Health Minister to enact control orders if he was "satisfied" that "incidence and transmission of COVID-19 in the community in Singapore constitutes a serious threat to public health" and the control order is "necessary or expedient" to supplement existing legislation

Table 12.1 Timeline of movement control/monitoring orders and legal frameworks used (early responses to Circuit Breaker).

Date	Movement control/Monitoring measures	Legal frameworks used
	2020	
27 Jan	Leave of absence (LOA) effected. Those on LOA should stay at home, minimize contact with other people in the home, and monitor their health closely. They may leave home briefly to get meals and necessities (gov.sg 2020b).	Infectious Diseases Act (Amendment to include COVID-19 (29 January)) (The Singapore Government 2020b)
28 Jan	Quarantine order (QO) effected. Issued to suspect cases and required isolation from other people in the home or in a suitable government facility. A QO is a directive with legal force. It has severe penalties for noncompliance (gov.sg 2020b).	Infectious Diseases Act
1 Feb	All visitors with recent travel history to mainland China not allowed entry into or transit through Singapore (Ministry of Health, Singapore 2020m).	Immigration Act
5 Feb	Large group and communal activities suspended in schools and social and elder-care facilities (Iskandar and Rosli 2020; National Council of Social Service 2020; Ang 2020a)	Infectious Diseases Act
7 Feb	Business continuity planning (BCP) and work-from-home guidelines issued by government agencies for respective sectors (Enterprise Singapore 2020; gov.sg 2020h).	
14 Feb	Doctors advised to issue 5 d medical leave to patients with respiratory symptoms (Elangovan 2020; Lai 2020).	
18 Feb	Stay-home notice (SHN) effected. Stricter than the LOA but one can stay with one's family members. Those on SHN must remain in their place of residence at all times during the SHN period and avoid interaction with other people in the home. (gov.sg 2020a)	Infectious Diseases Act (Amendment (26 Mar)) (Immigration and Checkpoints Authority 2020; The Singapore Government 2020d)
Mar	Denial of entry/transit of travellers, starting from Iran, Japan, and South Korea, then extending to Italy, France, Spain, and Germany.	Immigration Act
11 Mar	All social activities for seniors organized by government agencies suspended (Lim and Goh 2020).	Infectious Diseases Act (Section 20)
13 Mar	Health and manpower ministries urged employers to adopt telecommuting where feasible (Toh and Wong 2020).	
14 Mar	Enhanced measures in schools, preschools, and student care centers. All students and staff who returned from overseas between 14 and 20 Mar 2020 to be placed on a mandatory 14 d LOA (Ministry of Manpower, Singapore 2020k).	Infectious Diseases Act
14 Mar	Employers encouraged to impose LOA for employees returning to Singapore between 14 and 20 Mar (Ministry of Manpower, Singapore 2020k).	
20 Mar	All travellers entering Singapore were issued 14 d SHNs (Ministry of Health, Singapore 2020o).	Infectious Diseases Act
20 Mar	Suspension of events/gatherings with 250 or more participants (Baker 2020a). Retailers and food and beverage (F&B) operators to put in place visible markings and limit number of patrons to ensure sufficient physical distancing (at least 1 m apart) (Co and Tang 2020).	Infectious Diseases Act

Table 12.1 (Continued)

Date	Movement control/Monitoring measures	Legal frameworks used
20 Mar	Seniors to avoid crowded places, stay in well-ventilated areas when outdoors, and engage in more home-based activities (Ministry of Health, Singapore 2020p).	
20 Mar	TraceTogether launched as an application-based digital contact tracing tool. Use of TraceTogether was voluntary (Tang and Mahmud 2020).	
23 Mar	Denial of entry/transit of travellers from all countries.	Immigration Act
25 Mar	Doctors required to issue 5 d medical leave for individuals with respiratory symptoms. Patients issued with medical leave certificates for acute respiratory symptoms were asked to self-isolate at home for 5 d (Elangovan 2020).	Infectious Diseases Act (Enactment of the Infectious Diseases (COVID-19 – Stay Orders) Regulations 2020 (25 Mar)) (The Singapore Government 2020q)
26 Mar	*Tighter distancing measures: (*Ang 2020a*;* Baker 2020a*;* Ministry of Health, Singapore 2020f*)* **Social activities** – bars, night clubs, discos, cinemas, theatres, and karaoke outlets to close. All events and mass gatherings deferred or cancelled. Private celebrations/gatherings limited to 10 people or fewer. **Malls, museums, and attractions** – to reduce operating capacity to no more than one person per 16 sq m of usable space, with groups not exceeding 10 people. Shows, group tours, and open atrium sales suspended. **Tuition and enrichment centers** – classes suspended. **Religious services and congregations** – suspended. Places of worship could stay open for private worship/essential rites, subject to group sizes of less than 10 people at a time. **Funerals and wakes** – individuals to limit attendance as far as possible to family members only, and to gatherings of 10 people or fewer at any point.	Infectious Diseases Act (Enactment of the Infectious Diseases (Measures to Prevent Spread of COVID-19) Regulations 2020 (26 Mar))
1 Apr	Employers had to facilitate telecommuting by staff where possible and implement safe distancing measures within the workplace (Yong 2020).	Infectious Diseases Act (Enactment of the Infectious Diseases (Workplace Measures To Prevent Spread of Covid-19) Regulations 2020 (1 Apr))
7 Apr to 4 May	*Circuit Breaker measures*: (Mohan and Ang 2020; Channel News Asia 2020a) **Education** – schools and Institutes of higher learning to move to full home-based learning. Preschools and student-care centers to suspend services. (Schools, preschools, and student-care centers to provide limited services for children of parents working in essential sectors.) **Public** – members of the public strongly advised to stay home except to purchase necessities or seek essential services or urgent medical care. Reusable masks distributed to all Singapore residents. **Businesses/social activities** – all activities that could not be conducted via telecommuting from home to be suspended.	Enactment of the COVID-19 (Temporary Measures) Act 2020 (CTMA) Enactment of subsidiary legislation under CTMA – the COVID-19 (Temporary Measures) (Control Order) Regulations 2020 Infectious Diseases Act (Revocation of the Infectious Diseases (Measures to Prevent Spread of COVID-19) Regulations 2020 and the Infectious Diseases (Workplace Measures to Prevent Spread of COVID-19) Regulations 2020

(Continued)

Table 12.1 (Continued)

Date	Movement control/Monitoring measures	Legal frameworks used
	Attractions/recreation facilities – all attractions, theme parks, museums, casinos, and sports and recreation facilities to be closed. Restaurants/cafes/dining outlets to operate only for takeaways.	(10 Apr), and Amendment to the Infectious Diseases (COVID-19 – Stay Orders) Regulations 2020 (10 Apr)) (The Singapore Government 2020e)
	Essential sectors – essential services and those in economic sectors critical for local and global supply chains to remain open: • Health, social, and selected care services • Energy, petrol, and gas services • Public and private transport services, and logistics providers • Security, facilities management, and critical public infrastructure • Banking and finance, insurance and asset management; food retailers, supply and delivery (open for takeaway and delivery services only) • Water, waste, and environmental management • Information and communications services and providers • Manufacturing, pharmaceutical, and biomedical sciences Others: electricians, plumbers, vehicle repair, and veterinary services.	
	Across sectors – fiscal measures to support households and businesses under the Solidarity Package.	
	Masking – mandatory in public places.	
10 Apr	Employers in essential sectors to work out telecommuting arrangements where possible (Tan and Yong 2020).	COVID-19 (Temporary Measures) (Control Order) Regulations 2020 (Amendment (10 Apr)) (The Singapore Government 2020f)
15 Apr	For workplace premises that remained open, cross-deployment or movement of workers across different workplace premises disallowed (The Singapore Government 2020g).	COVID-19 (Temporary Measures) (Control Order) Regulations 2020 (Amendment (15 Apr)) (The Singapore Government 2020g)
21 Apr–1 Jun	*Extension of Circuit Breaker, with fewer businesses permitted to operate:* (gov.sg 2020i) **Less critical consumer services/businesses** – stand-alone outlets selling only beverages, packaged snacks, confectioneries or desserts, and hairdressing and barber services to close. Hairdressing and barber services to close. **Selected consumer-facing businesses** – businesses such as optician shops, pet supplies stores, and retail laundry services to operate by appointment only. Traditional Chinese Medicine (TCM) establishments allowed to open for consultation by appointment and dispensing of related medication. (gov.sg 2020j) **Visiting** – one to only enter another person's house to deliver essential goods/services, assist a senior/person with disability, or seek help in an emergency. One disallowed to "drop off" their children with their grandparents for childcare needs (exemptions made for essential service workers and HCWs).	Infectious Diseases (COVID-19 – Stay Orders) Regulations 2020 (Amendment (30 Apr)) (The Singapore Government 2020h) COVID-19 (Temporary Measures) (Control Order) Regulations 2020 (Amendment (1 May)) (The Singapore Government 2020i)

Table 12.1 (Continued)

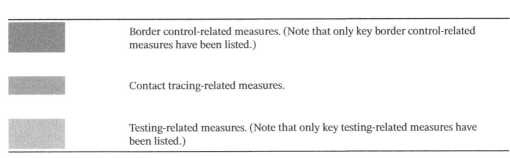

Date	Movement control/Monitoring measures	Legal frameworks used
23 Apr	SafeEntry is introduced and made mandatory at selected public venues and workplaces of essential services (gov.sg 2020k).	Infectious Diseases Act

	Border control-related measures. (Note that only key border control-related measures have been listed.)
	Contact tracing-related measures.
	Testing-related measures. (Note that only key testing-related measures have been listed.)

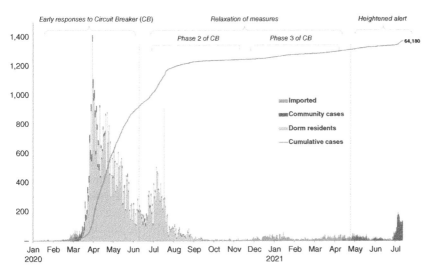

Figure 12.1 Singapore's epidemic curve of COVID cases. Source: Based on data from MOH websites. Data from March 2020 and prior from MOH press releases/past updates from https://www.moh.gov.sg/covid-19/past-updates Data from April 2020 onward from MOH Situation Reports from https://www.moh.gov.sg/covid-19/situation-report.

(The Singapore Government 2020a). Control orders can require people to stay at or in specified places, restrict contact between people, and prohibit or limit the conduct of businesses, events, or gatherings, with penalties for violation taken from the existing framework under the Infectious Diseases Act, including fines up to S$10,000 or imprisonment for up to six months or both and doubled for subsequent offences (Lee 2020; The Singapore Government 2021a).

Despite the sweeping powers involved, Singapore did not invoke emergency laws, where a "regime of exception" would be formed and ordinary legislative processes and constitutional liberties suspended. Instead, it adopted a "legislative model" of emergency powers and effected its COVID response through ordinary legislation, particularly the CMTA. Utilizing ordinary legislation means that all the usual protections under "normal" constitutional order remain intact and are implicitly understood to be compatible with the restrictions. The model was likely adopted as issuing emergency laws could provoke unnecessary public panic, and was also deemed legally unnecessary in Singapore's constitutional culture (Lee 2020; Neo and Lee 2020). Considering the range and details of control measures involved with the Circuit Breaker, the COVID-19 (Temporary Measures) (Control Order) Regulations 2020 was created with subsidiary legislation by the Minister for Health under powers conferred by the CMTA. The regulations defined the restrictions on population movement and activities and workplace management measures, such as permissible group gathering sizes, wedding solemnization restrictions, and work from home requirements (The Singapore Government 2021a).

A week into the Circuit Breaker, public transport usage and traffic volume dropped by more than 70%, foot traffic at popular parks and wet markets came down by nearly 50%, and close to 80% of the workforce were working from home (Ministry of Health, Singapore 2020a). On 23 April, the government announced an extension of the Circuit Breaker period (originally announced to end on 4 May) to 1 June 2020, tighter measures, and further closure of less essential workplaces to reduce the proportion of workers still commuting daily to work to around 15% (Ministry of Health, Singapore 2020a).

Unlike some countries where similar measures were met with protests and resistance, population compliance was generally good with little vocal opposition. Resort to judicial review of government action was rare, even though courts had made arrangements to review COVID measures during the Circuit Breaker and classified such applications as "essential and urgent" (Chua and Neo 2021; Lee 2020). While this has been largely attributed to the context of Singapore's governing philosophy and sociopolitical value system, the measured and open implementation approach of Singapore's COVID measures was noteworthy.

12.2.1 Enforcement Approach

Notwithstanding the legal legitimacy of the measures, policy and enforcement were marked by strong sensitivity to ground sentiment, individual freedoms, and civil rights principles. Physical distancing orders were introduced in varying levels of severity depending on the risk profiles of suspected infection cases (see Table 12.1), starting with the less restrictive (i) Leave of absence (LOA) from workplaces or schools and a (ii) stricter Quarantine order (QO) in late January, and then the (iii) "in-between" Stay-home notice (SHN) and (iv) mandatory five day stays for home medical leave in mid-February and March, the last three being directives with legal enforcement (Chen et al. 2020; gov.sg 2020a; gov.sg 2020b). The variegated approach pre-empted the more widespread impact and resentment an undifferentiated order may have caused. Enforcement of the orders was strong, with those in breach of QOs and SHNs being sentenced to imprisonment or subject to fines (Chen et al. 2020; Khalik 2020; Lam 2020a; Lam 2020b). Breaches of LOAs did not carry criminal penalties, but consequences included foreign work pass holders and their employers having their work passes and work pass privileges revoked, respectively (Ministry of Manpower, Singapore 2020a).

With the Circuit Breaker and more widespread applicability of control measures to the population with the general cessation of business activities and social gatherings, enforcement took on a more graduated and flexible stance. Even as nearly 3,000 enforcement officers and "ambassadors" from over 30 government agencies were deployed daily to public spaces across the island to ensure compliance to safe distancing measures a week into Circuit Breaker, and inspections were carried out at workplaces to check on compliance (Ministry of Health, Singapore 2020b), noncompliant cases were first issued advisories, followed by stern warnings, before being fined after the public had been given a few days to adjust to the updated rules (Heng 2020; Lee 2020; Channel News Asia 2020b).

Fines were also issued only after the government gazetted an amendment to the Control Order Regulations under the CMTA, providing for the composition of offences up to S$2,000, an amount far less than the maximum penalties permitted under the CMTA. It was clarified thereafter that members of the public found in breach of safe distancing measures would face a fine of S$300 for first-time offenders (Lee 2020; Ministry of Sustainability and the Environment, Singapore 2020).

Harder enforcement approaches were also coupled with flexibility in issuing penalties and softer methods of persuasion. For example, in the face of high numbers of noncompliance among the elderly at the start of the Circuit Breaker, the Prime Minister identified himself with the seniors and "appealed" to them to stay at home through a televised address (Prime Minister's Office Singapore 2020). The police were also keen to clarify that proactive enforcement was not practiced for some of the measures. They refuted rumors that checks were conducted at residential units on prohibited gatherings within homes and through roadblocks on safe distancing measures (Singapore Police Force 2020a; Singapore Police Force 2020b).

There was also responsiveness to feedback from the community on the Control Order Regulations issued during the Circuit Breaker. For example, criticisms of inconsistency that a ban on exercising and dog-walking was applied to common areas in condominiums but not to other similar public areas led to an amendment to the regulations (Krishnadas 2020). Similarly, negative feedback on the need to shut home-based food businesses and Traditional Chinese Medicine (TCM) retailers likely led to their being allowed to operate under restricted conditions in the lead up to the earliest phases of easing (Ng 2020; Tan 2020; Abdullah 2020a; Meah 2020a).

There were regular updates by the press on the types of incidents of noncompliance and the number of enforcement actions, which added to the communications around the restrictions and demonstrated that most of the population were complying with the measures and that only a minority were flagrantly breaching. Examples include news reporting of a woman who refused to wear a mask at a market and called herself a "sovereign" being fined and sentenced to jail, a British man who was arrested for refusing to wear a mask on a train, and self-employed individuals who made false declarations for fiscal aid being told to return aid pay-outs (Lam 2021; Phua 2021; Low 2021c). News reports on the woman who called herself a "sovereign" described how the incident caused a commotion at the market with people there telling her that she should be wearing a mask and offering her one while she shouted loudly in response. The narrative was very much one of a country coming together in a time of adversity, and the behaviors of those who resisted (or exploited) the Circuit Breaker measures were "denormalized" and frowned upon by the general population.

12.2.2 Financial and Other Supportive Resources

The use of supportive elements to facilitate compliance was noteworthy. Financial assistance was provided to individuals serving LOAs, SHNs, and QOs up until 7 April 2020 (Khalik 2020; National Trades Union Congress 2020; gov.sg 2020b), after which they ceased and were "replaced" by more systemic funding support to firms/employers in the forms of co-payment of employee wages, tax rebates, and cash-flow assisting schemes (Ministry of Finance, Singapore 2020a). Singapore's fiscal stimulus to cushion the economic impact on firms and livelihoods was computed as having one of the world's largest fiscal response ratios (Economic Policy Group Monetary Authority of Singapore 2020; Chen et al. 2021b).

Such funding support alleviated concerns on the impact to livelihood that could deter compliance to distancing orders. It was concurrently facilitated by the CMTA, which provided a framework for applying relief funding by firms, and the postponement of their contractual obligations where relevant as a result of the COVID situation (The Singapore Government 2020s). Similarly, the government's assurance of COVID-related inpatient treatment and the provision of subsidized consultations for acute respiratory infections (ARIs) at PHPCs since February 2020 encouraged those who are unwell to come forward (Chen et al. 2020; Goh 2020b).

MOH also encouraged healthcare institutions to commence teleconsultation services for follow-up care after issuing notice on their deferment of nonessential services at the start of the Circuit Breaker, facilitating the completion of government-mandated e-training and adherence to the National Telemedicine Guidelines for practitioners and use of healthcare subsidies and Medisave[1] for telemedicine consults (Lim 2020b; Ministry of Health, Singapore 2020c; Ministry of Health, Singapore 2020d; Chen et al. 2021a; Ministry of Health, Singapore 2021w). After masking in public areas became required by law in April 2020, the government and Temasek Foundation[2] distributed reusable and surgical masks to every Singapore resident on a bimonthly basis on average (Koh 2020; Temasek 2020; Co 2020a; gov.sg 2020c).

All in all, enforcement was calibrated and flexible, and at times somewhat participatory. Complementary structures were also instituted to enable ease of compliance. It can almost be said that the government facilitated compliance rather than strictly enforced it (Lee 2020).

12.2.3 Religion, Marriage, and Family Life

The rules pre-emptively addressed issues of rights pertaining to religion, marriage, and family life. Historically, the government's approach and relationship with mainstream religious groups have been one of cooperation, religious harmony being a key element in Singapore's social compact for survival. This approach goes beyond legislated rights for religion, where the freedom of religion is safeguarded in the Singapore Constitution and the Islamic Religious Council retains autonomy in its rulings on Muslim law for the Muslim community (The Singapore Government 2020t; The Singapore Government 2020u; Lee 2020).

Meetings were held between Ministers and religious leaders as early as February 2020 (Ministry of Health, Singapore 2020e). The Inter-Religious Organisation[3] and National Steering Committee on Racial and Religious Harmony[4] issued statements supporting government measures that may include suspension and cancellation of religious services/events in mid-March (Inter-Religious Oranisation Singapore 2021) before they were mandated later in the month (Ministry of Health, Singapore 2020f). Similarly, the Islamic Religious Council issued a ruling on Muslim law acknowledging the need for closure of mosques where necessary in February before it was later announced in March (Majlis Ugama Islam Singapura 2020; Office of the Mufti 2020). At the same time, consideration was given to the interests of religious communities, with places of worship permitted to conduct funeral rites subject to precautionary measures.

The fact that the National Steering Committee on Racial and Religious Harmony is chaired by a Minister (Prime Minister's Office Singapore 2021b), and the historical and strategic entrustment of the Muslim minister in Cabinet with the additional responsibility of overseeing Muslim affairs in Singapore, including the Administration of Muslim Law Act (Prime Minister's Office Singapore 2018a; Prime Minister's Office Singapore 2018b), is worth mentioning at this point.

---

1 MediSave is a compulsory individual savings scheme for Singapore citizens and permanent residents. It is used for one's healthcare expenditure, and workers and their employers contribute a specified percentage of monthly wages to it. It is mainly for use to cover hospitalization expenses, selected preventive care, and outpatient services and long-term care for certain chronic conditions.

2 Singapore-based nonprofit organization under the philanthropic arm of the Singapore State sovereign fund.

3 The Inter-Religious Organisation, Singapore (IRO) is a nongovernmental organization founded by leaders of diverse faiths to work together for religious harmony in Singapore (IRO 2021).

4 The National Steering Committee (NSC) on Racial and Religious Harmony is a national platform to build close relationships at the top level of community, government, and faith leaders (mccy 2021).

While rights to marriage and family life are not contained in the Singapore Constitution, their interests were also taken into account with the passing of the COVID-19 (Temporary Measures for Solemnization and Registration of Marriages) Act 2020 in May 2020 to facilitate virtual marriage solemnizations during the COVID pandemic (The Singapore Government 2020v). Such pre-emptive management of issues related to civil rights, whether based on the constitution or not, helped diffuse potential tensions that could arise, undertaking instead a communal and harmonious balancing of interests between self, communities, and nation.

12.2.4 Communications

Since the pandemic started, public health measures taken were accompanied by extensive communicative effort. Even though the CTMA already states that control orders and amendments thereof must be published beyond the legislative document to be made known to the public, itself a legal safeguard against abuse of emergency-like powers (The Singapore Government 2020w; Lee 2020), the government made concerted efforts to effect widespread dissemination and clear understanding of information on the control measures by the populace.

Apart from publishing the full text of the legislative documents on its website (The Singapore Government 2020s), and maintaining a webpage of the various amendments over time (Ministry of Health, Singapore 2020q), frequent press briefings and public announcements were made by ministers and the Prime Minister on public health measures as part of larger updates on pandemic developments and national strategic responses since the start of the pandemic. The press briefings and announcements were televised nationwide and streamed live on social media channels in the four official languages of English, Mandarin, Malay, and Tamil, with their content reported on print and digital news media platforms and as documents on government/government agency websites (Chen et al. 2020; Chen et al. 2021a; gov.sg 2021a).

Through WhatsApp messaging, a central source of information was also set up through which notifications and updates on COVID-related information and measures were disseminated directly and promptly (Chen et al. 2020). To date, 635,000 unique subscribers have signed up for the service (Smart Nation Singapore 2021a). Accompanying illustrated posters and explanations in the media by experts and experienced personnel became a common feature in Singapore's health communication. Media reports clarifying the details in enforcement and changes to measures are also regularly featured (see page 9).

Concurrently, clarifications on inaccurate news were frequently posted on the government's website and conveyed through the media, with a dedicated hotline for the public to call for information on the COVID-19 situation (Ministry of Health, Singapore 2021x; Chen et al. 2021a). Under the Protection from Online Falsehoods and Manipulation Act (POFMA), correction directions required parties to put up clarification notices for any falsehoods communicated. Several POFMA correction directions were issued to online sites for inaccurate representation of COVID public health measures, with accompanying media reporting on the misrepresentations (Chen et al. 2020; Kamil 2020; Singapore Legal Advice 2020; Channel News Asia 2020c; Channel News Asia 2020d). For example, a corrective direction was issued to an online site that asserted that the S$100 QO allowance was issued directly to foreign workers rather than their employers. This misrepresentation could potentially increase tensions between the foreign worker community and locals and affect trust between the latter and the government.

Carefully engineered health communications were used to build a collective sense of purpose, clarity, and direction of the evolving regulatory measures. It can be said that legislation themselves helped disseminate good knowledge and generated better consciousness about public health measures, with the POFMA complementarily suppressing misleading falsehoods. Such an approach protects civil rights by ensuring that one's freedom and ability to operate per the law is not limited by insufficient knowledge of the regulations.

12.3   Relaxation of Measures (June 2020–April 2021)

From mid-May 2020, with community infection rates generally stable, declining cases in the migrant worker dormitories, and no new large clusters emerging, Singapore started to exit gradually from Circuit Breaker. This was done in a tiered manner across two broadly categorized phases termed Phase 2 and Phase 3 of Circuit Breaker. Schools, workplaces, and selected attractions/recreational facilities were permitted to operate subject to stated capacity limits, while social gathering, dining-out, and cross-household visitations could take place under stated group size limits. The stated capacity and group size limits were increased across the two phases. Singapore shifted into Phase 2 of Circuit Breaker on 19 June 2020 (gov.sg 2020d). (See Table 12.2 for the timeline of movement control/monitoring orders and accompanying legal frameworks as Singapore exited from Circuit Breaker.) Community and dormitory cases peaked in August 2020 before subsequently dropping and maintaining at low single-digit ranges up until May 2021. Daily imported cases continued to occur during the gradual resumption of limited cross border travel but were managed with quarantine-test protocols (Ministry of Health 2020). (See Figure 12.1) Singapore progressed to exit into Phase 3 of Circuit Breaker in December 2020 with further relaxation of measures (Ministry of Health, Singapore 2020g).

As restrictions were relaxed into Phases 2 and 3 of Circuit Breaker, updated measures were legislated under amendments to the COVID-19 (Temporary Measures) (Control Order) Regulations 2020, and new subsidiary legislation such as that for performances and other activities (November 2020) (The Singapore Government 2021b) and major business events (April 2021) (The Singapore Government 2021c; The Singapore Government 2021d). As the migrant worker dormitories were progressively cleared of infections and measures instituted to facilitate the workers' safe resumption of work, updated measures were legislated under the COVID-19 (Temporary Measures) (Foreign Employee Dormitories – Control Order) Regulations 2020 (issued in September 2020) (The Singapore Government 2021e). (See section on "Migrant Worker Dormitories" for the measures legislated.)

The relaxation of measures was carried out with the same widespread and carefully engineered health communications, responsive and calibrated approach to policy and enforcement, and continued use of complementary interventions and persuasive methods to facilitate compliance. Similar to the moves allowing home-based food businesses and TCM retailers to operate before the Circuit Breaker ended, the government recognized that "parents and grandparents miss their children and grandchildren" amidst cross-household visitation restrictions during the Circuit Breaker and permitted limited household visits just before the start of Phase 2 (Toh 2020a; Goh 2020d).

Fiscal measures cushioning the impact of the Circuit Breaker for firms and employees were extended for sectors that had yet to reopen in the graduated exit process, tapered off gradually for recovering sectors, and took on an increasing focus to support a recalibration of business models and entrepreneurship in new sectors as the pandemic dragged on (Ministry of Finance, Singapore 2020b; Economic Development Board 2020a; Economic Development Board 2020b; Chen et al. 2021a). Continued reminders through Ministerial announcements and press briefings to stay vigilant accompanied announcements of relaxed restrictions. Minister Lawrence Wong announced prior that reopening into Phase 3 was conditional upon compliance with safe management measures by the population, emphasizing the necessary trade-off of certain individual freedoms

Table 12.2 Timeline of movement control/monitoring orders and legal frameworks used (relaxation of measures).

Date	Movement control/Monitoring measures	Legal frameworks used
	2020	
5 May	TCM establishments could resume businesses, with some therapies still disallowed (Teo 2020a).	COVID-19 (Temporary Measures) (Control Order) Regulations 2020
9 May	Requirements for safe management measures at the workplace issued, including work-from-home being the default mode of working, staggered start times and flexible workplace hours, and shift/split team arrangements (Ministry of Manpower, Singapore 2020l).	COVID-19 (Temporary Measures) (Control Order) Regulations 2020
12 May	*Gradual resumption of selected activities and services* (Baker 2020b): • Manufacturing and on-site preparation of all food • Retail outlets of food, including cakes, confectionery, and packaged snacks/desserts (for takeaway/deliveries only) • Home-based food businesses • Retail laundry services • Barbers and hairdressers (basic haircut services only) • Retail of pet supplies	COVID-19 (Temporary Measures) (Control Order) Regulations 2020
2 Jun	Students to resume school on a weekly rotation schedule (Ministry of Education, Singapore 2020). People, in groups of up to two visitors living in the same household per day, allowed to visit their parents/grandparents living elsewhere (Toh 2020c).	COVID-19 (Temporary Measures) (Control Order) Regulations 2020 (Amendment (2 Jun)) (The Singapore Government 2020j)
19 Jun	*Phase 2 of reopening:* **Social gatherings** – allowed to comprise up to 6 persons. Households allowed to receive up to five visitors per day (Kamil 2020). **Cinemas** – allowed to reopen from 13 Jul with safe distancing restrictions. **Tourism** – permitted to resume operations in stages from 1 Jul. Domestic tour operators, children recreation areas, and hotels (for staycation bookings) could apply to reopen. **Public libraries** – reopened from 1 Jul with shorter opening hours. **Places of worship** – permitted to resume congregational and other worship services from 26 Jun 2020, starting at 50 persons at a time and subject to safe management measures. **Public libraries** – reopened from 1 Jul with shorter opening hours (gov.sg 2020d). **Education** – students from all levels returned to school daily from 29 Jun 2020. Institutes of higher learning (IHLs) to progressively increase the number of students allowed back on campus at any one time for face-to-face learning, while maintaining a significant amount of online learning. Schools and campuses to continue to adhere to safe management measures (Ministry of Education, Singapore 2020).	COVID-19 (Temporary Measures) (Control Order) Regulations 2020 (Amendment (18 Jun)) (The Singapore Government 2020k)

(Continued)

Table 12.2 (Continued)

Date	Movement control/Monitoring measures	Legal frameworks used
	Dining out – diners allowed in groups of five or fewer at a table, with tables spaced 1 m apart (Co 2020b).	
	Key life events – marriage solemnizations/receptions could be held at places of worship and other external venues with a maximum of 20 persons (excluding the solemnizer).	
	Wakes and funerals – up to 30 persons present at any one time, subject to the venue's capacity limit based on safe management principles (gov.sg 2020o).	
	Visiting – one could visit their parents/grandparents, or "drop off" their children with their grandparents, subject to limit of up to two visitors from one household each day (Goh 2020d).	
Jun	Progressive resumption of some degree of restricted air travel through establishment of Reciprocal Green Lane arrangements with selected countries.	
1 Jul	Patients aged 13 yr and above with ARI and meeting the suspect case definition to undergo a COVID-19 PCR swab test. These patients would only be required to stay home until their swab test result was negative (Baker and Ang 2020).	Infectious Diseases (COVID-19 – Stay Orders) Regulations 2020 (Amendment (1 Jul)) (The Singapore Government 2020l)
4 Aug	*Expansion of permissible group size for certain activities* **Marriage solemnization/receptions** – could be held at a larger variety of venues (both indoor and outdoor) with a maximum of 10–50 persons depending on venue type and capacity limit based on safe management principles. **Wakes and funerals** – up to 30 persons could be present at any one time, subject to venue's capacity limit based on safe management principles.	COVID-19 (Temporary Measures) (Control Order) Regulations 2020 (Amendment (3 Aug)) (The Singapore Government 2020m)
1 Sep	Public facilities available for those conducting outdoor exercise classes, subject to class sizes of up to 50 people and with safe distancing measures (Goh 2020d).	COVID-19 (Temporary Measures) (Control Order) Regulations 2020
14 Sep	Nationwide distribution exercise of physical TraceTogether tokens (gov.sg 2020p; Smart Nation Singapore 2020; Baharudin 2020a).	
28 Sep	Enhanced safe management requirements for workplaces (Baker 2020b): • No more than 50% of employees permitted to return to the workplace at any time • Physical distance of at least 1 m between workers • No more than 5 people are allowed to gather for social or recreational purposes	COVID-19 (Temporary Measures) (Control Order) Regulations 2020 (Amendment (25 Sep)) (The Singapore Government 2020n)
28 Dec	*Phase 3 of reopening (*Ministry of Health, Singapore 2020g*):* **Social gatherings** – up to 8 persons permitted. Households could also receive up to 8 visitors at any point in time.	Enactment of the COVID-19 (Temporary Measures) (Performances and Other Activities – Control Order) Regulations 2020 (1 Nov)

(Continued)

Table 12.2 (Continued)

Date	Movement control/Monitoring measures	Legal frameworks used
	Retail and tourism – capacity limit increased from 10 sqm per person to 8 sqm per person. Attractions could apply to the Singapore Tourism Board to increase operating capacity from up to 50–65%. **Religious organizations** – capacity for congregational and other worship services increased to up to 250 persons (in zones of up to 50 persons for congregational services). **Marriage solemnization** – higher visitor limits for solemnizations held at home. **Live performances** – outdoor performances allowed up to 250 persons in zones of up to 50 persons.	COVID-19 (Temporary Measures) (Performances and Other Activities – Control Order) Regulations 2020 (Amendment (23 Dec)) (The Singapore Government 2020o) COVID-19 (Temporary Measures) (Control Order) Regulations 2020 (Amendment (23 Dec)) (The Singapore Government 2020p)
	2021	
15 Jan	Frequency of the RRT regime shortened from every 14 to 7 d for shore-based personnel in maritime sector going onboard ships (Ministry of Health, Singapore 2021g).	COVID-19 (Temporary Measures) (Control Order) Regulations 2021 (Amendment (13 January)) (The Singapore Government 2021j)
1-18 Jan	Travellers with recent travel history to **United Kingdom and South Africa** denied entry/transit into Singapore. Returning Singapore Citizens and Permanent Residents from the regions to undergo a 7 d self-isolation at their homes, following a 14 d SHN at SHN-dedicated facilities (Ministry of Health, Singapore 2021h).	Infectious Diseases Act Infectious Disease (COVID-19 – Stay Orders) Regulations 2020
24 Jan	All travellers, including Singapore Citizens and Permanent Residents, required to take a PCR test upon arrival in Singapore (Ministry of Health, Singapore 2021i).	Infectious Diseases Act
26 Jan	Tightening of measures in view of the upcoming Chinese New Year festive season (Ministry of Health, Singapore 2021j; The Singapore Government 2021k): • A cap of 8 distinct visitors per household per day • Individuals to visit at most 2 other households a day • Verbalization of messages accompanied by rituals not allowed Changes to live performances measures (The Singapore Government 2021k): • Attendees allowed to sit in groups of 8	COVID-19 (Temporary Measures) (Control Order) Regulations 2021 (Amendment (25 January)) (The Singapore Government 2021k) COVID-19 (Temporary Measures) (Performances and Other Activities – Control Order) Regulations 2021 (Amendment (25 January)) (The Singapore Government 2021k)
31 Jan	Short-term visitors entering Singapore required to purchase travel insurance covering COVID-19-related medical treatment and hospitalization costs (Ministry of Health, Singapore 2021i).	Infectious Diseases Act
1 Feb	Use of personal digital contact tracing data in criminal investigations legally restricted to the most serious offences (Smart Nation Singapore 2021d). Authorized police officers may request users to upload their TraceTogether data to support criminal investigations (Tham 2021).	Amendment bill moved under a Certificate of Urgency to give immediate legal force (Smart Nation Singapore 2021d). COVID-19 (Temporary Measures) Act 2020 (Amendment (1 Mar)) (The Singapore Government 2020a).

(Continued)

Table 12.2 (Continued)

Date	Movement control/Monitoring measures	Legal frameworks used
8–9 Feb	Free surveillance testing offered to stallholders, shop owners, and persons in the F&B industry with higher frequency of contact with the public during the festive season (Ministry of Health, Singapore 2021j).	
5 Apr	Loosening of workplace restrictions (Ministry of Health, Singapore 2021b): • Up to 75% of employees allowed to return to the workplace • Employers to stagger start times and implement flexible working hours • Split team arrangements no longer necessary • Workplace social gatherings of up to 8 persons allowed	COVID-19 (Temporary Measures) (Control Order) Regulations 2020 (Amendment (1 Apr)) (The Singapore Government 2021m)
19 Apr	SafeEntry Gateway Boxes deployed at venues with high footfall. Mandatory for selected malls, large stand-alone retails stores, cinemas, hospitals, polyclinics, and MICE venues (Ang 2021d; Smart Nation Singapore 2021e). Individuals can more conveniently check in by placing their TraceTogether tokens or their mobile phones installed with TraceTogether within 25 cm of the gateway devices.	Infectious Diseases Act
22 Apr	Travellers with recent travel history to the **United Kingdom** and **South Africa** allowed entry and transit into Singapore with test-quarantine protocols (Ministry of Health, Singapore 2021k).	Immigration Act Infectious Diseases Act
23 Apr	Travellers with recent travel history to India restricted from entering or transiting through Singapore. All travellers arrived from **India** and currently serving SHNs required to serve 21 d SHNs at dedicated SHN facilities (Ministry of Health, Singapore 2021k) (Ministry of Health, Singapore 2021l).	Immigration Act Infectious Disease (COVID-19 – Stay Orders) Regulations 2020
24 Apr	Selected activities/events could be scaled up with pre-event testing (PET) (Ministry of Health, Singapore 2021b): **Marriage solemnization/wedding receptions** – capacity limit increased from 100 to 250 attendees (in zones/timeslots of 50 attendees each) **Live performances** – capacity limit from 250 to 750 attendees **Pilot business-to-business events/pilot spectator sports events** – capacity limit from 250 to 750 attendees (in zones of 50 attendees each) **Wakes/funerals** – capacity limit from 30 to 50 attendees only on the day of burial/cremation Individuals who have completed the full vaccination regimen for more than 2 wk can be excluded from the PET.	COVID-19 (Temporary Measures) (Control Order) Regulations 2020 (Amendment (23 Apr 2021)) (The Singapore Government 2021n) COVID-19 (Temporary Measures) (Performances and Other Activities – Control Order) Regulations 2020 (Amendment (23 Apr 2021)) (The Singapore Government 2021o) COVID-19 (Temporary Measures) (Major Business Events – Control Order) Regulations 2021 (Amendment (24 Apr 2021)) Enactment of the COVID-19 (Temporary Measures) (Sporting Events and Activities – Control Order) Regulations 2021 (24 Apr 2021)

Table 12.2 (Continued)

Date	Movement control/Monitoring measures	Legal frameworks used
		Enactment of the Infectious Diseases (Antigen Rapid Test Providers) Regulations 2021 (24 Apr 2021)
		Enactment of the Infectious Diseases (Mass Gathering Testing for Coronavirus Disease 2019) Regulations 2021 (24 Apr 2021)
	Border control-related measures. (Note that only key border control-related measures have been listed.)	
	Contact tracing-related measures.	
	Testing-related measures. (Note that only key testing-related measures have been listed.)	

for larger societal ends and prompting continued compliance through suasion and nudging (Goh 2020e; gov.sg 2021b).

12.3.1 Prioritizing Sectors

The graduated exit from Circuit Breaker involved the calculated balancing of priorities between sectors and population groups. Schools were prioritized, and as school-based learning resumed progressively from June 2020, working from home remained the default mode of operation for nonessential sectors up until September 2020, when no more than 50% of employees were permitted to return to the workplace at any time, and then April 2021, when this was increased to 75%.

Meanwhile, sectors with higher risks of transmissions, such as nightclubs and karaoke joints, remained unopened (Chew 2020b; Mohan 2021; Toh 2021a). Similarly, tighter restrictive measures and other accompanying testing measures were instituted for certain at-risk populations, most notably for dormitory-based migrant workers. The isolation of migrant worker dormitories continued well into Phase 2. The workers are still carrying on under a restricted itinerary, reflecting the deliberated trade-offs between liberties of certain population groups and resumption of activities in the wider community and larger community societal functioning. (See the section on "Migrant Worker Dormitories" for a more detailed account and discussion on this issue.)

12.3.2 Strengthening Outbreak Control Capabilities

This phase in Singapore's pandemic history was also marked by strengthening surveillance structures, facilitating and working toward a less restrictive state of economic functioning and societal activities in what looked increasingly like a prolonged pandemic. Since April 2020, and spanning through Phases 2 and 3, diagnostic, technological, and infrastructural capabilities were incrementally scaled up to enable greater accuracy, speed, and breadth in detection, contact tracing, and quarantine and isolation efforts.

PCR testing, centrally managed under a national workflow system of approved laboratories and providers and initially only available in hospitals and selected PHPCs for suspect cases, has progressively extended to widespread accessibility across virtually all general practitioner clinics and other approved providers for a wide range of needs.

By June 2020, when PCR testing was available at most clinics, case management protocols changed to having patients presenting with ARI undergo a swab test and not needing to serve the rest of their five-day medical certificate leave once test results are reported as negative, alleviating earlier concerns of a prolonged medical leave affecting their income or job stability (Chen et al. 2020; Lai 2020; Goh 2020b). A broader PCR testing strategy was layered with rostered routine testing (RRT), rapid antigen tests, and serology tests for "higher risk" groups and specific use cases (Ministry of Health, Singapore 2021y; National Centre for Infectious Diseases 2020; Yuen 2020; Goh 2020f; Ministry of Health, Singapore 2020h; Ministry of Health, Singapore 2020i; Ministry of Health, Singapore 2020j; Ministry of Health, Singapore 2020k).

Technology was also leveraged. TraceTogether and SafeEntry (which was later integrated into the former) and a range of complementing apps were progressively introduced to monitor contact proximity and location information (see the section on "Leveraging Technology"). TraceTogether, the most widely applicable app, grew from an initial adoption rate of about 25% in June 2020 to more than 90% of Singapore residents by May 2021 (TraceTogether 2020; Cheng 2020; Baharudin and Yee 2020; Ang 2020b; Baharudin 2021a; The Straits Times 2021c). The reopening into Phase 3 was explained to be conditional not only on populace compliance with safe management measures, but also ramped-up PCR test capacity and higher adoption rates for TraceTogether. Phase 3 was later announced in December 2020 when these conditions were met (Goh 2020e; Ministry of Health, Singapore 2020g). TraceTogether was made mandatory for entry into most public venues from May 2021 (Ang 2021a).

Concurrently, efforts were made to repurpose spaces for quarantine or isolation while optimizing Singapore's limited land area (Tay 2020; The Straits Times 2020a; Chen et al. 2021a). Incremental efficiency in detection and contact tracing enabled corresponding reductions in movement restrictions over Phases 2 and 3 from a risk-calibrated approach, as the increased risk of community spread from increased physical contact and social mixing could be offset by more precise and faster detection and isolation (Thong et al. 2021).

Diagnostic and surveillance capabilities were at times scaled up and applied on a targeted basis to not only conserve resources and improve detection accuracy, but also to limit the inconvenience caused to fewer people. Prioritized, universal, or routine rostered testing of specified at-risk groups such as healthcare workers, nursing home staff, transport service drivers, and dormitory-based migrant workers, were conducted to enable rapid ringfencing of infection cases even as concurrent relaxation of measures increased the risk of new clusters (Crotty et al. 2020; Economic Development Board, Enterprise Singapore 2020; Toh 2020b).

Testing and surveillance capabilities also supported Singapore's progressive resumption of restricted air travel through established travel arrangements with select countries from June 2020. A nuanced border control approach was taken, with travellers from different countries fulfilling quarantine-test protocols and using TraceTogether of varying durations and intensity depending on their departing counties' relative importation risk for COVID (Chong 2020; Abdullah 2020b; Teo 2020b; Chen et al. 2021a; Immigration and Checkpoints Authority 2021a; Immigration and Checkpoints Authority 2021b).

Fiscal measures complemented the measures, with coverage for COVID-related care, which was withdrawn for residents who chose to travel from 24 March 2020 when Singapore just closed its borders, reinstated from 7 August 2020 when the resumption of essential travel was permitted (Goh 2020c; gov.sg 2020e). Similarly, from December 2020, the government provided vouchers to

Singaporeans to spend on local hotel stays, attraction tickets and tours to "rediscover" Singapore in an act to support local tourism businesses while concurrently addressing societal fatigue from prolonged border control restrictions (Tay and Lim 2020; Singapore Tourism Board 2021).

When COVID vaccines became available, the government announced its national vaccination strategy to enable all Singaporeans and long-term residents to be vaccinated for free by the end of 2021. Supplies for vaccines had been secured as early as June 2020 under advance purchase agreements. With authorizations granted by the Health Science Authority for their use from December 2020 (Health Sciences Authority 2020; gov.sg 2020f; Ministry of Health, Singapore 2020l), a national vaccination schedule was rolled out from December 2020, starting with the Prime Minister and Ministers, and then staff in healthcare institutions, followed by the elderly aged 70 years and above, and thereafter successively younger age-bands (Ministry of Health, Singapore 2020l; Awang 2021; Zhang 2021).

Streaming panel discussions and webinars held with MOH personnel and relevant experts helped bolster public confidence while expanding the network of vaccination centers improved accessibility (Zhang 2021). Like incremental testing capabilities, the vaccine's expected protection from severe disease and infection enabled less restrictive social inter-mixing. In April 2021, the government permitted increased capacity limits for events where pre-event testing was done and individuals who have completed vaccination could be excluded from the testing (Ministry of Health, Singapore 2021b).

12.3.3 General Elections 2020

Singapore organized a general election on 10 July 2020, in the middle of the pandemic. Here again, we see complementary use of legislation in the passing of the Parliamentary Elections (COVID-19 Special Arrangements) Act to facilitate safe conduct of elections within the limitations arising from the COVID situation, allowing political candidates to file nomination papers electronically, and letting voters under control orders to vote at facilities outside their electoral divisions (Chua and Neo 2021; Lee 2020). Legal academics have pointed to the elections as an opportunity for consolidation of the democratic legitimacy of Singapore's COVID response, where the elected government could be held to account for their successes or failures at the ballot box (Chua and Neo 2021; Lee 2020), reaffirming the peoples' sense of rights and participation in their country's legislative and policy response.

While PAP's election victory with 61.24% of votes and 83 out of 93 seats won is considered a high margin in other countries, the 10 seats won by the Workers' Party (the opposition party with the largest elected representation to date) is the highest number won by an opposition party in Singapore's post-independence history (Mohan and Phua 2020; Chew 2020a; Channel News Asia 2020e). Political analysts were generally of the view that while the vote slide was largely a continuation of a broader trending trajectory started decades ago, public unhappiness over how the pandemic had been handled with the migrant worker dormitory outbreaks, and over the public messaging around what was deemed by some as an opportunistic move to call for general elections during the pandemic, contributed partially to the results (Chua and Neo 2021; Hussain 2020; Lee 2020; Chew 2020a). Therefore, the election results can be said to be, in some part, a repudiation of the government's handling of the COVID-19 outbreak.

The implementation and framing of rules around Singapore's graduated exit from Circuit Breaker were characterized by continued sensitivity and attention to concepts of rights pertaining to family life, livelihood and social needs, more nuanced balancing and prioritization of these between groups, sectors, socioeconomic demands, and relative epidemiological risk, and more varied combinatory use of policy levers with incremental and an increasing range of tools and levers at the government's disposal. The intent was to achieve an acceptable level of livability, societal functioning, and economic activity while keeping the epidemic curve under control. At the same time, the start of the national vaccination programme paved the way for wider legislative and policy options in the future.

12.4   Heightened Alert (May 2021–June 2021)

As more transmissible variants emerged in other countries, imported cases and wider community transmission eventually emerged in May 2021 (see Figure 12.1). Despite stricter test-quarantine protocols for returning travellers and the denial of entry to wider groups of travellers from countries where the more contagious strains were circulating (National Council of Social Service 2020; gov.sg 2020b; The Singapore Government 2020b; Ministry of Health, Singapore 2020m), the Delta variant originating from India sparked two of the largest community clusters at that time (Tan 2021). Singapore went into Phase 3 Heightened Alert on 8 May 2021, and then into Phase 2 Heightened Alert on 16 May 2021 with further tightening of measures, in parallel with the earlier Phases 3 and 2 of exit from Circuit Breaker. (See Table 12.3 for a timeline of measures and legal frameworks.) Singapore stopped entry for all long-term pass holders and short-term visitors with recent travel history to India from 24 April 2021 (Ang 2021b).

Communications surrounding the Heightened Alert appealed once again to the communitarianism in the populace, seeking their cooperation to comply with the tightened measures, reminding all of how such communal efforts had stemmed epidemic spread before, and how letting their guard down can necessitate "more nasty, drastic measures" and another extensive Circuit Breaker would be a major setback for the nation (Ministry of Finance, Singapore 2021; Lai 2021a; Ng 2021; Channel News Asia 2021b).

By the time Phase 2 (Heightened Alert) was announced, the population was mentally prepared. As a newspaper article described, "most people's reactions were marked by readiness rather than alarm," with some having ran their errands at the hair salon or supermarkets over the past two weeks (Lin 2021). Home-based learning for schools was effected, two weeks prior to start of the national month-long school holiday, in view of several outbreaks in schools and how the Delta variant appears to affect children more (Lin 2021). Progress made in public health capabilities was emphasized, as well as how it enabled finer targeting of restrictions and surveillance efforts such as limiting closures and mass testing to affected institutions, geographic areas (e.g. neighborhoods), and services or subsectors involving mask-off indoor activities, instead of a broader sector-based approach (Lin 2021; Ministry of Finance, Singapore 2021; Ong 2021; Channel News Asia 2021c). Funding support for affected firms and employees could also, as a result, be extended more sustainably and in a more targeted way to smaller groups affected (Ministry of Finance, Singapore 2021).

With the epidemiologic spread from imported cases and subsequent entry into Heightened Alert, some Singaporeans expressed worries that other considerations, such as the economy, had been prioritized over the public's health (Mathews and Zainuddin 2021). National communications in the form of Ministerial briefings and commentary articles in mainstream media addressed these concerns, explaining the evidence-based and risk-calibrated approach behind Singapore's more porous but nuanced border policy, reinforcing the survivalist mentality as a small country and the impracticality of an impervious border, and cautioning against divisive xenophobic sentiments (Cook 2021; Khalik 2021; Mathews and Zainuddin 2021).

Antigen Rapid Tests (ART) was meanwhile rolled out on a widespread scale, complementing PCR testing of patients with ARI at clinics, mandated for staff involved in higher-risk mask-off

Table 12.3 Timeline of movement control/monitoring orders and legal frameworks used (Heightened Alert).

Date	Movement control/Monitoring measures	Legal frameworks used
	2021	
1 May	*Tightening of measures* (Ministry of Health, Singapore 2021m): **Malls and large standalone stalls** – operating capacity reduced to no more than one person per 10 sq.m. **Popular malls** – entry restriction on Sundays by odd and even numbers of one's National Registration Identification Card (NRIC) or Foreign Identification Number (FIN). **Outdoor barbecue pits and campsites** closed.	COVID-19 (Temporary Measures) (Control Order) Regulations 2020 (Amendment (30 Apr 2021)) (The Singapore Government 2021p)
1 May	Travellers with recent travel history to **Bangladesh, Nepal, Pakistan, and Sri Lanka** are restricted from entering or transiting through Singapore. Those arrived from these countries and currently serving SHNs required to serve 21 d SHNs at dedicated SHN facilities (Ministry of Health, Singapore 2021m).	Immigration Act Issued under the Infectious Diseases (COVID-19 – Stay Orders) Regulations 2020
7 May	Definition of recent travel history extended from 14 to 21 d when considering if border measures will apply to incoming travellers (Ministry of Health, Singapore 2021n). All travellers with recent travel history to **higher risk countries/regions** (all countries/regions except Australia, Brunei Darussalam, Mainland China, New Zealand, Taiwan, Hong Kong, and Macao) to serve 21 d SHNs at dedicated SHN facilities. (Ministry of Health, Singapore 2021n)	Issued under the Infectious Disease (COVID-19 – Stay Orders) Regulations 2020
8 May	*Phase 3 Heightened Alert (* gov.sg 2021c; The Singapore Government 2021p*):* **Social gatherings and interactions** – group sizes reduced from 8 to 5 persons. Up to 5 visitors per household per day is allowed. Individuals advised to keep to 2 or less social gatherings per day. **Workplace** – employees allowed to return to the workplace reduced from 75 to 50%. Group size for social gatherings reduced from 8 to 5 persons. **Congregational and worship services** – suspension of masked congregational singing. Up to 250 pax with PET, or up to 100 pax without PET. **Shopping malls and showrooms** – occupancy continues to be 1 person per 10 sqm of Gross Floor Area. **Attractions and shows** – operating capacity reduced from 65 to 50%. Shows (indoor and outdoor) to be capped at 100 pax with PET or 50 pax without PET. **Museums and public libraries** – operating capacity reduced from 65 to 50%. **Cinemas** – up to 250 pax with PET or up to 100 pax without PET. Safe distancing between groups of up to 5 pax. **Tour groups** – maximum group size reduced from 50 to 20 pax.	COVID-19 (Temporary Measures) (Control Order) Regulations 2021 (Amendment (7 May 2021)) (The Singapore Government 2021q) Infectious Diseases (Mass Gathering Testing for Coronavirus Disease 2019) Regulations 2021 (Amendment (7 May 2021)) (The Singapore Government 2021r) COVID-19 (Temporary Measures) (Performances and Other Activities – Control Order) Regulations 2021 (Amendment (7 May 2021)) (The Singapore Government 2021s) COVID-19 (Temporary Measures) (Sporting Events and Activities – Control Order) Regulations 2021 (Amendment (7 May 2021)) (The Singapore Government 2021f)

(Continued)

Table 12.3 (Continued)

Date	Movement control/Monitoring measures	Legal frameworks used
	Outdoor exercise facilities and classes – occupancy limit of 1 person per 10 sqm of Gross Floor Area or 50 persons, whichever is lower. Up to 30 pax per class subject to venue capacity limits, with 3 m between groups and 2 m between individuals. Group sizes of up to 5 pax allowed.	
	Indoor exercise facilities and classes – indoor gymnasiums and fitness studios closed.	
	Wedding solemnization and wedding reception – up to 250 pax with PET or 50 pax without PET.	
	Funerals – reduced from 50 to 30 pax for all days.	
	Sports events – all mass participation sports events suspended.	
	Live performances and pilot business-to-business events – number of attendees allowed reduced from 750 to 250 pax.	
	Cinemas – attendance reduced to 100 pax.	
15 May	Antigen rapid testing (ART) will be carried out together with the pre-existing PCR test for all who present with ARI symptoms to allow quicker contact tracing. Applicable to the Swab and Send Home Public Health Preparedness Clinics, polyclinics, emergency departments, and regional swab centers. Individuals who test positive on their ART will have to self-isolate until they receive a negative PCR test result. (gov.sg 2021d; Ministry of Health, Singapore 2021o)	Infectious Diseases Act Infectious Diseases (COVID-19 – Stay Orders) Regulations 2020 (Amendment (6 May 2021)) (The Singapore Government 2021i)
16 May	*Phase 2 Heightened Alert (*gov.sg 2021d*):* **Social gatherings and interactions** – group sizes reduced from 5 to 2 pax. Up to 2 visitors per household per day. Individuals are also recommended to keep to 2 social gatherings per person per day. The caring of grandchildren is not included in the number of household visitors or social gatherings per day. **Workplace** – work-from-home as the default. Cross-deployment and social gatherings are no longer allowed. **F&B, including hawker centers and food courts** – dining-in ceased. Only takeaway and delivery allowed. **Congregational and worship services** – no unmasking activities, including singing and the playing of wind and brass instruments. Up to 100 pax with PET or up to 50 pax without PET. **Shopping malls and showrooms** – occupancy reduced from 1 person per 10 sq.m of Gross Floor Area to 1 person per 16 sq.m of Gross Floor Area. **Attractions and shows** – operating capacity reduced to 25 from 50%. Shows (indoor and outdoor) to be capped at 100 pax with PET or 50 pax without PET.	COVID-19 (Temporary Measures) (Control Order) Regulations 2021 (Amendment (14 May 2021)) (The Singapore Government 2021t) Infectious Diseases (Mass Gathering Testing for Coronavirus Disease 2019) Regulations 2021 (Amendment (14 May 2021)) (The Singapore Government 2021u) COVID-19 (Temporary Measures) (Sporting Events and Activities – Control Order) Regulations 2012 (Amendment (14 May 2021)) (The Singapore Government 2021v) COVID-19 (Temporary Measures) (Performances and Other Activities – Control Order) Regulations 2021 (Amendment (14 May 2021)) (The Singapore Government 2021w)

Table 12.3 (Continued)

Date	Movement control/Monitoring measures	Legal frameworks used
	Museums and public libraries – operating capacity reduced to 25 from 50%.	
	Cinemas – up to 100 pax with PET or up to 50 pax without PET. Safe distancing between groups of 2 pax. No food and beverage to be consumed.	
	Massage establishments – services which require masks to be removed (e.g. facials and saunas) ceased.	
	Home-based businesses – allowed to operate on contactless delivery/collection.	
	Wedding solemnization – up to 100 pax with PET or 50 pax without PET. No wedding receptions allowed.	
	Funerals – reduced from 30 to 20 pax at any point in time.	
	MICE and live performances – up to 100 pax with PET or up to 50 pax without PET.	
17 May	*Mandatory TraceTogether-only SafeEntry commenced* (Chee 2021c; Ministry of Health, Singapore 2021n) SafeEntry can only be carried out through the TraceTogether token or phone application. Implemented across all venues with SafeEntry, including malls, eateries, offices, schools, and places of worship. Scanning of SafeEntry QR-codes with phone camera and SingPass App discontinued.	Infectious Diseases Act
29 May	Pre-departure COVID-19 PCR test for long-term pass holders and short-term visitors was extended to Singapore Citizens and Permanent Residents arriving from higher-risk regions (Ministry of Health, Singapore 2021p). Negative test results required for entry into Singapore.	Infectious Diseases Act
1 Jun	Household members of persons under quarantine required to self-isolate at home until the person under quarantine receives a negative COVID-19 PCR test result or is no longer under quarantine (Ministry of Health, Singapore 2021o). Household members should seek medical attention if they feel unwell during this period.	Infectious Diseases (COVID-19 – Stay Orders) Regulations 2020
14 Jun	*Gradual reopening to Phase 3 Heightened Alert* (gov.sg 2021e; Ministry of Health, Singapore 2021q): **Social gatherings and interactions** – group sizes up to 5 pax. Up to 5 visitors per household per day. Individuals are recommended to keep to 2 social gatherings per day. Grandchildren being cared for by grandparents need not be included in the number of household visitors or social gatherings per day. *(Same as 8 May 2021 – Phase 3 Heightened Alert)*	COVID-19 (Temporary Measures) (Control Order) Regulations 2021 (Amendment (11 Jun 2021)) (The Singapore Government 2021x) COVID-19 (Temporary Measures) (Performances and Other Activities – Control Order) Regulations 2021 (Amendment (11 Jun 2021)) (The Singapore Government 2021y)

(Continued)

Table 12.3 (Continued)

Date	Movement control/Monitoring measures	Legal frameworks used
	Congregational and worship services – up to 250 pax with PET or up to 50 pax without PET. May resume unmasking/singing/wind and brass instruments for live performances subject to relevant safe management measures.	COVID-19 (Temporary Measures) (Sporting Events and Activities – Control Order) Regulations 2021 (Amendment (11 Jun 2021)) (The Singapore Government 2021z)
	Cinemas – up to 250 pax with PET or up to 50 pax without PET. F&B service may resume if all customers are in groups of no more than 2 persons; if F&B service is not allowed, customers may be in groups of up to 5 persons.	Infectious Diseases (Mass Gathering Testing for Coronavirus Disease 2019) Regulations 2021 (Amendment (11 Jun 2021)) (The Singapore Government 2021g)
	Attractions and cruises – operating capacity increased from 25 to 50%.	
	MICE, live performances, and spectator sport events – events may resume. PET is required for events with 250 attendees and not required for events with 50 or fewer attendees.	
	Massage establishments – services which require masks to be removed (e.g. facials and saunas) allowed to resume, with prevailing safe management measures observed.	
	Home-based businesses – allowed to operate subject to prevailing safe management measures, e.g. up to 5 unique visitors a day.	
	In-person tuition and enrichment classes – resume with up to 50 pax per class in groups of up to 5 pax.	
	Hotels – group of up to 5 pax per room for staycations, except where individuals are all from the same household, subject to the room's maximum capacity.	
	Sports/exercise activities and classes provided by gyms/fitness studios – indoor mask-off activities at gyms/fitness studios may resume in groups of up to 2 pax. Indoor and outdoor classes capped at 30 pax (in groups of up to 5 pax for mask-on activities; in groups of no more than 2 pax for indoor mask-off activities). Safe distancing of at least 2 m between individuals and 3 m between groups must be maintained.	
	Wedding solemnization and wedding reception – up to 250 pax with PET or 50 pax without PET.	
	Funerals – up to 30 pax at any point in time on all days.	
16 Jun	ART self-test kits sold at retail pharmacies (Prime Minister's Office Singapore 2018a; Ministry of Health, Singapore 2021o). Suitable for individuals who do not have ARI symptoms but are concerned about COVID-19 exposure. The self-test kit complements rather than replaces a PCR test that remains necessary for individuals with ARI symptoms. Individuals with a positive ART Self-test kit result should visit a doctor for a PCR test.	

Table 12.3 (Continued)

Date	Movement control/Monitoring measures	Legal frameworks used
21 Jun	*Further reopening to Phase 3 (Heightened Alert)* (Ministry of Health, Singapore 2021r): **F&B, including hawker centers and food courts** – dine-in allowed with group sizes of up to 2 pax. **Wedding receptions** –50 attendees with PET for 20 attendees or up to 100 attendees with PET for all attendees. **Live performances** – unmasking and singing/playing of wind instruments for live performances allowed. Singing and playing of wind instruments may resume for live performances at congregational and worship services. **Gyms, fitness studios, and mask-off sports activities** – allowed to resume with safe distancing of at least 2 m between persons and at least 3 m between groups of up to 5 persons. Sports classes (both indoors and outdoors) capped at 30 persons, with groups of no more than 5 persons. Participants may unmask if they are engaging in strenuous activities, although they are strongly encouraged to remain masked where possible. **In-person tuition and enrichment classes (including those aged 18 and below)** – allowed to resume with enhanced safe management measures. Higher-risk arts and culture classes such as singing and wind instruments also allowed to resume. **Workplace** – work-from-home remains the default work arrangement. **Visits to residential care homes** – physical visits to residential care homes serving elderly can resume. Visitors need to take an ART at the home and test negative prior to entry.	COVID-19 (Temporary Measures) (Control Order) Regulations 2021 (Amendment (18 Jun 2021)) (The Singapore Government 2021h) COVID-19 (Temporary Measures) (Performances and Other Activities – Control Order) Regulations 2021 (Amendment (18 Jun 2021)) (The Singapore Government 2021aa) COVID-19 (Temporary Measures) (Sporting Events and Activities – Control Order) Regulations 2021 (Amendment (18 Jun 2021)) (The Singapore Government 2021ab)
21 Jun	Regular Fast and Easy Testing (FET) progressively rolled out for staff involved in higher-risk mask-off activities, starting from larger establishments (Singapore Food Agency 2021; Ministry of Health, Singapore 2021q). This includes staff in dine-in F&B establishments, personal care and appearance services, and gyms.	
23 Jun	SHNs for new travellers arriving from higher risk countries/regions will be reduced from 21 to 14 d at dedicated SHN facilities (Ministry of Health, Singapore 2021s).	Infectious Disease (COVID-19 – Stay Orders) Regulations 2020
27 Jun	All travellers required to test themselves regularly with the ART self-test kits on Days 3, 7, and 11 of their arrival in Singapore during their SHN, on top of pre-existing test protocols (Ministry of Health, Singapore 2021s).	Infectious Diseases Act
Early-Jul	"Health Alerts" to be sent via SMS to individuals who have visited places on the same days as infected persons. They will be required to undergo mandatory COVID-19 testing and stay isolated until they receive their results. Individuals who test negative will be given self-test kits to administer at home over subsequent days, advised to limit interactions, and restrict activities to essential ones (Ministry of Health, Singapore 2021r).	Infectious Diseases Act and the Infectious Diseases (COVID-19 – Stay Orders) Regulations 2021

(Continued)

Table 12.3 (Continued)

Date	Movement control/Monitoring measures	Legal frameworks used
Early-Jul	SafeEntry Gateway Check-out Boxes to be progressively deployed at venues with high footfall or high-risk mask-off activities (Ministry of Health, Singapore 2021r).	
12 Jul	*Updates to safe management measures in Phase 3 (Heightened Alert)* (Ministry of Culture, Community and Youth 2021; Ministry of Health, Singapore 2021t): **Group sizes at F&B establishments** – increased from 2 to 5 persons. **Live performances in congregational and other worship services** – performer group sizes increased from 2 to 5 persons. Capacity sizes for worship services also increased to 250 if carried out in places of worship or 50 if carried out in other places. **Wedding receptions** –no more than 250 persons allowed with PET (PET). **Indoor high-intensity/ mask-off sports/exercise activities** – gyms and fitness studios may conduct indoor mask-off sports/ exercise activities in group sizes of up to 5 persons. Sports and exercise classes allowed to continue in groups of no more than 5 persons, in classes of up to 50 persons. **Social gatherings at the workplace** – work-from-home remains the default. Employees who need to return to the workplace should have staggered start times and flexible working hours. Social and recreational gatherings of no more than 5 persons allowed.	COVID-19 (Temporary Measures) (Control Order) Regulations 2021 (Amendment (9 Jul)) (The Singapore Government 2021ac) COVID-19 (Temporary Measures) (Performances and Other Activities – Control Order) Regulations 2021 (Amendment (9 Jul)) (The Singapore Government 2021ad) COVID-19 (Temporary Measures) (Sporting Events and Activities – Control Order) Regulations 2021 (Amendment (9 Jul)) (The Singapore Government 2021ae) Enactment of the COVID-19 (Temporary Measures) (Religious Gatherings – Control Order) Regulations 2021 (12 Jul)
12–15 Jul	Travellers with recent travel history to Indonesia and Myanmar within the last 21 d denied entry/transit into Singapore (Ministry of Health, Singapore 2021u).	Infectious Diseases Act
15 Jul	FET made mandatory for all staff involved in higher-risk mask-off activities (Ministry of Health, Singapore 2021r; Ministry of Health, Singapore 2021t): • Dine-in F&B establishments • Personal care services • Gyms and fitness studios with unmasked clients ART will be made available at general retailers like supermarkets and convenience stores to increase ease of access.	Infectious Diseases Act

	Border control-related measures. (Note that only key border control-related measures have been listed.)
	Contact tracing-related measures.
	Testing-related measures. (Note that only key testing-related measures have been listed.)

activities, and indicated specifically in subsidiary legislation under powers conferred by the Infectious Diseases Act, thus further strengthening the existing testing regime (Ministry of Health, Singapore 2021c; Ministry of Health, Singapore 2021d; Ministry of Health, Singapore 2021e; The Singapore Government 2021f; The Singapore Government 2021g; The Singapore Government 2021h). The national vaccination programme continued to make headway, with the youngest eligible age band (from 12 to 39 years) able to register for vaccination from June 2021, and tweaking of the strategy to extend the interval between doses so that more people would be covered by at least one dose sooner (Mahmud 2021; Lai 2021b; Ang 2021c). As Singapore gradually reopened from Heightened Alert after the stabilization of community cases, close to 40% of the population had been fully vaccinated, with two-thirds of the population having received at least one dose (Baker 2021; Ministry of Health, Singapore 2021f). Communications also began to address the transition to a COVID-endemic world where the hitherto medicalized protocols for the disease that have worked well to protect an immunologically naïve population will transition to more home or community-based management with vaccination and better diagnostic and pharmaceutical options, permitting greater normality of life and greater freedom of movement, economic functioning, and the opening of borders (Cook and Hsu 2021; Gan et al. 2021).

This phase has seen the continued increase in sophistication of surveillance techniques and societal movement control calibration, enabling the flattening of the epidemic curve with less disruption to daily living as well as the acceleration of the vaccination plan. Strategic planning and public discourse have also taken on broader and longer term issues of national survival, prolonged fatigue, and transitioning to a new steady state of livability.

12.5 Leveraging Technology

Digital technologies feature strongly in the enablement of enforcement and compliance in Singapore's response and their calibration to facilitate greater degrees of freedom across response phases. This was most notable with the implementation and use of TraceTogether.

Conventional methods for contact tracing can be laborious, slow, incomplete, and prone to errors due to recall bias and false declarations (CNA 2020; Kretzschmar et al. 2020; Alkhatib 2021). Digital tools can thus help minimize delays and reduce gaps in contact identification, contact listing, and contact follow-up (Owusu 2020). TraceTogether and SafeEntry, developed by Singapore's Government Technology Agency (GovTech), were launched in March and April 2020, respectively, to support Singapore's contact tracing efforts. TraceTogether uses anonymized proximity information enabled by Bluetooth technology to track exchanges between individuals and identify past exposures to COVID-19. SafeEntry provides a complementary location check-in function when individuals enter buildings and public premises and serves as a digital visitor record system for businesses. Upon wide implementation, TraceTogether and SafeEntry helped to reduce the average time to quarantine of close contacts from 4 days to less than 1.5 days (Smart Nation Singapore 2021b).

Singapore's high digital baseline (having a mobile penetration of 148.2%[5] in 2020 (Department of Statistics Singapore 2021b)) enabled ease of TraceTogether's rollout. The country's pre-existing cultural tendency to trade liberal individualism for national interests (Government of Singapore 1991; Chua 2017), coupled with strengthening of the ethos of communitarianism over the course of the pandemic, has also made possible the virtually population-wide adoption of TraceTogether seen today.

---

5 Refers to mobile subscriptions over total population in Singapore, and indicating that some residents subscribe to more than one mobile line.

At the same time, quick recognition and resolution of barriers to uptake and appropriately timed announcements of a mandated approach helped nudge the necessary behavioral changes which facilitated the adoption process. The TraceTogether mobile application was initially launched as a voluntary opt-in measure. Limited uptake was noted for elderly and young children without or preferring not to use smartphones. Technical issues such as battery drain, low sensitivity (Huang et al. 2020), and the need for the TraceTogether app to run in the foreground to function on iPhones, further hampered the application's efficacy and uptake rates (Government Technology Agency 2020a; Baharudin 2020c). TraceTogether tokens, designed especially for elderly and young children, were distributed to all Singapore citizens and permanent residents for free at community centers from September 2020 (Meah 2020b), followed by an announcement in October that TraceTogether would become compulsory (Huang et al. 2021).

Meanwhile, continuous version updates addressed the application's technical issues without compromising cybersecurity (Government of Singapore 2021a). Between July and December 2020, a study found that the acceptance of TraceTogether increased from 65 to 89%, and 69 to 83% among older and younger adults respectively (Huang et al. 2021), achieving the near 70% adoption rate target set for relaxation of measures in Phase 3 Circuit Breaker (Tang 2020; Goh 2020e; Ministry of Health, Singapore 2020g). TraceTogether-only SafeEntry subsequently became mandatory at a wide range of settings, including workplaces, healthcare facilities, places of worships, malls, food and beverage outlets, cultural and entertainment venues, sports and fitness centers, country clubs, event venues, weddings, funeral events, and schools from 17 May 2021 (Low 2021a; Low 2021b), and adoption rates rose further to 92% in May 2021 (Baharudin 2021a). Legislation and policies were tweaked as incremental progress was made in technological infrastructure and behavioral acceptance.

Concurrently, the mandated approach and government data ownership are critical enablers of TraceTogether's success. Singapore's continued preference of BlueTrace-powered TraceTogether over alternatives such as the Exposure Notification (EN) feature on Android and iOS phones (rolled out since May 2020) was driven by its mandated directives, rather than relying on self-reporting of infections and individual social responsibility under EN. In contrast to TraceTogether, MOH also does not have access to data collected by these alternate applications for epidemiological investigations (Government Technology Agency 2020a).

Besides TraceTogether, other digital tools similarly augment traditional quarantine and social distancing enforcement measures (Mohan 2020). The Homer application has been used by all individuals issued with SHN and QOs to submit location reports and health status updates to authorities since January 2020 (Homer 2020). From 10 August 2020, it is also mandatory for travellers (aged 13 and above) to Singapore serving SHN at a place of residence outside of dedicated SHN facilities to wear an electronic wristband device and install a gateway device. Paired with a mobile phone app, StayHome@SG, Bluetooth, and global positioning system (GPS) signals alert authorities when individuals leave their place of residence during the SHN period (The Straits Times 2020b).

Organizations other than the government have also developed digital tools to improve detection and help monitor adherence to physical distancing measures and enforcement of national workplace measures. The uNivUS app, developed by the National University of Singapore, facilitates input and uploading of staff's temperature, ART test results, and vaccination status and enables users to check on the live status of crowding levels at the various dining places on the university campus.

Despite their wide deployment, technology remains complementary to manual checks and is not fully automated in Singapore. For example, the processing and filtering of TraceTogether signals based on the strength, duration, and setting of exposure are still required to identify close contacts (TraceTogether 2021). Manual intervention is driven by the need for human discretion in determining appropriate responses to changes in the epidemic situation and evolving technological capabilities. This discretionary balance between human intervention and automation helps ensure that automation does not perpetuate or magnify erroneous processes and fail to benefit from human insights.

12.5.1 Data Privacy, Security, and Governance

Individuals' data privacy interests are protected in Singapore under the 2012 Personal Data Protection Act and the 2002 Model Data Protection Code. However, these legislations apply solely to the private sector. The public sector adopts pre-existing laws and internal guidelines based on recommendations from the Public Sector Data Security Review Committee (Wong 2017; Smart Nation Singapore 2021c). The right to privacy is not contained in the Singapore Constitution (Privacy International 2015; Chok 2020; Lee 2020).

Unspoken cultural acceptance of privacy intrusions for the sake of other priorities, such as security, has not been uncommon (Han 2021a; Han 2021b). For example, quite interestingly, just in March 2021, Law and Home Affairs Minister K Shanmugam had shared positively the technological upgrades to the Singapore Police Force's surveillance capabilities and confirmed the installation of almost 90,000 police cameras island-wide (with "many more" to come) (Osman 2021; Han 2021b). In fact, Singapore's economic interest is the broader policy focus of data protection regulation under the Personal Data Protection Act (Wong 2017).

Despite this and the nonconstitution-based nature of privacy rights, the government has been eager to pre-emptively address privacy concerns with the technologies' rollout. To utilize SafeEntry and TraceTogether, users must agree to disclose and share their names, identification numbers, contact numbers, premise addresses, and entry and exit times with public sector agencies and third parties for purposes permissible under the CMTA (Government of Singapore 2020; GovTech (Government Technology Agency of Singapore) 2020). The launch of digital contact tracing tools was accompanied by frequent reassurance from the government about privacy safeguards. These include assurances that TraceTogether does not collect GPS data and track its users' every move. Data on exchanges with other TraceTogether devices is stored locally on users' devices in an encrypted format and uploaded manually only upon request by the Ministry of Health if an individual tests positive for COVID-19. Furthermore, Temporary IDs are anonymized and changed frequently, and mapping keys to identification details are kept in a secure server to prevent identity leaks. TraceTogether and SafeEntry data are also deleted automatically after 25 days (Government Technology Agency 2020b; Government of Singapore 2021b; Government of Singapore 2021c). For SHN monitoring devices, which cannot perform video and audio recordings and are discarded or returned after SHN, data are not stored on devices, and signals are sent via internal networks to ICA (Immigration and Checkpoints Authority 2021c). Privacy is thus protected by design (Goggin 2020).

There has been relatively little disquiet about the incremental use of digital contact tracing tools, even as the mandatory requirements for TraceTogether at a range of settings effectively limits the movement of individuals who choose to de-register from it (Baharudin 2021b; Government of Singapore 2021d). However, contrary to an initial announcement from the government that data collected from TraceTogether would only be used for contact-tracing purposes, it was revealed in January 2021 that the existing Criminal Procedure Code gives carte blanche to the police to access a wide range of data, not excepting the TraceTogether data which could then be used for criminal investigations. This triggered a public backlash. Some early adopters expressed their discontent by refusing or limiting their use of the digital contact tracing tool (Elangovan and Tan 2021a; Chee 2021b). In response to this, a COVID-19 (Temporary Measures) (Amendment) Bill was passed under a Certificate of Urgency in February 2021 (11 months after the introduction of

TraceTogether, and one month after the revelation (Chee 2021a)) limiting the use of TraceTogether data to investigations for seven categories of serious crimes (Government of Singapore 2021e). This incident reflects the government's continued sensitivity to privacy concerns in technological implementation, and the value placed by the populace on their longstanding relationship of trust with the government. It also serves as an example of an unintended collision of policies, or of a current policy with pre-existing legislation. As with some other countries, laws often do not keep pace with technology, leaving gaps in protections (Privacy International 1998) or points of disconnect between legislation and current practice.

Similarly, TraceTogether and SafeEntry data are not shared by GovTech with private companies, which developed their own contact tracing apps. A separate BluePass token and BlueGate device at construction sites (Tham 2020) was driven by an interest to rapidly detect and isolate emerging clusters and avoid more extensive business disruption. However, while organizations are permitted to collect personal data during emergencies such as the COVID-19 outbreak (Personal Data Protection Commission Singapore 2020), there is limited advice on the governance, concordance, and reconciliation of privately collected data with national data.

The continued success of digital technologies in supporting pandemic management is contingent on the government's abilities to not only access the data but also scope the limits of their collection and use, pre-empt and prevent data breaches, reassure the public, and safeguard the interests of the population. Updated and comprehensive legislation would support this.

12.5.2 What Next?

Even for a society that is relatively accustomed to surrendering private data to the government, TraceTogether's success signifies the ratcheting of state surveillance that has been glossed over in the exigent circumstances of the COVID fight. Some have pointed to the longer term and subtler implications of this trend (Chok 2020; Han 2021a).

The Leader of the Opposition in Parliament supported the Bill to restrict the use of personal contact tracing data for investigations into the most serious of crimes but probed its necessity considering the "abundance" of other law enforcement tools that are already in use for crime detection and securing convictions (Han 2021a). At the same time, despite concerns of mission creep, it has been argued that data access can enable more sophisticated policies such as the tiering of restrictions (instead of blanket curbs) which may paradoxically enable greater freedoms (Asher 2020). As with the emergence of large community-based clusters in May 2021, SMS alerts were sent to individuals who visited COVID-19 hotspots to register for compulsory testing during the Phase 3 (Heightened Alert) period. This enabled targeted monitoring, testing, and social distancing of large numbers of suspect COVID cases, instead of resorting to a nationwide Circuit Breaker where the entire community has to dial back on social mixing to stem community transmissions (Tang 2021). Beyond epidemiological control and criminal investigations, the unprecedented scale of data collection signifies enormous potential for data mining or modeling for urban development and other public policy purposes. It has been pointed out that "greater accountability and debate" about the potential trade-offs and benefits of such digital technologies, relative to traditional strategies, can potentially enable their socially optimal use on a broader scale (Chok 2020; Han 2021a).

12.6 Migrant Worker Dormitories

Singapore's labor market includes a large pool of low-wage migrant workers, facilitating lower-cost solutions and competitiveness in some labor-intensive industries (Phua and Chew 2020.; Teng

2014; Chin 2019; Chen et al. 2021b). As of December 2019, there were 1.43 million foreign workers in Singapore, nearly a quarter of the country's population of 5.7 million then. About 800,000 of this foreign workforce were in low-wage and low-skilled positions, mainly in the construction, marine shipyard, and process sectors and typically coming from developing countries such as India, Bangladesh, and Myanmar, with about 300,000 living in purpose-built dormitories and factory-converted dormitories across the island (Phua and Chew 2020; Government of Singapore 2020c; Government of Singapore 2021f; Neo 2015; Chen et al. 2020).

12.6.1 The Regulatory Regime

These low-wage workers are employed under the work permit regime, a temporary foreign worker programme for unskilled/low-skilled workers under a stratified visa scheme for foreigners working in Singapore. The work permit system involves tighter regulation on recruitment, mobility, and working conditions, as compared to the "employment pass scheme" available to professionals and mid-skilled workers (Ministry of Manpower, Singapore 2021c; Neo 2015). The system places marriage, pregnancy, and permanent residency restrictions that prevent work permit holders from socially integrating with the local population (Ministry of Manpower, Singapore 2021d; Yeoh 2006; Neo 2015). It also operates on a single-employer rule which enables strong employer control over the workers and renders them susceptible to exploitation, founded on their fears of repatriation and confounded by language or cultural barriers which prevent them from seeking redress (Neo 2015; Fillinger et al. 2017).

It has been argued that the "developmentalist philosophy" underlying Singapore's work permit regime gives businesses ease of access to affordable manpower while separating the workers' social interests and the potential "burdens" they may place from the larger Singapore society (Parliament Singapore 2004; Neo 2015; Fillinger et al. 2017). Similarly, pre-COVID, work permit holders are under a different health provision and financing scheme where employers are mandated to provide medical insurance coverage of at least S$15,000 annually for worker inpatient and surgery fees, and bear the costs of their outpatient medical treatment (Ministry of Manpower, Singapore 2021a). This cost burden and the rational motive to keep labor costs low provide a disincentive for employers to help the workers receive care (Yip et al. 2021), and consequently, for the workers to seek care (Lee et al. 2014; Yip et al. 2021). The migrant worker group is also excluded from official statistics on health outcomes as they are considered a transitory population.

Due to the cost of space in Singapore and the natural incentive for employers to turn to cost-saving solutions, migrant workers tend to live in reportedly cramped, unsanitary, and suboptimally ventilated conditions. Some 10–20 workers share one 45–90 square meter room, with at least 80 people sharing one bathroom (Yea 2020). Meals received also tend to be low in cost and nutritionally insufficient (SCMP 2019).

12.6.2 The Dormitory Outbreaks

By early April, there were rising clusters in the community and large outbreaks started to emerge in migrant worker dormitories. When Singapore entered the Circuit Breaker, the dormitory clusters took the government and general populace by surprise despite warnings sounded in some quarters prior (Sadarangani et al. 2017; Abdullah and Kim 2020; SCMP 2020; Yap et al. 2020; Zhang 2020). After the reporting of four dormitory-related cases on 30 March 2020, reported dormitory cases rose rapidly, shifting from double-digit figures to triple ones and reaching over 54,000 cases at over 90% of Singapore's reported cases by the end of the dormitory outbreaks in November 2020 (Ministry of Health, Singapore 2020r; Mcdonald 2021).

Dormitories were progressively circumscribed as isolation areas to prevent transmission in the community (TODAYonline 2020a; Channel News Asia 2020f). The interagency taskforce set up to provide a more dedicated effort to contain the outbreak situation adopted a three-pronged strategy, viz to contain the spread in dormitories, to enforce safe distancing measures on the premises, and to move uninfected workers in essential services to other facilities to minimize further cross-infection (Phua and Ang 2020; gov.sg 2020g). Rapid response teams provided medical support and mass testing services, ensured food distribution, cleanliness, and hygiene at the dormitories (Ministry of Manpower, Singapore 2020b), and instituted measures such as staggering the use of common facilities and stopping the intermixing of workers between blocks (Ministry of Manpower, Singapore 2020c), while facilities were repurposed to serve as isolation and care facilities for patients with mild symptoms or alternative accommodation for uninfected workers (Ministry of Health, Singapore 2020c; Ministry of Manpower, Singapore 2020d). (See Table 12.4 for the movement control/monitoring measures and accompanying legal frameworks for the dormitory-based foreign worker population.)

Progressively, as the outbreak situation was managed and gradually improved, a multilayered and broad-based testing strategy involving serology and RRT was developed to understand the epidemiological spread in dormitories better and systematically permit workers who no longer pose risks of transmission to resume work (Economic Development Board, Enterprise Singapore 2020; Ministry of Manpower, Singapore 2020e; Chen et al. 2021a). Resumption of work was also conditional on informational updates in the Ministry of Manpower's database, acceptance of prevailing testing routines, and the use of TraceTogether and BluePass (Ministry of Manpower, Singapore 2021e; Kurohi 2020; Baharudin 2020b; Ministry of Manpower, Singapore 2020f; Ministry of Manpower, Singapore 2020g; Chen et al. 2021a).

By August 2020, all dormitory-based workers had been tested at least once, and 89% were permitted to resume work. This increased to 98% by November 2020. Since October 2020, the number of new infections detected in the dormitories has remained very low (Ministry of Manpower, Singapore 2020e). More recently, Singapore has been vaccinating migrant workers who have not been previously infected. Migrant workers' vaccination in their home countries are currently not recognised and are pending evaluation from the Ministry of Health (Kok 2021a). As of 31 May 2021, 55,000 (around 20%) of the workers have received both doses of the COVID-19 vaccine, and another 67,000 have received their first dose (Lim and Kok 2021).

Even as the rest of Singapore exited gradually from Circuit Breaker from June 2020, dormitory dwelling migrant workers continue to be mostly confined to the dormitories even a year on. Their movement outside the dormitories remains limited to workplaces and recreational centers demarcated for their use, while movement into the community is restricted to the running of essential errands, subject to employers' approval (Transient Workers Count Too 2020; Ministry of Manpower, Singapore 2020h; Elangovan 2021b).

12.6.3 Reflections

Public health measures instituted at the dormitories since the start of the outbreak in April 2020 till today have met with little overt resistance from the migrant worker population. This is unsurprising considering the power differential defined by pre-existing structures that are set against them.

Notwithstanding the lack of resistance from the said community, as with the practice of quarantine of any population contained in high-density accommodation settings within an outbreak facility (Nakazawa et al. 2020; Pougnet et al. 2020; Yap et al. 2020; Zhang et al. 2020), there were ethical considerations and trade-offs involved in the circumscribing of the dormitories as isolation areas in April 2020, as heightened risks of infection for the workers were weighed against objectives

Table 12.4 Timeline of movement control/monitoring orders and legal frameworks used for dormitory-based migrant worker population.

Date	Movement control/Monitoring measures	Legal frameworks used
	2020	
5–22 Apr	Dormitories with clusters of cases progressively gazetted as isolation areas, eventually totaling 21 gazetted dormitories (TODAYonline 2020a; Channel News Asia 2020f).	Infectious Diseases Act
9 Apr	Distancing measures as part of "dedicated strategy" by Inter-Agency Taskforce, with staff from the government assisting dormitory operators to: • Implement safe distancing measures • Reduce the number of workers in each dorm • Arrange for uninfected workers working in essential services to be temporarily housed separately in other accommodation (Phua and Ang 2020).	Enactment of the COVID-19 (Temporary Measures) (Control Order) Regulations 2020 (7 April 2020)
21 Apr	Daily movement of workers in and out of all dormitories no longer allowed (gov.sg 2020l).	Infectious Diseases (COVID-19 – Stay Orders) Regulations 2020 (Amendment (10 April 2020)) (The Singapore Government 2020e) COVID-19 (Temporary Measures) (Control Order) Regulations 2020 (Amendment (10 and 15 April 2020)) (The Singapore Government 2020f; The Singapore Government 2020g)
20 Apr–4 May	180,000 construction work permit and S pass holders (and their dependents) placed on mandatory SHN (Phua and Ang 2020).	Infectious Diseases (COVID-19 – Stay Orders) Regulations 2020
27 May	The FWMOMCare mobile application launched for migrant workers to self-monitor their health and access telemedicine services. Employers to encourage workers to register to download the application.	Not mandatory (Ministry of Manpower, Singapore 2020m)
9 Jun	Migrant workers cleared of virus and fulfilled requirements permitted to resume work (Baharudin 2020b). Movement to and from dormitories were subject to employers' approval and strictly for medical or emergency purposes (The Singapore Government 2020c).	COVID-19 (Temporary Measures) (Control Order) Regulations 2020 (Amendment (1 Jun 2020)) (The Singapore Government 2020j) Employment of Foreign Manpower (Work Passes) Regulations 2012 (Amendment (1 Jun 2020)) (The Singapore Government 2020c)
19 Jun	All work permit and S Pass holders in the construction, marine shipyard and process sectors, and all dormitory-based workers to download and activate TraceTogether before resumption of work (Wong 2020).	Infectious Diseases Act

(Continued)

Table 12.4 (Continued)

Date	Movement control/Monitoring measures	Legal frameworks used
1 Aug	Workers staying in dormitories, workers in the construction, marine and process sectors, and personnel who go into worksites to undergo PCR RRT every 14 d. This does not apply to recovered workers. Individuals who have not done so will not be allowed to resume work (Ministry of Manpower, Singapore 2020n).	Infectious Diseases Act
1 Aug (in Phase 2)	Workers cleared of COVID-19 infections allowed to run errands outside their dorms during staggered rest days and time slots, and with necessary submission of errands/location details by employers/dormitory operators (Ministry of Manpower, Singapore 2020o).	COVID-19 (Temporary Measures) (Control Order) Regulations 2020 Employment of Foreign Manpower (Work Passes) Regulations 2012
Sep	Several semipermanent Quick Build Dormitories with improved living standards for migrant workers completed (TODAYonline 2020b; gov.sg 2020m). This has: • Reduced density of workers by having no more than 10 beds per room (from 12 to 16 beds), and at least 6 sq.m of living space per resident (from 4.5 sq.m) • Improved hygiene by having an ensuite toilet, sink, and shower for every 5 beds and 15 sick bay beds per 1,000 bed spaces • Improved safe living measures by segregating the dormitory into six clusters that do not intermix More permanent dormitories with better living standards will continue to be built in the next few years.	Not applicable
18 Oct	BluePass tokens (compact, water-resistant, and purpose-built for the dormitory and worksite environment) to facilitate contact tracing distributed to all migrant and local workers living or working in dormitories as well as those in the construction, marine shipyard, and process sectors (Ministry of Manpower, Singapore 2020g).	Infectious Diseases Act
18 Oct–15 Nov	ART piloted for migrant workers as part of RRT. ART given every 7 d, complementing 14 d RRT (Ministry of Manpower, Singapore 2020p).	Infectious Diseases Act
4 Nov	Recovered workers can be exempted from RRT, as well as from quarantine if they are identified as close contacts of COVID-19 cases within 180 d of infection. However, recovered workers with ARI symptoms will be tested for COVID-19 within 90 d of infection (Ministry of Manpower, Singapore 2020q).	Infectious Diseases Act and the Infectious Diseases (COVID-19 – Stay Orders) Regulations 2020

Table 12.4 (Continued)

Date	Movement control/Monitoring measures	Legal frameworks used
28 Dec (Phase 3)	Preparations made to allow workers to visit migrant worker recreational centers more often in a safe and regulated manner (Ministry of Manpower, Singapore 2020e; gov.sg 2020n). Only 50 individuals are allowed at an event each time.	Enactment of the COVID-19 (Temporary Measures) (Foreign Employee Dormitories – Control Order) Regulations 2020 (14 Sep 2020)
	2021	
9 Jan	All workers in the marine sector to undergo RRT every 7 d (Health Promotion Board 2021).	Infectious Diseases Act
8 Mar	Vaccinated migrant workers permitted to undergo RRT at reduced frequency of every 28 d instead of every 14 d (Channel News Asia 2021d).	Infectious Diseases Act
15 Mar	All newly arrived migrant workers from the construction, marine, and process sectors from higher-risk countries/regions to complete SHN, an enhanced medical examination and Settling-In Programme (SIP) at a one-stop pilot Migrant Worker Onboarding Centre (MWOC) at dedicated Quick Build Dormitories (Ministry of Manpower, Singapore 2021b).	Infectious Diseases (COVID-19 – Stay Orders) Regulations 2020
24 Apr	The maximum capacity of approved events in migrant worker recreational centers increased from 50 individuals to 250 individuals, inclusive of staff and performers (The Singapore Government 2021af).	COVID-19 (Temporary Measures) (Foreign Employee Dormitories – Control Order) Regulations 2020 (Amendment (23 Apr 2021)) (The Singapore Government 2021af)
29 Apr	Recovered dormitory workers and migrant workers in the construction, marine, and process sectors no longer exempted from RRT after 270 d post COVID-19 infection (Ministry of Health, Singapore 2021v). Newly arrived migrant workers with a serology positive result (indicating previous infection) will also be enrolled onto the 14 d RRT and have to undergo SHN at a SHN-dedicated facility before an additional testing regime at the MWOC.	Infectious Disease Act and the Infectious Diseases (COVID-19 – Stay Orders) Regulations 2020
16 May	The maximum capacity of approved events in migrant worker recreational centers reduced from 250 individuals to 100 individuals.	COVID-19 (Temporary Measures) (Foreign Employee Dormitories – Control Order) Regulations 2020 (Amendment (15 May 2021)) (The Singapore Government 2021ag)

(Continued)

Table 12.4 (Continued)

Date	Movement control/Monitoring measures	Legal frameworks used
18 May	All visitors to construction sites to undergo RRT of 7 or 14 d frequencies depending on risk levels. This includes vaccinated migrant workers who will no longer be allowed to have longer RRT frequency intervals of 14 or 28 d, respectively (The Singapore Contractors Association Limited 2021; Kok 2021b).	Infectious Disease Act
30 May	Use of ART self-test kits piloted among non-dormitory-based migrant workers working in construction sites, as part of RRT. Frequency of tests to vary, depending on workers' RRT frequency and vaccination status (Sin 2021).	Infectious Disease Act

of preventing disease spread to and maintaining socioeconomic activity in the larger community. While the migrant workers have been described as generally young, displaying mild symptomology, and less likely to suffer severe disease of COVID, studies have pointed to implications of long-term health effects of COVID for them (Fan et al. 2021; Yee et al. 2021). Concerns have also been expressed in some media articles and by NGOs that the prolonged movement restrictions in dormitories are taking a toll on the workers' mental health (Channel News Asia 2020g; Yee et al. 2021).

Concerns include the post-Circuit Breaker amendments to the Employment of Foreign Manpower (Work Passes) Regulations which disproportionately strengthen the legal frameworks they are subject to for COVID measures vis-à-vis other residents. Apart from complying with national baseline restrictions on mask-wearing and social distancing, migrant workers are expected to keep their living spaces clean, practice good personal hygiene and "peaceably" undergo medical examinations. In addition, their movement to and from the dormitories is subject to employers' permission (Kaur-Gill 2020; Transient Workers Count Too 2020; The Singapore Government 2020c; The Singapore Government 2021e; The Singapore Government 2021i). The epidemiological relevance of continued tightened restrictions for the community, considering that 47% of workers in dormitories have been infected with COVID, and herd immunity effects, was also discussed (Ministry of Manpower, Singapore 2020e; Elangovan 2021b). Consciousness of the cost and trade-offs for dormitory-based migrant workers in Singapore's COVID response policy framing has been comparatively more limited, raising concerns from interest groups and parts of society.

The emergence of large outbreaks in the dormitories should not have been unforeseen, considering that the first dormitory COVID case was reported as early as 10 February 2020 (SCMP 2020), there were early warning signs of inadequate medical support for migrant workers (Zhang 2020), and there had been experiences of disease outbreaks among the population group prior (Sadarangani et al. 2017; Abdullah and Kim 2020).

The country's model of political governance that predominantly focuses on economic survival, while driving much of the efficient management of the pandemic curve amidst national functionality needs, had ironically also blindsided the state to the "black elephant" event, preventing pre-emptive "awareness of the cramped and unsanitary living conditions that many foreign workers were made to live in by the employers" (Woo 2020). The dormitories outbreak revealed the vulnerabilities inherent in socioeconomic structures that framed the workers' accommodation and community networks (Chen et al. 2020; Yi et al. 2021), which ironically led to "burdens" the very structures were meant to prevent – a heavy burden of disease and response operations, and severe impairment to economic productivity in related sectors, during the pandemic (Neo 2015; Economic Policy Group Monetary Authority of Singapore 2020; Chen et al. 2021b; Ministry of Trade and Industry 2021). The event signifies the importance of a more integrationist approach for minor or vulnerable populations in public health security.

There have been shifts toward a more inclusive approach since. These include progressive efforts to improve standards of living spaces for migrant workers (Lim 2020c; Sin 2021; Elangovan 2021b), establishment of a more comprehensive medical support system for the population group from August 2020, with longer term plans to set up a primary care ecosystem from July 2021 (Ministry of Manpower, Singapore 2020i; Ministry of Health, Singapore 2020n; Chia and Tan 2021; Kok and Ng 2021), and formation of a multiparty taskforce to enhance mental healthcare support for them (Ministry of Manpower, Singapore 2020j). Beyond this, however, the ongoing calls for more urgent review of the disproportionate burden of restrictions they are facing are a reminder that the "costs" borne by any population group, even when done with resilience and seeming acceptance, should not be taken for granted. These should continually take a central place in the national discourse, and policy framing and deliberation.

12.7 Discussion

Singapore's experience reflects how legislation is but one of the many policy levers available to the government in a public health security crisis, and the value of a trust-motivated and whole-of-society approach (as opposed to a coercive enforcement or adversarial approach), as well as how sensitivity to the felt liberties of the people is central to the efficacy of the country's response.

The need for dramatic, drastic, and sometimes draconian measures to contain the epidemic has placed many governments in quandaries, having to balance their pandemic measures with economic realities, the populace's expected "way of life," and the obverse health consequences of the measures themselves. Options available to governments vary depending on a wide range of constraints and enablers, which can perhaps be simply described in the PESTLE framework (political, economic, sociological, technological, legal, and environmental) often used in business strategic planning.

All six elements can be discerned in the following description of Singapore's policy response to the pandemic. The government's longstanding political dominance, its social contract with the people, and the relatively contained and urban environment of a small city-state enabled legislative responses that curtailed personal freedoms that might be untenable in other communities. The ability to rapidly implement technological applications limited the need for even more restrictive policies. The economic resources of the country also enabled interventional and fiscal measures that mitigated much of the effects of both the outbreak and its restrictions, which in turn sustained the population's general acceptance of the measures taken, including the use of technological applications.

Singapore's unique governance model, constitutionalism, and societal culture enabled the relatively unchallenged implementation of broad-scale movement control orders in its COVID response. The longstanding trust between the people and the government, and a communal philosophy of nation or society before self, facilitated pragmatic social acceptance of greater degrees of trade-offs in personal space for the sake of national security. There was a continuing focus on the compromises and intrusions placed on the conveniences and livelihoods of the larger populace. Despite the widespread powers and discretion accorded to Ministers with the emergency legislation, and the nonconstitutional limitation of certain liberties and rights, sensitivity to such rights remained central in Singapore's approach to policy and enforcement. Community cohesion was reinforced through the experience of the pandemic, and the community generally ridiculed or rebuked transgressors of public health measures, e.g. distancing or masking measures transgressors (Alkhatib 2020; Chua 2021; Toh 2021b).

A wide range of policy tools, including fiscal levers, public education, technological innovation, and diagnostic and biomedical interventions, were deployed and their combinatory use was anticipated and adjusted as the extent and sophistication of capabilities were stepped up or scaled down to conserve resources. This facilitated greater acceptance of trade-offs and enabled greater degrees of freedom and economic functioning in the larger community while maintaining epidemiological control in more defined groups, to sustain a tolerable level of livability and security.

An academic article pointed out that the limitations of constitutional safeguards against violations of rights and abuse of power in Singapore's legislation signify the importance of "the ability and willingness of the people in power to carry themselves as 'honourable men (and women)'" in the system (Lee 2020). The public backlash upon discovering technically legal but initially unrealized potential use of TraceTogether's data for criminal investigations is a stark reminder that the people's trust in the government to do the right thing should not be taken for granted.

More notably, the blindsiding of the government and larger populace to the migrant worker dormitory outbreaks follows on a socioeconomic regulatory regime that has for decades supported the sequestering of migrant workers from the wider society (Neo 2015; Chen et al. 2021b). The dormitories outbreak shows that neat delineation between the interests of minority or vulnerable populations and the larger populace is not possible as their interests are intertwined economically, socially, and physically, and the attempt can lead to broader consequences. While there have been calls for a more inclusive and integrationist approach, the continued subjection of dormitory-based migrant workers to more onerous controls has, however, met relatively little societal unease (Chua and Neo 2021).

As the pandemic progresses, the lessons learnt should not be forgotten. Issues around accountability, transparency, and fundamental human rights and justice and their harmonization with other societal or national aims, such as public security or economic expedience, should not be glossed over. These include the deeper implications of expanding state surveillance capabilities, the epidemiological relevance of a continuing two-tiered system of movement control orders between dormitory-based migrant workers and the larger populace, as well as other foundational questions involving personal liberties amid public objectives as pandemic development and response strategies evolve.

12.8 Conclusion

Singapore's unique model of governance and constitutional culture has made possible a broad-scale and calibrated public health response implementation that was relatively unchallenged. Her experience has also demonstrated technocratic expertise and administrative capability on the part of the government, seen in its orchestrated deployment of multiple policy and infrastructural levers to achieve a delicate balancing of livability, functionality, and epidemiological risk control. While this model may not be easily replicable elsewhere, countries can similarly avail themselves to a wide range of tools, dialing up or down the PESTLE elements as appropriate for their own circumstances, to attain the balance around competing needs while maintaining the standards of ethics and equity as expected by their populations.

Acknowledgements

We would like to thank Lim Su Xin and Loo Min Shuen for their assistance in the search and collation of relevant content for sections in this chapter, as well as for their hard work in developing the timelines of public health measures and legal frameworks used.

References

Abdullah Z. Home-based food businesses can resume operations from May 12 with strict measures in place. CNA [Internet]. 2020a May 2 [cited 2021 Jul 6]; Available from: https://www.channelnewsasia.com/news/singapore/home-based-food-businesses-restrictions-lifted-may-12-covid-19-12696528

Abdullah Z. Fast lane, green lane, air travel bubble: What you need to know about Singapore's COVID-19 travel measures. CNA [Internet]. 2020b Oct 13 [cited 2021 Jul 6]; Available from: https://www.channelnewsasia.com/news/singapore/singapore-covid-19-fast-lane-green-lane-travel-arrangements-13271974

Abdullah WJ, Kim S. Singapore's responses to the COVID-19 outbreak: a critical assessment. *Am Rev Public Adm.* 2020 Aug;50(6–7):770–6.

Alkhatib S. "Sovereign" woman accused of failing to wear mask in public faces two additional charges. The Straits Times [Internet]. 2020 May 19 [cited 2021 Jul 16]; Available from: https://www.straitstimes.com/singapore/courts-crime/sovereign-woman-accused-of-failing-to-wear-mask-in-public-faces-two

Alkhatib S. Jail for housewife from Safra Jurong Covid-19 cluster who did not disclose meetings with male friend, Courts & Crime News & Top Stories. The Straits Times [Internet]. 2021 May 3 [cited 2021 Aug 7]; Available from: https://www.straitstimes.com/singapore/courts-crime/jail-for-housewife-with-covid-19-who-failed-to-disclose-meetings-with-male

Ang J. Coronavirus: Assemblies, large group activities in S'pore schools to be suspended. The Straits Times [Internet]. 2020a Feb 5 [cited 2021 Jul 14]; Available from: https://www.straitstimes.com/singapore/coronavirus-assemblies-and-other-large-group-activities-in-schools-and-pre-schools-to-be

Ang B. A-Z inventions of Covid-19: TraceTogether and SafeEntry programmes. The Straits Times [Internet]. 2020b Dec 20 [cited 2021 May 3]; Available from: https://www.straitstimes.com/life/tracetogether-and-safeentry-programmes

Ang Q. TraceTogether token or app mandatory at malls, workplaces, schools from June 1, Singapore News & Top Stories – The Straits Times. The Straits Times [Internet]. 2021a Apr 22 [cited 2021 Jul 6]; Available from: https://www.straitstimes.com/singapore/mandatory-use-of-tracetogether-token-or-app-for-checking-in-at-malls-workplaces-schools-to

Ang HM. COVID-19: Singapore to stop entry for all long-term pass holders, short-term visitors with recent travel history to India. CNA [Internet]. 2021b Apr 22 [cited 2021 Jul 16]; Available from: https://www.channelnewsasia.com/news/singapore/covid-19-travel-history-to-india-cannot-enter-singapore-14672986

Ang HM. Children aged 12 to 15 to receive Pfizer-BioNTech COVID-19 vaccine in Singapore. CNA [Internet]. 2021c May 18 [cited 2021 Jul 9]; Available from: https://www.channelnewsasia.com/news/singapore/covid-19-pfizer-biontech-vaccine-children-singapore-12-15-14833074

Ang HM. New SafeEntry Gateways to be set up at malls, cinemas, supermarkets and more public places. CNA [Internet]. 2021d Mar 16 [cited 2021 Jul 15]; Available from: https://www.channelnewsasia.com/news/singapore/safeentry-gateways-deployed-malls-cinemas-supermarkets-14418004

Asher S. TraceTogether: Singapore turns to wearable contact-tracing Covid tech. BBC News [Internet]. 2020 Jul 4 [cited 2021 Aug 7]; Available from: https://www.bbc.com/news/technology-53146360

Awang N. PM Lee receives Covid-19 vaccine, says it's 'painless, effective and important'. TODAYonline [Internet]. 2021 Jan 8 [cited 2021 Jul 16]; Available from: https://www.todayonline.com/singapore/pm-lee-receives-covid-19-vaccine-says-its-painless-effective-and-important

Baharudin H. Distribution of TraceTogether tokens starts; aim is for 70% participation in contact tracing scheme [Internet]. The Straits Times. 2020a [cited 2021 Jul 15]; Available from: https://www.straitstimes.com/singapore/government-aiming-for-70-participation-in-tracetogether-programme-says-vivian-on-first-day

Baharudin H. 5,500 migrant workers from 40 dorms approved to resume work in Singapore. The Straits Times [Internet]. 2020b Jun 10 [cited 2021 Jul 14]; Available from: https://www.straitstimes.com/singapore/5500-migrant-workers-from-40-dorms-approved-to-resume-work-here

Baharudin H. Coronavirus: Contact tracing app update fixes battery drain in iPhones. The Straits Times [Internet]. 2020c Jul 7 [cited 2021 Aug 7]; Available from: https://www.straitstimes.com/singapore/contact-tracing-app-update-fixes-battery-drain-in-iphones

Baharudin H. More than 1,100 users have deregistered from TraceTogether: Vivian. The Straits Times [Internet]. 2021a May 11 [cited 2021 Aug 7]; Available from: https://www.straitstimes.com/singapore/more-than-1100-users-have-deregistered-from-tracetogether-vivian

Baharudin H. 1,155 have asked to opt out of TraceTogether programme. The Straits Times [Internet]. 2021b May 12 [cited 2021 Aug 7]; Available from: https://www.straitstimes.com/singapore/1155-have-asked-to-opt-out-of-tracetogether-programme

Baharudin H, Yee YW. Coronavirus: 25% of TraceTogether users update app to latest version. The Straits Times [Internet]. 2020 Jun 10 [cited 2021 Aug 7]; Available from: https://www.straitstimes.com/tech/25-of-tracetogether-users-update-app-to-latest-version

Baker JA. COVID-19 temporary measures: Gatherings outside of school and work limited to 10 people, entertainment venues to close. CNA [Internet]. 2020a Mar 24 [cited 2021 Jul 14]; Available from: https://www.channelnewsasia.com/news/singapore/covid-19-bars-cinemas-entertainment-venues-closed-gatherings-12571538

Baker JA. Singapore to start gradual easing of circuit breaker measures as COVID-19 community cases decline. CNA [Internet]. 2020b May 2 [cited 2021 Jul 14]; Available from: https://www.channelnewsasia.com/news/singapore/covid19-some-businesses-to-resume-from-may-5-12696134

Baker JA. People fully vaccinated under national programme may be able to gather in groups of 8 from end-July. CNA [Internet]. 2021 Jul 7 [cited 2021 Jul 9]; Available from: https://www.channelnewsasia.com/news/singapore/covid-19-fully-vaccinated-differentiated-measures-group-size-8-15172038

Baker JA, Ang HM. COVID-19: From Jul 1, patients aged 13 and above with acute respiratory infection to undergo testing once they visit a doctor. Channel News Asia [Internet]. 2020 Jun 25 [cited 2021 Jul 16]; Available from: https://www.channelnewsasia.com/news/singapore/covid-19-patients-13-above-testing-acute-respiratory-infection-12870046

Bloomberg. Singapore Has a S$100 Billion Plan for Adapting to Climate Change – Bloomberg [Internet]. 2020 [cited 2021 May 8]. Available from: https://www.bloomberg.com/news/features/2020-02-25/singapore-has-a-100-billion-plan-for-adapting-to-climate-change

Chan SK. Judicial review – from angst to empathy. *Singap Acad Law J [Internet].* 2010 Sep [cited 2021 Jun 23]; Available from: https://search.informit.org/doi/abs/10.3316/informit.406479249611653

Chang WC, Sivam R-W. Constant vigilance: Heritage values and defensive pessimism in coping with severe acute respiratory syndrome in Singapore. *Asian J Soc Psychol.* 2004;7(1):35–53.

Channel News Asia. PM Lee on COVID-19 situation: At a glance | Video – CNA [Internet]. 2020a [cited 2021 Jul 6]. Available from: https://www.channelnewsasia.com/news/singapore/pm-lee-on-covid-19-situation-at-a-glance-video-12608020

Channel News Asia. 8 stores given warnings for not complying with COVID-19 safe distancing measures. CNA [Internet]. 2020b Apr 7 [cited 2021 Jul 16]; Available from: https://www.channelnewsasia.com/news/singapore/covid19-stores-warnings-compliance-safe-distancing-12617164

Channel News Asia. Health Minister orders POFMA correction directions to States Times Review, Facebook over COVID-19 post. CNA [Internet]. 2020c Feb 14 [cited 2021 Jul 16]; Available from: https://www.channelnewsasia.com/news/singapore/coronavirus-covid19-pofma-states-times-review-facebook-12435898

Channel News Asia. Wuhan virus: POFMA Office issues correction direction to Facebook over posts claiming Woodlands MRT closure. CNA [Internet]. 2020d Jan 28 [cited 2021 Jul 16]; Available from: https://www.channelnewsasia.com/news/singapore/wuhan-virus-moh-pofma-correction-direction-facebook-12361810

Channel News Asia. GE2020: PAP wins with 61.24% of vote; WP claims two GRCs including new Sengkang GRC – CNA. 2020e Jul 11 [cited 2021 Aug 11]; Available from: https://www.channelnewsasia.com/singapore/ge2020-general-election-final-result-pap-wp-952471

Channel News Asia. COVID-19: Two more foreign worker dormitories declared as isolation areas. CNA [Internet]. 2020f Apr 23 [cited 2021 Jul 14]; Available from: https://www.channelnewsasia.com/news/singapore/covid-19-foreign-worker-dormitories-isolation-homestay-changi-12668236

Channel News Asia. COVID-19: No spike in number of migrant worker suicides, says MOM – CNA. Channel News Asia [Internet]. 2020g Apr 20 [cited 2021 Aug 11]; Available from: https://www.channelnewsasia.com/singapore/migrant-workers-mental-health-suicides-covid-19-mom-608621

Channel News Asia. In full: Lawrence Wong's ministerial statement on whole-of-government response to COVID-19. CNA [Internet]. 2021b May 11 [cited 2021 Jul 8]; Available from: https://www.channelnewsasia.com/news/singapore/lawrence-wong-full-ministerial-statement-covid-19-government-14786936

Channel News Asia. Jewel Changi Airport, Terminals 1 and 3 to be closed to public as COVID-19 testing continues. CNA [Internet]. 2021c May 12 [cited 2021 Jul 8]; Available from: https://www.channelnewsasia.com/news/singapore/covid-19-jewel-changi-airport-terminals-1-3-closed-free-test-14795582

Channel News Asia. Singapore to vaccinate migrant workers against COVID-19, starting with 10,000 dormitory residents. CNA [Internet]. 2021d Mar 8 [cited 2021 Jul 14]; Available from: https://www.channelnewsasia.com/news/singapore/covid-19-vaccination-migrant-workers-dormitories-moh-14360202

Charlton E. Singapore crowned world's most open and competitive economy [Internet]. World Economic Forum. 2019 [cited 2021 Jul 13]. Available from: https://www.weforum.org/agenda/2019/10/competitiveness-economy-best-top-first-singapore-secret-consistency/

Chee K. Bill introduced to make clear TraceTogether, SafeEntry data can be used to look into only 7 types of serious crimes. The Straits Times [Internet]. 2021a Feb 1 [cited 2021 Aug 7]; Available from: https://www.straitstimes.com/singapore/proposed-restrictions-to-safeguard-personal-contact-tracing-data-will-override-all-other

Chee K. Vivian Balakrishnan says he "deeply regrets" mistake on TraceTogether data. The Straits Times [Internet]. 2021b Feb 2 [cited 2021 Aug 7]; Available from: https://www.straitstimes.com/singapore/vivian-balakrishnan-says-he-deeply-regrets-mistake-on-tracetogether-data-first-realised-it

Chee K. TraceTogether check-in starts May 17: Can ID cards still be used for SafeEntry? The Straits Times [Internet]. 2021c May 5 [cited 2021 Jul 15]; Available from: https://www.straitstimes.com/

tech/tech-news/askst-can-id-cards-still-be-used-for-safeentry-when-compulsory-tracetogether-check-in

Chen JI-P, Yap JC-H, Hsu LY, Teo YY. COVID-19 and Singapore: from early response to circuit breaker. *Ann Acad Med Singapore.* 2020 Aug 30;49(8):561–72.

Chen JI-P, Ko KC, Mei-li AYL, Yap JC, Lim J. COVID-19 health system response monitor: Singapore [Internet]. World Health Organization. Regional Office for South-East Asia; 2021a [cited 2021 Jun 25]. Available from: https://apps.who.int/iris/handle/10665/341403

Chen JI-P, Teo YY, Yap JC-H. Policy Foundations in Singapore: Resilience in the Face of COVID [Internet]. Saw Swee Hock School of Public Health, National University of Singapore; 2021b. (Research Submission to The Reform for Resilience Call for Evidence). Available from: https://www.r4rx.org/research-submissions

Cheng I. About 25,000 close contacts of COVID-19 cases identified using TraceTogether: Gan Kim Yong. CNA [Internet]. 2020 Nov 2 [cited 2021 May 3]; Available from: https://www.channelnewsasia.com/news/singapore/tracetogether-app-tokens-close-contacts-cases-identified-covid19-13442296

Chew P. Islands and national identity: the metaphors of Singapore. *Int J Sociol Lang.* 2000;143(1):121–37.

Chew HM. Leader of the Opposition: A turning point but also a "double-edged sword", say analysts. Channel News Asia [Internet]. 2020a Jul 29 [cited 2021 Aug 4]; Available from: https://www.channelnewsasia.com/news/singapore/leader-of-opposition-pritam-singh-double-edged-sword-analysts-12972250

Chew HM. With no prospect of reopening, KTV lounge owners say industry has been "forsaken". CNA [Internet]. 2020b Oct 22 [cited 2021 Jul 7]; Available from: https://www.channelnewsasia.com/news/singapore/karaoke-teo-heng-havefun-entertainment-nightlife-shut-covid19-13331426

Chia HX, Tan SY. Commentary: New primary healthcare plan for migrant workers can mitigate risk of disease outbreaks. CNA [Internet]. 2021 Jul 6 [cited 2021 Jul 21]; Available from: https://www.channelnewsasia.com/news/commentary/migrant-workers-covid-19-welfare-healthcare-needs-15158320

Chin C. Precarious work and its complicit network: migrant labour in Singapore. *J Contemp Asia.* 2019 Aug 8;49(4):528–51.

Chok L. The policy black box in Singapore's digital contact tracing strategy [Internet]. LSE Southeast Asia Blog. 2020 [cited 2021 Jul 22]; Available from: https://blogs.lse.ac.uk/seac/2020/09/22/the-policy-black-box-in-singapores-digital-contact-tracing-strategy/

Chong C. Which places are open for travel and what are the rules? The Straits Times [Internet]. 2020 Oct 31 [cited 2021 Jul 6]; Available from: https://www.straitstimes.com/singapore/which-places-are-open-for-travel-and-what-are-the-rules

Chotirmall SH, Wang L-F, Abisheganaden JA. Letter from Singapore: The clinical and research response to COVID-19. Respirol Carlton Vic [Internet]. 2020 [cited 2021 Apr 13]; Available from: https://www.ncbi.nlm.nih.gov/pmc/articles/PMC7461090/

Chua BH. Liberalism Disavowed: Communitarianism and State Capitalism in Singapore [Internet]. Cornell University Press; 2017 [cited 2021 Aug 7]. Available from: https://www.jstor.org/stable/10.7591/j.ctt1zkjz35

Chua N. Woman at MBS tells SDA: "You have no right to ask me to do anything" [Internet]. 2021 [cited 2021 Jul 16]. Available from: https://mothership.sg/2021/05/mbs-woman-sda-badge/

Chua S, Neo JL. COVID-19 as an Opportunity for Democratic Consolidation? [Internet]. Verfassungsblog. 2021 Feb 24 [cited 2021 Jul 8]. Available from: https://verfassungsblog.de/covid-19-as-an-opportunity-for-democratic-consolidation/

CNA. COVID-19: Two to be charged with giving false information to MOH during contact tracing. CNA [Internet]. 2020 Feb 26 [cited 2021 Aug 7]; Available from: https://www.channelnewsasia.com/singapore/covid19-coronavirus-charged-false-info-moh-contact-tracing-780626

Co C. COVID-19: Singapore to distribute improved reusable masks via vending machines, community centres from May 26. CNA [Internet]. 2020a May 21 [cited 2021 Jul 16]; Available from: https://www.channelnewsasia.com/news/singapore/covid-19-coronavirus-where-collect-reusable-mask-improved-12757066

Co C. Households with more than 5 people may book more than 1 table in F&B outlets; more exercise classes in open spaces – CNA. Channel News Asia [Internet]. 2020b Aug 21 [cited 2021 Jul 15]; Available from: https://www.channelnewsasia.com/news/singapore/covid-19-mtf-households-more-than-5-may-book-more-than-1-table-13042178

Co C, Tang SK. Safe distancing rules still a work in progress for some businesses days after announcement. CNA [Internet]. 2020 Mar 22 [cited 2021 Jul 14]; Available from: https://www.channelnewsasia.com/news/singapore/safe-distancing-rules-retailers-cafes-covid-19-coronavirus-12565234

Cook AR. Commentary: Why Singapore's travel restrictions will keep changing for a while more. CNA [Internet]. 2021 Apr 29 [cited 2021 May 8]; Available from: https://www.channelnewsasia.com/news/commentary/singapore-travel-restrictions-india-hong-kong-bubble-latest-14709690

Cook AR, Hsu LY. Commentary: In Singapore's bold plan to reopen, these are the hard-nosed decisions society must make. CNA [Internet]. 2021 Jun 25 [cited 2021 Jul 9]; Available from: https://www.channelnewsasia.com/news/commentary/covid-19-case-cluster-phase-2-3-vaccine-test-quarantine-travel-15082680

Criminal Law (Temporary Provisions) Act (Cap 67, 2000 Rev Ed Sing) [CLTPA].

Crotty F, Watson R, Lim WK. Nursing homes: the titanic of cruise ships – will residential aged care facilities survive the COVID-19 pandemic? *Intern Med J.* 2020 Sep;50(9):1033–6.

Dan YY, Tambyah PA, Sim J, Lim J, Hsu LY, Chow WL, et al. Cost-effectiveness analysis of hospital infection control response to an epidemic respiratory virus threat. *Emerg Infect Dis.* 2009 Dec;15(12):1909–16.

Department of Statistics, Singapore. Latest Data [Internet]. Base. 2021a [cited 2021 Jul 13]. Available from: http://www.singstat.gov.sg/whats-new/latest-data

Department of Statistics Singapore. InfoComm and Media – Latest Data [Internet]. InfoComm and Media. 2021b [cited 2021 Aug 7]. Available from: http://www.singstat.gov.sg/find-data/search-by-theme/industry/infocomm-and-media/latest-data

eca International. Singapore named the most liveable location in the world for 15th year in a row [Internet]. 2021 [cited 2021 Jul 10]. Available from: https://www.eca-international.com/News/January-2021/Singapore-named-the-most-liveable-location-in-the

Economic Development Board. Singapore's Solidarity Budget for workers and businesses affected by COVID-19 [Internet]. 2020a [cited 2021 Jul 5]. Available from: https://www.edb.gov.sg/content/dam/edb-en/insights/headquarters/singapore-budget-2020-covid-19-relief-measures-for-singaporeans-and-businesses--/EDB_SG%20Solidarity%20Budget%20(Final).pdf

Economic Development Board. EDB_SG Fortitude Budget_Summary Infographic.pdf [Internet]. 2020b [cited 2021 Jul 6]. Available from: https://www.edb.gov.sg/content/dam/edb-en/insights/headquarters/singapore-budget-2020-covid-19-relief-measures-for-singaporeans-and-businesses--/EDB_SG%20Fortitude%20Budget_Summary%20Infographic.pdf

Economic Development Board, Enterprise Singapore. Advisory For Rostered Routine Testing For The Marine & Offshore Sector [Internet]. 2020 [cited 2021 Jul 6]; Available from: https://covid.gobusiness.gov.sg/guides/AdvisoryRRTfornonMO.pdf

Economic Policy Group Monetary Authority of Singapore. Macroeconomic Review [Internet]. 2020 Oct [cited 2021 Apr 14]. Available from: https://www.mas.gov.sg/monetary-policy/MAS-Macroeconomic-Review

Economic Policy Group Monetary Authority of Singapore. Macroeconomic Review [Internet]. 2020 Oct [cited 2021 Apr 14]; Available from: https://www.mas.gov.sg/monetary-policy/MAS-Macroeconomic-Review

Elangovan N. Covid-19: Jail, fine for those who leave home while on five-day MC, doctors say tougher stance is needed. TODAYonline [Internet]. 2020 Mar 27 [cited 2021 Jul 14]; Available from: https://www.todayonline.com/singapore/jail-fine-those-who-leave-home-while-five-day-mc-doctors-say-tougher-stance-needed

Elangovan N. The Big Read: A year after the first COVID-19 outbreak in dorms, how has life changed for foreign workers? CNA [Internet]. 2021b Mar 29 [cited 2021 Jul 22]; Available from: https://www.channelnewsasia.com/news/singapore/the-big-read-covid-19-outbreak-dormitories-foreign-workers-14504974

Elangovan N, Tan YL. Some TraceTogether users upset with Govt's revelation on police access to data, say they'll use it less – TODAY. 2021a Jan 7 [cited 2021 Aug 7]; Available from: https://www.todayonline.com/singapore/some-tracetogether-users-upset-govts-revelation-police-access-data-say-theyll-use-it-less

Enterprise Singapore. Guide on business continuity planning for 2019 novel coronavirus [Internet]. 2020 [cited 2021 Jul 14]. Available from: https://www.enterprisesg.gov.sg/covid-19

Fan BE, Umapathi T, Chua K, Chia YW, Wong SW, Tan GWL, et al. Delayed catastrophic thrombotic events in young and asymptomatic post COVID-19 patients. *J Thromb Thrombolysis.* 2021 May 1;51(4):971–7.

Fillinger T, Harrigan N, Chok S, Amirrudin A, Meyer P, Rajah M, et al. Labour protection for the vulnerable: An evaluation of the salary and injury claims system for migrant workers in Singapore. 2017 p. 124. (Research Collection School of Social Sciences).

Friedrich CJ. *Limited Government: A Comparison.* Englewood Cliffs, N.J.: Prentice-Hall; 1974.

Gan KY, Wong L, Ong YK. Living normally, with Covid-19: Task force ministers on how S'pore is drawing road map for new normal. The Straits Times [Internet]. 2021 Jun 24 [cited 2021 Jul 9]; Available from: https://www.straitstimes.com/opinion/living-normally-with-covid-19

Giffard, H.S. *Halsbury's Laws of Singapore.* Vol. 1. Butterworths Asia; 1999.

Gill SS, Swah S, Sook Lin & Bok LLP. Legal systems in Singapore: overview [Internet]. Practical Law. 2021 [cited 2021 Jul 10]. Available from: http://uk.practicallaw.thomsonreuters.com/w-008-9647?transitionType=Default&contextData=(sc.Default)&firstPage=true

Goggin G. COVID-19 apps in Singapore and Australia: reimagining healthy nations with digital technology. *Media Int Aust.* 2020 Nov;177(1):61–75.

Goh T. Wuhan virus: First Singaporean case confirmed; she was on Scoot flight from Wuhan. The Straits Times [Internet]. 2020a Jan 31 [cited 2021 Jul 10]; Available from: https://www.straitstimes.com/singapore/health/wuhan-virus-first-singaporean-confirmed-to-have-virus-she-was-on-scoot-flight-from

Goh T. Coronavirus: More patients with respiratory symptoms at PHPCs, but some afraid 5-day MC will affect income, Health News & Top Stories – The Straits Times. The Straits Times [Internet]. 2020b Feb 24 [cited 2021 Jul 6]; Available from: https://www.straitstimes.com/singapore/health/more-patients-with-respiratory-symptoms-at-phpcs-but-some-afraid-5-day-mc-will

Goh YH. Singapore residents who continue to travel abroad will pay full hospital charges if warded for coronavirus. The Straits Times [Internet]. 2020c Mar 24 [cited 2021 Jul 7]; Available from: https://www.straitstimes.com/singapore/singapore-residents-who-continue-to-travel-will-pay-full-hospital-charges-if-warded-for

Goh YH. Limited visits to parents or grandparents to be allowed from June 2 after circuit breaker. The Straits Times [Internet]. 2020d May 19 [cited 2021 Jul 6]; Available from: https://www.straitstimes.com/singapore/limited-visits-to-parents-or-grandparents-to-be-allowed-from-june-2-seniors-urged-to-stay

Goh T. Singapore's phase 3 will go ahead if 3 conditions met, including having 70% TraceTogether take-up rate. The Straits Times [Internet]. 2020e Nov 10 [cited 2021 Jul 6]; Available from: https://www.straitstimes.com/singapore/health/phase-3-will-go-ahead-if-3-conditions-are-met-including-achieving-70-per-cent

Goh T. Approved private clinics now offer PCR tests to anyone. The Straits Times [Internet]. 2020f Dec 1 [cited 2021 Jul 6]; Available from: https://www.straitstimes.com/singapore/health/approved-private-clinics-now-offer-pcr-tests-to-anyone

gov.sg. What are the racial proportions among Singapore citizens? [Internet]. 2019 [cited 2021 Jul 13]. Available from: http://www.gov.sg/article/what-are-the-racial-proportions-among-singapore-citizens

gov.sg. Everything you need to know about Stay-Home Notice [Internet]. 2020a [cited 2021 Jul 14]. Available from: http://www.gov.sg/article/everything-you-need-to-know-about-the-stay-home-notice

gov.sg. What's the difference between a Leave of Absence and a Quarantine Order? [Internet]. 2020b [cited 2021 Jul 14]. Available from: http://www.gov.sg/article/whats-the-difference-between-a-leave-of-absence-and-a-quarantine-order

gov.sg. Mask Go Where [Internet]. 2020c [cited 2021 Jul 16]. Available from: https://mask.gowhere.gov.sg/

gov.sg. Moving into phase 2: What activities can resume [Internet]. 2020d [cited 2021 Jul 5]. Available from: http://www.gov.sg/article/moving-into-phase-2-what-activities-can-resume

gov.sg. Further steps towards a new COVID normal [Internet]. 2020e [cited 2021 Jul 7]. Available from: http://www.gov.sg/article/further-steps-towards-a-new-covid-normal

gov.sg. gov.sg | How Singapore is ensuring access to COVID-19 vaccines [Internet]. 2020f [cited 2021 Jul 16]; Available from: https://www.gov.sg/article/how-singapore-is-ensuring-access-to-covid-19-vaccines

gov.sg. Containing COVID-19 spread at foreign worker dormitories [Internet]. 2020g [cited 2021 Jul 22]; Available from: http://www.gov.sg/article/containing-covid-19-spread-at-foreign-worker-dormitories

gov.sg. COVID-19: Advisories for Various Sectors [Internet]. 2020h [cited 2021 Jul 27]; Available from: http://www.gov.sg/article/covid-19-sector-specific-advisories

gov.sg. What you can and cannot do during the circuit breaker period [Internet]. 2020i [cited 2021 Jul 14]; Available from: http://www.gov.sg/article/what-you-can-and-cannot-do-during-the-circuit-breaker-period

gov.sg. Circuit Breaker extension and tighter measures: What you need to know [Internet]. 2020j [cited 2021 Jul 14]; Available from: http://www.gov.sg/article/circuit-breaker-extension-and-tighter-measures-what-you-need-to-know

gov.sg. Digital contact tracing tools required for all businesses and services operating during circuit breaker [Internet]. 2020k [cited 2021 Jul 14]; Available from: http://www.gov.sg/article/digital-contact-tracing-tools-for-all-businesses-operating-during-circuit-breaker

gov.sg. Tackling transmissions in migrant worker clusters [Internet]. 2020l [cited 2021 Jul 14]; Available from: http://www.gov.sg/article/tackling-transmissions-in-migrant-worker-clusters

gov.sg. Improved standards of new dormitories for migrant workers [Internet]. 2020m [cited 2021 Jul 14]. Available from: http://www.gov.sg/article/improved-standards-of-new-dormitories-for-migrant-workers

gov.sg. Moving into phase 3 of re-opening on 28 Dec 2020 [Internet]. 2020n [cited 2021 Jul 14]; Available from: http://www.gov.sg/article/moving-into-phase-3-of-re-opening-on-28-dec-2020

gov.sg. Phase Two: Easing of restrictions on key life events [Internet]. 2020o [cited 2021 Jul 15]; Available from: http://www.gov.sg/article/phase-two-easing-of-restrictions-on-key-life-events

gov.sg. Token Go Where – FAQ [Internet]. 2020p [cited 2021 Jul 15]; Available from: https://token .gowhere.gov.sg/faq

gov.sg. COVID-19 Resources [Internet]. 2021a [cited 2021 Jul 16]. Available from: http://www.gov.sg/ article/covid-19-resources

gov.sg. Stay vigilant in Phase 2 [Internet]. 2021b [cited 2021 Jul 6]. Available from: http://www.gov.sg/ article/stay-vigilant-in-phase-2

gov.sg. Heightened alert to minimise risk of community spread [Internet]. 2021c [cited 2021 Jul 15]; Available from: http://www.gov.sg/article/heightened-alert-in-the-fight-against-covid-19

gov.sg. Additional restrictions under Phase 2 (Heightened Alert) to minimise transmission [Internet]. 2021d [cited 2021 Jul 15]; Available from: http://www.gov.sg/article/additional-restrictions-under-phase-2--heightened-alert

gov.sg. (Updated 18 Jun 2021) Gradual re-opening to Phase 3 (Heightened Alert) from 14 June 2021 [Internet]. 2021e [cited 2021 Jul 16]; Available from: http://www.gov.sg/article/gradual-re-opening-to-phase-3-heightened-alert-from-12-july

Government of Singapore. Shared values [Internet]. 1991 Jan [cited 2021 Aug 7]. Available from: http://eservice.nlb.gov.sg/item_holding.aspx?bid=5809358

Government of Singapore. SafeEntry – National digital check-in system [Internet]. General. 2020 [cited 2021 Aug 7]. Available from: https://www.safeentry.gov.sg/terms_of_use

Government of Singapore. App Release Notes – TraceTogether [Internet]. TraceTogether FAQs. 2021a [cited 2021 Aug 7]; Available from: https://support.tracetogether.gov.sg/hc/en-sg/articles/ 360046481013-App-Release-Notes

Government of Singapore. How does TraceTogether work? [Internet]. TraceTogether FAQs. 2021b [cited 2021 Aug 7]; Available from: https://support.tracetogether.gov.sg/hc/en-sg/articles/ 360043543473-How-does-TraceTogether-work-

Government of Singapore. Are there data safeguards in place when using SafeEntry? [Internet]. Team SafeEntry. 2021c [cited 2021 Aug 7]; Available from: https://support.safeentry.gov.sg/hc/en-us/ articles/900000702546-Are-there-data-safeguards-in-place-when-using-SafeEntry-

Government of Singapore. How can I de-register from the TraceTogether Programme? [Internet]. TraceTogether FAQs. 2021d [cited 2021 Aug 7]; Available from: https://support.tracetogether.gov.sg/ hc/en-sg/articles/360043735713-How-can-I-de-register-from-the-TraceTogether-Programme-

Government of Singapore. Amendments In Covid-19 (Temporary Measures) Act On The Use Of Personal Digital Contact Tracing Data [Internet]. 2021e Feb [cited 2021 Aug 7]; Available from: https://www.smartnation.gov.sg/whats-new/press-releases/amendments-in-covid-19-temporary-measures-act--on-the-use-of-personal-digital-contact-tracing-data

Government of Singapore. Foreign workforce numbers [Internet]. Ministry of Manpower. 2021f [cited 2021 Apr 19]; Available from: https://www.mom.gov.sg/documents-and-publications/foreign-workforce-numbers

Government Technology Agency. Two reasons why Singapore is sticking with TraceTogether's protocol [Internet]. 2020a [cited 2021 Aug 7]; Available from: https://www.tech.gov.sg/media/technews/two-reasons-why-singapore-sticking-with-tracetogether-protocol

Government Technology Agency. 9 geeky myth-busting facts you need to know about TraceTogether [Internet]. 2020b [cited 2021 Aug 7]; Available from: https://www.tech.gov.sg/media/technews/ geeky-myth-busting-facts-you-need-to-know-about-tracetogether

Government of Singapore. Ministerial Statement by Mrs Josephine Teo, Minister for Manpower, 4 May 2020 [Internet]. Ministry of Manpower. 2020c [cited 2021 Apr 19]; Available from: https://www .mom.gov.sg/newsroom/parliament-questions-and-replies/2020/0504-ministerial-statement-by-mrs-josephine-teo-minister-for-manpower-4-may-2020

GovTech (Government Technology Agency of Singapore). Your TraceTogether app works in the background now! [Internet]. 2020 [cited 2021 Aug 7]; Available from: https://www.facebook.com/GovTechSG/photos/a.411947277510/10157076929317511

Han K. COVID app triggers overdue debate on privacy in Singapore | Civil Rights News | Al Jazeera [Internet]. 2021a [cited 2021 Jul 22]; Available from: https://www.aljazeera.com/news/2021/2/10/covid-app-triggers-overdue-debate-on-privacy-in-singapore

Han K. In Singapore, Covid vs privacy is no contest [Internet]. 2021b [cited 2021 Jul 22]; Available from: https://www.lowyinstitute.org/the-interpreter/singapore-covid-vs-privacy-no-contest

Health Promotion Board. Rostered Routine Testing (RRT) [Internet]. Rostered Routine Testing (RRT). 2021 [cited 2021 Jul 14]; Available from: https://www.hpb.gov.sg/rrt

Health Sciences Authority. Monitoring the safety profile of COVID-19 vaccines [Internet]. HSA. 2020 [cited 2021 Jul 16]; Available from: https://www.hsa.gov.sg/announcements/dear-healthcare-professional-letter/monitoring-the-safety-profile-of-covid-19-vaccines

Heng M. Coronavirus: 8 establishments warned for non-compliance with safe distancing measures. The Straits Times [Internet]. 2020 Apr 7 [cited 2021 Jul 12]; Available from: https://www.straitstimes .com/singapore/coronavirus-8-establishments-warned-for-non-compliance-with-safe-distancing-measures

Homer. Stay home, stay safe with Homer [Internet]. Homer. 2020 [cited 2021 Aug 7]. Available from: https://homer.gov.sg/

Hong J. Singapore Is Now the World's Best Place to Be During Covid. Bloomberg.com [Internet]. 2021 Apr 27 [cited 2021 Jul 10]; Available from: https://www.bloomberg.com/news/newsletters/2021-04-27/singapore-is-now-the-world-s-best-place-to-be-during-covid

Huang Z, Guo H, Lee Y-M, Ho EC, Ang H, Chow A. Performance of digital contact tracing tools for COVID-19 response in Singapore: cross-sectional study. *JMIR MHealth UHealth*. 2020 Oct 29;8(10):e23148.

Huang Z, Guo H, Lim HY, Chow A. Awareness, acceptance, and adoption of the national digital contact tracing tool post COVID-19 lockdown among visitors to a public hospital in Singapore. *Clin Microbiol Infect Off Publ Eur Soc Clin Microbiol Infect Dis.* 2021 Jul;27(7):1046–8.

Huff WG. The developmental state, government, and Singapore's economic development since 1960. *World Dev.* 1995 Aug 1;23(8):1421–38.

Hussain Z. GE2020 results signal a return to the norm, or start of a new normal? The Straits Times [Internet]. 2020 Jul 19 [cited 2021 Aug 4]; Available from: https://www.straitstimes.com/politics/a-return-to-the-norm-or-start-of-a-new-normal

Immigration & Checkpoints Authority. Stay Home Notice (SHN) [Internet]. 2020 [cited 2021 Jul 14]; Available from: https://safetravel.ica.gov.sg/health/shn

Immigration & Checkpoints Authority. Overview [Internet]. 2021a [cited 2021 Jul 6]; Available from: https://safetravel.ica.gov.sg/rgl/overview

Immigration & Checkpoints Authority. Travelling to Singapore [Internet]. 2021b [cited 2021 Jul 6]; Available from: https://safetravel.ica.gov.sg/arriving/overview

Immigration & Checkpoints Authority. SHN Electronic Monitoring Device [Internet]. 2021c [cited 2021 Aug 7]. Available from: https://safetravel.ica.gov.sg/health/shn-monitoring

Internal Security Act (Cap 143, 1985 Rev Ed) [ISA].

Inter-Religious Oranisation Singapore. Interfaith Leaders Support Efforts By Religious Communities to Deal with COVID-19 Situation – Inter-Religious Organisation, Singapore [Internet]. 2021 [cited 2021

Jul 16]. Available from: https://iro.sg/press-release/interfaith-leaders-support-efforts-by-religious-communities-to-deal-with-covid-19-situation-2/

IRO. Inter-Religious Organisation, Singapore [Internet]. 2021 [cited 2021 Aug 11]. Available from: https://iro.sg/

Iskandar H, Rosli TM. Coronavirus: Large group activities in schools suspended. The New Paper [Internet]. 2020 Feb 5 [cited 2021 Jul 14]; Available from: https://www.tnp.sg/news/singapore/coronavirus-large-group-activities-schools-suspended

Kamil A. Health Minister asks Pofma office to issue correction direction to States Times Review over Covid-19 post – TODAY. TODAYonline [Internet]. 2020 Feb 14 [cited 2021 Jul 16]; Available from: https://www.todayonline.com/singapore/health-minister-asks-pofma-office-issue-correction-direction-states-times-review-over

Kamil A. Covid-19: Cinemas to reopen from July 13 after being closed since late March – TODAY. Today Online [Internet]. 2020 Jul 3 [cited 2021 Jul 15]; Available from: https://www.todayonline.com/singapore/covid-19-cinemas-reopen-july-13-after-being-closed-late-march

Kanagaratnam K. Singapore: the national family planning program. *Stud Fam Plann.* 1968;1(28):1–11.

Kaur-Gill S. The COVID-19 Pandemic and Outbreak Inequality: Mainstream Reporting of Singapore's Migrant Workers in the Margins. Front Commun [Internet]. 2020 [cited 2021 Aug 11];0. Available from: https://www.frontiersin.org/articles/10.3389/fcomm.2020.00065/full

Khalik S. Wuhan virus: $100 a day for those quarantined; severe penalties for people who flout quarantine orders. The Straits Times [Internet]. 2020 Jan 28 [cited 2021 Jul 16]; Available from: https://www.straitstimes.com/singapore/health/100-a-day-for-those-quarantined-severe-penalties-for-people-who-flout-quarantine

Khalik S. Unlike large resource-rich countries, Singapore cannot afford to close its borders for long: Lawrence Wong. The Straits Times [Internet]. 2021 May 4 [cited 2021 Jul 9]; Available from: https://www.straitstimes.com/singapore/health/unlike-large-resource-rich-countries-singapore-cannot-afford-to-close-its-borders

Koh F. Collection exercise for reusable masks kicks off in latest step in coronavirus battle. The Straits Times [Internet]. 2020 Apr 5 [cited 2021 Jul 16]; Available from: https://www.straitstimes.com/singapore/collection-exercise-for-reusable-masks-kicks-off-in-latest-step-in-coronavirus-battle

Kok Y. 30,000 migrant workers across 30 dorms to get Covid-19 jabs as next phase of vaccination drive begins, Singapore News & Top Stories – The Straits Times. The Straits Times [Internet]. 2021a Mar 26 [cited 2021 Aug 11]; Available from: https://www.straitstimes.com/singapore/30000-migrant-workers-across-30-dorms-to-get-covid-19-jabs-as-next-phase-of-inoculation

Kok Y. All visitors to construction sites must undergo routine Covid-19 testing: BCA. The Straits Times [Internet]. 2021b May 18 [cited 2021 Jul 14]; Available from: https://www.straitstimes.com/singapore/all-visitors-to-construction-sites-here-must-undergo-routine-covid-19-testing-bca

Kok Y, Ng KG. New healthcare system to be set up for migrant workers in S'pore; 6 medical centres planned. The Straits Times [Internet]. 2021 Jun 30 [cited 2021 Jul 21]; Available from: https://www.straitstimes.com/singapore/health/new-healthcare-system-to-be-set-up-for-migrant-workers-in-spore-6-medical-centres

Kretzschmar ME, Rozhnova G, Bootsma MCJ, Boven M van, Wijgert JHHM van de, Bonten MJM. Impact of delays on effectiveness of contact tracing strategies for COVID-19: a modelling study. *Lancet Public Health.* 2020 Aug 1;5(8):e452–9.

Krishnadas D. BCA's ban on exercise and dog-walking in condominiums makes no sense [Internet]. TODAYonline. 2020 [cited 2021 Jul 14]. Available from: https://www.todayonline.com/voices/bcas-ban-exercise-and-dog-walking-condominiums-makes-no-sense

Kuguyo O, Kengne AP, Dandara C. Singapore COVID-19 pandemic response as a successful model framework for low-resource health care settings in Africa? *Omics J Integr Biol.* 2020 Aug;24(8):470–8.

Kurohi R. Coronavirus: MOM outlines new measures for workers resuming work after June 1, including staggered rest days in Phase 2 of reopening. The Straits Times [Internet]. 2020 May 30 [cited 2021 Jul 22]; Available from: https://www.straitstimes.com/singapore/manpower/coronavirus-mom-outlines-new-measures-for-workers-resuming-work-after-june-1

Lai L. Coronavirus: Docs to give 5-day medical leave to patients with respiratory symptoms; subsidised rates for S'poreans at designated clinics. The Straits Times [Internet]. 2020 Feb 14 [cited 2021 Jul 6]; Available from: https://www.straitstimes.com/singapore/health/coronavirus-docs-to-give-5-day-medical-leave-to-patients-with-respiratory-symptoms

Lai L. No dining in, social gatherings capped at 2 people from May 16 as S'pore tightens Covid-19 rules. The Straits Times [Internet]. 2021a May 15 [cited 2021 Jul 8]; Available from: https://www.straitstimes.com/singapore/health/no-dining-in-social-gatherings-capped-at-2-people-from-may-16-as-spore-tightens

Lai L. S'pore delays 2nd Covid-19 vaccine dose to 6–8 weeks later; those aged 40-44 can register for jabs from Wednesday. The Straits Times [Internet]. 2021b May 18 [cited 2021 Jul 9]; Available from: https://www.straitstimes.com/singapore/spore-delays-2nd-vaccine-dose-to-6-8-weeks-later-those-aged-40-44-can-register-for-jabs

Lam L. China couple charged under Infectious Diseases Act for obstructing COVID-19 containment work. CNA [Internet]. 2020a Feb 28 [cited 2021 Jul 16]; Available from: https://www.channelnewsasia.com/news/singapore/covid19-coronavirus-china-couple-charged-infectious-diseases-act-12480170

Lam L. Jail for man who breached stay-home notice to eat bak kut teh at hawker centre, run errands – CNA. Channel News Asia [Internet]. 2020b Apr 23 [cited 2021 Jul 16]; Available from: https://www.channelnewsasia.com/news/singapore/covid-19-breach-stay-home-notice-bak-kut-teh-jail-12668182

Lam L. Woman who made "sovereign" remark, refused to wear mask gets jail and fine. CNA [Internet]. 2021 May 7 [cited 2021 Aug 11]; Available from: https://www.channelnewsasia.com/singapore/woman-sovereign-remark-refuse-mask-shunfu-market-jail-fine-1347696

Lee D. Covid-19 in Singapore: "Responsive communitarianism" and the legislative approach to the 'most serious crisis' since independence. *Singap J Leg Stud [Internet]*. 2020 Jan [cited 2021 Jun 23]; Available from: https://search.informit.org/doi/abs/10.3316/informit.622713918075496

Lee W, Neo A, Tan S, Cook AR, Wong ML, Tan J, et al. Health-seeking behaviour of male foreign migrant workers living in a dormitory in Singapore. *BMC Health Serv Res*. 2014 Jul 10;14:300.

Lim J. SINGAPORE'S EXPERIENCE- COVID-19 | LinkedIn [Internet]. 2020a [cited 2021 Aug 12]. Available from: https://www.linkedin.com/pulse/singapores-experience-covid-19-jeremy-lim/

Lim J. Coronavirus: More doctors attending to patients through video call, Health News & Top Stories – The Straits Times. The Straits Times [Internet]. 2020b May 4 [cited 2021 Jul 16]; Available from: https://www.straitstimes.com/singapore/health/more-doctors-attending-to-patients-through-video-call

Lim YL. Lessons from high-density dorms spark new approach, Singapore News & Top Stories – The Straits Times. The Straits Times [Internet]. 2020c Aug 3 [cited 2021 Aug 11]; Available from: https://www.straitstimes.com/singapore/lessons-from-high-density-dorms-spark-new-approach

Lim MZ, Goh YH. Coronavirus: Govt agencies to suspend activities for seniors for 14 days to cut risk of transmission. The Straits Times [Internet]. 2020 Mar 10 [cited 2021 Jul 14]; Available from: https://www.straitstimes.com/singapore/health/govt-agencies-to-suspend-activities-for-seniors-for-14-days-starting-march-11-to

Lim MZ, Kok Y. One in five migrant workers in dorms fully vaccinated against Covid-19: MOM, Singapore News & Top Stories – The Straits Times. The Straits Times [Internet]. 2021 Jun 8 [cited

2021 Aug 11]; Available from: https://www.straitstimes.com/singapore/one-in-five-of-migrant-workers-in-dorms-fully-vaccinated-against-covid-19-mom

Lin S. Commentary: Some pain even as Singapore rises to the challenge of tighter COVID-19 measures. CNA [Internet]. 2021 May 18 [cited 2021 Jul 8]; Available from: https://www.channelnewsasia.com/news/commentary/rules-tightened-singapore-circuit-breaker-covid-19-fatigue-14831062

Liow ED. The neoliberal-developmental state: Singapore as case study. *Crit Sociol.* 2012 Mar 1;38(2):241–64.

Low Z. TraceTogether-only SafeEntry required from Jun 1 at all higher-risk venues. CNA [Internet]. 2021a Apr 22 [cited 2021 Aug 7]; Available from: https://www.channelnewsasia.com/singapore/tracetogether-safeentry-malls-workplace-jun-1-app-token-covid-19-236826

Low Z. Mandatory TraceTogether-only SafeEntry brought forward to May 17. CNA [Internet]. 2021b May 4 [cited 2021 Aug 7]; Available from: https://www.channelnewsasia.com/singapore/covid19-tracetogether-safeentry-may-17-brought-forward-token-app-1358126

Low Z. Man seen without mask on train charged with failing to wear mask outside State Courts. CNA [Internet]. 2021c Jul 20 [cited 2021 Aug 11]; Available from: https://www.channelnewsasia.com/singapore/covid-19-benjamin-glynn-train-no-mask-outside-state-courts-2046101

Lum LH, Badaruddin H, Salmon S, Cutter J, Lim AY, Fisher D. Pandemic preparedness: nationally-led simulation to test hospital systems. *Ann Acad Med Singapore.* 2016;45(8):6.

Mahmud AH. Singaporeans aged 12 to 39 can register for COVID-19 vaccination from Jun 11. CNA [Internet]. 2021 Jun 10 [cited 2021 Jul 9]; Available from: https://www.channelnewsasia.com/news/singapore/covid-19-vaccination-age-12-to-39-recovered-single-dose-14986126

Mahmud AH, Yong M. What we know about the locally transmitted coronavirus cases in Singapore. CNA [Internet]. 2020 Feb 4 [cited 2021 Jul 10]; Available from: https://www.channelnewsasia.com/news/singapore/wuhan-coronavirus-singapore-virus-new-cases-local-transmission-12390118

Majlis Ugama Islam Singapura. Media Statement on Temporary Closure of Mosques and Suspension of Mosque Activities [Internet]. 2020 [cited 2021 Jul 16]. Available from: https://www.muis.gov.sg/Media/Media-Releases/12-Mar-20-Media-Statement-on-Temporary-Closure-of-Mosques

Mathews M, Zainuddin S. Commentary: Worries over rising COVID-19 cases are fuelling racially charged comments. CNA [Internet]. 2021 May 2 [cited 2021 Jul 9]; Available from: https://www.channelnewsasia.com/news/commentary/covid-19-racist-remarks-racially-charged-xenophobia-14718848

mccy. MCCY – Community Sector-National Steering Committee on Racial and Religious Harmony [Internet]. 2021 [cited 2021 Aug 11]. Available from: https://www.mccy.gov.sg/sector/initiatives/national-steering-committee-on-racial-and-religious-harmony

Mcdonald T. Singapore has COVID-19 well under control – but its migrant workers still face year-old restrictions [Internet]. Fortune. 2021 [cited 2021 Aug 11]; Available from: https://fortune.com/2021/04/07/singapore-covid-migrant-workers-restrictions-dormitories/

Meah N. Some shuttered home-based F&B businesses lament lost Ramadan, Hari Raya bumper sales – TODAY. TODAYonline [Internet]. 2020a Apr 27 [cited 2021 Jul 6]; Available from: https://www.todayonline.com/singapore/home-based-fb-businesses-face-income-crunch-just-some-would-usually-enjoy-strongest-sales

Meah N. Contact tracing solutions being developed for elderly and young without smartphones: Lawrence Wong. TODAYonline [Internet]. 2020b May 4 [cited 2021 Aug 7]; Available from: https://www.todayonline.com/singapore/contact-tracing-solutions-being-developed-elderly-and-young-without-smart-phones-lawrence

Menon S (n.d.). Executive power: rethinking the modalities of control. *Int LAW.* 29: 29.

Ministry of Culture, Community and Youth. Phase Three (Heightened Alert) – Precautionary measures for religious activities [Internet]. 2021 [cited 2021 Jul 16]; Available from: http://www.mccy.gov.sg/

about-us/news-and-resources/press-statements/2021/jul/phase-three-heightened-alert-precautionary-measures-religious-activities

Ministry of Education, Singapore. Arrangements for Schools and Institutes of Higher Learning in Phase Two [Internet]. Base. 2020 [cited 2021 Jul 14]; Available from: http://www.moe.gov.sg/news/press-releases/20200617-arrangements-for-schools-and-institutes-of-higher-learning-in-phase-two

Ministry of Finance, Singapore. fy2020_solidarity_budget_statement.pdf [Internet]. 2020a [cited 2021 Jul 16]. Available from: https://www.mof.gov.sg/docs/librariesprovider3/budget2020/statements/fy2020_solidarity_budget_statement.pdf

Ministry of Finance, Singapore. FY2020_ministerial-statement-oct 2021 [Internet]. 2020b [cited 2021 Jul 6]. Available from: https://www.mof.gov.sg/docs/librariesprovider3/budget2020/statements/fy2020_ministerial-statement-oct.pdf

Ministry of Finance, Singapore. Ministerial Statement – Jul 2021 [Internet]. Budget. 2021 [cited 2021 Jul 8]. Available from: https://www.mof.gov.sg/singaporebudget/ministerial-statements/ministerial-statement-jul-2021

Ministry of Foreign Affairs. Foreign Policy [Internet]. 2021 [cited 2021 May 8]. Available from: http://www.mfa.gov.sg/Overseas-Mission/Dubai/About-Singapore/Foreign-Policy

Ministry of Health. MOH | Situation Report [Internet]. Ministry of Health, Singapore. 2020 [cited 2021 May 4]. Available from: https://www.moh.gov.sg/COVID-19/situation-report

Ministry of Health, Singapore. MOH | News Highlights [Internet]. Strong National Push to Stem Spread of COVID-19. 2020a [cited 2021 Jul 16]. Available from: https://www.moh.gov.sg/news-highlights/details/strong-national-push-to-stem-spread-of-covid-19

Ministry of Health, Singapore. MOH | News Highlights [Internet]. Continued Stringent Implementation & Enforcement Of Circuit Breaker Measures. 2020b [cited 2021 Jul 16]. Available from: https://www.moh.gov.sg/news-highlights/details/continued-stringent-implementation-enforcement-of-circuit-breaker-measures

Ministry of Health, Singapore. MOH | News Highlights [Internet]. Comprehensive Medical Strategy for COVID-19. 2020c [cited 2021 Jul 16]. Available from: https://www.moh.gov.sg/news-highlights/details/comprehensive-medical-strategy-for-covid-19

Ministry of Health, Singapore. MOH | News Highlights [Internet]. Continuation Of Essential Healthcare Services During Period Of Heightened Safe Distancing Measures. 2020d [cited 2021 Jul 16]. Available from: https://www.moh.gov.sg/news-highlights/details/continuation-of-essential-healthcare-services-during-period-of-heightened-safe-distancing-measures

Ministry of Health, Singapore. MOH | News Highlights [Internet]. Minister For Health And Minister For Culture, Community & Youth Meet Church Leaders On Covid-19. 2020e [cited 2021 Jul 16]. Available from: https://www.moh.gov.sg/news-highlights/details/minister-for-health-and-minister-for-culture-community-youth-meet-church-leaders-on-covid-19

Ministry of Health, Singapore. MOH | News Highlights [Internet]. Tighter measures to minimise further spread of Covid-19. 2020f [cited 2021 Jul 14]. Available from: https://www.moh.gov.sg/news-highlights/details/tighter-measures-to-minimise-further-spread-of-covid-19

Ministry of Health, Singapore. MOH | News Highlights [Internet]. Moving into phase three of re-opening. 2020g [cited 2021 Jul 6]. Available from: https://www.moh.gov.sg/news-highlights/details/moving-into-phase-three-of-re-opening

Ministry of Health, Singapore. MOH | Regulations, Guidelines and Circulars [Internet]. Co-Ordination Of Testing Resources For Coronavirus Disease 2019 (Covid-19). 2020h [cited 2021 Jul 6]. Available from: https://www.moh.gov.sg/licensing-and-regulation/regulations-guidelines-and-circulars/details/co-ordination-of-testing-resources-for-coronavirus-disease-2019-(covid-19)

Ministry of Health, Singapore. MOH | News Highlights [Internet]. Scaling up of Covid-19 testing. 2020i [cited 2021 Jul 6]; Available from: https://www.moh.gov.sg/news-highlights/details/scaling-up-of-covid-19-testing

Ministry of Health, Singapore. MOH | News Highlights [Internet]. Safeguarding lives and livelihoods. 2020j [cited 2021 Jul 6]; Available from: https://www.moh.gov.sg/news-highlights/details/safeguarding-lives-and-livelihoods

Ministry of Health, Singapore. MOH Circular: Availability of Covid-19 Serology Testing For Determination of Previous Covid-19 Infection in the Outpatient Setting. 2020k.

Ministry of Health, Singapore. MOH | News Highlights [Internet]. Government Accepts Recommendations Of Expert Committee On Covid-19 Vaccination. 2020l [cited 2021 Jul 16]. Available from: https://www.moh.gov.sg/news-highlights/details/government-accepts-recommendations-of-expert-committee-on-covid-19-vaccination

Ministry of Health, Singapore. MOH | News Highlights [Internet]. Extension of precautionary measures to minimise risk of community spread in singapore. 2020m [cited 2021 Jul 14]. Available from: https://www.moh.gov.sg/news-highlights/details/extension-of-precautionary-measures-to-minimise-risk-of-community-spread-in-singapore

Ministry of Health, Singapore. MOH Circular: Medical Support for Migrant Workers After Clearance of Dormitories. 2020n.

Ministry of Health, Singapore. MOH | News Highlights [Internet]. Additional measures for travellers to reduce further importation of Covid-19 cases. 2020o [cited 2021 Jul 14]; Available from: https://www.moh.gov.sg/news-highlights/details/additional-measures-for-travellers-to-reduce-further-importation-of-covid-19-cases

Ministry of Health, Singapore. MOH | News Highlights [Internet]. Advisory on precautionary measures for seniors. 2020p [cited 2021 Jul 14]; Available from: https://www.moh.gov.sg/news-highlights/details/advisory-on-precautionary-measures-for-seniors

Ministry of Health, Singapore. MOH | COVID-19 (Temporary Measures) Act 2020 – Control Orders [Internet]. 2020q [cited 2021 Jul 16]. Available from: https://www.moh.gov.sg/policies-and-legislation/covid-19-(temporary-measures)-(control-order)-regulations

Ministry of Health, Singapore. MOH | COVID-19 Situation Report [Internet]. 2020r [cited 2021 Jul 6]; Available from: https://www.moh.gov.sg/covid-19/situation-report

Ministry of Health, Singapore. MOH | Past Updates on COVID-19 Local Situation [Internet]. 2021a [cited 2021 Jul 10]. Available from: https://www.moh.gov.sg/covid-19/past-updates

Ministry of Health, Singapore. MOH | News Highlights [Internet]. Expansion of vaccination programme; further easing of community measures. 2021b [cited 2021 Jul 8]; Available from: https://www.moh.gov.sg/news-highlights/details/expansion-of-vaccination-programme-further-easing-of-community-measures

Ministry of Health, Singapore. MOH | News Highlights [Internet]. Updates on border measures for travellers from Vietnam. 2021c [cited 2021 Jul 15]; Available from: https://www.moh.gov.sg/news-highlights/details/updates-on-border-measures-for-travellers-from-vietnam

Ministry of Health, Singapore. MOH | News Highlights [Internet]. Updates on border measures for travellers from Australia and Guangdong province, Mainland China. 2021d [cited 2021 Jul 16]. Available from: https://www.moh.gov.sg/news-highlights/details/updates-on-border-measures-for-travellers-from-australia-and-guangdong-province-mainland-china

Ministry of Health, Singapore. MOH | News Highlights [Internet]. Updates on border measures for travellers from Fiji and Israel. 2021e [cited 2021 Jul 15]; Available from: https://www.moh.gov.sg/news-highlights/details/updates-on-border-measures-for-travellers-from-fiji-and-israel

Ministry of Health, Singapore. MOH | COVID-19 Vaccination [Internet]. 2021f [cited 2021 Jul 9]; Available from: https://www.moh.gov.sg/covid-19/vaccination

Ministry of Health, Singapore. MOH | News Highlights [Internet]. Measures taken to safeguard health and safety of shore-based personnel in maritime sector. 2021g [cited 2021 Jul 16]. Available from: https://www.moh.gov.sg/news-highlights/details/MPA2Jan

Ministry of Health, Singapore. MOH | News Highlights [Internet]. Updates on border measures for travellers from South Africa. 2021h [cited 2021 Jul 15]; Available from: https://www.moh.gov.sg/news-highlights/details/updates-on-border-measures-for-travellers-from-south-africa

Ministry of Health, Singapore. MOH | News Highlights [Internet]. Updates on border measures and travel insurance. 2021i [cited 2021 Jul 16]; Available from: https://www.moh.gov.sg/news-highlights/details/updates-on-border-measures-and-travel-insurance

Ministry of Health, Singapore. MOH | News Highlights [Internet]. Tightening safe management measures and update on vaccination plans. 2021j [cited 2021 Jul 16]; Available from: https://www.moh.gov.sg/news-highlights/details/tightening-safe-management-measures-and-update-on-vaccination-plans

Ministry of Health, Singapore. MOH | News Highlights [Internet]. Updates on border measures for travellers from India, Hong Kong, United Kingdom and South Africa. 2021k [cited 2021 Jul 14]; Available from: https://www.moh.gov.sg/news-highlights/details/updates-on-border-measures-for-travellers-from-india-hong-kong-united-kingdom-and-south-africa

Ministry of Health, Singapore. MOH | News Highlights [Internet]. Updates on border measures for travellers from India, Westlite Woodlands dormitory cluster and additional precautions for recovered persons. 2021l [cited 2021 Jul 16]; Available from: https://www.moh.gov.sg/news-highlights/details/updates-on-border-measures-for-travellers-from-india-westlite-woodlands-dormitory-cluster-and-additional-precautions-for-recovered-persons

Ministry of Health, Singapore. MOH | News Highlights [Internet]. Updates on local situation, border measures for Bangladesh, Nepal, Pakistan, Sri Lanka, and Thailand and precautionary measures to minimise transmission from Tan Tock Seng Hospital cluster. 2021m [cited 2021 Jul 14]; Available from: https://www.moh.gov.sg/news-highlights/details/updates-on-local-situation-border-measures-for-bangladesh-nepal-pakistan-and-sri-lanka-thailand-and-precautionary-measures-to-minimise-transmission-from-tan-tock-seng-hospital-cluster

Ministry of Health, Singapore. MOH | News Highlights [Internet]. Updates on local situation, border measures and shift to heightened alert to minimise transmission. 2021n [cited 2021 Jul 15]; Available from: https://www.moh.gov.sg/news-highlights/details/updates-on-local-situation-border-measures-and-shift-to-heightened-alert-to-minimise-transmission_4May2021

Ministry of Health, Singapore. MOH | News Highlights [Internet]. Updates on local situation and vaccination programme. 2021o [cited 2021 Jul 15]; Available from: https://www.moh.gov.sg/news-highlights/details/updates-on-local-situation-and-vaccination-programme

Ministry of Health, Singapore. MOH | News Highlights [Internet]. Updated pre-departure testing requirements. 2021p [cited 2021 Jul 15]; Available from: https://www.moh.gov.sg/news-highlights/details/updated-pre-departure-testing-requirements

Ministry of Health, Singapore. MOH | News Highlights [Internet]. Maintaining heightened alert to minimise risk of transmission as we re-open safely. 2021q [cited 2021 Jul 14]; Available from: https://www.moh.gov.sg/news-highlights/details/maintaining-heightened-alert-to-minimise-risk-of-transmission-as-we-re-open-safely

Ministry of Health, Singapore. MOH | News Highlights [Internet]. Calibrated reopening to keep our community safe. 2021r [cited 2021 Jul 15]; Available from: https://www.moh.gov.sg/news-highlights/details/calibrated-reopening-to-keep-our-community-safe

Ministry of Health, Singapore. MOH | News Highlights [Internet]. Updates on border measures for travellers from higher risk countries/regions. 2021s [cited 2021 Jul 15]; Available from:

https://www.moh.gov.sg/news-highlights/details/updates-on-border-measures-for-travellers-from-higher-risk-countries-regions

Ministry of Health, Singapore. MOH | News Highlights [Internet]. Updates on phase 3 (heightened alert) measures. 2021t [cited 2021 Jul 16]; Available from: https://www.moh.gov.sg/news-highlights/details/updates-on-phase-3-(heightened-alert)-measures-7Jul

Ministry of Health, Singapore. MOH | News Highlights [Internet]. Updates on border measures for travellers from Indonesia. 2021u [cited 2021 Jul 16]; Available from: https://www.moh.gov.sg/news-highlights/details/updates-on-border-measures-for-travellers-from-indonesia_10Jul2021

Ministry of Health, Singapore. MOH | News Highlights [Internet]. Updates on border measures for travellers from india, westlite woodlands dormitory cluster and additional precautions for recovered persons. 2021v [cited 2021 Jul 14]. Available from: https://www.moh.gov.sg/news-highlights/details/updates-on-border-measures-for-travellers-from-india-westlite-woodlands-dormitory-cluster-and-additional-precautions-for-recovered-persons

Ministry of Health, Singapore. MOH | Time-limited Extension of CHAS Subsidy and Use of MediSave for Follow up of Chronic Conditions through Video Consultations in view of COVID-19 [Internet]. 2021w [cited 2021 Jul 16]. Available from: https://www.moh.gov.sg/covid-19/vc

Ministry of Health, Singapore. MOH | Clarifications on Misinformation regarding COVID-19 [Internet]. 2021x [cited 2021 Jul 16]. Available from: https://www.moh.gov.sg/covid-19/clarifications

Ministry of Health, Singapore. MOH | Updates on COVID-19 (Coronavirus Disease 2019) Local Situation [Internet]. 2021y [cited 2021 Jul 6]; Available from: https://www.moh.gov.sg/covid-19

Ministry of Manpower, Singapore. More workers and employers taken to task for breaching leave of absence requirements [Internet]. Ministry of Manpower Singapore. 2020a [cited 2021 Jul 16]. Available from: https://www.mom.gov.sg/newsroom/press-releases/2020/0224-more-workers-and-employers-taken-to-task-for-breaching-loa

Ministry of Manpower, Singapore. Food Distribution, Cleanliness and Hygiene Standards at Sungei Tengah Lodge and Tampines Dormitory Stabilised within 48 hours [Internet]. Ministry of Manpower Singapore. 2020b [cited 2021 Aug 11]. Available from: https://www.mom.gov.sg/newsroom/press-releases/2020/0411-food-distribution-cleanliness-and-hygiene-standards-at-stl-and-td-stabilised-within-48-hours

Ministry of Manpower, Singapore. Comprehensive Approach to Take Care of the Well-Being of Foreign Workers Living in Dormitories [Internet]. Ministry of Manpower. 2020c [cited 2021 Aug 11]; Available from: https://www.mom.gov.sg/newsroom/press-releases/2020/0501-comprehensive-approach-to-take-care-of-the-well-being-of-foreign-workers-living-in-dormitories

Ministry of Manpower, Singapore. Speech by Minister Josephine Teo at Supplementary Budget Debate [Internet]. Ministry of Manpower Singapore. 2020d [cited 2021 Aug 11]; Available from: https://www.mom.gov.sg/newsroom/speeches/2020/0406-speech-by-minister-josephine-teo-at-suplementary-budget-debate

Ministry of Manpower, Singapore. Measures to contain the COVID-19 outbreak in migrant worker dormitories [Internet]. 2020e [cited 2021 Jul 14]; Available from: https://www.mom.gov.sg/newsroom/press-releases/2020/1214-measures-to-contain-the-covid-19-outbreak-in-migrant-worker-dormitories

Ministry of Manpower, Singapore. Workers in Dormitories Returning to Work and Updates on AccessCode [Internet]. Ministry of Manpower Singapore. 2020f [cited 2021 Jul 22]; Available from: https://www.mom.gov.sg/newsroom/press-releases/2020/0610-workers-in-dormitories-returning-to-work-and-updates-on-accesscode

Ministry of Manpower, Singapore. Joint mom-bca-edb press release on enabling targeted quarantining through contact-tracing devices for more than 450,000 workers [Internet]. Ministry of Manpower

Singapore. 2020g [cited 2021 Jul 14]; Available from: https://www.mom.gov.sg/newsroom/press-releases/2020/1016-enabling-targeted-quarantining-through-contact-tracing-devices

Ministry of Manpower, Singapore. Eligible Migrant Workers will be able to visit Recreation Centres on Rest Days from 31 Oct 2020 [Internet]. Ministry of Manpower Singapore. 2020h [cited 2021 Aug 11]; Available from: https://www.mom.gov.sg/newsroom/press-releases/2020/1028-eligible-migrant-workers-will-be-able-to-visit-recreation-centres-on-rest-days-from-31-oct-20

Ministry of Manpower, Singapore. Advisory on continued medical support for migrant workers [Internet]. Ministry of Manpower Singapore. 2020i [cited 2021 Jul 22]; Available from: https://www.mom.gov.sg/covid-19/advisory-on-continued-medical-support-for-migrant-workers

Ministry of Manpower, Singapore. New Taskforce to Enhance Mental Health Care Support for Migrant Workers [Internet]. Ministry of Manpower Singapore. 2020j [cited 2021 Jul 21]; Available from: https://www.mom.gov.sg/newsroom/press-releases/2020/1106-new-taskforce-to-enhance-mental-health-care-support-for-migrant-workers

Ministry of Manpower, Singapore. Companies Encouraged to Impose Leave of Absence for Employees Returning Between 14 and 20 March 2020 [Internet]. 2020k [cited 2021 Jul 14]; Available from: https://www.mom.gov.sg/newsroom/press-releases/2020/0320-companies-encouraged-to-impose-loa-for-employees-returning-between-14-and-20-march-2020

Ministry of Manpower, Singapore. Requirements for Safe Management Measures at the workplace [Internet]. 2020l [cited 2021 Jul 14]; Available from: https://www.mom.gov.sg/covid-19/requirements-for-safe-management-measures

Ministry of Manpower, Singapore. New resources to provide better care for migrant workers [Internet]. 2020m [cited 2021 Jul 14]; Available from: https://www.mom.gov.sg/newsroom/press-releases/2020/0527-new-resources-to-provide-better-care-for-migrant-workers

Ministry of Manpower, Singapore. Employers To Ensure Workers Go Through Rostered Routine Testing [Internet]. 2020n [cited 2021 Jul 14]; Available from: https://www.mom.gov.sg/newsroom/press-releases/2020/0818-employers-to-ensure-workers-go-through-rostered-routine-testing

Ministry of Manpower, Singapore. Advisory for dormitory operators to submit essential errands form for migrant workers to carry out essential errands [Internet]. 2020o [cited 2021 Jul 14]; Available from: https://www.mom.gov.sg/covid-19/advisory-for-dorm-operators-to-submit-essential-errands

Ministry of Manpower, Singapore. Pilot of antigen rapid tests for quicker detection of COVID-19 infection among migrant workers [Internet]. 2020p [cited 2021 Jul 14]; Available from: https://www.mom.gov.sg/newsroom/press-releases/2020/1025-pilot-of-antigen-rapid-tests-for-quicker-detection-of-covid-19-infection-among-migrant-workers

Ministry of Manpower, Singapore. Update on rostered routine testing policy for Migrant workers recovered from covid-19 [Internet]. 2020q [cited 2021 Jul 14]; Available from: https://www.mom.gov.sg/newsroom/press-releases/2020/1106-update-on-rostered-routine-testing-policy-for--migrant-workers-recovered-from-covid-19

Ministry of Manpower, Singapore. Medical insurance requirements for foreign worker [Internet]. Ministry of Manpower Singapore. 2021a [cited 2021 Aug 11]; Available from: https://www.mom.gov.sg/passes-and-permits/work-permit-for-foreign-worker/sector-specific-rules/medical-insurance

Ministry of Manpower, Singapore. MOM pilots one-stop onboarding centre for newly-arrived migrant workers [Internet]. Ministry of Manpower Singapore. 2021b [cited 2021 Jul 14]; Available from: https://www.mom.gov.sg/newsroom/press-releases/2021/0303-mom-pilots-one-stop-onboarding-centre-for-newly-arrived-migrant-workers

Ministry of Manpower, Singapore. Employment Pass [Internet]. Ministry of Manpower Singapore. 2021c [cited 2021 Jul 22]; Available from: https://www.mom.gov.sg/passes-and-permits/employment-pass

Ministry of Manpower, Singapore. Work Permit conditions [Internet]. Ministry of Manpower Singapore. 2021d [cited 2021 Jul 22]; Available from: https://www.mom.gov.sg/passes-and-permits/work-permit-for-foreign-worker/sector-specific-rules/work-permit-conditions

Ministry of Manpower, Singapore. Work passes [Internet]. Ministry of Manpower Singapore. 2021e [cited 2021 Aug 11]; Available from: https://www.mom.gov.sg/passes-and-permits

Ministry of Sustainability and the Environment, Singapore. Stiffer Penalties for Breach of Safe Distancing Measures from 12 April 2020 [Internet]. 2020 [cited 2021 Jul 16]. Available from: https://www.mse.gov.sg/resource-room/category/2020-04-11-press-release-on-stiffer-fines-for-breach-of-safe-distancing-measures/

Ministry of Trade and Industry. MTI Maintains 2021 GDP Growth Forecast at "4.0 to 6.0 Per Cent" [Internet]. 2021 Feb [cited 2021 Apr 14]; Available from: https://www.mti.gov.sg/Newsroom/Press-Releases/2021/02/MTI-Maintains-2021-GDP-Growth-Forecast-at-4_0-to-6_0-Per-Cent

Mohan M. More than 3,500 electronic wristband devices issued to travellers serving stay-home notices: ICA. CNA [Internet]. 2020 Sep 12 [cited 2021 Aug 7]; Available from: https://www.channelnewsasia.com/singapore/electronic-wristband-devices-stay-home-notice-ica-covid-19-699176

Mohan M. Nightlife, karaoke businesses still see a future despite the ongoing COVID-19 challenges. CNA [Internet]. 2021 May 30 [cited 2021 Jul 7]; Available from: https://www.channelnewsasia.com/news/singapore/covid-entertainment-nightlife-karaoke-club-bar-singapore-14904416

Mohan M, Ang HM. COVID-19: Singapore makes "decisive move" to close most workplaces and impose full home-based learning for schools, says PM Lee – CNA. Channel News Asia [Internet]. 2020 Apr 3 [cited 2021 Jul 6]; Available from: https://www.channelnewsasia.com/news/singapore/covid19-decisive-move-workplaces-closed-lee-hsien-loong-12606614

Mohan M, Phua R. GE2020: PAP wins with 61.24% of vote; WP claims two GRCs including new Sengkang GRC [Internet]. Channel News Asia. 2020 [cited 2021 Aug 4]. Available from: https://www.channelnewsasia.com/news/singapore/ge2020-general-election-final-result-pap-wp-12922882

Moss D. Singapore's Covid Success Isn't Easily Replicated. Bloomberg.com [Internet]. 2021 Jan 3 [cited 2021 Jul 10]; Available from: https://www.bloomberg.com/opinion/articles/2021-01-03/singapore-s-covid-success-isn-t-easily-replicated

Nakazawa E, Ino H, Akabayashi A. 2020 Chronology of COVID-19 Cases on the Diamond Princess Cruise Ship and Ethical Considerations: A Report From Japan. Disaster Med Public Health Prep.: 1–8.

National Centre for Infectious Diseases. SEROEPIDEMIOLOGICAL STUDIES_FOR RELEASE FINAL_UPDATED.pdf [Internet]. 2020 [cited 2021 Jul 6]; Available from: https://www.ncid.sg/News-Events/News/Documents/SEROEPIDEMIOLOGICAL%20STUDIES_FOR%20RELEASE%20FINAL_UPDATED.pdf

National Council of Social Service. Enhanced precautionary measures for residential and community-based facilities against COVID-19 (Coronavirus Disease 2019 [Internet]. NCSS. 2020 [cited 2021 Jul 14]. Available from: https://www.ncss.gov.sg/press-room/advisory/past-covid-19-advisories

National Trades Union Congress. Media Release – Tripartite Care Package for Quarantined Taxi and Private Hire Vehicle Drivers.pdf [Internet]. 2020 [cited 2021 Jul 16]. Available from: https://www.lta.gov.sg/content/dam/ltagov/industry_innovations/pdf/Media%20Release%20-%20Tripartite%20Care%20Package%20for%20Quarantined%20Taxi%20and%20Private%20Hire%20Vehicle%20Drivers.pdf

Neo JL. Riots and rights: law and exclusion in Singapore's migrant worker regime. *Asian J Law Soc.* 2015 May;2(1):137–68.

Neo JL, Lee D. Singapore's Legislative Approach to the COVID-19 Public Health 'Emergency' [Internet]. Verfassungsblog. 2020 Apr 18 [cited 2021 Jul 14]; Available from: https://verfassungsblog.de/singapores-legislative-approach-to-the-covid-19-public-health-emergency/

Ng CK. Why shut TCM retailers during circuit breaker? TODAYonline [Internet]. 2020 Apr 21 [cited 2021 Jul 16]; Available from: https://www.todayonline.com/voices/why-shut-tcm-retailers-during-circuit-breaker

Ng JS. Don't let guard down on Covid-19, another lockdown would be major setback to economic recovery: PM Lee. TODAYonline [Internet]. 2021 May 1 [cited 2021 Jul 8]; Available from: https://www.todayonline.com/singapore/dont-let-guard-down-covid-19-another-lockdown-would-be-major-setback-economic-recovery-pm

Office of the Mufti. Muis: Office of the Mufti [Internet]. Fatwa On Precautionary Measures In Dealing With The Covid-19. 2020 [cited 2021 Jul 16]. Available from: https://www.muis.gov.sg/officeofthemufti/Fatwa/Fatwa-Covid-19-English

Ong J. Half of the cases at largest Covid-19 cluster in Bukit Merah View not vaccinated. The Straits Times [Internet]. 2021 Jun 24 [cited 2021 Jul 8]; Available from: https://www.straitstimes.com/singapore/half-of-the-cases-at-largest-covid-19-cluster-in-bukit-merah-view-not-vaccinated

Osman D. Almost 90,000 police cameras installed, more to come: Shanmugam [Internet]. yahoo!news. 2021 [cited 2021 Jul 22]; Available from: https://sg.news.yahoo.com/90000-police-cameras-installed-singapore-shanmugam-102536548.html?guccounter=1

Ovais S. Singapore retains top spot as world's most competitive economy. The Straits Times [Internet]. 2020 Jun 16 [cited 2021 Jul 13]; Available from: https://www.straitstimes.com/business/economy/singapore-retains-top-spot-as-worlds-most-competitive-economy

Owusu PN. Digital technology applications for contact tracing: the new promise for COVID-19 and beyond? *Glob Health Res Policy.* 2020 Aug 3;5(1):36.

Parliament Singapore. Singapore Parliamentary Reports [Internet]. Marriage Restriction Policy (Column 665). 2004 [cited 2021 Jul 22]; Available from: https://sprs.parl.gov.sg/search/topic?reportid=015_20040921_S0007_T0009

Perry M, Kong L, Yeoh BSA. Singapore: A Developmental City State. Res Collect Sch Soc Sci [Internet]. 1997 Jan 1; Available from: https://ink.library.smu.edu.sg/soss_research/1825

Personal Data Protection Commission Singapore. Advisories on Collection of Personal Data for COVID-19 Contact Tracing and Use of SafeEntry [Internet]. 2020 [cited 2021 Aug 7]. Available from: https://www.pdpc.gov.sg/Help-and-Resources/2020/03/Advisory-on-Collection-of-Personal-Data-for-COVID-19-Contact-Tracing

Phua R. 1,000 self-employed individuals asked to return COVID-19 SIRS payouts due to erroneous declarations. CNA [Internet]. 2021 Jan 5 [cited 2021 Aug 11]; Available from: https://www.channelnewsasia.com/singapore/self-employed-person-income-relief-scheme-erroneous-declarations-386201

Phua R, Ang HM. 'Dedicated strategy' to break COVID-19 spread in dormitories, including housing healthy workers in army camps. CNA [Internet]. 2020 Apr 9 [cited 2021 Jul 14]; Available from: https://www.channelnewsasia.com/news/singapore/covid-19-foreign-worker-dormitories-range-of-measures-12625624

Phua R, Chew HM. Can Singapore rely less on foreign workers? It's not just about dollars and cents, say observers – CNA. 2020 [cited 2021 Apr 21]; Available from: https://www.channelnewsasia.com/news/singapore/singapore-foreign-workers-reliance-challenges-12806970

Pougnet R, Pougnet L, Dewitte J-D, Lucas D, Loddé B. COVID-19 on cruise ships: preventive quarantine or abandonment of patients? *Int Marit Health.* 2020;71(2):147–8.

Prime Minister's Office Singapore. PMO | Valedictory Letter from Prime Minister Lee Hsien Loong to Mr Abdullah Tarmugi [Internet]. Prime Minister's Office Singapore. Prime Minister's Office Singapore; 2018a [cited 2021 Jul 16]. Available from: https://www.pmo.gov.sg/Newsroom/valedictory-letter-prime-minister-lee-hsien-loong-mr-abdullah-tarmugi

Prime Minister's Office Singapore. PMO | Valedictory Letter from PM Lee Hsien Loong to Dr Yaacob Ibrahim [Internet]. Prime Minister's Office Singapore. \Anonymous; 2018b [cited 2021 Jul 16]. Available from: https://www.pmo.gov.sg/Newsroom/valedictory-letter-pm-lee-hsien-loong-dr-yaacob-ibrahim

Prime Minister's Office Singapore. PMO | PM Lee Hsien Loong on the COVID-19 situation in Singapore on 10 April 2020 [Internet]. Prime Minister's Office Singapore. katherine_chen; 2020 [cited 2021 Jul 16]. Available from: https://www.pmo.gov.sg/Newsroom/PM-Lee-Hsien-Loong-on-the-COVID-19-situation-in-Singapore-on-10-April-2020

Prime Minister's Office Singapore. PMO | The Government [Internet]. Prime Minister's Office Singapore. katherine_chen; 2021a [cited 2021 Jul 10]. Available from: https://www.pmo.gov.sg/The-Government

Prime Minister's Office Singapore. PMO | Mr Edwin TONG [Internet]. Prime Minister's Office Singapore. chua_cheng_gee; 2021b [cited 2021 Jul 16]. Available from: https://www.pmo.gov.sg/The-Cabinet/Mr-Edwin-TONG

Privacy International. Privacy and Human Rights – Overview [Internet]. Global Internet Liberty Campaign. 1998 [cited 2021 Jul 22]; Available from: http://gilc.org/privacy/survey/intro.html

Privacy International. The Right to Privacy in Singapore [Internet]. 2015 Jun [cited 2021 Jul 22]. (Universal Periodic Review Stakeholder Report: 24th Session, Singapore). Available from: https://www.privacyinternational.org/sites/default/files/2017-12/Singapore_UPR_PI_submission_FINAL.pdf

Sadarangani SP, Lim PL, Vasoo S. Infectious diseases and migrant worker health in Singapore: a receiving country's perspective. *J Travel Med [Internet]*. 2017 Jul 1 [cited 2021 Aug 11];24(4). Available from: https://doi.org/10.1093/jtm/tax014

Schein EC. *Strategic Pragmatism: The Culture of Singapore's Economics Development Board [Internet]*. Vol. 1, MIT Press Books. The MIT Press; 1996 [cited 2021 May 8]. Available from: https://ideas.repec.org/b/mtp/titles/0262193671.html

SCMP. In rich Singapore, why must migrant workers go hungry? [Internet]. South China Morning Post. 2019 [cited 2021 Jul 30]. Available from: https://www.scmp.com/week-asia/health-environment/article/3004901/rich-singapore-why-must-migrant-workers-go-hungry

SCMP. How did migrant worker dorms become Singapore's biggest Covid-19 cluster? [Internet]. South China Morning Post. 2020 [cited 2021 Jul 30]; Available from: https://www.scmp.com/week-asia/explained/article/3080466/how-did-migrant-worker-dormitories-become-singapores-biggest

Sin Y. All dorms to be regulated under Foreign Employee Dormitories Act: MOM. The Straits Times [Internet]. 2021 Mar 3 [cited 2021 Jul 22]; Available from: https://www.straitstimes.com/singapore/all-dorms-to-be-regulated-under-a-single-law-the-foreign-employee-dormitories-act-mom

Sin Y. DIY Covid-19 test kits being piloted at construction worksites. The Straits Times [Internet]. 2021 Jun 2 [cited 2021 Jul 14]; Available from: https://www.straitstimes.com/singapore/diy-covid-19-test-kits-to-be-piloted-at-construction-worksites

Singapore Food Agency. Mandatory Fast and Easy Testing (FET) regime for all outlet employees at dine-in F&B establishments [Internet]. 2021 [cited 2021 Jul 15]; Available from: https://www.sfa.gov.sg/covid-19/mandatory-fast-and-easy-testing-(fet)-regime-for-all-outlet-employees-at-dine-in-f-b-establishments

Singapore Legal Advice. Singapore Fake News Laws: Guide to POFMA (Protection from Online Falsehoods and Manipulation Act) [Internet]. SingaporeLegalAdvice.com. 2020 [cited 2021 Jul 16]. Available from: https://singaporelegaladvice.com/law-articles/singapore-fake-news-protection-online-falsehoods-manipulation/

Singapore Police Force. Police Do Not Conduct Road Blocks To Enforce Elevated Safe Distancing Measures [Internet]. Singapore Police Force. 2020a [cited 2021 Jul 16]. Available from: http://www

.police.gov.sg/Media-Room/News/20200413_OTHERS_-Police_Do_Not_Conduct_Road_Blocks_
To_Enforce_OpsTP

Singapore Police Force. Singapore Police Force [Internet]. Police Do Not Conduct Checks At
Residential Units To Enforce Elevated Safe Distancing Measures. 2020b [cited 2021 Jul 16]. Available
from: https://www.facebook.com/singaporepoliceforce/posts/10159695384084408

Singapore Tourism Board. STB unveils targeted measures to support tourism businesses affected by
2019-nCoV | STB [Internet]. 2020 [cited 2021 Jul 10]. Available from: https://www.stb.gov.sg/
content/stb/en/media-centre/media-releases/stb-unveils-
targetedmeasurestosupporttourismbusinessesaffectedby.html.html

Singapore Tourism Board. SingapoRediscovers Vouchers | STB [Internet]. 2021 [cited 2021 Jul 7];
Available from: https://www.stb.gov.sg/content/stb/en/trade-events-and-resources/
SingapoRediscovers-Vouchers.html

Smart Nation Singapore. TraceTogether Tokens to be distributed at the constituency level [Internet].
Default. 2020 [cited 2021 Jul 15]; Available from: https://www.smartnation.gov.sg/whats-new/
press-releases

Smart Nation Singapore. SNDGO | Press Releases – Building A Smart Nation with Tangible Benefits
For Our Citizens and Businesses [Internet]. 2021a [cited 2021 Aug 12]. Available from: https://www
.smartnation.gov.sg/whats-new/press-releases/building-a-smart-nation-with-tangible-benefits--
for-our-citizens-and-businesses

Smart Nation Singapore. Factsheet on Digital Contact Tracing Tools [Internet]. 2021b Feb [cited 2021
Aug 7]. Available from: https://www.smartnation.gov.sg/docs/default-source/press-release-
materials/factsheet-on-digital-contact-tracing-tools_1-feb-final.pdf?sfvrsn=9269785a_2

Smart Nation Singapore. Government's Personal Data Protection Initiatives [Internet]. Government's
Personal Data Protection Initiatives. 2021c [cited 2021 Aug 7]; Available from: https://www
.smartnation.gov.sg/why-Smart-Nation/secure-smart-nation/pdp-initiatives

Smart Nation Singapore. Press Releases [Internet]. Amendments in Covid-19 (temporary measures) act
on the use of personal digital contact tracing data. 2021d [cited 2021 Jul 16]; Available from:
https://www.smartnation.gov.sg/whats-new/press-releases

Smart Nation Singapore. Press Releases [Internet]. SafeEntry Gateway for an improved and seamless
check-in experience. 2021e [cited 2021 Jul 15]; Available from: https://www.smartnation.gov.sg/
whats-new/press-releases

Tan S-A. Coronavirus: Home bakers cannot operate under circuit breaker rules. The Straits Times
[Internet]. 2020 Apr 26 [cited 2021 Jul 6]; Available from: https://www.straitstimes.com/business/
home-bakers-cannot-operate-under-circuit-breaker-rules

Tan A. 550 Covid-19 cases infected with Delta variant detected in Singapore so far. The Straits Times
[Internet]. 2021 Jun 9 [cited 2021 Jul 8]; Available from: https://www.straitstimes.com/singapore/
health/550-out-of-about-62000-covid-19-cases-in-singapore-infected-with-delta-variant

Tan C, Yong C. Coronavirus: Call for firms to be sensitive to fears of older staff working outside,
Transport News & Top Stories – The Straits Times. The Straits Times [Internet]. 2020 Apr 15 [cited
2021 Jul 14]; Available from: https://www.straitstimes.com/singapore/transport/call-for-firms-to-
be-sensitive-to-fears-of-older-staff-out-working

Tang SK. 70% of Singapore residents participating in TraceTogether programme: Vivian Balakrishnan.
CNA [Internet]. 2020 Dec 23 [cited 2021 Aug 7]; Available from: https://www.channelnewsasia
.com/singapore/covid-19-tracetogether-adoption-singapore-crosses-70-percent-500596

Tang SK. SMS alerts, mandatory testing for people who visited COVID-19 hotspots on same days as
confirmed cases. CNA [Internet]. 2021 Jun 18 [cited 2021 Aug 7]; Available from: https://www
.channelnewsasia.com/singapore/sms-alerts-mandatory-testing-individuals-covid-19-hotspots-
1959901

Tang SK, Mahmud AH. Singapore launches TraceTogether mobile app to boost Covid-19 contact tracing efforts. CNA [Internet]. 2020 Mar 20 [cited 2021 Jul 14]; Available from: https://www.channelnewsasia.com/news/singapore/covid19-trace-together-mobile-app-contact-tracing-coronavirus-12560616

Tay TF. More than half of Singapore's hotel rooms used in Covid-19 battle, not all can reopen for staycations: STB chief. The Straits Times [Internet]. 2020 Jul 22 [cited 2021 Jul 6]; Available from: https://www.straitstimes.com/singapore/more-than-half-of-singapores-hotel-rooms-used-in-covid-19-battle-not-all-can-reopen-for

Tay C, Lim J. Who will get SingapoRediscovers Vouchers and what can you do with them? The Straits Times [Internet]. 2020 Nov 23 [cited 2021 Jul 7]; Available from: https://www.straitstimes.com/singapore/consumer/faq-who-will-get-singaporediscovers-vouchers-and-what-can-you-do-with-them

Temasek. A Pair of Reusable Antibacterial Masks Free For Each Singapore Resident [Internet]. Temasek Corporate Website English. 2020 [cited 2021 Jul 16]. Available from: https://www.temasek.com.sg/en/news-and-views/news-room/news/2020/a-pair-of-reusable-antibacterial-masks-free-for-each-singapore-resident

Teng YM. Chapter 10: Singapore's System for Managing Foreign Manpower. 2014 p. 21. (Managing International Migration for Development in East Asia).

Teo. What to know about circuit breaker rules in Singapore (updated as the situation changes). TODAYonline [Internet]. 2020a May 5 [cited 2021 Jul 14]; Available from: https://www.8days.sg/seeanddo/thingstodo/what-to-know-about-circuit-breaker-rules-in-singapore-updated-as-12704248

Teo G. Singapore to unilaterally lift border restrictions to travellers from Taiwan from Dec 18. CNA [Internet]. 2020b Dec 11 [cited 2021 Jul 6]; Available from: https://www.channelnewsasia.com/news/singapore/covid-19-singapore-open-up-to-travellers-from-taiwan-ong-ye-kung-13750320

Tham I. Coronavirus: New contact tracing device and check-in system on trial at worksite. The Straits Times [Internet]. 2020 Jul 17 [cited 2021 Aug 7]; Available from: https://www.straitstimes.com/singapore/new-contact-tracing-device-and-check-in-system-on-trial-at-worksite

Tham Y-C. Police can access TraceTogether data only through person involved in criminal probe: Vivian Balakrishnan. The Straits Times [Internet]. 2021 Jan 5 [cited 2021 Jul 16]; Available from: https://www.straitstimes.com/singapore/politics/police-can-access-tracetogether-data-only-through-person-involved-in-criminal

The Singapore Contractors Association Limited. Mandatory Rostered Routine Testing (rrt) for anyone entering the worksite [Internet]. Mandatory Rostered Routine Testing (RRT) For Anyone Entering The Worksite. 2021 [cited 2021 Jul 14]; Available from: https://www.scal.com.sg/government-circulars/mandatory-rostered-routine-testing-rrt-for-anyone-entering-the-worksite

The Singapore Government. COVID-19 (Temporary Measures) (Amendment) Act 2021 – Singapore Statutes Online [Internet]. Mar 1, 2020a. Available from: https://sso.agc.gov.sg/Acts-Supp/6-2021/Published/20210301?DocDate=20210301

The Singapore Government. Infectious Diseases Act (Amendment of First and Second Schedules) Notification 2020 – Singapore Statutes Online [Internet]. Jan 29, 2020b. Available from: https://sso.agc.gov.sg/SL-Supp/S68-2020/Published/20200128?DocDate=20200128

The Singapore Government. Employment of Foreign Manpower (Work Passes) (Amendment) Regulations 2020 – Singapore Statutes Online [Internet]. 2020c [cited 2021 Jul 14]; Available from: https://sso.agc.gov.sg/SL-Supp/S427-2020/Published/20200601?DocDate=20200601

The Singapore Government. Infectious Diseases (COVID-19 – Stay Orders) (Amendment) Regulations 2020 – Singapore Statutes Online [Internet]. Mar 26, 2020d. Available from: https://sso.agc.gov.sg/SL-Supp/S184-2020/Published/20200326?DocDate=20200326

The Singapore Government. Infectious Diseases (COVID-19 – Stay Orders) (Amendment No. 3) Regulations 2020 – Singapore Statutes Online [Internet]. Apr 10, 2020e. Available from: https://sso.agc.gov.sg/SL-Supp/S263-2020/Published/20200410?DocDate=20200410

The Singapore Government. COVID-19 (Temporary Measures) (Control Order) (Amendment No. 2) Regulations 2020 – Singapore Statutes Online [Internet]. Apr 10, 2020f. Available from: https://sso.agc.gov.sg/SL-Supp/S262-2020/Published/20200410?DocDate=20200410

The Singapore Government. COVID-19 (Temporary Measures) (Control Order) (Amendment No. 3) Regulations 2020 – Singapore Statutes Online [Internet]. Apr 15, 2020g. Available from: https://sso.agc.gov.sg/SL-Supp/S273-2020/Published/20200415?DocDate=20200415

The Singapore Government. Infectious Diseases (COVID-19 – Stay Orders) (Amendment No. 4) Regulations 2020 – Singapore Statutes Online [Internet]. Apr 30, 2020h. Available from: https://sso.agc.gov.sg/SL-Supp/S358-2020/Published/20200430?DocDate=20200430

The Singapore Government. COVID-19 (Temporary Measures) (Control Order) (Amendment No. 6) Regulations 2020 – Singapore Statutes Online [Internet]. May 1, 2020i. Available from: https://sso.agc.gov.sg/SL-Supp/S357-2020/Published/20200430?DocDate=20200430

The Singapore Government. COVID-19 (Temporary Measures) (Control Order) (Amendment No. 8) Regulations 2020 – Singapore Statutes Online [Internet]. Jun 2, 2020j. Available from: https://sso.agc.gov.sg/SL-Supp/S428-2020/Published/20200601?DocDate=20200601

The Singapore Government. COVID-19 (Temporary Measures) (Control Order) (Amendment No. 9) Regulations 2020 – Singapore Statutes Online [Internet]. Jun 18, 2020k. Available from: https://sso.agc.gov.sg/SL-Supp/S473-2020/Published/20200618?DocDate=20200618

The Singapore Government. Infectious Diseases (COVID-19 – Stay Orders) (Amendment No. 7) Regulations 2020 – Singapore Statutes Online [Internet]. Jul 1, 2020l. Available from: https://sso.agc.gov.sg/SL-Supp/S535-2020/Published/20200701?DocDate=20200701

The Singapore Government. COVID-19 (Temporary Measures) (Control Order) (Amendment No. 11) Regulations 2020 – Singapore Statutes Online [Internet]. Aug 3, 2020m. Available from: https://sso.agc.gov.sg/SL-Supp/S669-2020/Published/20200803?DocDate=20200803

The Singapore Government. COVID-19 (Temporary Measures) (Control Order) (Amendment No. 15) Regulations 2020 – Singapore Statutes Online [Internet]. Sep 25, 2020n. Available from: https://sso.agc.gov.sg/SL-Supp/S816-2020/Published/20200925?DocDate=20200925

The Singapore Government. COVID-19 (Temporary Measures) (Performances and Other Activities – Control Order) (Amendment No. 2) Regulations 2020 – Singapore Statutes Online [Internet]. Dec 23, 2020o. Available from: https://sso.agc.gov.sg/SL-Supp/S1071-2020/Published/20201223?DocDate=20201223

The Singapore Government. COVID-19 (Temporary Measures) (Control Order) (Amendment No. 20) Regulations 2020 – Singapore Statutes Online [Internet]. Dec 23, 2020p. Available from: https://sso.agc.gov.sg/SL-Supp/S1070-2020/Published/20201223?DocDate=20201223

The Singapore Government. COVID-19 – (Stay Orders) Regulations 2020 – Singapore Statutes Online [Internet]. Mar 25, 2020q [cited 2021 Jul 16]. Available from: https: https://sso.agc.gov.sg/SL-Supp/S182-2020/Published/20200325?DocDate=20200325

The Singapore Government. Constitution of the Republic of Singapore, Art. 25(1) – Singapore Statutes Online [Internet] 2020r Revised Edition [cited 2022 May 17]. Available from: https: https://sso.agc.gov.sg/Act/CONS1963?WholeDoc=1#pr25-

The Singapore Government. COVID-19 (Temporary Measures) Act 2020 – Singapore Statutes Online [Internet]. 2020s [cited 2021 Jul 16]. Available from: https://sso.agc.gov.sg/Act/COVID19TMA2020

The Singapore Government. Constitution of the Republic of Singapore – Singapore Statutes Online [Internet]. Article 15. 2020t [cited 2021 Jul 16]. Available from: https://sso.agc.gov.sg/Act/CONS1963?ProvIds=P1IV-

The Singapore Government. Administration of Muslim Law Act – Singapore Statutes Online [Internet]. 2020u [cited 2021 Jul 16]. Available from: https://sso.agc.gov.sg/Act/AMLA1966

The Singapore Government. COVID-19 (Temporary Measures for Solemnization and Registration of Marriages) Act 2020 – Singapore Statutes Online [Internet]. 2020v [cited 2021 Jul 16]. Available from: https://sso.agc.gov.sg/Act/COVID19TMSRMA2020

The Singapore Government. COVID-19 (Temporary Measures) Act 2020 – Singapore Statutes Online [Internet]. note 6, s 34(6). 2020w [cited 2021 Jul 16]. Available from: https://sso.agc.gov.sg/Act/COVID19TMA2020

The Singapore Government. COVID-19 (Temporary Measures) (Control Order) Regulations 2020 – Singapore Statutes Online [Internet]. Jul 5, 2021a. Available from: https://sso.agc.gov.sg/SL/COVID19TMA2020-S254-2020?DocDate=20210113w

The Singapore Government. COVID-19 (Temporary Measures) (Performances and Other Activities – Control Order) Regulations 2020 – Singapore Statutes Online [Internet]. Jul 5, 2021b. Available from: https://sso.agc.gov.sg/SL/COVID19TMA2020-S927-2020?DocDate=20210611

The Singapore Government. COVID-19 (Temporary Measures) (Major Business Events – Control Order) Regulations 2021 – Singapore Statutes Online [Internet]. Jul 5, 2021c. Available from: https://sso.agc.gov.sg/SL/COVID19TMA2020-S278-2021?DocDate=20210611

The Singapore Government. COVID-19 (Temporary Measures) (Sporting Events and Activities – Control Order) Regulations 2021 – Singapore Statutes Online [Internet]. Jul 5, 2021d. Available from: https://sso.agc.gov.sg/SL/COVID19TMA2020-S277-2021?DocDate=20210611

The Singapore Government. COVID-19 (Temporary Measures) (Foreign Employee Dormitories – Control Order) Regulations 2020 – Singapore Statutes Online [Internet]. Jul 5, 2021e. Available from: https://sso.agc.gov.sg/SL/COVID19TMA2020-S781-2020?DocDate=20210515

The Singapore Government. COVID-19 (Temporary Measures) (Sporting Events and Activities – Control Order) (Amendment) Regulations 2021 – Singapore Statutes Online [Internet]. May 7, 2021f; Available from: https://sso.agc.gov.sg/SL-Supp/S307-2021/Published/20210507?DocDate=20210507

The Singapore Government. Infectious Diseases (Mass Gathering Testing for Coronavirus Disease 2019) (Amendment No. 3) Regulations 2021 – Singapore Statutes Online [Internet]. Jun 11, 2021g; Available from: https://sso.agc.gov.sg/SL-Supp/S367-2021/Published/20210611?DocDate=20210611

The Singapore Government. COVID-19 (Temporary Measures) (Control Order) (Amendment No. 11) Regulations 2021 – Singapore Statutes Online [Internet]. Jun 18, 2021h. Available from: https://sso.agc.gov.sg/SL-Supp/S379-2021/Published/20210619?DocDate=20210619

The Singapore Government. Infectious Diseases (COVID-19 – Stay Orders) (Amendment) Regulations 2021 – Singapore Statutes Online [Internet]. May 6, 2021i. Available from: https://sso.agc.gov.sg/SL-Supp/S303-2021/Published/20210505?DocDate=20210505

The Singapore Government. COVID-19 (Temporary Measures) (Control Order) (Amendment) Regulations 2021 – Singapore Statutes Online [Internet]. Jan 13, 2021j. Available from: https://sso.agc.gov.sg/SL-Supp/S16-2021/Published/20210113?DocDate=20210113

The Singapore Government. COVID-19 (Temporary Measures) (Control Order) (Amendment No. 2) Regulations 2021 – Singapore Statutes Online [Internet]. 2021k [cited 2021 Jul 16]. Available from: https://sso.agc.gov.sg/SL-Supp/S40-2021/Published/20210125?DocDate=20210125

The Singapore Government. COVID-19 (Temporary Measures) (Performances and Other Activities – Control Order) (Amendment) Regulations 2021 – Singapore Statutes Online [Internet]. Jan 25, 2021k. Available from: https://sso.agc.gov.sg/SL-Supp/S41-2021/Published/20210125?DocDate=20210125

The Singapore Government. COVID-19 (Temporary Measures) (Control Order) (Amendment No. 4) Regulations 2021 – Singapore Statutes Online [Internet]. Apr 1, 2021m. Available from: https://sso .agc.gov.sg/SL-Supp/S238-2021/Published/20210401?DocDate=20210401

The Singapore Government. COVID-19 (Temporary Measures) (Control Order) (Amendment No. 5) Regulations 2021 – Singapore Statutes Online [Internet]. Apr 23, 2021n. Available from: https://sso .agc.gov.sg/SL-Supp/S275-2021/Published/20210423?DocDate=20210423

The Singapore Government. COVID-19 (Temporary Measures) (Performances and Other Activities – Control Order) (Amendment No. 3) Regulations 2021 – Singapore Statutes Online [Internet]. Apr 23, 2021o. Available from: https://sso.agc.gov.sg/SL-Supp/S276-2021/Published/ 20210423?DocDate=20210423

The Singapore Government. COVID-19 (Temporary Measures) (Control Order) (Amendment No. 6) Regulations 2021 – Singapore Statutes Online [Internet]. Apr 30, 2021p. Available from: https://sso .agc.gov.sg/SL-Supp/S299-2021/Published/20210430?DocDate=20210430

The Singapore Government. COVID-19 (Temporary Measures) (Control Order) (Amendment No. 7) Regulations 2021 – Singapore Statutes Online [Internet]. May 7, 2021q. Available from: https://sso .agc.gov.sg/SL-Supp/S309-2021/Published/20210507?DocDate=20210507

The Singapore Government. Infectious Diseases (Mass Gathering Testing for Coronavirus Disease 2019) (Amendment) Regulations 2021 – Singapore Statutes Online [Internet]. May 7, 2021r. Available from: https://sso.agc.gov.sg/SL-Supp/S310-2021/Published/20210507?DocDate=20210507

The Singapore Government. COVID-19 (Temporary Measures) (Performances and Other Activities – Control Order) (Amendment No. 4) Regulations 2021 – Singapore Statutes Online [Internet]. May 7, 2021s. Available from: https://sso.agc.gov.sg/SL-Supp/S306-2021/Published/ 20210507?DocDate=20210507

The Singapore Government. COVID-19 (Temporary Measures) (Control Order) (Amendment No. 8) Regulations 2021 – Singapore Statutes Online [Internet]. May 14, 2021t. Available from: https://sso .agc.gov.sg/SL-Supp/S329-2021/Published/20210515?DocDate=20210515

The Singapore Government. Infectious Diseases (Mass Gathering Testing for Coronavirus Disease 2019) (Amendment No. 2) Regulations 2021 – Singapore Statutes Online [Internet]. May 14, 2021u. Available from: https://sso.agc.gov.sg/SL-Supp/S324-2021/Published/20210515?DocDate=20210515

The Singapore Government. COVID-19 (Temporary Measures) (Sporting Events and Activities – Control Order) (Amendment No. 2) Regulations 2021 – Singapore Statutes Online [Internet]. May 14, 2021v. Available from: https://sso.agc.gov.sg/SL-Supp/S326-2021/Published/ 20210515?DocDate=20210515

The Singapore Government. COVID-19 (Temporary Measures) (Performances and Other Activities – Control Order) (Amendment No. 5) Regulations 2021 – Singapore Statutes Online [Internet]. May 14, 2021w. Available from: https://sso.agc.gov.sg/SL-Supp/S327-2021/Published/ 20210515?DocDate=20210515

The Singapore Government. COVID-19 (Temporary Measures) (Control Order) (Amendment No. 10) Regulations 2021 – Singapore Statutes Online [Internet]. Jun 11, 2021x. Available from: https://sso .agc.gov.sg/SL-Supp/S371-2021/Published/20210611?DocDate=20210611

The Singapore Government. COVID-19 (Temporary Measures) (Performances and Other Activities – Control Order) (Amendment No. 6) Regulations 2021 – Singapore Statutes Online [Internet]. Jun 11, 2021y. Available from: https://sso.agc.gov.sg/SL-Supp/S370-2021/Published/ 20210611?DocDate=20210611

The Singapore Government. COVID-19 (Temporary Measures) (Sporting Events and Activities – Control Order) (Amendment No. 3) Regulations 2021 – Singapore Statutes Online [Internet]. Jun 11, 2021z. Available from: https://sso.agc.gov.sg/SL-Supp/S369-2021/Published/ 20210611?DocDate=20210611

The Singapore Government. COVID-19 (Temporary Measures) (Performances and Other Activities – Control Order) (Amendment No. 7) Regulations 2021 – Singapore Statutes Online [Internet]. Jun 18, 2021aa. Available from: https://sso.agc.gov.sg/SL-Supp/S378-2021/Published/20210619?DocDate=20210619

The Singapore Government. COVID-19 (Temporary Measures) (Sporting Events and Activities – Control Order) (Amendment No. 4) Regulations 2021 – Singapore Statutes Online [Internet]. Jun 18, 2021ab. Available from: https://sso.agc.gov.sg/SL-Supp/S377-2021/Published/20210619?DocDate=20210619

The Singapore Government. COVID-19 (Temporary Measures) (Control Order) (Amendment No. 12) Regulations 2021 – Singapore Statutes Online [Internet]. 2021ac [cited 2021 Jul 16]. Available from: https://sso.agc.gov.sg/SL-Supp/S508-2021/Published/20210709?DocDate=20210709

The Singapore Government. COVID-19 (Temporary Measures) (Performances and Other Activities –Control Order) (Amendment No. 8) Regulations 2021 – Singapore Statutes Online [Internet]. Jul 9, 2021ad. Available from: https://sso.agc.gov.sg/SL-Supp/S510-2021/Published/20210709?DocDate=20210709

The Singapore Government. COVID-19 (Temporary Measures) (Sporting Events and Activities – Control Order) (Amendment No. 5) Regulations 2021 – Singapore Statutes Online [Internet]. Jul 9, 2021ae. Available from: https://sso.agc.gov.sg/SL-Supp/S511-2021/Published/20210709?DocDate=20210709

The Singapore Government. COVID-19 (Temporary Measures) (Foreign Employee Dormitories – Control Order) (Amendment) Regulations 2021 – Singapore Statutes Online [Internet]. Apr 23, 2021af. Available from: https://sso.agc.gov.sg/SL-Supp/S274-2021/Published/20210423?DocDate=20210423

The Singapore Government. COVID-19 (Temporary Measures) (Foreign Employee Dormitories – Control Order) (Amendment No. 2) Regulations 2021 – Singapore Statutes Online [Internet]. May 15, 2021ag. Available from: https://sso.agc.gov.sg/SL-Supp/S328-2021/Published/20210515?DocDate=20210515

The Straits Times. NUS student facility latest site to be chosen for quarantine. The Straits Times [Internet]. 2020a Jan 27 [cited 2021 Jul 6]; Available from: https://www.straitstimes.com/singapore/nus-student-facility-latest-site-to-be-chosen-for-quarantine

The Straits Times. Coronavirus: Monitoring devices for travellers on stay-home notice outside of facilities do not store personal data or record video, audio. The Straits Times [Internet]. 2020b Aug 4 [cited 2021 Aug 7]; Available from: https://www.straitstimes.com/singapore/devices-do-not-store-personal-data-or-record-video-audio

The Straits Times. Forum: With higher TraceTogether adoption, can alcohol now be served till midnight? The Straits Times [Internet]. 2021c Apr 24 [cited 2021 Jul 6]; Available from: https://www.straitstimes.com/opinion/forum/forum-with-higher-tracetogether-adoption-can-alcohol-now-be-served-till-midnight

Thio L. The Theory and Practice of Judicial Review of Administrative Action in Singapore: Trends and Perspectives. SAL Conf 2011 – Singap Law Dev 2006–2010 [Internet]. 2011 [cited 2021 Jun 23]; Available from: https://www.academia.edu/935298/The_Theory_and_Practice_of_Judicial_Review_of_Administrative_Action_in_Singapore_Trends_and_Perspectives

Thong G, Ooi SP, Araral E, Wu AM. How Singapore is handling the pandemic [Internet]. Policy Forum. 2021 [cited 2021 Jul 5]. Available from: https://www.policyforum.net/how-singapore-is-handling-the-pandemic/

TODAYonline. Punggol, Toh Guan dorms gazetted as 'isolation areas,' almost 20,000 foreign workers under quarantine. TODAYonline [Internet]. 2020a Apr 5 [cited 2021 Jul 14]; Available from:

https://www.todayonline.com/singapore/punggol-toh-guan-dorms-gazetted-isolation-areas-almost-20000-foreign-workers-under

TODAYonline. New dorms with 'better standards' to be built for 100,000 foreign workers in coming years: Lawrence Wong. TODAYonline [Internet]. 2020b Jun 1 [cited 2021 Jul 14]; Available from: https://www.todayonline.com/singapore/new-dorms-better-standards-be-built-100000-foreign-workers-coming-years-lawrence-wong

Toh WL. Coronavirus: Allowing people to visit relatives after June 1 under cautious study. The Straits Times [Internet]. 2020a May 13 [cited 2021 Jul 6]; Available from: https://www.straitstimes.com/singapore/allowing-people-to-visit-relatives-after-june-1-under-cautious-study

Toh TW. More workers in essential services getting tested for Covid-19, Health News & Top Stories – The Straits Times. The Straits Times [Internet]. 2020b Apr 28 [cited 2021 Jul 6]; Available from: https://www.straitstimes.com/singapore/health/more-workers-in-essential-services-getting-tested-for-covid-19

Toh TW. Coronavirus: How rules on social gatherings have changed since circuit breaker. The Straits Times [Internet]. 2020c Jul 22 [cited 2021 Jul 14]; Available from: https://www.straitstimes.com/singapore/health/how-rules-on-social-gatherings-have-changed-since-circuit-breaker

Toh C. Pilot to reopen nightclubs, karaoke joints put on hold amid increase in Covid-19 community cases. The Straits Times [Internet]. 2021a Jan 19 [cited 2021 Jul 7]; Available from: https://www.straitstimes.com/singapore/pilot-plans-to-reopen-nightclubs-and-karaoke-joints-put-on-hold-mti-mha

Toh Z. YouTuber Royce Lee's Spot On Parody Of The Woman Who Refused To Wear A Mask At MBS Is Absolutely Hilarious. TODAYonline [Internet]. 2021b May 18 [cited 2021 Jul 16]; Available from: https://www.8days.sg/sceneandheard/celebrities/youtuber-royce-lee-s-spot-on-parody-of-the-woman-who-refused-to-14833130

Toh TW, Wong L. Firms urged to stagger work hours, let staff work from home. The Straits Times [Internet]. 2020 Mar 14 [cited 2021 Jul 14]; Available from: https://www.straitstimes.com/singapore/firms-urged-to-stagger-work-hours-let-staff-work-from-home

Tortajada C. Water Management in Singapore. *Int J Water Resour Dev.* 2006 Jun 30;22:227–40.

TraceTogether. How do TraceTogether and SafeEntry work together? Is SafeEntry still required since there is TraceTogether? [Internet]. TraceTogether FAQs. 2020 [cited 2021 May 3]. Available from: https://support.tracetogether.gov.sg/hc/en-sg/articles/360052744534-How-do-TraceTogether-and-SafeEntry-work-together-Is-SafeEntry-still-required-since-there-is-TraceTogether-

TraceTogether. I'm home alone – why are there Bluetooth exchanges with other TraceTogether users? [Internet]. TraceTogether FAQs. 2021 [cited 2021 Aug 7]. Available from: https://support.tracetogether.gov.sg/hc/en-sg/articles/360050088633-I-m-home-alone-why-are-there-Bluetooth-exchanges-with-other-TraceTogether-users-

Transient Workers Count Too. Post-Covid law makes migrant workers prisoners of employers [Internet]. TWC2. 2020 [cited 2021 Aug 11]; Available from: http://twc2.org.sg/2020/06/29/post-covid-law-makes-migrant-workers-prisoners-of-employers/

Vaswani K. Coronavirus: The detectives racing to contain the virus in Singapore. BBC News [Internet]. 2020 Mar 19 [cited 2021 Aug 12]; Available from: https://www.bbc.com/news/world-asia-51866102

White Paper on Shared Values (Paper Cmd No 1 of 1991), para 52.

Wong YongQuan B. Data privacy law in Singapore: the Personal Data Protection Act 2012. *Int Data Priv Law.* 2017 Nov 1;7(4):287–302.

Wong L. All foreign workers have to download and activate TraceTogether app by June 19: MOM, Singapore News & Top Stories – The Straits Times. The Straits Times [Internet]. 2020 Jun 16 [cited 2021 Jul 14]; Available from: https://www.straitstimes.com/singapore/all-foreign-workers-have-to-download-and-activate-tracetogether-app-by-june-19-mom

Wong T, Yeoh BSA. 2003 Fertility and the Family: An Overview of Pro-natalist Population Policies in Singapore. ASIAN METACENTRE Res Pap Ser No 12.:27.

Woo JJ. Policy capacity and Singapore's response to the COVID-19 pandemic. *Policy Soc.* 2020 Jul 2;39(3):345–62.

Yap JC-H, Ang IYH, Tan SHX, Chen JI-P, Lewis RF, Yang Q, et al. COVID-19 Science Report: Containment Measures [Internet]. 2020 Feb [cited 2021 Jul 22]. Available from: https://scholarbank .nus.edu.sg/handle/10635/164815

Yea S. This is why Singapore's coronavirus cases are growing: a look inside the dismal living conditions of migrant workers [Internet]. The Conversation. 2020 [cited 2021 Jul 30]; Available from: http://theconversation.com/this-is-why-singapores-coronavirus-cases-are-growing-a-look-inside-the-dismal-living-conditions-of-migrant-workers-136959

Yee K, Peh HP, Tan YP, Teo I, Tan EUT, Paul J, et al. Stressors and coping strategies of migrant workers diagnosed with COVID-19 in Singapore: a qualitative study. *BMJ Open.* 2021 Mar 19;11(3):e045949.

Yeoh B. Bifurcated labour: The unequal incorporation of transmigrants in Singapore. *Tijdschr Voor Econ En Soc Geogr.* 2006 Feb 1;97:26–37.

Yi H, Ng ST, Farwin A, Pei Ting Low A, Chang CM, Lim J. Health equity considerations in COVID-19: geospatial network analysis of the COVID-19 outbreak in the migrant population in Singapore. *J Travel Med [Internet].* 2021 Mar 1 [cited 2021 Jul 22];28(2). Available from: https://doi.org/10.1093/ jtm/taaa159

Yip W, Ge L, Ho AHY, Heng BH, Tan WS. Building community resilience beyond COVID-19: The Singapore way. *Lancet Reg Health – West Pac.* 2021 Feb;7:100091.

Yong M. COVID-19: Jail, fines for employers who do not allow employees to work from home where possible. CNA [Internet]. 2020 Apr 2 [cited 2021 Jul 14]; Available from: https://www .channelnewsasia.com/news/singapore/covid-19-work-from-home-singapore-jail-fines-coronavirus-12602224

Yuen S. More private clinics, labs will be able to do PCR tests, Health News & Top Stories – The Straits Times. The Straits Times [Internet]. 2020 Nov 11 [cited 2021 Jul 6]; Available from: https://www .straitstimes.com/singapore/health/more-private-clinics-labs-will-be-able-to-do-pcr-tests

Zhang J. S'porean doc who sees migrant workers: If we don't look after the weakest link, we all pay the price [Internet]. Mothership. 2020 [cited 2021 Jul 15]. Available from: https://mothership.sg/2020/ 03/singapore-migrant-workers-doctor-covid-19/

Zhang J. S'pore seniors aged 60-69 to get Covid-19 vaccines from end-March 2021 – Mothership.SG – News from Singapore, Asia and around the world. Mothership [Internet]. 2021 Feb 19 [cited 2021 Jul 16]; Available from: https://mothership.sg/2021/02/covid-19-vaccine-seniors/

Zhang Y, Jiang B, Yuan J, Tao Y. The impact of social distancing and epicenter lockdown on the COVID-19 epidemic in mainland China: A data-driven SEIQR model study. 2020. (Preprint).

Section 4

Countries Focused on Fostering Popular Trust in Government, Emphasizing Social Welfare, and Limiting Sanctions and Restrictions

13

Sweden and Covid-19: A (Mainly) Recommendary Approach

Iain Cameron and Anna Jonsson Cornell

Department of Law, Uppsala University, Uppsala, Sweden

13.1 Introduction

This chapter analyzes the Swedish legal frameworks and policy approaches which were taken in order to counter the Covid-19 pandemic in Sweden. We examine, inter alia the social distancing measures that were introduced, testing, contact tracing as well as the Swedish legislators' and Swedish authorities' efforts to balance civil liberties with effective public health measures. The Swedish response to the pandemic has differed from that taken by the majority of other states. This chapter attempts to explain why this is so, and the impact that the constitution and the existing legal framework for dealing with pandemics has had on policy choices in Sweden. For reasons that will be explained in this chapter, Sweden did not declare a constitutional state of emergency. Rather, it largely relied on the ordinary law dealing with contagious diseases and a policy that builds on trust between the authorities and citizens, on the one hand, and between citizens, on the other. Before we move into the constitutional and legal details, we provide a brief description of how events unfolded and the Swedish policies designed to counter the spread of Covid-19.[1]

13.2 Setting the Stage – The Initial Swedish Response to the Pandemic

The World Health Organization (WHO) declared the pandemic on March 11 2020.[2] More than a month before the WHO-statement, the Swedish Government had classified the SARS-Cov2 virus as "dangerous to society" (2 February 2020), which meant that all the mandatory measures provided by the Swedish Contagious Diseases Prevention Act (*Smittskyddslagen*, 2004:168, hereinafter, SSL) could be used. However, the main Swedish policy response was to rely upon recommendations and voluntary measures. There are several explanations for this approach. Above all, it is necessary to recognize the decisive role played by the responsible administrative agency, the Public Health Authority (*Folkhälsomyndigheten*, FHM). FHM early on took the view that responding to the virus

---

1 We should note that we have written previously about this issue, inter alia in "Dealing with Covid-19 in Sweden", in J. Grogan and A. Donald (eds), *The Routledge Handbook on Law and the COVID-19 Pandemic*, August 2021.
2 https://www.who.int/director-general/speeches/detail/who-director-general-s-opening-remarks-at-the-media-briefing-on-covid-19---11-march-2020, last accessed on 11 August 2021.

Impacts of the Covid-19 Pandemic: International Laws, Policies, and Civil Liberties, First Edition. Edited by Nadav Morag.
© 2023 John Wiley & Sons, Inc. Published 2023 by John Wiley & Sons, Inc.

would be a marathon rather than a sprint and that in order for measures to be sustainable they needed to be voluntary, and considered relevant and proportionate by the public.

The Swedish strategy, formulated by FHM, was containment, not eradication of the virus. Achieving herd immunity was not FHM's official policy, although there is much that indicates that this was the underlying idea. FHM considered that effective vaccines would not be available for a while, and the virus was not likely to be fatal for the large majority of the population. The main priority was thus stated to be the protection of the elderly over the age of 70 and other risk groups. FHM issued recommendations to the public to maintain social distancing, especially in all public places and on public transport, and underlined the importance of everyone taking a personal responsibility not to spread contagion, so as to ensure that hospital services (particularly the limited number of intensive care beds) were not overwhelmed. Employers were requested to ask workers, where possible, to work from home. No shops, gyms, or other businesses were ordered to be closed (this power at the time was not part of SSL), but licensed premises (restaurants, bars, etc.) were only to allow table service and all businesses were requested to take steps to reduce overcrowding.[3] A raft of economic measures was adopted speedily by the government, providing for financial support to businesses, particularly to furlough employees.[4] Some local authorities introduced a ban on visiting care homes. This was later – too late according to some critics – supplemented by a national ban issued by the government, acting under the SSL.

Anonymized metadata surveys of mobile phones showed that there was a high level of compliance with the work at home and social distancing recommendations.[5] A significant part of the Swedish economy is employed in "white collar" work, and most such businesses switched relatively effectively to distance working. The economic support provided to businesses meant that large employers in different industries (vehicle production, etc.) were able to furlough employees. Nonetheless, the virus spread quickly in March and April of 2020, particularly in Stockholm. There appear to be several reasons for this. Many Swedes had been abroad during the winter break (end of February), on skiing and other holidays. FHM had not, however, made any recommendations on self-isolation of returning holiday-makers. Although WHO recommended extensive testing and tracking, FHM considered this of limited use with the argument that the virus had already reached the pandemic stage. Moreover, the regions – which had the physical capabilities and responsibilities to organize testing and tracing – considered they had insufficient resources to do so, and therefore saw this as a low priority. Elderly people in care homes, who are the frailest section of society, usually over 85 and generally in poor health, began dying in large numbers.[6] Particularly significant here is the fact that the Swedish workforce for elderly care is drawn partly from part-time workers from socially deprived areas, which have high levels of crowded accommodation and intergenerational living. Part-time workers did not have security of tenure, and so there were incentives to go to work even if they suspected they might be infected. Moreover, in these areas many people work in small businesses and service professions and could not easily go over to distance work. As a consequence, these areas have suffered disproportionally from the pandemic.

---

3 This was originally in the form of recommendations, backed up by a coercive power to shut, temporarily, premises.
4 Some 400 government decisions were registered between February and September 2020, many of which concerned economic measures Agency for Public Management, (*Statskontoret*), *Förvaltningsmodellen under coronapandemin*, 2020.
5 See statistics provided by the FHM at https://www.folkhalsomyndigheten.se/smittskydd-beredskap/utbrott/ aktuella-utbrott/covid-19/statistik-och-analyser/analys-och-prognoser/rapport-om-rorelse--och-resematt/, last accessed on 26 October 2021.
6 Another explanation advanced by FHM for the relatively high death rates of the elderly was the fact that the previous years' influenza death rates had been unusually low in Sweden.

Another important factor in the initial high death rate in Sweden was the lack of protective personal equipment (PPE), and, initially, of reliable quick tests for staff working in care homes, and for those providing meals and cleaning for elderly still living in their own homes. As is now known, people infected with Sars-Cov2 may not have significant symptoms, and the virus can also be transmissible before a person develops symptoms. At the beginning of the crisis, almost all regions and municipalities did not have a sufficient contingency stock of PPE despite having a legal duty to prepare for emergencies.[7] However, the law provides for no central supervisory powers to check that the municipalities and regions are fulfilling their duties in this regard, and does not impose any sanctions.

Testing and contact tracing were introduced after the summer of 2020. The regions had refused to take the costs of testing people other than hospital personnel, since they did not consider it to be health care as defined in the legislation. The regions only agreed to introduce large-scale testing and tracking when the government agreed to underwrite the costs of this. As is well known, a "second wave"[8] of the virus hit many states during the autumn of 2020. In Sweden, deaths peaked again in November 2020. Intensive care facilities were badly stretched, but not overwhelmed. However, health-care workers were (very understandably) showing signs of fatigue.

Public confidence in FHM had been relatively high during the first nine months of 2020 but it began to fall thereafter, presumably because FHM had predicted that the most likely scenario during the autumn was local outbreaks of the virus, not the widespread outbreak which actually occurred. The government began introducing a number of binding and nonbinding measures, such as early closing of restaurants and recommending wearing of masks on public transport during peak hours even though FHM had earlier considered these to be of questionable value. The WHO was from the outset clear on the importance of testing, contact tracing, and isolation of contagious individuals. For reasons that will be elaborated below, testing and contact tracing failed at the beginning of the pandemic in Sweden. This together with social and economic factors contributed to the spread of the disease in Sweden and the dire consequences it had for the most vulnerable part of the population living on elderly care facilities.

13.3 The Constitutional Context

The first thing which can be noted here as regards the Swedish constitutional context is that there is no provision in the Swedish constitution for the declaration of a state of emergency in peacetime, only in war or where there is an imminent danger of war (RF Chapter 15).[9] Nor is there a general law on public emergencies. There are two main explanations for this, the first being Sweden's peaceful history (200 years without a war), the second being Sweden's parliamentary system and the primacy given to the parliament in the constitution.[10] Instead, the Swedish crisis management systems rest on the idea of "anticipatory statutorification," which means that emergency provisions in sector-specific statutes (covering accidents, natural disasters, etc.) provide delegations to the government to exercise certain powers (and to subdelegate these to administrative agencies) as well

---

7 Health and Hospital Care Act (2017:30) Chapter 7, section 2, Act (2006:544) on local authorities' and regions' measures before and during extraordinary events in peacetime, Chapter 2, section 1. References to statutes and ordinances in force, Svensk författningssamling, SFS, are by year and statute/ordinance number.

8 References to "waves" can be misleading, as it can refer to mutations of the virus.

9 A Jonsson Cornell, J Salminen, "Emergency laws in comparative constitutional law," German Law Journal, 233–249 (2019).

10 A commission of inquiry recommended including provisions for peacetime emergencies, but the political parties thought that there was no reason to change the present system. Proposition [Bill] 2009/10:80, En reformerad grundlag, 207.

as powers and responsibilities for regional and local authorities. The terms used for describing when these embedded provisions can be triggered vary considerably ("war," "heightened preparedness," "serious peacetime crisis," etc.) as do the thresholds for triggering these powers.[11] Where these sector-specific regulations turn out to be inadequate, the solution is to rely upon the parliament's willingness and capacity to act swiftly when needed (called *konstitutionell beredskap* "constitutional readiness") and enact new powers.

Second, Sweden has collective rather than ministerial government,[12] and central public administration is performed by semiautonomous administrative agencies. These agencies have a duty to obey government directives (RF 12:1) as long as such directives do not involve the application and interpretation of the law in specific cases (RF 12:2). This means, among other things, that individual ministers cannot order their department and/or administrative agencies to take certain measures. This also applies in a time of crisis. However, administrative agencies can be generally steered by the government (as a collective) in a number of different ways, for example by ordinances which specify in more detail statutory requirements, by budgetary means, by setting goals that the administrative agency is expected to meet, etc. Importantly, when it comes to handling a crisis like the pandemic, the bulk of specialist knowledge is in the administrative agencies and the regions rather than the (small) government departments. In addition, administrative authorities are not in any hierarchical position vis-a-vis one another except in cases where they are specifically given oversight or appeal functions. This constitutional setting has created a culture in which ministers and political leadership in general, tend to have a "hands-off" approach toward the agencies which are under the supervision and control of their departments, reacting only when problems with political dimensions emerge. During the pandemic, politicians have constantly referred to the need to follow the advice of their "expert administrative agencies." In normal times, the Swedish system of governance has a number of advantages. It can prevent political partisanship, improve transparency, and foster rational and effective administration. However, in a situation of a peace time crisis it runs the risk, at least in the short term, of being a slow, inefficient, and fragmentized system of governance, where no one takes a holistic responsibility. It was clear to the Swedish public that the FHM was the main actor, but according to the Swedish administrative model, administrative agencies do not answer either to the public, or politicians when it comes to decisions in individual cases and interpretation of laws. This might be perceived as the democratic chain of representation being broken, but the system is more complicated. Ultimately, it is the politicians who set the legal and economic frame for the agencies.

Third, to this should be added that the bulk of the public services for schooling, elderly care, and social services in general are delivered by the 290 local authorities (*kommuner*) and, in the areas of transport, hospitals and primary public health care, by 20 county regional authorities (*regioner*). Moreover, regional and local self-governance is part of the constitution.[13] This is, however, not a residual competence, such as that provided for by the Tenth Amendment to the US Constitution. It rather expresses a constitutional convention, resting on the idea of subsidiarity, which means that central government should not interfere in local autonomy without good reason.[14] Each local and regional authority has an elected assembly from which the governing body is chosen. They

---

11 Some 16 different terms have been identified, J Hirschfeld, O Petersson, *Rättsregler i kris* (Diagolos, 2020).
12 See RF 7:3. References to the Swedish constitution, the Instrument of Government (*Regeringsformen*, RF), are to chapter and section number. For details, see T Bull, I Cameron, "Sweden," in A von Bogdandy, (ed), *Ius Publicum Europaeum - Constitutional Foundations, Evolution and Gestalt of European Constitutions*, forthcoming, https://papers.ssrn.com/sol3/papers.cfm?abstract_id=3782353.
13 The constitution provides that restrictions made by the parliament in local authority autonomy "*ought* not to go further than are necessary" (RF 14:3) (our emphasis).
14 MPs in the parliament are often drawn from the ranks of local politicians, and there is considerable reluctance to legislate against the wishes of the collective of local authorities, even if it is clear that it is the parliament which has

thus have their own democratic legitimacy. Many of the tasks of regional and local authorities are nonetheless regulated to a greater or lesser extent in national statutes. There are also, in the areas of schooling, health care, and care of the elderly, national supervisory bodies, which can receive complaints from the public. During the early 1990s, a wave of deregulation of public services occurred and some public services, in education, primary health care, and care of the elderly, are nowadays provided by private actors which have been procured by the local or regional authorities. Local authorities vary widely in size, as well as population, the largest being Stockholm. Thus, the Swedish public service system, including health-care services, is heavily decentralized which in a time of crisis brings considerable challenges.

Fourth, the Swedish system for crisis management can be described as collaborative instead of hierarchical. It is guided by three principles: (i) responsibility, (ii) parity, and (iii) proximity.[15] Sweden thus differs from many other countries which have a more hierarchical and centralized approach to emergencies. This decentralized approach is in fact relatively new for Sweden. During the Cold War, when the main threat was perceived as nuclear war and/or invasion from the Soviet Union, Sweden had parallel command structures for civil defense where decision-making power over most issues, including law and order, in the event of a crisis were to be devolved to regional governors.[16] This system was abandoned following the end of the Cold War. Instead, the idea, now referred to as the principle of responsibility was developed. It means that the actor responsible for a given activity under normal conditions should also be responsible for that activity during a crisis. This is based on the position that it is difficult to shift a modern networked administration into a hierarchical and centralized command and control mode in the event of a crisis.[17] Where coping with a crisis involves several local authorities and/or administrative agencies, these are expected to cooperate with each other and sectoral legislation seldom provides for a "lead" agency, giving it control over other agencies. The disadvantage with the collaborative process is that it can be time-consuming, and that it can be unclear, both to the public and to the administrative agencies involved, who has the main responsibility. It can also impair initiative-taking, as administrative agencies, and local authorities, tend to resist taking on new responsibilities which they consider lie outside of their primary mandate, or if they involve increasing costs (even if within their primary mandate). The multiplicity of actors on different levels, including even private actors means that responsibility can become very diffuse, and thus there can also be problems afterward in seeking accountability for action or inaction. For example, as pointed out above, the regions, but also local authorities, failed to secure sufficient stocks of PPE during the first part of 2020, which undoubtedly contributed to the initial high death toll in Sweden among the elderly. Maintaining stockpiles of equipment and having regular cooperative/integrated training exercises cost money, and this is easily deprioritized in times of budget restraints. The parity principle follows on from the responsibility principle and provides that, as far as possible, the same structures, resources, and organization of activities should apply as applied under normal conditions. The proximity principle provides that a crisis should primarily be handled where it occurs, by those who are (geographically) closest to it.

the final word (see, e.g. U. Strandberg, "Kommunal självstyre," in I Mattson, O Petersson (eds), *Svensk författningspolitik*, 5th ed., Studentlitteratur, 2020).

15 P Bergling, M Wimelius, J Engberg, M Naarttijärvi, E Wennerström, *Krisen, myndigheterna och lagen: Krishantering i rättens gränsland* (Gleerups, 2015).

16 For the historical background, see Swedish Defence College, *Förutsättningar för krisberedskap och totalförsvar i Sverige*, 2019.

17 P Becker, F Bynander, "The System for Crisis Management in Sweden: Collaborative, Conformist, Contradictory," in CN Madu & C-H Kuei (eds), *Handbook of Disaster Risk Reduction and Management* (World Scientific Publishing, Singapore, 2017).

There is a central government agency tasked with the function of preparing for civil contingencies (*Myndigheten för samhällsskydd och beredskap*, MSB). MSB has a limited operative capability, it functions primarily as a supporting and coordinating body for local authorities and government agencies which have more primary responsibilities in dealing with crises, e.g. by maintaining depots for supplies and equipment for dealing with natural disasters (pumps, fire-fighting equipment, tents, etc.). MSB warned, at an early stage, of the need for regions and local authorities to secure much greater supplies of PPE, but these warnings appear to have been largely ignored.[18] It has no epidemiological competence, and the role it has played in the Covid-19 pandemic has been both limited and diffuse.

In conclusion, the Swedish constitutional context for handling peace time crisis is characterized by constitutional silence on peace time emergencies, anticipatory statutorification, a fragmentized, decentralized, and nonhierarchical system for providing public services, and a decentralized crisis management system which relies on collaboration between the involved actors.

13.4 The Legislative Procedure, Delegation of Powers, and Rights Protection

The fact that the Swedish constitution is silent on peace time crisis means that the ordinary legislative procedure as a main rule applies also during a crisis. In general, an emergency that is characterized by quickly changing circumstances, the need for fairly drastic measures, flexibility and speed, often entails shifting regulatory power from the parliament to the government. In the Swedish context, provision for such shifting of regulatory powers in both normal and crisis situations is made in sectoral legislation. However, one of the challenges with this approach is that not all forms of crisis and emergencies can be predicted. In order to handle such unpredicted circumstances, or needs, the legislative procedure can be speeded up, although this undoubtedly affects the quality of the procedure and the product, i.e. the statute.

RF Chapter 8 § 2 contains a list of areas of law which as a main rule requires regulation by statute. Among these areas are civil law, criminal law, and procedural law. Moreover, in principle, any public law norms entailing obligations for natural or legal persons vis-a-vis the state must also be in the form of statute (RF 8:2 p. 2), as must rules concerning the basic structure and competence of local and regional authorities (RF 8:2 p. 3). However, in both these areas, RF 8:3 provides that the parliament may, by statute, delegate power to the government to issue ordinances (*förordningar*). Moreover, parliament may authorize the government to subdelegate this power to administrative agencies or local authorities (RF 8:10). Where a statute provides for subdelegation, only fines, not imprisonment, can be provided for as a penalty for breaches of that subdelegated rule. Under RF 8:7 and 8:11, the government also has an independent power to issue ordinances in areas not specifically reserved for statutes and may subdelegate this power to administrative agencies.

The Swedish system for preparation of laws is good in international comparison in that the government is required by the constitution to consult administrative agencies and local authorities when preparing new statutes. Moreover, other actors such as civil society organizations, the bar association, law faculties, etc., frequently submit their opinions on drafts, and these opinions are taken into consideration. Proposals for legislation are either made by public commissions of inquiry or come from within a department (often borrowing expertise from an administrative agency). In both cases, the proposal is published and time is given for consultation with a variety of public

---

18 KU hearing with Dan Eliasson 26 March, 2021. https://www.riksdagen.se/sv/sa-funkar-riksdagen/riksdagens-uppgifter/kontrollerar-regeringen/ku-utfragningar-om-granskningsarenden-2021/.

bodies and civil society (a requirement in the constitution, RF 7:2). Draft laws are also submitted to the Council on Legislation that consists of judges temporarily seconded from the Supreme Court and the Supreme Administrative Court. The Council checks the constitutionality of the proposal and performs a quality control function over it (RF 8:22).[19] The constitutionally protected principle of access to official documents, together with a constitutional requirement to prepare adequately governmental decisions (including statutes) means that the Swedish legislative procedure and policy making in general have a high level of transparency.[20] The emphasis in the Swedish system is firmly on avoiding conflict of norms and difficulties in the interpretation and application of the law by preparing laws well in the first place. The Swedish courts – all the Swedish courts – have a power of judicial review (RF 11:14), but in practice this has been used sparingly.[21]

Acts of parliament (statutes) are generally necessary to limit constitutional rights. The rights most relevant during the Covid-19 pandemic are the freedoms of assembly (RF 2:1, p. 3) and demonstration (RF 2:1 p. 4), freedom of movement (RF 2:8), the protection of personal integrity and against arbitrary detention (RF 2:6), and the right to protection of private property (RF 2:15). These are all relative rights which can be limited by statute (RF 2:20-24). For all of these rights, necessity and proportionality tests apply. The Swedish courts apply the three parts of the "classic" proportionality: namely effectiveness or suitability, necessity in the sense of the least intrusive means, and proportionality stricto sensu, i.e. the balancing of what can be gained against the intrusion it entails into protected interests. The material content of the right of property is formulated narrowly, and limitations are easier to justify, but also here a proportionality test has to be satisfied. For some rights, limitations may only be made for specific purposes stated in the constitution. The freedoms of assembly and demonstration are two such rights. In these cases, such a specific purpose includes measures to combat an epidemic (RF 2:24). Sweden has ratified the ECHR, which is also fully incorporated into Swedish law by statute. This has had an important impact on the interpretation of Swedish constitutional law and the protection of rights in particular. It has also contributed to strengthening the principle of proportionality as a general constitutional principle. Overall, the role of courts has been fortified when it comes to rights protection due to the impact of binding European human rights law.

13.5 The Public Health Agency and the Act on Protection Against Contagious Diseases

As noted in the Introduction, FHM has had a dominant role in determining the Swedish response to the Covid-19 pandemic. FHM has a general mandate to promote better public health. Until recently, Sweden had a specialist epidemiological agency, the Institute of Prevention of Contagious Diseases in addition to FHM. In 2014, this agency was amalgamated with FHM. FHM thus has the main responsibility to follow epidemiological developments, prescribe or recommend measures to be taken in the event of an epidemic, and advise the government on what other measures might be necessary. The other agency in the area of health care, the National Board of Health and Welfare (*Socialstyrelsen*), was left with more general standard-setting functions, and a new body, the Health and Social Care Inspectorate (*Inspection för vård och omsorg*, IVO) was created to receive complaints

---

19 See generally T Bull, "Judges without a court: judicial preview in Sweden," in T Campbell, K Ewing, A Tomkins (eds) *The Legal Protection of Human Rights; Sceptical Essays*, (OUP, 2011).
20 See, e.g. T Bull, I Cameron, "Legislative review for human rights compatibility: a view from Sweden," in M. Hunt, H.J. Hooper, and PW Yowell, *Parliaments and Human Rights: Redressing the Democratic Deficit*, (Hart, 2015).
21 Ibid.

and make inspections of health care and elderly care facilities. There were two consequences of these institutional changes as far as epidemiology was concerned. Although FHM is bound by its instruction to base any measures it might take on scientific research, the close link which the previous Institute had with academic research in epidemiology, virology, and immunology was de-prioritized. The second consequence was that all nonacademic expertise in epidemiology was concentrated in a single agency, and that this agency was given both operative (prescribing) and advisory functions.

As previously mentioned, the main legislation applicable to prevent the spreading of Covid-19 is the Act on Protection Against Contagious Diseases (SSL). According to the SSL, all measures taken should build on science, be evidence based and proportional, as well as respect the principle of equality and protect the personal integrity of individuals (SSL 1:4). Under SSL 2:1, all individuals have a responsibility to take measures to avoid infecting others. SSL imposes a duty on each health region to appoint a "prevention of contagion" doctor (*smittskyddsläkare*) with the powers to inter alia order quarantine of infected people (SSL 3:9) or *smaller* areas (e.g. a household or block) where the disease is spreading, and the source of the disease or the level of contagion unknown (SSL 3:10). Chapter 5 of the SSL regulates isolation of individuals who are contagious. A decision to order isolation of an individual is taken by the administrative court upon a request by the prevention of contagion doctor. Administrative courts deal only with matters of public law and when there is a dispute between an individual/company and (local and state) administrative agencies. In extreme cases, thus, individuals can be subjected to mandatory isolation. Individuals subject to such decisions have a right to judicial review. However, the Act places emphasis firmly on the human rights of people who are, or are suspected, of being contagious. It is apparent from the travaux préparatoires to the SSL that the Act was influenced by the view that the measures adopted to counter the spread of HIV-Aids were an overreaction, and at times, not in accordance with human freedom and personal integrity.[22] SSL further provides that the government, or the administrative agency specified by the government, may issue the additional regulations required for an effective protection against contagion and for the protection of individuals (SSL 9:4). The government has subdelegated this authority to FHM.[23]

The government's classification of the SARS-Cov2 virus as "dangerous to society" on 2 February 2020 meant that all the measures, including quarantine and isolation provisions, available in the SSL could be put in use. Quarantine, testing, and contract tracing was not, however, used in the beginning of the pandemic. People who suspected they were ill were simply requested to stay at home. In this context, it should also be noted that prevention of contagion doctors have the legal authority to examine and if needed quarantine individuals that enter Sweden from a country with widespread contagious diseases (SSL 3:8, 9). These powers have not, to our knowledge, been used in Sweden in relation to Covid-19. Sweden did, however, introduce entry requirements for non-EU residents in March 2020, and for non-Swedish citizens and residents in December 2020. These remained in force until March 2022, in different forms, and imposing different requirements on citizens and residents in the Nordic states, EU states, and other states. In conclusion, the SSL does not provide for explicit powers to isolate healthy people, to protect them from contagion, or for a general and total lockdown.[24]

---

22 Prop. 2003/04:30 Ny Smittskyddslag. In this respect, it can be noted that another important historical experience which has influenced the restrained Swedish response was the Swine Flu (H1N1) epidemic in 2009. To contain Swine Flu, Sweden embarked on a mass vaccination programme, which was by many seen as an overreaction to what was a mild virus. Although this programme probably saved some lives, a relatively large number of people (perhaps as much as 4,000, many of them young) suffered life-long side effects from the vaccine.
23 Smittskyddsförordning (2004:255) section 12.
24 It states only that "In a "peacetime crisis that has a significant impact on the possibilities of maintaining effective infection protection" the government may issue "other measures" if "there is a need for coordinated

Another factor which should be mentioned here is that the Swedish state can be described as having a low coercive capacity. Police numbers per head of population in Sweden, indeed in all the Nordic states, are comparatively low. Sweden also has a small army and a small territorial army/national guard. This makes it, practically speaking, difficult to impose a drastic lockdown, unless such a measure is generally perceived by the population as legitimate.

13.6   Legal Measures Taken to Counter the Spread of Covid-19

The picture given in the media in some countries that Sweden imposed no restrictions at all is not accurate. Early on, the existing powers under the Public Order Act (*Ordningslagen*, 1993:1617, OL) allowing restrictions as to the number of participants in public meetings and events (including religious services) were put to use.[25] Initially the limit was set to 500 people, later on 29 March 2020, the number was set to 50 and on 24 November 2020, the number was reduced to eight people. In February 2020, universities and high schools were ordered to go over to remote teaching. Nurseries and primary/lower secondary schools (ages 6–15) were kept open on the basis that the risks the virus posed to children were relatively small, and counterbalanced by the major disruption that this would entail for society, particularly for essential workers with small children. As schools fall within the area of competence of local authorities, authorization to the government to close high schools required the parliament to enact, quickly, a temporary Act (SFS 2020:148). This Act granted the government this power, which was framed more generally to include, if necessary in the future, also closing nurseries, basic schools, and other learning facilities, as well as for ordering provision for day care/schooling of the children of essential workers. Interestingly, and a good illustration of the lack of Swedish preparedness for emergencies generally, there were no such pre-existing lists of categories of essential workers. Eventually, MSB produced such lists, although as schools were never shut, these did not have to enter into force.

However, the powers under OSL only applied to public meetings and public events. There were no powers generally to close down, or regulate, the public space generally (parks, etc.). Nor were there any powers to regulate private gatherings (e.g. parties in a person's house).

On 4 April 2020, the government submitted to the parliament, in great haste, an amending bill to the SSL providing for certain temporary executive powers to issue ordinances to close or regulate malls, venues, and transportation.[26] The proposal was simultaneously sent for consultation for a very short – 24 hours – period, to a considerable limited number of public bodies. The bill was not considered to unduly infringe upon constitutional rights. The Council of legislation made constructive proposals for amendments, including the need to submit subsequently any ordinances adopted immediately to the parliament for approval. The parliament's Committee on the Constitution (Konstitutionsutskottet, KU), to which bills raising constitutional issues are referred, stated that the power to issue government ordinances only be exercised where there was a clear need for speed in each particular case and that the government must always make a proportionality assessment when issuing ordinances. The government accepted all the concrete criticisms made and reformulated the provisions accordingly. This procedure illustrates that "constitutional preparedness" actually works.

---

national measures or from a national perspective of other specific measures in the field of infection protection" (SSL 9:6). In some countries, such a vague general power might be seen as sufficient to take sweeping measures, in a crisis but not in Sweden.

25 OL 2:15. (SFS 2020:114), (SFS 2020:115).
26 Prop. 2019/20:155. SFS 2020:241.

However, after having forced through this amendment, the new powers were never used. This can probably be put down to FHM's preference for voluntary measures, and the fact that voluntary measures were having a clear effect, even if there were still relatively high rates of infection in society. These new provisions in SSL expired on 30 June 2020.

This date also saw the government appointment of a commission of inquiry, the "Corona Commission."[27] The government initially wished to leave all issues of accountability until after the pandemic was over. However, the opposition parties insisted on the appointment of an independent inquiry headed by a retired senior judge, rather than a parliamentary inquiry. Bearing in mind the fact that responsibility for the pandemic response is split between central, regional, and local government, this was sensible. The Corona Commission was given a very large number of factual and policy issues to consider, and was tasked to submit two partial reports and its final report by February 2022, seven months before the next parliamentary election.[28]

In November, the government used an existing delegation in the Alcohol Act (2010:1622) to forbid the selling of alcohol in licensed premises after 20.00. Shortly after, in December 2020, a new bill was also submitted to parliament, again in a hurry, supplementing the SSL and containing more far-reaching powers (compared to the changes made in April). The new Covid-19 Act (2021:4) was adopted on 8 January 2021, and entered into force on 10 January. The Covid-19 Act is a temporary law, and it was originally supposed to apply until the end of September 2021. On 12 August 2021, the government proposed that the Act be prolonged to the end of January 2022.[29] The Act finally expired in March 2022. The Covid-19 Act gave the government powers to regulate shopping malls, gyms, and public transport. Moreover, powers were given to ban spontaneous private assemblies in specified areas, and to shut off access to parks and similar public spaces, where such powers are proportional and there are objective grounds for fearing that social distancing guidelines cannot or will not be upheld. These powers, both to issue rules and to take decisions in individual cases, could be delegated to administrative agencies and local authorities, opening up for potential problems of legal certainty. However, the new powers stopped short of banning access to all public places. The law provided for administrative fines up to 2000 SKR (200 Euros) for violations of regulations issued under the law. Figures are not yet available on how often the fines have been imposed, but these have been relatively rare. We analyze the Swedish legal measures from the perspective of rule of law indicators below.

13.7 Vaccination and Exit Strategies

Deaths declined in Sweden even before the vaccination program was rolled out in the beginning of 2021. However, infection levels remained at a moderately high level. Vaccination priorities are by age group, something which is facilitated by the fact that all Swedish citizens and residents have a unique personal identification number. Groups especially at medical risk, together with hospital and care personnel received priority.[30] Following scares during the spring of serious side effects with the Astra Zeneca vaccine (albeit extremely rare), FHM decided that this vaccine should only be given to people over 65 years old. The regions are responsible for handling vaccination, again with financial support from central government. Vaccination is not mandatory, though historically speaking, Sweden was one of the countries which made vaccination mandatory for a variety of

---

27 Coronakommissionen dir. 2020:74.
28 Sverige under pandemin, SOU 2022:10.
29 Prop 2020/21:219. The government proposed in August 2021 to renew the period of validity of the law to the end of January 2022, but there was insufficient support for this in the Riksdag.
30 School teachers unions protested several times about the fact that they were not given priority, but there were no strikes called.

illnesses. It is generally recognized that Sweden has high levels of trust and social capital,[31] and a consequence of this is high levels of voluntary vaccination. There has been little discussion, so far, of introducing measures for those refusing to vaccinate themselves, e.g. by limiting their right to visit restaurants or use public transport. Sweden has largely avoided the anti-vaccination protests which have occurred during the summer of 2021 in countries such as France. This is not to say that there are no problems in Sweden. Vaccination skepticism has increased and the negative experience of narco-epilepsy following the general vaccination program for swine influenza has had an effect. Available figures up to 20 August 2021 indicate levels of over 80% (first dose) and 60% (both doses) in the country as a whole.[32] Statistics which differentiate on the basis of ethnicity are not available in Sweden, but some indications can be obtained by comparing vaccination rates from area to area, and they appear to be much lower (c. 60%) in poorer (immigrant dominated) areas,[33] something which is causing frustration particularly in medical staff working in intensive care.[34]

It would be constitutionally possible to introduce some vaccination "carrots and sticks" policies in Sweden. The right to personal integrity (RF 2:6) is a relative right, and it can be limited by statute, assuming that the proportionality test is satisfied, which in turn requires objective scientific justification. Such justification is easier to provide for some situations than others. One could, for example, contemplate a mandatory vaccination requirement for (continued) employment as a caregiver in a care home for the elderly. It is likely that some private care homes, in particular, wanted to introduce such a requirement for its staff. This would be easier to introduce for new rather than existing staff. Dismissing an employee for refusing to take vaccine would be more difficult, because the employer would have to show that this new requirement was reasonable, and there were no alternative tasks (not involving contact with the elderly) which the employee could perform. In Sweden, such terms of employment issues have traditionally been left to collective negotiations between the trade unions and employers' associations. The unions are likely to oppose introducing such requirements by means of legislation. With the omikron variant being so contagious, the debate on whether or not to introduce some element of compulsion largely disappeared.

With increased vaccination availability from March 2021, and a relatively efficient level of vaccination, Sweden began "opening up." Beginning in 1 June, licensing hours for establishments selling alcohol were extended to 22.00, later to 24.00. The new regulations differentiated between different types of public meetings as regards to the dangers they are presumed to pose for the spreading of the virus. Permitted numbers of participants in public meetings and events were increased.[35] All restrictions were finally removed in March 2022.

13.8 Putting the Swedish Soft Power Strategy in Context

As already noted, it is incorrect to say that there were no restrictions at all in operation in Sweden. Nonetheless, it is evident that Sweden, for most of 2020, put most of its faith in voluntary measures. Even after November 2020, when more legally binding measures were introduced, the policy was still largely based on recommendations and voluntary measures, with the legal powers being used

---

31 At least according to the World Values Survey, www.worldvaluessurvey.org, and the Gothenburg-based Quality of Government project, https://www.gu.se/en/quality-government.
32 https://www.folkhalsomyndigheten.se/folkhalsorapportering-statistik/statistikdatabaser-och-visualisering/vaccinationsstatistik/statistik-for-vaccination-mot-covid-19/. More recent figures are 71% with three doses, https://covid19-country-overviews.ecdc.europa.eu/countries/Sweden.html#vaccine-uptake.
33 See, e.g. https://www.svt.se/nyheter/lokalt/stockholm/farre-an-40-procent-har-vaccinerat-sig-i-alby-bland-65-plussare.
34 See e.g. Dagens Nyheter, 1 September 2021.
35 Socialdepartementet PM S2021/05005.

as "back-up." The other Nordic states epidemiological agencies initially had a similar policy of containment,[36] as did, for example, the United Kingdom. However, in all these states, politicians abandoned this policy, in the United Kingdom after the publication of the Imperial College study indicating that as many as 500,000 people in the United Kingdom could die of Covid-19.[37] Sweden did not. There are various explanations for this. The first, and most important, is that FHM did not consider that the death rates would be nearly as high as 1% of the population.[38] In other countries, either the government believed these much higher estimates, or considered that it should be on the safe side, or considered that even lower levels of excess mortality justified taking more sweeping, lockdown, measures.

The Swedish government did not overrule its epidemiological agency, FHM. Why not? The main reason is the Swedish governmental culture of indirect leadership and the hands-off approach described above. To this should be added the lack of sweeping powers in the existing legal framework which could be put into operation without parliamentary approval. Of course, it would have been possible for the government to ask the parliament for new powers, as happened in both Norway and Denmark (Finland already had powers under the constitution and statute to declare a state of emergency). But the balance of political power in the parliament probably affected the government's decision. There was no guarantee that the parliament would give the minority government new powers, especially if these were sweeping.[39]

In times of national crisis, Swedish politicians have traditionally sought consensus, and at least during the first nine months of 2020, the leaders of all the political parties were united behind the "soft" approach. Besides, more cynically, the "china shop" rule would apply to any attempt by the government to change the policy (i.e. if you break it, it's yours). FHM, with the State Epidemiologist as a leading figure, was unequivocally, and publicly, against shutting down society. The State Epidemiologist, in fact, famously expressed the view that the rest of the world seemed to have gone mad.[40] If the government disagreed, it would have to take responsibility for acting against its expert administrative agency. In April 2020, a group of academics in epidemiology and related disciplines had expressed harsh criticism of FHM's predictions and policies. They advocated some sort of shut down to win time, particularly for PPE and testing and tracing resources to be built up, and in order to understand better how the virus was spreading and how it could be countered, epidemiologically and medically.[41] There was, however, no consensus in the academic community,[42] and as noted above, the Swedish government had no other public agency expertise besides the FHM to rely upon.[43] Unlike, e.g. the United Kingdom or the United States, there is no post of "chief medical/scientific officer" to the government. FHM's broader mandate to promote public

---

36 See the report to the Danish Parliament, Folketinget, *Håndteringen af covid-19 i foråret 2020 – Rapport afgivet af den af Folketingets Udvalg for Forretningsordenen nedsatte udredningsgruppe vedr. håndteringen af covid-19*, January 2021.

37 NM Ferguson, D Laydon, G Nedjati-Gilani et al. "Impact of non-pharmaceutical interventions (NPIs) to reduce COVID-19 mortality and healthcare demand." https://www.imperial.ac.uk/media/imperial-college/medicine/sph/ide/gida-fellowships/Imperial-College-COVID19-NPI-modelling-16-03-2020.pdf, 16 March 2020, (1 December 2020).

38 F Anderberg, *Flocken* (Bonniers, Stockholm 2021).

39 At the present time, the Swedish government is a minority government consisting of a coalition between the Social Democratic and Green parties, ruling with the tacit support of three other parties.

40 https://sverigesradio.se/artikel/7501940.

41 Published in the newspaper Dagens Nyheter, 14 April 2020.

42 The independent Royal Academy of Sciences (KvA) recommended that FHM appointed a reference group, to broaden its expertise and proposed a list of possible candidates. The divisions between FHM and parts of the academic community seemed confirmed, when FHM appointed a reference group, but not any of the candidates proposed by KvA.

43 The most relevant expertise would be the regional network of contagion doctors. We are not aware if they had a different view at the time (April 2020) from that of FHM, but presumably not.

health probably influenced its approach: shutting down schools would result in long-term damage to pupils' learning. Mental illness and obesity problems and domestic violence would probably increase. Moreover, FHM considered that the virus would spread anyway, at least in urban areas, as essential services, public transport, etc., would continue to run. With the virus already present in most countries in the world, closing borders would do little to stop its spread. What might also have influenced the government is that, throughout the spring of 2020, there were clearly high levels of public confidence in FHM.

However, it is clear that Sweden was not so successful when it came to achieving one of the main stated goals of the government and FHM, namely the protection vulnerable groups.[44] The structural deficiencies in Swedish care of the elderly were well known, and it was strange that no one in the parliament, or the media, at the time (February–April 2020), raised any questions about what effects the government's Covid-19 strategy, or lack of it, was likely to have on this group. Deaths and numbers of people needing intensive care in hospital peaked in April–May 2020 and again in November 2020. Eventually, the death rates of the elderly, particularly in November 2020, had the effect that public pressure to do *something* mounted. This, the prospect of vaccines arriving soon and the fact that by November 2020 hospital staff were much more exhausted, can explain why Sweden partially departed from its recommendatory approach and enacted new legal measures, as described above.

13.9 Evaluating the Swedish Measures from a Rule of Law Perspective

During the pandemic, a number of different indicators, trackers, and evaluative criteria have been proposed by different bodies to assess the legal measures taken to respond to the virus. The Council of Europe advisory body on constitutional law, the Venice Commission,[45] has formulated six principles for dealing with public emergencies: respect for the overarching principle of the rule of law, necessity, proportionality, temporariness, effective judicial control and political accountability, and loyal cooperation between state institutions, central and local/regional government. We consider that these principles provide a useful basis for evaluating the Swedish measures.[46] We emphasize, however, that when it comes to the question of whether a state has "complied" or not with a principle, there is usually a *spectrum of compliance*, rather than a simple binary conclusion "comply/not comply."

The first principle, "legality" can be seen in a broad or narrow sense. In a broad sense, it refers to the entirety of the VC's own Rule of law checklist,[47] which concretizes the vague concept of the "rule of law," breaking it down into a number of components. Sweden has shown a relatively high respect for the principle of legality. Existing powers have not been subjected to dubious extensive interpretations. There has been no retroactive legislation. However, some criticisms can still be made with regard to this principle, in relation to the Swedish approach. The first point is that, where the constitution requires limitations in rights to be in the form of a statute, then proceeding by means of recommendations can short-circuit judicial review. There is no legal norm to review. A policy or recommendation can also, in practice, undermine a legal rule. One particularly

---

44 See below, section 13.9 (Corona Commission report finding).
45 See generally I Cameron, "The role of the venice commission in strengthening the rule of law," in A B Engelbrekt, A Moberg, J Nergelius (eds) *Rule of Law in the EU 30 Years After the Fall of the Berlin Wall* (Hart, 2021).
46 Venice Commission, Respect for Democracy, Human Rights and Rule of Law during States of Emergency: Reflections, CDL-AD(2020)014, 19 June 2020. We should note that Iain Cameron was part of the Venice Commission working group which produced the "Reflections" document.
47 CDL-AD(2016)007.

problematic example can be mentioned here. When deciding whether or not to give a patient intensive care, a prognosis has to be made about the likelihood that the patient will survive intensive care, and make a full, or at least, some sort of, recovery. A difficult ethical dilemma arises when intensive care facilities are scarce. Accusations have been levelled at some regions that during the first wave, a policy was put in place which in practice established levels of prioritization. IVO concluded[48] – disputed by the regions – that doctors on several occasions did not visit the elderly care homes, that they were not familiar with the persons and their medical journals, and that they instead had made standardized assessments, relying on non-medically trained staff at the care homes. The law on the other hand clearly specifies that an individual assessment of medical care needs is required and that people who have greater needs should receive priority over people with lesser needs. The consequence was that some – it is unclear how many – elderly patients received palliative care, instead of hospital care.

Another criticism relates to the legislative process. As noted above, the two central pieces of legislation granting increased powers to the government were hurried through the parliament. For a state which relies on the legislative process being thorough, and unhurried, there is a problem in relying upon "constitutional preparedness." Many of the advantages of the Swedish system of preparation of legislation are lost if the government submits a bill in a hurry, and parliament passes it in a hurry. The logical conclusion is that the post hoc review function of the courts becomes more important something which is not in line with the main principle applicable in Swedish constitutional law, parliamentary supremacy. These two episodes did not give a very inspiring picture of government competence, even if the legislation did not, at least in comparison to almost all other European states, involve too sweeping powers. A lesson to be learned is that if one wishes to maintain the value of the legislative process (and maintain the subsidiary role of the courts), then draft legislation should be prepared in advance, and be published and discussed by the parliament in advance too. While it might not be possible to foresee exactly all the new powers which might be necessary for future crises, parliament and the public should know the general types of powers which are likely to be put in place, and the balances which are to be drawn between different competing interests.

Emergency powers, according to the Venice Commission, should be temporary. Their sole raison d'être is to enable the return of normalcy. In Sweden, the two new acts which provide for considerable delegation of powers to the government were made temporary; meaning that parliament's approval for their extension must be sought. Otherwise, as already noted, the Swedish system rests upon emergency provisions "embedded" in ordinary legislation. Some writers have been against this idea, and have argued that emergency legislation be kept quite separate from ordinary legislation.[49] The main difficulty with embedded legislation is that it potentially blurs the boundary between normalcy and an emergency, and/or normalizes an emergency. As noted, some of the embedded provisions give the government the power to trigger special powers. However, in the Swedish system, the parliament is still primary, and all the existing mechanisms for securing government accountability to the parliament continue to apply. Thus, the democratic risks are limited. Another argument is that separation makes it easier to identify, and so repeal, emergency powers when the situation calling for exceptional powers has come to an end. This is not a problem in Sweden either. However, a third argument is strong in the Swedish context, namely the lack of coherence between disparate crisis rules in different pieces of legislation and difficulty of obtaining an overview of emergency powers. Foreseeability is a fundamental part of the rule of law.

---

48 https://www.ivo.se/publicerat-material/nyheter/2020/ingen-region-har-tagit-fullt-ansvar-for-individuell-vard/.
49 See e.g. R. Cormacain, "Keeping Covid-19 emergency legislation socially distant from ordinary legislation: principles for the structure of emergency legislation," *The Theory and Practice of Legislation*, (2020) https://doi.org/10.1080/20508840.2020.1786272.

As regards the necessity and proportionality principles, whereas in most countries, the public discussion has been about unwarranted executive aggrandizement, in Sweden it has rather been the opposite, namely whether government should have taken, or exercised, *more* powers. This is a suitable place to say something about proportionality as regards rights restrictions in particular. In our view, among the largest interferences in human rights which have occurred in many countries, responses to Covid-19 have been the long-term closures of the public space as such, i.e. requiring people to remain in their homes except when they have a specified permissible reason for leaving these, and fining them if they are unable to justify being outside. In many countries, large numbers of fines have been issued. Such confinements have disproportionally affected poor people who live in cramped accommodation. It is one thing to introduce a short local curfew, when this is timed right, and is the only way to prevent a deadly pandemic. But a democratic Rechtsstaat (state that follows the rule of law) cannot lock up its entire population for any length of time. Moreover, the *immediate* death toll is only one element in measuring success and failure of the Covid response, albeit a crucial one. Long-term problems exacerbated by severe lockdowns mean a *future* death toll, or at least, loss of life expectancy.[50]

Another serious interference, which we also consider difficult to justify objectively speaking, is obligatory collection of identifiable personal data, i.e. requiring people to download apps on mobile phones which monitor their movements. From this perspective, the Swedish legal response does not involve major limitations of constitutional rights. No tracking apps, not even voluntary apps, were introduced. MSB was initially told by the government to develop such an app, but FHM vetoed this on personal integrity grounds.[51] FHM considered that the concrete benefit of such an app was limited: it could only be voluntary, but it anyway entailed a restriction in private integrity. Other aspects of the Swedish strategy also score reasonably on the necessity and proportionality principles. Although under the Covid-19 Act public spaces such as parks can be temporarily closed, and even private gatherings in public spaces which have not been closed can be dispersed, any such measures must comply with proportionality requirements, and there are rights of judicial review.

Having said this, we accept that more critical assessments can be made of the Swedish responses from a rights perspective. Three rights can be mentioned here. First, the right to life, and the state's positive duties to protect life. In Eurostat's comparisons per head of population, death rates in Sweden are around the middle.[52] However, it is very clear that it has fared much less well compared to its Nordic neighbors. The main structural failure has been as regards care of the elderly, something we deal with under another principle – loyal cooperation (below). Second, as already noted, care homes were the subject of a national visiting ban, which was kept in place for a long period irrespective of local conditions (i.e. the extent of the spreading of the virus in the locality or region). For elderly people who were physically unable to leave these care homes, this ban meant that they had no physical contact with relatives. The government later delegated this power to FHM and allowed it to introduce local bans. Third, the right to gather publicly and demonstrate was also affected. During the second and third waves, some people have been fined for taking part in public demonstrations, and a few such demonstrations in Stockholm have been broken up. In particular, the fact that the ban on public meetings was imposed on all types of meeting meant that even

---

50 Having said this, Covid-19 appears to have long-term effects in a percentage of those infected. This should also be taken into account on the other side of the scale.

51 This is another example of the autonomy of administrative agencies, the lack of coordination between government departments and the lead role which FHM took. MSB had in accordance with the government instruction, contracted software developers to produce the app. When FHM vetoed the idea, MSB had to pay contractual penalties. "MSB betalar miljoner för stoppad 'corona-app'," Ny Teknik, 25 May 2020.

52 https://ec.europa.eu/eurostat/statistics-explained/index.php?title=Excess_mortality_-_statistics#Excess_mortality_in_the_European_Union_between_January_2020_and_June_2021

religious services were covered. For religious congregations, this meant an almost total ban on celebrating church services together. At a later stage during the pandemic, the government made an exception for funerals, raising the number of individuals to be allowed from eight to 20. Our overall assessment is that the Swedish responses to the virus, even after the enactment of the Covid-19 law, satisfy the necessity/proportionality principles. This assessment is shared by the Oxford University "stringency index," where Sweden is rated relatively low.[53]

As regards legislative and judicial oversight, Parliament continued to operate, as a result of voluntary agreement between the political parties, with a reduced physical presence of 55 MPs (down from 349). Meetings of committees and other parliamentary work were held online. It seems likely that the quality of this work suffered. The wisdom of relying upon voluntary agreements between the political parties during a crisis can be questioned. There should be rules agreed in an advance. The parliament has established a committee of inquiry to look into both issues.[54] But defects in parliamentary scrutiny had, on the whole, less serious consequences in Sweden compared with many other countries, where parliaments, with little debate, agreed to giving their governments sweeping powers. As most Swedish government measures were recommendations, at least initially, there was no provision for parliamentary scrutiny or confirmation. As noted, the new, binding, executive powers provided for by statute in April and November 2020 were made subject to parliamentary confirmation, largely due to the intervention of KU and the Council on Legislation. Both these bodies have been fully operative during the pandemic and KU held a series of public hearings in spring 2021 with government, administrative agencies, and local authority. KU was unanimous, but relatively mild, in its criticism of six issues handled by the government response.[55]

As regards judicial scrutiny, the courts continued to function, usually operating remotely. In some areas, they have actually increased their productivity.[56] There have, of course, been concerns regarding the quality of justice/fair trial in criminal and migration cases where video equipment has been used. As regards cases concerning legal responses to Covid-19, for most of 2020, the courts only received relatively minor issues to rule on. A few cases concerned the legality of local authority bans on visiting elderly care homes (these were overturned, but they had anyway been replaced with a national ban issued by the government). Another set of cases has concerned the legality of local authority decisions not to provide home assistance to elderly resident in one local authority visiting holiday homes situated in another local authority (overturned).

The Covid-19 Act passed in November contained powers to shut down shops, etc. The political opposition demanded that general orders to shut shops, gyms, etc., would result in compensation. The compromise which was reached in the Act was that shops, etc., subject to a ban would be compensated for their standing costs (rent, utilities, etc.) but not (speculative) loss of profits. However, as malls, etc., were not in fact shut down, and shops generally followed the restrictions, there have not been many cases submitted to the courts. The situation was tougher for certain types of business, theatres, cinemas, amusement parks, the operation of which was made more or less impossible by the restrictions imposed on the number of participants in public events. However, these have benefited from furloughing rules. The same can be said for bars and restaurants which

---

53 https://covidtracker.bsg.ox.ac.uk/stringency-scatter. The same can be said for the comparative survey made by Democracy Reporting International Extraordinary or extralegal responses? The rule of law and the COVID-19 crisis, May 2021, https://democracy-reporting.org/uploads/publication/15175/document/extraordinary-or-extralegal-respons-61028d04eeabd.pdf. However, as we were the Swedish correspondents in this survey, we cannot cite this as independent support for our own views.

54 In December 2020, Parliament convened and tasked a cross-party Committee with a review of the work of the parliament and its administration during the pandemic.

55 KU betänkande 2020/21:20, granskningsbetänkande.

56 Some concern has been expressed about the difficulty of evaluating oral testimony delivered via video link.

were forced to close at 20.00 for several months, but as they were not totally shut down, they have not benefited from the compensation provisions in the Covid-19 Act.

However, another category of cases has taken up much of the time of the administrative courts from the second half of 2020, onward, namely appeals regarding denial of assistance for furloughing of employees, and other types of economic relief granted to companies. As noted earlier, the Swedish government was quick to put in place a raft of economic measures for businesses to ameliorate the effects of the economic crisis which came in the wake of the pandemic. A relatively small agency, the Agency for Economic and Regional Growth, was given the task of handing out this money. The speed in which these rules had been put in place had a deleterious effect on their quality, leaving inter alia, room for inflated claims for compensation. The process for applying for money was complicated, something which favored big companies, who could afford good accountants and lawyers. The responsible Agency had limited resources, and limited experience in this area. Moreover, it attempted to minimize the room for abuse of the rules with narrow interpretations of the rules. The rules themselves were changed several times. The upshot of all this is that there have been many appeals from many small businesses, which are not incorporated as companies, against negative decisions, and many complaints that there have been major delays in paying out economic assistance and contributions toward furloughing employees, with the result that some of these businesses have been bankrupted.

The final Venice Commission principle is that of "loyal cooperation" between central, regional, and local government. As indicated above, this has not been without difficulties. The first report of the Corona Commission (mentioned above), on care of the elderly, is important for the future debate on allocation of competence between central government, the regions, and local authorities. Communication channels between central government and local authorities must be improved. The main finding in the report is that local authorities' care of the elderly (to a considerable extent outsourced to private actors) must be reformed by requiring a much greater presence of medically qualified staff and by management reforms. The sharp division between health care and care of the elderly has not worked. There must therefore be improved coordination between the regions and local authorities as regards care of the elderly (who often suffer from multiple illnesses). Improving pay and conditions for workers and having more permanently employed staff in nursing homes is also important. While a significant number of local authorities have failed to deliver safe standards of care, the Corona Commission states clearly that the overall legal and political responsibility for this failure lies with the present, and former, central governments, who have failed for many years to deal with these known problems. This report should revive a discussion in Sweden as to how to organize the public administration of the health service. There is already such a discussion, but it is largely focused on how to create regions with sufficiently large (and sufficiently equal) tax bases to afford high-quality (and nationally comparable) care to the inhabitants of the region. The question – a very large question, beyond the scope of the present chapter – is whether it is meaningful to have regional health authorities at all, and whether their existing responsibilities should be split between primary health care (for local authorities) and advanced hospital care (for central government).

13.10 Concluding Remarks

We are not setting out to examine the "success" or "failure" of the Swedish policies, which is something which should be done by a broad spectrum of expertise, and only after more time has elapsed. It is evident that FHM made several mistakes. It did not think that the virus would reach Europe. It did not recommend early enough limiting the size of public meetings and events. It did not recommend that people entering the country from places where the contagion existed to self-isolate or get tested. It thought that the virus would spread like influenza, rather than in clusters and so it greatly overestimated the numbers of people who had been infected, and who had antibodies. It considered that, after summer 2020, only partial local outbreaks would occur. The Corona Commission criticized all these errors and the relative inactivity of the government, except in the field of economic support. Whether or not it was a mistake not to apply a "principle of precaution" and recommend a partial lockdown of society as occurred in other Nordic states is something which is still being discussed but the Corona Commission considered it was correct not to impose a total lock-down of society (something which would anyway have required asking the parliament to grant the government extensive new legal powers). As already noted, these steps would have required the parliament to pass very speedy legislation and would potentially have had negative effects on schools, mental health, etc. It is impossible to know if a partial lockdown, if imposed at the right time (in March/April 2020), would have saved more people. The Danish experience does indicate that, at least, it *might* have been possible to limit the spreading of the virus which in turn would have meant that the – at the early stages very limited – testing and tracing capacity could have been used, and thus, in turn, the spread of the virus limited still further. We would, however, argue that the second wave of the virus shows that there is no simple relationship between the severity of lockdown measures taken in many European states and the death toll from the virus. Amending SSL to provide for greater lockdown powers should certainly be discussed, but we argue, strongly, that a lockdown should not be available as a substitute for having a sufficiently large, and properly funded and equipped, public health service, and a functioning crisis management system in the first place.

On imposing political accountability for failures afterward, we are not optimistic. The consensus in the parliament during most of 2020, as well as the division of responsibilities between central government, regions, and local authorities, will make it more difficult to impose any accountability for failures and shortcomings in the responses to the crisis. Accountability in the sense of backward-looking imposition of political or legal responsibility is, generally speaking, relatively weak in Sweden. The idea is that it is more important with forward-looking accountability, i.e. learning from failures and doing better in the future. The final report of the Corona-Commission contains strong criticism, but this is spread relatively equally among politicians at all three levels (central, regional, and local). Various commissions of inquiry have started investigating improvements in SSL and crisis managment legislation generally, and some of the revealed defects will probably be corrected. However, the structural problems in a "multi-level" approach based on the "principle of responsibility" are likely to remain.

In our view, the Coronavirus has shown that Sweden needs to expand the "legal armory" of measures available for dealing with pandemics as well as seriously reappraise its model for political governance of peace-time crises generally. Crises are characterized by fast-changing circumstances which in turn require speedy, multisector, proactive responses. The present decentralized, fragmented, and coordination-based model has its merits, but there are obvious disadvantages too. We would argue that it is necessary to consider if the principle of responsibility should be modified, or rather, partially abolished, by introducing some form of a hierarchical decision-making process in a crisis. If regions are to be retained, then one should consider if, in a crisis, some form of decision-making body with power to bind all the regions should be created, i.e. a new layer above the regions, e.g. composed of a representative from each of these. The alternative is to give such a power to a central body, though this would involve the creation of a new agency, as FHM's competence is at present limited to epidemiological matters, and so too narrow. At the central level, one can consider having "lead" agencies with the power to bind other agencies (and reallocate their resources) as regards different types of societal threat (fires, floods, pandemics, etc.). The existing fragmented legislative picture should be examined with the aim of improving coherence between the different legal frameworks for dealing with different types of peace time crisis. And finally, one of the main lessons of the pandemic for Sweden is the need to provide high, or at least, higher, quality care of the elderly generally. This requires allocating larger resources, and more input of medical competence, to local authority elderly care.

14

Administrative Guidance in Coronavirus Special Measures Act in 2021 in Japan

Yuichiro Tsuji

Meiji University Graduate School of Law

14.1 The 2020 CSMA

After experiencing the runaway power of the government before World War II, the current constitution has been concerned about the abuse of government power.[1] The Constitution of Japan does not contain any provisions on emergencies. Laws enacted by the Diet have been used to deal with emergencies such as national defense[2] or natural disaster.[3]

In 2020, the Diet amended the Influenza Special Measures Act.[4] Originally prepared as the Influenza Special Measures Act (ISMA) targeting influenza, the law was partially amended to address COVID-19. Hereafter, the revised ISMA in 2020 means the 2020 CSMA (Coronavirus Special Measures Act).

The 2020 CSMA applied to COVID-19 for a certain period in the Supplementary Provisions.[5] In the text, COVID-19 was defined as a new strain of influenza.[6] As a result, the CSMA is now permanently applied to COVID-19. Hereafter, the term "new strains of influenza" includes COVID-19.

14.1.1 2021 CSMA and Administrative Guidance

On 7 January 2021, Prime Minister Yoshihide Suga declared a state of emergency in one metropolis and three prefectures of Tokyo, Chiba, Saitama, and Kanagawa.[7] Under Article 32[8] of the CSMA, the head of the Government Response Headquarters (prime minister) may declare a state of emergency. When issuing a state of emergency declaration, the head shall announce the duration, area, and outline of the state of emergency and report it to the Diet. On 13 January 2021, the government added Tochigi Prefecture to the list of areas to be declared a state of emergency.

1 Tsuji, Y, Godzilla and the Japanese Constitution: A Comparison Between Italy and Japan, *3 Italian Law Journal*, No. 2, 451-477 (2017).
2 Jiei tai hō [Self Defense Act], Act No. 165 of 1954, Art.76,78.
3 Saigai taisaku kihon hō [Basic Act on Disaster Management], Act No.223 of 1961, Art.105,106(Japan).
4 supra note 1, CSMA (amended ISMA). The ISMA was originally enacted in 2011 in light of the Avian Influenza (A/H1N1) outbreak.
5 Supplementary provision of CSMA. See also, Order for Enforcement of the Act on Special Measures against Influenza, Ordinance No. 122 of 2013 (Japan).
6 Art.2(1) of the 2021 CSMA.
7 Prime Minister's office of Japan, Shingata koronauirusukansenshō ni kansuru Suga naikakusōri daijin kisha kaiken [Prime Minister Kan's press conference on the new coronavirus infection] (7 January 2021). Available at: https://www.kantei.go.jp/jp/99_suga/statement/2021/0107kaiken.html.
8 Art.32 of the CSMA.

Impacts of the Covid-19 Pandemic: International Laws, Policies, and Civil Liberties, First Edition. Edited by Nadav Morag.

To declare a state of emergency, the prime minister must recognize a situation in which the outbreak of a new strain of influenza has occurred in Japan and is likely to have an enormous impact on the lives of the people and the national economy due to its rapid, nationwide spread, or likelihood to spread, as specified by a Cabinet Order.

On 2 February 2021, Prime Minister Suga decided to extend the state of emergency to 7 March in nine prefectures (Saitama, Chiba, Tokyo, Kanagawa, Gifu, Kyoto, Osaka, Hyogo, and Fukuoka) except Tochigi Prefecture,[9] declaring that it would be lifted ahead of schedule if the situation improved.[10] He continued to request that restaurants do not operate post 8 p.m., and continued to request voluntary restraint from going out unnecessarily, including during the day. He also called for a 70% reduction in the number of employees coming to work by encouraging businesses to provide teleworking opportunities to their employees. He further decided to continue with restrictions on events, such as limiting them to 5,000 people or less. Tochigi Prefecture lifted the restriction on 7 February, and despite this, requests for shorter working hours and restrictions on events were maintained, and then eased in stages.

Following the advice of the Subcommittee on Countermeasures for New Coronavirus Infections under the Cabinet Secretariat,[11] the government has divided the state of emergency into four stages which are determined by six indicators.[12] These indicators are (i) the availability of hospital beds, (ii) the number of patients under treatment, (iii) the PCR positivity rate, (iv) the number of newly infected patients, (v) the comparison of the last week with the previous week, and (vi) the percentage of unknown routes of infection.[13]

The government's subcommittee defined Stage 3 as when 25% or more of the beds that are currently reserved are occupied, and 20% or more of the maximum available beds are occupied, and Stage 4 when half or more are occupied, assuming that the maximum number of beds can be secured. The government will determine the stage in each of the two categories: overall and for critically ill patients.

The number of patients to be treated is determined from the combined figures of those hospitalized and those treated at home or in hotels. If this number is 15 or more per 100,000 population, the state of emergency is at Stage 3, and if it is 25 or more, it is at Stage 4. In Stage 3, the number of newly infected persons is 15 or more per 100,000 population in one week, and in Stage 4 it is 25 or more per 100,000 population in one week.

Every week, the Ministry of Health, Labor, and Welfare (MHLW) publishes the status of healthcare delivery systems, surveillance systems, and infections for each prefecture.[14] The government

---

9 Tochigi prefecture, 2021. *Kinkyū jitai sochi-go no kansen kakudai bōshi ni muketa chiji messēji (2 tsuki 4-nichi)* [Governor's message to prevent the spread of infection after emergency measures] (4 February 2021). Available at: https://www.pref.tochigi.lg.jp/e04/20210204chijimesse-ji.html.

10 Prime Minister's office of Japan, Shingata koronauirusukansenshō ni kansuru Suga naikakusōri daijin kisha kaiken [Prime Minister Kan's press conference on the new coronavirus infection] (2 February 2021). Available at: https://www.kantei.go.jp/jp/99_suga/statement/2021/0202kaiken.html.

11 Cabinet Secretariat (2021). Subcommittee on Countermeasures for New Coronavirus Infections under the Cabinet Secretariat. Available at: https://www.cas.go.jp/jp/seisaku/ful/yusikisyakaigi.html.

12 Director, Office for Promotion of Countermeasures to Combat Novel Coronavirus Infections, Cabinet Secretariat (2021). *Indicators and guidelines for the implementation of countermeasures in response to future changes in the infection situation Indicators and guidelines for the implementation of countermeasures* (7 August 2020). Available at: https://corona.go.jp/news/pdf/jimurenraku_0811.pdf.

13 Id.

14 Ministry of Health, Labor, and Welfare (MHLW) (2021. *Todōfuken no iryō teikyō taisei-tō no jōkyō (iryō teikyō taisei-tō no fuka kansen no jōkyō) ni tsuite* [Status of medical care delivery system, etc., in prefectures (medical care delivery system, surveillance system, and status of infection). Available at: https://www.mhlw.go.jp/stf/seisakunitsuite/newpage_00035.html.

has set a guideline for lifting the declaration as the six indicators of the infection situation indicate a drop from Stage 4 to Stage 3.[15]

In Tokyo and three other prefectures, the government continued to ask restaurants to stop operating beyond 8 p.m. The government continued to limit the number of people at large-scale events to a maximum of 5,000 and a capacity of 50% or less.

On 21 March 2021, the government lifted the declaration of a state of emergency in Tokyo and three other prefectures. The requirement for lifting this was that "necessary measures will be continued until the state of emergency is reduced to Stage 2 or lower according to the government subcommittee's index." However, according to the Asahi Shimbun 30 March, five of the six indicators of the government's subcommittee, which indicate the status of the spread of infection and the tightness of medical care, indicate that Osaka Prefecture is at Stage 3. Therefore, Osaka Governor Yoshimura has asked the government to apply priority measures to curb the spread of the disease.

14.1.2 How CSMA was Amended

The lack of compensation provisions in the 2020 CSMA has been highlighted by Social Networking Services as a major flaw, but compensation provisions do exist for certain businesses and regulatory regimes.[16] There is no compensation provision for violations of requests to shorten business hours made to restaurants, bars, night clubs, and so on.

Only Article 63-2 of the CSMA encourages government financially support businesses, but does not define what business is.

Article 62[17] provides for the obligation of the government to compensate for damages incurred when carrying out the following acts. Article 29 (5)[18] (use of facilities for hospitals or clinics or accommodation facilities), Article 31-3[19] (use of land, etc., to establish temporary medical facilities), Article 49[20] (use of land or houses), or Article 55(2)[21] (request for sale of goods), paragraph 3[22] (transport operators) or paragraph 4[23] (excluding the part pertaining to paragraph 1 of the same Article).

According to Article 62(2),[24] the national and prefectural governments shall reimburse the actual costs of medical personnel who respond to requests pursuant to Article 31(1) or (2),[25] or who provide medical care to patients in accordance with instructions pursuant to Article 31(3),[26] in accordance with standards specified by a Cabinet Order.

The 2020 CSMA has no sanctions for violations of requests of reducing business hours for non-medical businesses.

---

15 Cabinet Secretariat (2021). Subcommittee on Countermeasures for New Coronavirus Infections under the Cabinet Secretariat. Available at: https://www.cas.go.jp/jp/seisaku/ful/yusikisyakaigi.html. Director, Office for Promotion of Countermeasures to Combat Novel Coronavirus Infections. 6 indicators (1. the urgency of the hospital bed, 2. number of the patients, 3. PCR positive rates, 4. number of new reports, 5. comparison between the latest week and the week before that, 6. percentage of cases where the route of infection is unknown).
16 Id. Art.62 of 2020 CSMA.
17 Id.
18 Id. Art. 29(5).
19 Id. Art.31-3.
20 Id. Art. 49.
21 Id. Art.55(2).
22 Id. Art.55(3).
23 Id. Art.55(4).
24 Id. Art.62(2).
25 Id. Art.31(1), (2).
26 Id. Art.31(3).

14.1.3 How CSMA was Amended, and Why

The 2020 CSMA was amended by the Diet on 3 February and came into effect on 13 February 2021. The 2021 CSMA has established new priority measures (Priority Measures to Prevent Spread) to prevent the spread of the disease,[27] which can be issued before a state of emergency in Article 32[28] is declared.

The requirement for implementing the prevention measures is when there is a risk of an enormous impact on people's lives and the economy. The implementation does not require nationwide spread as in the case of a declaration of a state of emergency; it is sufficient that the disease is spreading in a limited area.[29]

The Basic Response Policy[30] in the 2021 CSMA sets out the requirements for the implementation of the Priority Measures to Prevent Spread. The requirements consider whether the infection is likely to spread from the specified area of the prefecture to a wider area, and whether there is a risk that the healthcare provision system would be disturbed. The government has designated priority areas for preventing the spread of the disease. Prefectural governors can request or order businesses to shorten their business hours.

In accordance with the amendment of the 2021 CSMA, the antivirus task force has revised its basic response policy to state that the implementation of priority measures to prevent the spread of the disease[31] depends upon whether the infection situation is equivalent to Stage 3 (rapid increase in infection).

14.1.4 Legalization of the Self-restraint Order

The 2021 CSMA priority measures to prevent the spread of infectious diseases stipulate sanctions against certain types of businesses that do not comply with the request of shortening business hours.[32] Businesses that do not comply with the government's request can be ordered to comply, and a fine of up to 200,000 yen will be imposed for violation of the order when the new priority measures are implemented.[33]

First, the government may seek advice from the Subcommittee on Countermeasures for New Coronavirus Infections when requesting and issuing orders to shorten business hours,[34] and when it issues an order, it may publicize the purpose and intent of the order.[35] The prefectural governor is granted the authority to collect reports and conduct on-site inspections and other investigations when issuing orders.[36]

Second, the 2021 CSMA has upgraded "instructions" to "orders" for businesses that do not comply with requests to restrain business operations based on emergency declarations,[37] and can impose a non-penal (administrative) fine of up to 300,000 yen for violations of orders during

---

27 Art.31-4 of the 2021 CSMA.
28 Id. Art.32.
29 Id. Art.31-4.
30 Art. 18 of the 2021 CSMA. The Government Response Headquarters shall formulate a basic policy for dealing with new strains of influenza, etc. (hereinafter referred to as the "Basic Response Policy") based on the Government Action Plan. The Basic Response Policy shall include: (i) the facts concerning the situation of the outbreak of new strains of influenza, (ii) the general policy for dealing with such new strains of influenza, and (iii) important matters concerning the implementation of countermeasures against new strains of influenza.
31 Art. 31-4 of the 2021 CSMA.
32 Id. Art. 31-6(1).
33 Id. Art. 80.
34 Id. Art. 31-6(4).
35 Id. Art. 31-6(5).
36 Id. Art. 72.
37 Id. Art. 45(3).

a state of emergency.[38] In issuing a request to shorten business hours based on a declaration of emergency, the government is required to listen to the advice of academic experts and announce the purpose and intent of the order. In issuing this order, the government is granted the authority to conduct on-site inspections of businesses, which can also be done under the new priority measures.

Third, the national and local governments shall effectively provide financial support to those affected by the new strains of influenza, and to businesses affected by the preventive measures.[39] Under the 2021 CSMA, the government is obligated to provide financial support and can respond to the spread of the disease in an effective manner.[40]

Fourth, the governor requests that "the person in question should not go out of their residence or equivalent place without permission, except when it is necessary for the maintenance of daily life."[41] This is a request based on Article 45(1). However, this is only a request, and no order or penalty is imposed on the violator.

14.1.5   Sanctions, not Penal but Administrative

In both the declaration of a state of emergency and the new measures to prevent the spread of the disease, the government can impose a non-penal (administrative) fine on businesses that violate the shortened business hours order. Under Article 45(3)[42] of the 2021 CSMA, prefectures may order businesses that do not respond to requests to shorten their business hours and take "appropriate measures" to enforce compliance with such requests.

When the government declares a state of emergency[43] and implements the priority measures,[44] businesses that fail to comply with the order "without justifiable reason" will be subject to a non-penal (administrative) fine of up to 300,000 yen[45] for violating the order during a declaration of a state of emergency. A non-penal fine of not more than 200,000 yen[46] will be imposed for violation of an order during the implementation of the Priority Measures to Prevent Spreading.

A non-penal (administrative) fine under the CSMA is a penalty for the violation of an administrative duty and does not imply social condemnation. Unlike a non-penal (administrative) fine, a fine as a criminal penalty is a penalty for having committed a socially reprehensible act, and carries a criminal record. Since the provisions of the 2021 CSMA are socially preventive measures to prevent the spread of the disease, they are limited to a non-penal (administrative) fine.

When the new priority measures are in effect, the governor requests that individuals do not enter stores, restaurants, and so on, where shortened business hours are requested.[47] This request does not restrict individuals from going out, and there are no orders or sanctions against violators.

Finally, during a state of emergency, the governor requests individuals to "refrain from going out of their residences or other places equivalent to their residences, except when it is necessary for the maintenance of their lives."[48] This, again, is only a request, and no order or penalty is imposed on the violator.

---

38 Id. Art. 79.
39 Id. Art. 63-2.
40 Id.
41 Id. Art. 45(1).
42 Id. Art.45(3).
43 Id. Art. 45(3).
44 Id. Art. 31-6.
45 Id. Art. 79.
46 Id. Art. 80.
47 Id. Art. 31-6(2).
48 Id. Art.45(1).

14.1.6 Revision of the Infectious Diseases Act

The Infectious Diseases Act,[49] which was amended in 2021, is a statute that stipulates the response and medical care during an outbreak of an infectious disease, while the CSMA is designed to prevent the spread of infectious diseases in society.

The revised Infectious Diseases Act clearly defines COVID-19 as a new type of influenza and other infectious diseases in law.[50] As a result, the Infectious Diseases Act is now permanently applied to COVID-19.

Under the 2020 Infectious Diseases Act, if a suspected infected person refuses to be hospitalized, there is a specific danger that the infected person will be free to go out and spread the disease. For example, a person with COVID-19 who remains mildly ill or asymptomatic may go out of their home or residential treatment facility and visit establishments such as restaurants or spas. Under the 2021 Infectious Diseases Act, if this is found to be the case, restaurants and other facilities must cease operations and conduct disinfection work.[51]

If a suspected infected person does not comply with hospitalization measures or flees from the hospital, a non-penal (administrative) fine of up to 500,000 yen is imposed. In revising the Infectious Diseases Act, the Diet was concerned that patients do not always voluntarily declare the place to be visited. Although some posit that refusing hospitalization should be fined as a criminal penalty when it risks spreading infection, the 2021 amendment only imposes a non-penal (administrative) fine.[52]

The revised Infectious Diseases Act makes active epidemiological investigations, which investigate infection routes and clusters, more effectively.[53] Under the revised Act, if a patient refuses to cooperate with active epidemiological investigations, it is possible to order them to cooperate.[54]

Here, the term "patient" includes patients with pseudo-symptoms who can be reasonably suspected of being infected, as well as asymptomatic pathogen carriers.[55]

When the prefectural governor or the MHLW orders cooperation, they must deliver a document that describes the necessary compliance measures.[56] Patients who violate the order without justifiable reason shall be subject to a non-penal (administrative) fine of not more than 300,000 yen.[57]

Further, the revised Infectious Diseases Act amended the hospitalization measures.[58] Among patients with COVID-19, hospitalization is recommended for those who are likely to become seriously ill, such as the elderly.[59] Those who do not comply with the recommendation for hospitalization may be forcefully hospitalized.[60]

For other patients, the prefectural governor may request the cooperation of the patient to receive treatment at a facility or at home.[61] For those who do not comply with the request for cooperation in medical treatment at an accommodation facility or at home, a recommendation for hospitalization and hospitalization measures may be imposed.[62]

---

49 Kansenshō no yobō oyobi kansenshō no kanja ni taisuru iryō ni kansru hō [Act on the Prevention of Infectious Diseases and Medical Care for Patients with Infectious Diseases], Act No. 114 of 1998, art. 19 (revised in 2021). [hereinafter, Infectious Diseases Act].
50 Id. Art.6(7)(3).
51 Id. Art. 27.
52 Id. Art.80.
53 Id. Art.15(8).
54 Id.
55 Id. Art. 8(2), (3).
56 Id. Art.15(10), (11).
57 Id. Art.81.
58 Id. Art.19.
59 Id. Art.19(1) as applied mutatis mutandis by Art. 26(2) of the same Act.
60 Id. Art.19(3) as applied mutatis mutandis by Art. 26 (2) of the same Act.
61 Id. Art.44-3(2).
62 Id. Art.26(2).

If a patient escapes during hospitalization, or if they fail to be hospitalized against hospitalization measures without justifiable reasons, a non-penal (administrative) fine of up to 500,000 yen will be imposed.[63]

Lastly, the revised Infectious Diseases Act strengthened the authority of the MHLW and prefectural governors. Article 16-2[64] of the revised Infectious Diseases Act, prior to the revision in 2021, originally provided for the authority of the MHLW and prefectural governors to request cooperation from medical personnel.

The revised Act adds private laboratories for infectious diseases to the list of those who are subject to cooperation requests,[65] and states that if a subject who has received a "cooperation request" fails to cooperate without a valid reason, a "recommendation" can be made,[66] and if the recommendation is not followed, this fact can be made public.[67]

Article 16-3 is the basis for requesting private hospitals to accept COVID-19 patients and revealing those that do not comply to the public.

In reality, it is unlikely that a unilateral recommendation will be made to hospitals that do not have the facilities or personnel to accept patients with COVID-19.

A non-penal (administrative) fine of up to 300,000 yen[68] will be imposed if a person refuses, without justifiable reason, an epidemiological survey by a public health center to identify persons who have had close contact with COVID-19 infected persons.[69]

The court imposes this administrative fine on the violator. In this procedure, the prefecture notifies the district court. In this notice, the prefectures specify the article of the Infectious Diseases Act (Article 80 or 81) on which the administrative fine is based and the amount of the fine. In addition, the reasoning behind the imposition of the administrative fine should be clarified. The details of the violation and the time at which it occurred should be clearly stated to avoid a double fine for the same violation. If the violator provides a reason for not responding to hospitalization measures or active epidemiological investigations, the prefectural government should clearly state the reason why it does not fall under the category of "justifiable reason" under Article 80 or 81 of the Infectious Diseases Act if that is indeed the case.[70]

14.2 Administrative Guidance and COVID-19 in 2021

Authoritarian government may be at the root of the reason that administrative guidance has been used so much in Japan. The fact that administrative guidance has been used so often shows that there is a deep-rooted mentality in Japan that respects the government and despises the private sector. Administrative guidance shows the peculiarity of Japanese society, which has tried to continue the relationship between the government and citizens in a consensual rather than confrontational way.

Administrative guidance is a form of law that attempts to achieve administrative objectives based on the voluntary or consensual consent of the other party.[71] It is a factual act, not a legal act, which should be carried out within the scope of the administrative agency's jurisdiction.

----

63 Id. Art.80.
64 Id. Art.16-2.
65 Id.
66 Id. Art.16-3(2).
67 Id. Art.16-3(3).
68 Id. Art. 80.
69 Id. Art. 15(8).
70 MHLW (2021). *Administrative handling of administrative penalties associated with the enforcement of the "Act for Partial Revision of the Act on Special Measures against Influenza, etc. of a New Type"* (related to the Infectious Diseases Act) (10 February 2021). Available at: https://www.mhlw.go.jp/content/000737654.pdf.
71 Gyōsei tetuduki hō [Administrative procedure Act], Act No. 88 of 1993, art.2(6)(Japan).

The provisions on administrative guidance in the Administrative Procedure Act (APA)[72] apply not only to administrative guidance for which there are statutory grounds but also for those that do not need statutory grounds. Administrative organs may provide such guidance to achieve certain administrative objectives within the scope of their duties or affairs under their jurisdiction, despite there being no explicit provisions for this.

14.2.1 Traditional Theory in Japanese Administrative Law

Traditionally, Japanese administrative law has been largely influenced by German law. After World War II, as the constitution of Japan was established, American law has also had an influence. It has three principles for administrative activity.

First, government must have the basis and authority of law to operate. Second, the law is superior to administrative activity, and all administrative activities shall not violate the law. Third, norms regarding the rights and duties of citizens are established by law only through the Diet. Only the statute can create new laws and regulations, and the government cannot create laws without the delegation of the law-making power.

There are several viewpoints on whether or not administrative activities require a legal basis. Generally, administrative activities that restrict people's rights and impose obligations require a legal basis.[73]

Since administrative guidance does not necessarily require a legal basis, there is a danger that the rule of law may be substantially hollowed out in the name of voluntary acts of private citizens. Under the principle of administration by law, administrative guidance that violates the law is prohibited (supremacy of law). Therefore, the APA regulates (i) administrative guidance regarding application[74] and (ii) administrative guidance regarding authority such as permission and approval,[75] based on the idea that a legal basis is necessary for administrative guidance that places significant pressure on the citizens.

14.2.2 Legal Control of Administrative Guidance

In administrative jurisprudence, the following requirements are necessary for administrative guidance. (i) The administrative guidance must have a basis in the law of administrative organization. (ii) It must be aimed at realizing certain administrative objectives. (iii) It must be for a specific person. (iv) It must be voluntary in principle for the other party.[76]

APA disciplines administrative guidance in procedure. Article 32(1)[77] of APA demands persons imposing administrative guidance carefully consider their actions so that they do not exceed, even in the slightest degree, the scope of the duties or processes under the jurisdiction of the administrative organ concerned. Further, the administrative guidance should be, to the utmost degree, realized based solely upon the voluntary cooperation of the subject party. Article 32(2)[78] of APA states that "persons imposing Administrative Guidance must not treat the subject party disadvantageously owing to their non-compliance with the Administrative Guidance in question."

In order to operate a restaurant, a permit from the public health center and notification to the fire department are generally required, although there are some differences depending on the

---

72 Id.
73 Sakurai, K. and Hashimoto, H. (2017) *GYŌSEIHŌ* [Administrative law], 5th ed., Japan: Kōbundo, p. 12.
74 Art. 5 of APA.
75 Id. Art.12.
76 Sakurai and Hashimoto (2017, p. 179).
77 Art. 31(1) of APA.
78 Id. Art. 32(2).

type of business. Restaurants that serve alcoholic beverages late at night need to notify the police. Government agencies have requested restaurants to shorten their business hours to prevent the spread of COVID-19. If they do not comply with this request, Article 34 further states that the administrative organ with the authority to grant licenses to restaurants and other permits "must not engage in conduct such as compelling a subject party to comply with the Administrative Guidance in question by deliberately suggesting that they are capable of exercising the authority."[79]

If the administrative organ issues an order to many restaurants to reduce their hours of operation, it shall establish the Administrative Guidance Guideline to achieve a common administrative aim in advance, and make such guideline known to the public.[80]

Since such guidance is intended to achieve certain administrative objectives through the voluntary cooperation of the other party, it does not necessarily require specific provisions in the statute. However, there are two types of administrative guidance: those that are based on statutes and those that are not. The cases based on statutes include Article 15 of the Noise Regulation Law, the warning in Article 4 regarding the Law Concerning the Regulation of Stalking, and the recommendation in Article 34 regarding the Environmental Impact Assessment Law.

14.2.3   Art. 33 of APA When a Citizen does not Follow Administrative Guidance

If a law stipulates that when a citizen does not follow an administrative guidance, the administrative organ may issue a suborder for compliance (an administrative act that creates an obligation of action, inaction, benefit, or acceptance to the citizen) or publicize the name of the individual or restaurant; Article 32(2)[81] of the APA on prohibition of disadvantageous treatment does not apply here. Administrative guidance does not have to involve a legal basis, and if a statute stipulates that the administrative organ may publicize the fact that a citizen or businesses are not following a recommendation and the contents of the recommendation, then doing so will not violate Article 32(2)[82] of the APA.

When citizens or businesses express their intention not to comply with the administrative guidance of a government organ, the administrative organ may not obstruct the citizen's exercise of their rights by conduct such as imposing the guidance forcefully.[83]

In reality, administrative organs provide administrative guidance under the purview of their regulatory authority and with the intention of invoking said authority if such guidance is not followed. Therefore, citizens have no choice but to accept such guidance, and administrative organs are well aware of this and try to enforce guidance.

However, an administrative organ with the authority to grant some permissions, or to render dispositions pertaining to some permission, is not allowed to compel a subject party to comply with the administrative guidance in question by deliberately suggesting that they are capable of exercising the said authority.[84]

The procedure for requesting the cessation of illegal administrative guidance and requesting administrative guidance was legally established in APA[85] in 2014.

If a citizen who has received administrative guidance to correct a violation of the law believes that such guidance does not conform to the requirements of the law, they may appeal to the

---

79 Id. Art. 34.
80 Id. Art. 36.
81 Id. Art.32(2).
82 Id.
83 Id. Art.33.
84 Id. Art.34.
85 Id. Art. 36-2.

administrative body. Such administrative guidance shall not be suspended until the administrative agency confirms that the guidance complies with the relevant legal requirements.

14.2.4 Public Announcement

Article 27(1) of the Public Assistance Act[86] and Article 24[87] of the National Land Use Planning Act provide for public announcements when administrative guidance is not followed. The Public Assistance Act and the National Land Use Planning Act are cases where there is a legal basis for administrative guidance, and some ordinances passed in the local assembly also have provisions for public announcement.[88] If such laws or ordinances exist, the interpretation of the purpose and intent of the laws and regulations on which the administrative guidance is based can be used as a clue to examine the legality of a guidance. Administrative guidance cannot violate the substantive and procedural rules set forth by the laws and regulations on which it is based (supremacy of law).

It is not in conflict with Article 32[89] of the APA (prohibition of adverse treatment) to issue administrative guidance and then suspend business or take other measures when the business does not comply with such guidance. If the administrative agency issues a guidance and the permit holder does not comply and hence violates the permit authority, thus meeting certain requirements for punishment as stipulated in the law, the permit authority may take measures such as suspending business or revoking the permit. In principle, public announcements are informational and do not restrict the rights and interests of citizens, so they do not need a legal basis. However, public announcements can be classified into "provision of information" or "violation of administrative duty." If we take the theory of legal basis of infringement, public announcement whose main cause is "violation of a duty" needs a legal basis.

14.2.5 Public Announcement in TMG

Public announcements have the function of providing information to the general public as well as encouraging the fulfillment of obligations by those whose names are announced. In Japanese administrative law, it has traditionally been explained as a function of providing information to citizens. Recently, it concerns the effectiveness of administrative guidance. Strictly speaking, publication itself does not compel the fulfillment of obligations (i.e. that citizens are obligated to do something). However, some municipalities have started to publish the names, addresses, and other necessary matters of municipal tax delinquents in their ordinances. This brings us to the issue of the Tokyo Metropolitan Government's (TMG) ordinance.

The TMG publicizes the names of businesses if they do not comply with the metropolitan government's request to shorten business hours. This follows Section 24(9)[90] of the CSMA, which requires requesting restaurants to cooperate. Then, pursuant to Section 45(2)and (3)[91] of the CSMA, the name of the restaurant to whom the request was made will be made public. The name of

---

86 Seikatsu hogo hō [Public Assistance Act], Act No. 144 of 1950, Art.27(1)(Japan). (A public assistance administrator may provide a public assistance recipient with guidance or instructions necessary for maintaining or improving their livelihood or otherwise achieving the purpose of public assistance.)
87 Kokudo riyō keikaku hō [National Land Use Planning Act], Act No.92 of 1974, Art.24 (Japan).
88 Nihon-Koku Kenpō [CONSTITUTION], Art. 94, translated in (The Constitution of Japan) [JAPANESE LAW TRANSLATION]. Available at: http://www.japaneselawtranslation.go.jp/law/detail/?id=174&vm=04&re=01& new=1 (Japan).
89 Art. 32 of APA.
90 Art.24(9) of the 2021 CSMA.
91 Id. Art.45(2),(3).

the restaurant, its location, the content of the request, and the reason for the instruction will be published on the website of each prefecture.[92]

Public announcements during emergencies[93] and during the implementation of the new measures to prevent the spread of the disease[94] are not sanctions; they are intended to help citizens change their behaviors in a rational manner. It is therefore necessary to consider the impact of such public announcements because they may damage the reputation of the businesses. Article 45(5)[95] of the 2021 CSMA has just been amended from "must be made public" to "may be made public." In such cases, it should be noted that the information may not be made public.

14.2.6 Merits and Demerits of Administrative Guidance

Administrative guidance has both good and bad aspects. The bad aspect is that it may circumvent law since it does need to have a legal basis. The good aspect, however, is that it allows for flexible and immediate responses to changing issues to protect the lives of the people. It functions as a type of preliminary procedure to encourage the other party to comply voluntarily before the administrative agency invokes its regulatory authority. Therefore, the APA should follow the prescribed procedures when issuing administrative guidance.

Although administrative guidance is an act of seeking the voluntary cooperation of the other party, liability for damages under Article 1 of the State Redress Act[96] may apply in relation to such guidance. For example, if it is administered under pressure that exceeds the acceptable limit, it may be possible for the person to claim damages for mental distress, even if they did not ultimately follow the administrative guidance.[97]

In a State Redress Act lawsuit, a causal relationship is required between the administrative guidance and the damage. When contesting an administrative act, administrative disposition litigation (Kōkoku Soshō)[98] may be filed under the Administrative Case Litigation Act (ACLA). As a general rule, administrative guidance is not recognized as a disposition because the citizens can choose whether to follow it or not. Even if the causal relationship between administrative guidance and damage is denied, the citizen who received such guidance can file a lawsuit based on Article 4[99] of the ACLA to confirm that the person who received the guidance is not obligated to follow the guidance in light of their rights and obligations. This is referred to as a public law-related action (Tōjisha Soshō, TS).[100] However, the "benefit of confirmation" is necessary for this litigation. In some cases, administrative guidance may be recognized as a disposition.

The Supreme Court[101] in 2004 ruled that a notice given by an administrative body constitutes an administrative disposition.

Consequently, the Ministry of Health and Welfare (pre-MHLW) shall, when receiving a notification of import of food or other items prescribed in Article 16[102] of the Food Sanitation Act (prior to amendment by Act No. 55 of 2003), determine whether said food violates the said Act based on the

92 Sakurai and Hashimoto (2017, p. 140).
93 Art.45(5) of the 2021 CSMA.
94 Id. Art.31-6(1),(3).
95 Id. Art.45(5) of the 2021 CSMA.
96 Kokka baishou hō [State Redress Act], Act No. 22 of 1947, art. 1 (Japan).
97 Saiko Saibansho [Sup. Ct.] July 10, 1980, Showa 52 (o) no. 405, 130 SAIKŌ SAIBANSHO MINJI HANREISHŪ [MINSHŪ] 131.
98 Gyōsei jiken soshou hō [Administrative Case Litigation Act], Act No. 139 of 1962, Art. 3 (Japan).
99 Id. Art.4.
100 Id.
101 Saiko Saibansho [Sup. Ct.] April 26, 2004, Hei 15 (gyo hi) no. 206, 58(4) SAIKŌ SAIBANSHO MINJI HANREISHŪ [MINSHŪ] 989. Available at: https://www.courts.go.jp/app/hanrei_jp/detail2?id=52393.
102 Shokuhin eisei hō [Food Sanitation Act] (prior to amendment by Act No. 55 of 2003), Art. 16 (Japan).

said Article. The person who made the notification shall be notified whether the said foods do or do not violate the said Act. Based on Article 16 of the Food Sanitation Act before the amendment, the quarantine station chief notified the person who notified the importation of the food prescribed in the said Article that the food violated the said Act. The Supreme Court ruled that this notice constituted and was subject to an administrative disposition. The Supreme Court explained that as a result of the notification by the quarantine station chief, the import license under the Customs Act could no longer be obtained.

14.2.7 How to Impose Administrative Fine Procedural Requirement

A notice regarding a non-penal (administrative) fine under Section 80(1)[103] of the 2021 CSMA was issued to businesses who failed to comply with an order under Section 31-6(3)[104] of the CSMA.[105] Since the 2021 CSMA does not contain any special provisions on the procedure for the imposition of a non-penal (administrative) fine, such fine is imposed by a court trial under Article 119[106] of the Act on Non-Contentious Case Procedures.

In cases where the prefectural government determines that the violation cannot be overlooked in terms of administrative order, the prefectural government shall fill out the form without omission and notify the district court.

The court initiates the procedure for the trial of the non-penal (administrative) fine ex officio, and the trial is conducted after hearing the opinion of the public prosecutor and the statements of the parties.

The court, which has the authority to initiate proceedings ex officio, is usually not in a position to know the facts of the breach of duty that may entail a non-penal (administrative) fine. Therefore, it is often the case that the prefectural government notifies the court of the breach of duty, which marks the beginning of the proceedings.[107] The notice from the prefecture to the court is de facto, without any legal basis. The prefecture is not obligated to file a petition or to notify the court. There may be a basis for notification in a statute, but not in the 2021 CSMA.[108]

14.2.8 APA Ordinance and TMG

The APA does not apply to administrative guidance by the metropolitan government; Article 3(3)[109] of the APA excludes administrative guidance by local government agencies. It is now necessary to review the APA ordinance established in the local government.

Tomin First, the party supporting Governor Yuriko Koike, was attempting to impose an administrative penalty (a fine of up to 50,000 yen) by amending the metropolitan ordinance on countermeasures against novel coronavirus infections. Its bill includes cases where (i) when an infected person infects others by failing to comply with a request to restrict work or refrain from going out,

103 Art. 80(1) of the 2021 CSMA.
104 Id. Art. 31-6(3).
105 Tokyo to inshoku 4 shisetsuni karyō tetuduki jitan meirei sitagawazu [Tokyo Metropolitan Government begins procedures to impose administrative fine on four restaurants that fail to comply with short-time orders], *Nikkei Shimbun*, 29 March 2021. Available at: https://www.nikkei.com/article/DGXZQODG296SY0Z20C21A3000000/.
106 Hisho jiken tetsuduki hō [Act on Non-Contentious Case Procedures], Act No. 51 of 2011, Art.119 (Japan).
107 Director, Office for Promotion of Countermeasures to Combat Novel Coronavirus Infections, Cabinet Secretariat, *Promulgation of the "Act for Partial Revision of the Act on Special Measures against Influenza of a New Type" and the "Cabinet Order Concerning the Establishment of Relevant Cabinet Orders in Connection with the Enforcement of the Act for Partial Revision of the Act on Special Measures against Influenza of a New Type"*, (12, February2021). Available at: https://corona.go.jp/news/pdf/sekoutuuchi_20210212.pdf.
108 Usui, M. A Study of Civil Penalties Imposed by Local Government, *Meiji Law School Review*, Vol. 16, p.49 (2015). Available at: https://m-repo.lib.meiji.ac.jp/dspace/bitstream/10291/17409/1/houkadaigakuinronshu_16_49.pdf.
109 Art.3(3) of the APA.

(ii) when a business fails to comply with a request to close or shorten business hours and infects more than a certain number of people, and (iii) when a person suspected of being infected refuses to take a test without a valid reason.

As per the revised Infectious Diseases Act, infected people can be asked to cooperate in prevention efforts by not going out, but there are no penalties for refusal. The TMG's draft ordinance aimed to make the inspections more effective by penalizing those in close contact with the infected who did not agree to the inspections.

Under Article 22[110] of the Constitution, restaurants enjoy the freedom to operate to businesses such as restaurants. The constitutionality of restrictions on the freedom to operate requires a detailed examination of the means to achieve the goal of protecting the health and lives of citizens.[111]

The public announcement is to provide information to citizens and does not restrict the rights and interests of restaurants under administrative guidance. However, it must be noted that in Japan, where peer pressure is strong, public announcement in a way restricts the freedom to operate businesses. When comparing the public interest of protecting the health and lives of the people with the freedom of business, we must not ignore the possibility that the public interest will inevitably deny the freedom of business.[112]

Global Dining Inc. filed a lawsuit against the Tokyo Metropolitan Government, claiming that the order to shorten business hours is unconstitutional and illegal. In May 2022, the Tokyo District Court ruled that the reduced business hours order was illegal. However, the court did not find state liability against TMG. The court focused on whether TMG had a reasonable basis for issuing the order four days before the emergency declaration was lifted.

14.3 Conclusion

In the 2020 CSMA, the government asked businesses to shorten their operating hours and there was no provision for sanctioning the request. Strong peer pressure in Japan resulted in many businesses shortening their hours of operation, but despite this, the prime minister was forced to re-extend the state of emergency in major cities.

This study examines the CSMA as amended in 2021. There are two main aspects of this amendment. The first is the addition of new measures to prevent the spread of infection,[113] and the second is the imposition of sanctions for violating the order to reduce business hours.[114] The new measures intend to prevent the spread of the disease by limiting the avenues of infection.[115]

The Infectious Diseases Act has also been amended to impose a non-penal (administrative) fine of up to 500,000 yen on patients who refuse to be hospitalized, and a non-penal fine of up to 300,000 yen on those who refuse to be investigated by the public health center. Both the CSMA[116] and the Infectious Diseases Act provided for non-penal administrative penalties, not criminal penalties.

In Japan, administrative guidance, which does not necessarily require a legal basis, was an extremely useful tool for responding to the spread of infection in a flexible manner prior to the

---

110 Nihon-Koku Kenpō [CONSTITUTION], Art. 22, translated in (The Constitution of Japan) [JAPANESE LAW TRANSLATION]. Available at: http://www.japaneselawtranslation.go.jp/law/detail/?id=174&vm=04&re=01& new=1 (Japan).
111 Moto, H., ed. (2018). *KENPŌKŌGI* (2nd ed.), Japan: Nihonhyōronsha, p. 298.
112 Koyama, G., Legal Issues in a Corona-disrupted Society (5) Voluntary Restraint, Compensation, and Publicity: Informal Regulatory Methods. *Hanrei jiho*, Vol. 2460, p. 145 (2021). (Koyama implies that even the informal regulatory such as public announcement can violate the principle of proportionality.)
113 Art.31-4 of 2021 CSMA.
114 Id. Art. 80.
115 Id. Art.31-4.
116 Id. Art.79, 80. Art.80, 81 of the Infectious Diseases Act.

2021 CSMA amendment. However, administrative guidance is a measure that expects citizens to act voluntarily and cannot solve all problems. To ground the activities of the government in law, the political sector is required to amend the law to cope with the spread of COVID-19.

Administrative guidance, if enforced more strictly than the law permits, may result in a liability in the State Redress Act.[117] In addition, the APA stipulates that the government shall not treat citizens unfavorably for not following the administrative guidance.[118]

Although the APA does not apply to the administrative guidance provided by the TMG, the TMG has enacted an Administrative Procedure Ordinance. The TMG's attempt to impose sanctions on infected individuals who infect others by failing to comply with requests to restrict work or refrain from going out, and on businesses that infect more than a certain number of people by failing to comply with requests to close or shorten business hours, has failed.

Under the 2021 amendment to the CSMA, the name of the business and the restaurant will be made public[119] if the order to shorten business hours is not obeyed.

The public announcement[120] of the request or order to change the opening hours may be key in preventing the spread of the disease because it can influence the general public's behavior. Therefore, it is necessary to consider the impact of such public announcements because they may prove counterproductive in preventing the spread of infection or cause slanderous behavior. In addition, publishing the name of a restaurant may attract too much attention and result in too many visitors, and the government may not publish the name if it cannot expect citizens to behave reasonably.

Under the Constitution, restaurants are granted the freedom to do business, and the purpose that supersedes their freedom to do business is the protection of life and health of the people. The means of achieving this purpose must be examined to determine if they properly serve this purpose.

In Japanese administrative jurisprudence, public announcement is considered to be a provision of information to citizens, not a restriction on their rights or the imposition of obligations. If the degree of disadvantage caused by a public announcement is too extensive, it is considered illegal in light of the principle of proportionality.

References

[Books]

Sakurai, K., and Hashimoto, H., (2017) *GYŌSEIHŌ* [Administrative law], 5th ed. Japan:Kōbundo
Moto, H., ed. (2018). *KENPŌKŌGI*, 2nd ed. Japan: Nihonhyōronsha.

[Government Sources]

Cabinet Secretariat (2021). *Subcommittee on Countermeasures for New Coronavirus Infections under the Cabinet secretariat.* https://www.cas.go.jp/jp/seisaku/ful/yusikisyakaigi.html.
Director, Office for Promotion of Countermeasures to Combat Novel Coronavirus Infections, Cabinet Secretariat (2021). *Indicators and guidelines for the implementation of countermeasures in response to future changes in the infection situation Indicators and guidelines for the implementation of countermeasures* (7 August 2020).

---

117 Kokka baishou hō [State Redress Act], Act No. 22 of 1947, Art. 1 (Japan).
118 Art.32(2) of APA.
119 Art.31-6(1), (3) of the 2021 CSMA.
120 Id. Art.45 (state of emergency is declared). Art.31-6(1),3 (measures to prevent the spread of infection are in effect).

Director, Office for Promotion of Countermeasures to Combat Novel Coronavirus Infections, Cabinet Secretariat (2021). *Promulgation of the "Act for Partial Revision of the Act on Special Measures against Influenza of a New Type" and the "Cabinet Order Concerning the Establishment of Relevant Cabinet Orders in Connection with the Enforcement of the Act for Partial Revision of the Act on Special Measures against Influenza of a New Type"* (12 February 2021). https://corona .go.jp/news/pdf/sekoutuuchi_20210212.pdf.

Ministry of Health, Labor, and Welfare (MHLW) (2021). *Todōfuken no iryō teikyō taisei-tō no jōkyō (iryō teikyō taisei-tō no fuka kansen no jōkyō) ni tsuite* [Status of medical care delivery system, etc., in prefectures (medical care delivery system, surveillance system, and status of infection). https://www.mhlw.go.jp/stf/seisakunitsuite/newpage_00035.html.

MHLW (2021). *Administrative handling of administrative penalties associated with the enforcement of the "Act for Partial Revision of the Act on Special Measures against Influenza, etc. of a New Type" (related to the Infectious Diseases Act)* (10 February 2021). https://www.mhlw.go.jp/ content/000737654.pdf.

Prime Minister's office of Japan (n.d.), Shingata koronauirusukansenshō ni kansuru Suga naikakusōri daijin kisha kaiken [Prime Minister Kan's press conference on the new coronavirus infection] (7 January 2021). https://www.kantei.go.jp/jp/99_suga/statement/2021/0107kaiken .html (2 February 2021).

Tochigi prefecture (2021). *Kinkyū jitai sochi-go no kansen kakudai bōshi ni muketa chiji messēji (2 tsuki 4-nichi)* [Governor's message to prevent the spread of infection after emergency measures] (4 February 2021). https://www.pref.tochigi.lg.jp/e04/20210204chijimesse-ji.html.

[Constitution and statutes]

Nihon-Koku Kenpō [CONSTITUTION], Art. 94, translated in (The Constitution of Japan) [JAPANESE LAW TRANSLATION]. http://www.japaneselawtranslation.go.jp/law/detail/? id=174&vm=04&re=01&new=1 (Japan).

(Statutes)

Gyōsei jiken soshou hō [Administrative Case Litigation Act], Act No. 139 of 1962, Art. 3(Japan).

Gyōsei tetuduki hō [Administrative procedure Act], Act No. 88 of 1993, art.2(6)(Japan).

Hisho jiken tetsuduki hō [Act on Non-Contentious Case Procedures], Act No. 51 of 2011, Art.119(Japan).

Jiei tai hō [Self Defense Act], Act No. 165 of 1954, Art.76,78.

Kansenshō no yobō oyobi kansenshō no kanja ni taisuru iryō ni kansru hō [Act on the Prevention of Infectious Diseases and Medical Care for Patients with Infectious Diseases], Act No.114 of 1998, art. 19. [hereinafter, Infectious Diseases Act].

Kokka baishou hō [State Redress Act], Act No. 22 of 1947, art. 1 (Japan).

Kokudo riyō keikaku hō [National Land Use Planning Act], Act no.92 of 1974, Art.24(Japan).

Saigai taisaku kihon hō [Basic Act on Disaster Management], Act No.223 of 1961, Art.105,106(Japan).

Seikatsu hogo hō [Public Assistance Act], Act No. 144 of 1950, Art.27(1)(Japan).

Shingata influenza tō taisaku tokbetsu sochi hō [Coronavirus Special Measures Act], Act No. 31 (revised as Act No. 4 of 2020). Available at: https://elaws.e-gov.go.jp/search/elawsSearch/ elaws_search/lsg0500/de-tail?lawId=424AC0000000031 (Japan) [hereinafter CSMA].

Supplementary provision of CSMA. See also, Order for Enforcement of the Act on Special Measures against Influenza, Ordinance No. 122 of 2013 (Japan).

[Judicial decisions]

Saiko Saibansho [Sup. Ct.] July 10, 1980, Showa 52 (o) no. 405, 130 SAIKŌ SAIBANSHO MINJI HANREISHŪ [MINSHŪ] 131.

Saiko Saibansho [Sup. Ct.] April 26, 2004, Hei 15 (gyo hi) no. 206, 58(4) SAIKŌ SAIBANSHO MINJI HANREISHŪ [MINSHŪ] 989. Available at: https://www.courts.go.jp/app/hanrei_jp/detail2?id=52393.

[Articles]

Tsuji, Y, Japanese Government Actions against COVID-19 under the Directives of Constitutional and Administrative Law, *Cardozo Journal of International and Comparative Law (JICL)*, Vol. 4, No. 1, pp. 1–34 (2021).

Tsuji, Y, Godzilla and the Japanese Constitution: A Comparison Between Italy and Japan, *3 Italian Law Journal*, No. 2, 451–477 (2017).

Usui, M., A Study of Civil Penalties Imposed by Local Government, *Meiji Law School Review*, Vol.16, pp. 49 (2015). https://m-repo.lib.meiji.ac.jp/dspace/bitstream/10291/17409/1/houkadaigakuinronshu_16_49.pdf.

Koyama, G., Legal Issues in a Corona-disrupted Society (5) Voluntary Restraint, Compensation, and Publicity: Informal Regulatory Methods, *Hanrei jiho1*, Vol. 2460, p. 45 (2021).

[Newspaper article]

Tokyo to inshoku 4 shisetsuni karyō tetuduki jitan meirei sitagawazu (2021). [Tokyo Metropolitan Government begins procedures to impose administrative fine on four restaurants that fail to comply with short-time orders]. *Nikkei Shimbun* (29 March). https://www.nikkei.com/article/DGXZQODG296SY0Z20C21A3000000/.

15

Canada's Fight Against COVID-19: Constitutionalism, Laws, and the Global Pandemic

Iffath U. Syed

Health Policy & Administration, Pennsylvania State University, Sharon, PA, USA

In this chapter, I will discuss major events, focusing on policies which occurred during the course of Canada's fight against COVID-19, starting from January 2020. The sources of this chapter include government websites, technical reports, mass media, and other gray literature. Given that significant media coverage occurred in some of the highest populated provinces, such as the Ontario, Quebec, and British Columbia, this chapter will include many examples from these provinces, especially the Province of Ontario, which also contains Canada's capital, Ottawa.

Canada had previously experienced an outbreak of Severe Acute Respiratory Sydnrome (SARS) in 2003. It was a significant event and there were a number of hard lessons learned from it. First, it crippled Toronto's economy, which included the loss of frontline healthcare workers. It also led to the fit-testing of N-95 respirators that were deemed to be appropriate personal protective equipment (PPE) for battling SARS along with other measures. Although Canada had previous experience of a coronavirus epidemic (i.e. SARS), the country's response to the recent strain of the novel form of the coronavirus has demonstrated inadequacy in preventing unnecessary hospital visits, research funding, and supervision of unreliable media reports. According to the *Learning from SARS* report by David Naylor and other Canada's top epidemic control experts, about 80% of Dr. Naylor's recommendations were implemented (Webster 2020; Yu et al. 2020).

During the contemporary novel coronavirus (COVID-19) pandemic, Canada has demonstrated a flexible approach in combating the spread of COVID-19. There have been a number of strengths in its approach to manage the COVID-19 pandemic, but also significant vulnerability. Canada is geographically close in proximity and economic exchange with the United States, the latter of which has been one of the hardest hit nations in the world with over 30 million cases and over half a million deaths, followed by Brazil, India, France, Russia, and the United Kingdom as of March 2021 (Coronavirus Resource Center 2021). Given Canada's geography, as well as the fact that it receives a large share of global migration, it is in a vulnerable position with respect to infectious disease.

Canada is said to be moderately hit by the spread of COVID-19 that originated from Wuhan, China. Canada's first case of COVD-19 was recorded on 25 January 2020, referred to as Patient Zero, who was a 56-year-old male who had returned from Wuhan, China to Toronto, Ontario (Bronca 2020; Silverstein et al. 2020). Patient Zero's wife also tested positive for COVID-19 but was asymptomatic. During this time, Canada issued a travel advisory against nonessential travel to China due to the outbreak, including a regional travel advisory to avoid all travel to the province of Hubei (Government of Canada 2020).

Impacts of the Covid-19 Pandemic: International Laws, Policies, and Civil Liberties, First Edition. Edited by Nadav Morag.
© 2023 John Wiley & Sons, Inc. Published 2023 by John Wiley & Sons, Inc.

After a few weeks, on 6 February 2020, Dr. David Williams, Ontario's public health chief, said that they would begin testing patients with symptoms who had come from other Chinese cities outside the quarantined Wuhan area (Bronca 2020), which meant that positive cases would be required to self-quarantine. On 26 February, Federal Minister of Health Patty Hajdu recommended that citizens should stockpile food and medication, noting that it was "good to be prepared because things can change quickly [in any emergency]" (Bharti 2020). This recommendation faced criticism from provincial politicians. For example, the Manitoba health minister Cameron Friesen and the Ontario health minister Christine Elliott both felt that there was no need for such aggressive stockpiling (Hayes and Patton 2020; Reimer 2020), and recommended against such bulk purchases in order to avoid the strain on supply chains. Despite heightened vigilance about the new and emerging coronavirus infectious disease, and despite new screening measures for those who were reporting being ill, a mining conference was held in Toronto which took place 2–5 March 2020 and attracted about 25,000 attendees from around the world, which resulted in confirmed positive cases (Bronca 2020).

The global COVID-19 pandemic drastically worsened in early March 2020 due to its rapid spread into Europe, North America, and other parts of Asia. Canadians travelling abroad were urged to return home. Some perceived this as irrational, since calling travelers home would likely spread the coronavirus more rapidly in the domestic context in Canada. For teaching staff and students below the senior high school level, all travel/leave out of Canada was prohibited except under exceptional circumstances until the end of June (Cho and Kurpierz 2020). Quebec was the only province that had banned travel between internal regions (on 28 March) (Cho and Kurpierz 2020).

Testing was a crucial early response that Canada did not diligently utilize until months into the pandemic (Yu et al. 2020). Despite its flaws, viral DNA detection was the primary testing method in Canada. Another area of concern was the passivity of testing. The first testing device was approved at the end of March 2020 and was slowly made available to the public (Yu et al. 2020). Testing was also initially limited to individuals who had contact with confirmed cases or recommended by a physician after presenting with at least one symptom of COVID-19 (Yu et al. 2020).

15.1 Non-Pharmaceutical Intervention (NPI) Measures

Canada was relatively delayed in implementing lockdown procedures and non-pharmaceutical intervention (NPI) measures, i.e. facemask recommendations (Yu et al. 2020). Ontario announced lockdown procedures on 17 March 2020 (Yu et al. 2020), comparatively late to when WHO announced COVID-19 as a worldwide pandemic on 11 March (Yu et al. 2020). As part of the interventions, leaders at the federal and provincial levels advised the community to follow the advice provided by public health officials (Walsh 2020h). Every province declared a state of emergency, closed primary and secondary schools, and many in-person university classes were also suspended. Every province shut down restaurants (except for take-out), and closed bars (Cho and Kurpierz 2020). A pause was even made on the scheduling of elective surgeries as a means of preventing transmission of COVID-19 given the more than 500 daily COVID-19 cases experienced in Ontario in April 2020 (Walsh 2020h). Almost all the provinces closed gyms (except British Columbia), imposed fines for ignoring social distancing (except Saskatchewan), and imposed fines for ignoring self-isolation protocols (except Manitoba) (Cho and Kurpierz 2020). Cinemas, surprisingly, were not shut down all across Canada. For example, Quebec allowed some cinemas to remain open; although later they were closed (Pringle 2021); whereas in Ontario, they were closed from the beginning of the first wave. British Columbia's lockdown was relatively light, allowing nonessential businesses to stay open provided they "…adapt [their] services and workplace to the orders and recommendations of the provincial health officer" (Cho and Kurpierz 2020) but as of 1 June had experienced fewer cases than Ontario, Quebec, or Alberta. Every province also restricted visits to nursing homes (Cho and Kurpierz 2020). Canadian hospitals efficiently adapted to the numerous stresses brought by the pandemic. For instance, Canadian hospitals have quickly restructured their emergency departments (ED) to facilitate an increase in health-care delivery (Yu et al. 2020). Amidst these closures, community gardens were opened in April 2020 as they provided an essential source of food, particularly for families and individuals facing food insecurity (Walsh 2020i). Prior to reopening the community gardens, however, safeguards for physical distancing and the cleaning and disinfecting of surfaces were first ensured (Walsh 2020i). To further support families, the federal government increased tax-free support under the Child Canada Benefit (CCB) program, increasing the benefit to $6,765 per child under age 6, and $5,708 per child aged 6 through 17 (Walsh 2020y). The increase in the benefit was introduced as further to the one-time payment of $300 earlier in May 2020 (Walsh 2020y).

Mandating indoor mask wear in public places is another powerful policy measure to slow the spread of COVID-19, with little associated economic disruption at least in the short run (Karaivanov et al. 2020). As early as February, numerous officials in Asian countries recommended wearing face masks as a means of self-protection, whereas recommendations in Canada were given at a much later date (Yu et al. 2020). The Chief Public Health Officer advised Canadians to wear a nonmedical face mask on 6 April in locations where social distancing is difficult to maintain (Yu et al. 2020). On 17 April, the Federal Minister of Transport announced measures requiring all air passengers to have a nonmedical mask or face coverings during travel and came into effect on 20 April 2020 (Yu et al. 2020). These delayed actions suggested that Canada was not diligent in taking action during the early stages of the pandemic which may have been crucial in drastically reducing viral transmission (Yu et al. 2020). However, research shows that despite this, mask mandates were associated with an average reduction of 25–31% in the weekly number of newly diagnosed COVID-19 cases in Ontario, Canada, and 36–46% reduction in weekly cases (Karaivanov et al. 2020). Mask mandates also increased self-reported mask usage in Canada by 30 percentage points, suggesting that the policy has a significant impact on behavior (ibid). Restrictions on businesses and gatherings were associated with a decrease of 48–57% in weekly cases, compared to a lack of such restrictions (ibid).

With the continued flattening of the curve, discussions for reopening were presented in April 2020. To address the mental health impact of COVID-19, in May 2020, Premier Ford presented expanded access to virtual and online mental health supports (Walsh 2020o). The increased supports included internet-based cognitive behavior therapy (iCBT) and virtual mental health services (Walsh 2020o). Specific services for children and youth and frontline workers experiencing anxiety, burnout, or post-traumatic stress disorder were also incorporated within the plan for expanded virtual mental health services (Walsh 2020o). For nonmedical manufacturing companies in Ontario, $50 million in funding was provided through the Ontario Together Fund to provide essential nonmedical supplies and services (Walsh 2020y). With the reopening of Ontario's economy, face-covering recommendations and additional recommendations for public transit were presented for the protection of both passengers and staff (Walsh 2020z).

15.2 COVID-19 Special Acts for Relief and Compensatory Measures

A number of policy measures were implemented in order to manage the outbreak and assist Canadians. Two measures, the Canada Emergency Wage Subsidy (CEWS) and the Canada Emergency Response Benefit (CERB), together comprised $109 billion of the $169 billion slated for use (Finance Canada and Parliamentary Budget Office, 2020; Cho and Kurpierz 2020). Every province froze evictions (Cho and Kurpierz 2020).

On 6 March 2020, the Federal Minister of Finance Bill Morneau stated that the next federal budget would include measures in response to the outbreak, including an increase to the risk adjustment provision and to support Canadians who were quarantined due to coronavirus (Tunney 2020). Days later, on 11 March 2020, the World Health Organization (WHO) declared the COVID-19 outbreak a pandemic (WHO 2020). Exactly another day later, it was confirmed that Canada's Prime Minister, Justin Trudeau's wife, Sophie Grégoire Trudeau tested positive for COVID-19 after returning from a speaking engagement in London, England, and she and the Prime Minister went into self-isolation (Slaughter and Bogart 2020). In addition to these events, various provincial governments across Canada became vigilant and implemented public school closures, announcing that students would not return to in-person instruction after the March break for at least several weeks (DeClerq 2020a). School closures, together with other measures such as travel restrictions were associated with a large decrease in weekly case-growth (Karaivanov et al. 2020).

On 13 March, Canada's Prime Minister, Justin Trudeau, announced that the federal government was preparing a stimulus package to address those affected by the pandemic (Russell and Connolly 2020). The federal government also announced a formal border-exit control policy and advised Canadians to avoid all nonessential travel and urged Canadians who were outside of Canada to return home promptly (Hansen and Cyr 2020). During the same day, various postsecondary schools across Canada banned in-person classes (Rodrigues 2020). A few days later, on 16 March, Federal Minister of Foreign Affairs, François-Philippe Champagne, also announced that for citizens who are still abroad, the country would provide emergency loans of up to $5,000 to cover travel costs or basic needs until they are able to return (Aiello 2020). The same day, the federal government announced that there would be new entry restrictions that would be implemented shortly after midnight ET on 18 March, restricting entry into the country to only Canadian citizens and permanent residents and their immediate families (Harris 2020). By this time, every province has declared a state of emergency in Canada. For example, on 17 March 2020, Ontario's Premier, Doug Ford, declared Ontario's first state of emergency following the death of a Barrie man (Tubb 2021).

Effective 18 March 2020, the federal government of Canada announced that all foreign nationals entering Canada and all returning Canadians and international arrivals would be funneled through airports in Toronto, Vancouver, Montreal, and Calgary (Bronca 2020). Initially, travelers from the United States were excepted from this policy but on 18 March 2020, they were also banned in a mutual agreement with the US government (with exceptions in place for family members, for essential employees who commute across the border and for to ensure continued exchange of goods) (Harris 2020). In addition to these travel restrictions, the Federal Minister of Foreign Affairs François-Philippe Champagne also announced that for citizens who are still abroad, the country would provide emergency loans of up to $5,000 to cover travel costs or basic needs until they are able to return (Aiello 2020).

In late March, various provincial governments started implementing policies across Canada. For example, the Ontario government implemented a mandatory closure of all nonessential workplaces in order to fight the spread of COVID-19 (Government of Ontario 2020a). However, to assist essential workers, the provincial government of Ontario issued an emergency order directing certain childcare centers to reopen with fewer children to allow for physical distancing (Government of Ontario 2020b). These included shut down of restaurants (except for take-out), closed bars, frozen evictions, and restricted visits to nursing homes (Cho and Kurpierz 2020). All but one province has closed gyms (British Columbia allowed them to remain open), while some of the remainder of the provinces also imposed fines for ignoring social distancing (in Saskatchewan for instance), or imposed fines for ignoring self-isolation protocols (e.g. Manitoba) (Cho and Kurpierz 2020). On the same day, Toronto mayor John Tory declared a state of emergency due to the COVID-19 pandemic (Katawazi 2020).

On 24 March 2020, a small number of MPs from each party met in the House of Commons to vote on an $82-billion emergency spending legislation, known as Bill C-13 (Connolly 2020; Corbella 2020). The passage of the bill was stalled due to the federal government's proposed clauses that gave the finance minister the right to spend money and raise taxes without the approval of Parliament until 31 December 2021 (ibid). After criticism from the Official Opposition over the minority government's "power grab" which was considered undemocratic, a revised bill was agreed upon the next day that would permit the government six months of special spending powers until 30 September 2020, with oversight from a Parliamentary committee (BNN Bloomberg 2020; Corbella 2020).

By the end of March 2020, Quebec was the only province that had banned travel between internal regions (on 28 March 2020) and one of only four provinces that had banned travel between provinces – but it also experienced some of the worst infectious spread of any province (Cho and Kurpierz 2020). It has also implemented curfews from 8 p.m. and 5 a.m., and anyone who violates the curfew would be fined between $1,000 and $6,000 (Pringle 2021). The curfews were delayed on 17 March 2021 and started at 9:30 p.m. (Riga 2021), but then rolled back to 8:00 p.m. again after case counts increased (Montpetit 2021). In contrast, British Columbia's lockdown was relatively light, allowing nonessential businesses to stay open provided they "…adapt [their] services and workplace to the orders and recommendations of the provincial health officer" (Cho and Kurpierz 2020).

At the federal level, as of April 2020, the Canadian government also offered Federal Aid Programs of which included a CAD $73B wage subsidy bill that was passed by the Senate and received Royal Assent, as well as CAD $50M in federal support for farmers to help with farm labor shortages and cover any costs of mandatory quarantine for foreign workers coming into Canada (Walsh 2020a). By mid-April, the total number of COVID-19 cases in Canada was 25,663, with approximately 780 deaths (Walsh 2020a). Furthermore, almost six million Canadians applied for financial support under the Canadian Emergency Response Benefit (CERB) (Walsh 2020a). The federal Employment and Workforce Development Minister Carla Qualtrough had urged the provinces not to claw back the CERB benefit from recipients of provincial social assistance. Although British Columbia followed this recommendation and exempted social assistant recipients from benefit-claw back, other provincial governments, such as Ontario's conservative government under Premier Doug Ford, did not initially do this and indicated that it would review CERB and its impact on recipients of social assistance (Walsh 2020a). The Canadian Armed Forces (CAF) and the Canadian Rangers were also deployed to help in the territories of Nunavut and northern Quebec in the fight against COVID-19 (Walsh 2020b). On 18 April, the federal government announced Supports for Medical Research while the Ontario government along with the provincial Minister of Colleges and Universities announced investment of $20 million to advance medical research and develop tools and resources to combat COVID-19 and other infectious diseases through its Rapid Research Fund (Walsh 2020d). By the end of April 2020, the federal government also included a CEWS program for small and large businesses in order to encourage them to rehire laid off employees or to hire new employees (Walsh 2020e). CEWS offered businesses a maximum of $847 per employee per week, for a period of 12 weeks dating back to 15 March and ending on 6 June, with no limit on the total subsidy amount that an eligible employer may claim (Alini and D'Amore 2020; Walsh 2020e).

The federal government also announced various measures for students. For example, it announced a $9B support package for postsecondary students and recent graduates which included launching Canada Emergency Student Benefit (CESB), which would provide support to students and new graduates who are not eligible for the CERB and to provide $1,250 per month for eligible students or $1,750 per month for eligible students with dependents or disabilities from May to August 2020 (Walsh 2020f). It also launched various grants to help students gain valuable work experience and skills in national services to assist in their communities during the COVID-19 pandemic; and provide up to $5,000 for their education in the fall (Walsh 2020f), and enhancement of the Canada Student Loans Program and opportunities for graduate students and postdoctoral fellows through the National Research Council of Canada (Walsh 2020f). In May 2020, Prime Minister Justin Trudeau announced student eligibility for the CESB in which students could receive $1,250 a month from May to August 2020 and an additional $1,750 for students caring for a dependent and students with disabilities (Walsh 2020v). Students making less than $1,000 a month remained eligible for the CESB benefit. Additionally, the doubling of funding for student grants was announced by the federal government providing up to $6,000 for full-time students and $3,600 for part-time students (Walsh 2020v). Graduate research scholarships and postdoctoral fellowships and the extension of federal research grants were also announced, funded by $291 million for federal granting councils (Walsh 2020v). By the end of May 2020, the Ontario government announced the reduction of financial barriers for full-time postsecondary students through a six-month deferral of the Ontario Student Assistance Program (OSAP), effective from 30 May through 30 September 2020 (Walsh 2020z).

In addition to supporting individual students, on 15 May 2020, the Prime Minister announced $450 million in funding to support the academic research community during the pandemic (Walsh 2020x). The purpose of these funds was to support the wages of and retain staff at Canada's research institutes and those funded by industry or philanthropic sources impacted by COVID-19 (Walsh 2020x). A wage subsidy of up to 75% per individual was provided to ensure the continuation of essential research (Walsh 2020x).

The freezing of evictions by all provinces earlier in 2020 led to the development of the Ontario-Canada Emergency Commercial Rent Assistance Program (OCECRA) to provide relief to landlords and small businesses (Walsh 2020h). The $241 million program offered forgivable loans to commercial property owners that were impacted by the inability of small business owners to pay the cost of their rental (Walsh 2020h). The plan was initially aimed to provide reduced rental costs to small business tenants by 75% in April, May, and June 2020 (Walsh 2020h). The Canada Emergency Commercial Rental Assistance (CECRA) similarly provided a lowered rent by 75% for small businesses, nonprofit organizations, and charitable organizations impacted by COVID-19 (Walsh 2020h). CECRA was made eligible for tenants paying less than $50,000 per month in rent and experiencing an at least 70% drop in revenue due to COVID-19 (Walsh 2020h). The program was to be available for April, May, and June 2020, with tenants expected to pay 25% of the rent (Walsh 2020h). Commercial property owners would then be responsible for covering 25% of the rent, with the federal government and provinces covering the remaining 50% of the rent (Walsh 2020h). Landlords became eligible for applying for benefits through CECRA beginning on 25 May 2020 (Walsh 2020z). At the end of May, the Prime Minister again announced the need to present additional measures to support larger companies (Walsh 2020z). Service hotlines were established to further support small and vulnerable businesses on their path to recovery (Walsh 2020ad).

The federal government also provided additional supports to e-commerce entities through the Canadian Agricultural Partnership given the spike in online shopping during COVID-19 (Walsh 2020h). The funding streams from the $2.5 million investment included the ability of organizations and businesses to apply for a grant of up to $5,000 to support e-business and marketing as well as an option for cost-share funding of up to $75,000 for the implementation of high-impact projects (Walsh 2020h). Along with the announcements for OCECRA, CECRA, and the investments of the Canadian Agricultural Partnership, Prime Minister Trudeau also announced additional support for small businesses within federal developments, highlighting small businesses as the "backbone of our community" (Walsh 2020h).

Prime Minister Trudeau announced additional funding for fish and seafood processors in April 2020 in the form of $62.5 million (Walsh 2020i). As fish and seafood processors served as a key source of food for the public, the funds were aimed to keep processors and their workers safe through the purchase of PPE and the implementation of additional health protocols to support social distancing measures (Walsh 2020i). Additionally, support was offered to fish harvesters in May 2020 due to the decreased demand and declining prices for Canadian fish and seafood products experienced by Canadian fishers (Walsh 2020w). The support from the government came in the form of $267.6 million in income support for self-employed fish harvesters through the Fish Harvester Benefit and an additional $201.8 million to provide $10,000 grants in the Fish Harvester Grant program (Walsh 2020w). Also in May 2020, the Prime Minister announced additional support for Canada's agriculture industry in response to a request from the Canadian Federation of Agriculture for $2.6 billion in aid (Walsh 2020o). The initial amount offered was $252 million to support farmers and food processors safely operate during the COVID-19 pandemic (Walsh 2020o). An additional $2.2 million was introduced to support the protection of employees at licensed meat processing plants (Walsh 2020r).

Beyond providing financial support for businesses and individual renters, Premier Ford also announced additional temporary pandemic pay for frontline workers that were placing their lives at risk to care for those in long-term care (LTC) homes, retirement homes, emergency shelters, supportive housing, social services congregate care centers, corrections institutions and youth justice facilities, Indigenous healing and wellness facilities and shelters, home and community care, and some hospital staff (Walsh 2020i). Eligible frontline workers received a pay increase of four dollars per hour to their hourly wages for an initial period of 16 weeks (Walsh 2020i). Eligible frontline workers that worked more than 100 hours per month also received an additional $250 per month over the 16-week period (Walsh 2020i). In May 2020, additional pay increases were discussed due to a call for additional support of frontline and marginalized workers (Walsh 2020q).

Additional support for Indigenous communities was announced on 14 May 2020, including $360 million in interest-free loans and contributions to Indigenous businesses; $75 million to First Nations, Inuit, and Métis students in need of support in finding a job within their community; and $10 million for emergency shelters to house Indigenous women and children fleeing violence (Walsh 2020w). On 21 May 2020, Prime Minister Trudeau announced an additional $75 million on top of the $15 million announced in March to support organizations in addressing the critical needs of Indigenous people living in both urban centers and off-reserve (Walsh 2020aa). On 29 May 2020, a new investment of $650 million was announced to support healthcare, income, and shelter initiatives within indigenous communities (Walsh 2020ah).

On Monday, 27 April, applications for the Canadian Emergency Wage Subsidy (CEWS) program, a $73 billion wage subsidy program, were provided to prevent businesses and nonprofit organizations from laying off their employees (Walsh 2020j). The first payments were expected to arrive by 7 May 2020 (Walsh 2020j). The restrictions for the program were that individuals were eligible to apply for either CEWS or the Canadian Emergency Relief Benefit (Walsh 2020j). In May 2020, an extension of the CEWB beyond June 2020 was announced in response to the revelation by Statistics Canada that approximately two million people in Canada lost their jobs in April due to COVID-19 (Walsh 2020r). The purpose of the extension of CEWB was to encourage businesses to apply for the subsidy and keep their employees on their payroll (Walsh 2020r).

By 13 May 2020, more than 120,000 employers were approved to receive CEWS to support approximately two million workers (Walsh 2020v). The extension of CEWB was also to serve as an alternative to CERB (Walsh 2020r). Also in May 2020, the Large Employer Emergency Financing Facility (LEEFF) program was introduced to maintain employees on the payroll through government-supported loans and financing (Walsh 2020t). With the effects of COVID-19 ongoing, on 15 May 2020, the extension of CEWS until 29 August and the broadening of eligibility criteria were announced (Walsh 2020x). The Canadian Emergency Business Account (CEBA) program was similarly extended and expanded to further support Canadian employers to include businesses with sole proprietors, businesses that rely on contractors, and family-owned businesses that issue payments through dividends (Walsh 2020y).

15.3 Long-Term Care Crisis

Although Canada maintained a considerably low number of confirmed cases at this time compared to the United States, the number of deaths in particular sectors of work, such as in LTC homes, had exceeded the average of the Organization for Economic Cooperation and Development (OECD) (Grant 2020; Syed and McLaren 2021). The federal government, through the Public Health Agency of Canada (PHAC), also introduced new interim guidelines in April 2020 for LTC infection prevention and control of COVID-19 for LTC homes (PHAC 2020a). The guidelines complemented provincial efforts, and ensured proper training on the use of PPE and identifying suspected or confirmed cases of COVID-19 in staff, residents, and any essential visitors. Unfortunately, many provinces, such as Ontario also attempted to identify and limit staff from working in more than one LTC home (Walsh 2020c), which resulted in a catastrophic deficiency of staff. Eventually, the CAF were brought into LTC homes in Ontario and Quebec, where the worst of the pandemic hit elderly residents (Walsh 2020ae). The particularly hardest hit provinces included Ontario and Quebec, for which the Red Cross trained the military and the CAF entered LTC homes to assist with the pandemic (Armstrong 2020). On 26 May 2020, the Province of Ontario released a 14 May 2020 report by the CAF and the province asked the federal government of Canada for assistance and CAF to extend their stay in the LTC homes (Walsh 2020ae; Canadian Military Family Magazine 2020). A day later, the Province of Ontario announced they would be taking over five LTC homes in Toronto and the Greater Toronto Area (GTA) following the CAF report that had cited neglect and abuse in LTC homes (Walsh 2020af). The CAF announced that they would remain at least until 12 June 2020 to manage outbreaks within the LTC homes (Walsh 2020af). Three of the five LTC homes were located in Toronto: Eatonville Care Centre, Hawthorne Place Care Centre, and Altamont Care Community (Patton 2020). In response to these issues, the Ontario government adopted an emergency order allowing the government to take control of the management of LTC facilities facing challenges due to COVID-19, including those facing a high number of COVID-19 cases, deaths, and staff shortages (Walsh 2020v). An independent inquiry into LTC homes was announced along with a mandate for incident management to deal with staffing levels, infection management, and resources during COVID-19 (Walsh 2020ag).

The COVID-19 Action Plan for Vulnerable People was introduced to bring long-term solutions to vulnerable populations (Walsh 2020g). The COVID-19 Action Plan for Vulnerable People included new measures for mental health and addictions agencies, providing such organizations with extra part-time, temporary, and contract staff to facilitate redeployment (Walsh 2020g). In alignment with long-term planning, the COVID-19 Action Plan for Vulnerable People was aimed at those in LTC facilities, including homes serving individuals with developmental disabilities, shelters for survivors of gender-based violence and human trafficking, and children in residential settings (Walsh 2020g). For seniors, a one-time payment of $500 was offered to eligible seniors to assist with unexpected living expenses incurred due to COVID-19 (Walsh 2020t).

Testing within LTC settings became a priority, with Health Minister Elliott announcing on 14 May 2020, that all LTC home residents had been tested, with testing expanding to congregate settings (Walsh 2020w). By 19 May 2020, an independent commission into the LTC system in Ontario was announced for launch in September 2020 (Walsh 2020y).

15.4 Research and Vaccine Development Initiatives

Along with the global initiative to develop a vaccine against COVID-19, Canada invested in research and vaccine development (Walsh 2020g). In April 2020, the Canadian national strategy included more than $1 billion, which was more than triple the previously announced $275 million for COVID-19 research and medical countermeasures (Walsh 2020g). The breakdown of the funds introduced in the national strategy included $40 million for the development of host genome sequencing efforts; $23 million for the acceleration of vaccine development against COVID-19; $29 million for the production of vaccines for testing in clinical trials and the associated infrastructure and operations for vaccine development; $600 million for vaccine and therapy clinical trials; $10 million for the development of a national data monitoring initiative for data sharing and coordination; $10.3 million for the ongoing support of vaccine research, clinical trials, and monitoring; $114.9 million for medical and social countermeasures against the spread of COVID-19; and $675,000 for research on clinical trials in the use of potential cell therapy to explore how cells in the airway and brain are affected by COVID-19 (Walsh 2020g). Clinical trials were first approved at the Canadian Center for Vaccinology at Dalhousie University in May 2020 (Walsh 2020y).

Beyond research and vaccine development, a COVID-19 Immunity Task Force was developed to establish priorities and support oversight of testing (Walsh 2020g). Such an initiative was necessary for tracking the virus long-term, with an initially anticipated timeline of two years from April 2020 (Walsh 2020g). A specific emphasis was placed on monitoring specific risk groups such as health-care workers and the elderly (Walsh 2020g). In May 2020, Canada also committed $850 million toward global COVID-19 efforts and presented the new integrated laboratory system in Ontario used to support COVID-19 testing targets (Walsh 2020n). In Ontario, the government partnered with the Medical Innovation Xchange (MIX) to provide free support to nonmedical manufacturing companies to provide essential supplies and equipment to health-care facilities during COVID-19, building upon the support provided through the Ontario Together Fund (Walsh 2020y). To support rapid research, Ontario announced $20 million toward the Ontario COVID-19 Rapid Research Fund for the discovery of COVID-19 vaccines and treatments (Walsh 2020aa). At the time of the announcement, Ontario was leading the country in COVID-19 clinical trials and treatments at 22 clinical trials (Walsh 2020aa).

With advancements in clinical trials and efforts to reopen the economy, Prime Minister Trudeau announced on 22 May 2020, three focus areas for safely reopening the economy (Walsh 2020ab). The three focus areas were (i) scaling up testing and identifying and isolating new cases, (ii) accelerating capacity for contact tracing, and (iii) improving the sharing of information across jurisdictions (Walsh 2020ab).

15.5 Other Policies and Governmental Actions to Dampen the Pandemic

In April 2020, efforts to reopen Ontario and Quebec were introduced (Walsh 2020j). These efforts aimed to ease restrictions implemented in response to COVID-19 (Walsh 2020j). The plans for reopening by Ontario as one of the two largest provinces in Canada was introduced through A Framework for Reopening out Province, which includes advice from Ontario's Chief Medical Officer of Health on the measures needed to support the safe, gradual reopening of businesses, services, and public spaces (Walsh 2020j). Within these plans for reopening, Premier Doug Ford emphasized that the plan was to serve as a roadmap of guiding principles rather than a calendar for the reopening of the province (Walsh 2020j). The plan introduced the gradual reopening to occur in the form of stages for the reopening of Ontario (Walsh 2020j). In Stage 1, workplaces that could meet public health guidelines, limited essential gatherings, and some outdoor spaces would be permitted to opening (Walsh 2020j). Within Stage 1, continued protections for vulnerable populations were to be provided and hospitals would be opened to some nonurgent and scheduled services and other health-care services (Walsh 2020j). In Stage 2, additional workplaces, public spaces, and larger public gatherings would be permitted, again with continued protections (Walsh 2020j). Stage 3 was the final stage to allow for the reopening of all workplaces and reduced restrictions for public gatherings, with ongoing protection for vulnerable populations (Walsh 2020j). However, even in the final stage, large gatherings in the form of concerts and sporting events were still expected to be restricted (Walsh 2020j). Each of the three stages presented by Ford was contingent on the spread and containment of COVID-19, health system capacity, public health system capacity, and incidence tracking capacity (Walsh 2020j). In response to this proposal for reopening Ontario, Chief Medical Officer of Health, Dr. Williams, noted that the province was still in a pandemic phase as of April 2020 and still had a "ways to go" before reopening (Walsh 2020j). With the reopening still further away, Ontario Jobs and Recovery Committee continues with recovery plans for the providence to revive the economy (Walsh 2020j).

In response to the reopening provincial economies and Ontario in particular, Prime Minister Trudeau explained that the federal government would provide support to the provinces as they considered reopening (Walsh 2020j). Efforts for reopening were to involve collaborations on shared guidelines to ensure adequate medical capacity, sufficient testing, and customized guidelines for specific sectors (Walsh 2020j). Through agreement among federal, provincial, and territorial governments, a set of guiding principles was developed for restarting the Canadian economy to ensure control of transmission and adequate capacity upon reopening (Walsh 2020k). Government officials began to announce a path toward reopening, coinciding with the flattening of the curve (Walsh 2020l). On this path, the Premier presented guidelines to support workplace safety additional guidance specific to individual sectors (Walsh 2020l). The Premier announced that in Ontario, certain businesses would be allowed to reopen on 4 May 2020, following the strict guidelines introduced, which was presented as a sign of hope for reopening after the pandemic (Walsh 2020m). Ontario continued to reduce restrictions, with additional opening of retail stores and essential construction between 8 May and 11 May 2020 (Walsh 2020p). On 9 May, the opening of provincial parks and conservation was reserved for restricted use (Walsh 2020s). Plans to support the reopening of schools were also developed, including plans for support from the government to provide funding to childcare agencies for when parents returned to work (Walsh 2020s). The rollout of the reopening of provinces was approached with caution due to concerns surrounding reopening too soon (Walsh 2020s). The reopening of the economy was associated with more potential outbreaks and deaths associated with COVID-19, particularly in LTC facilities (Walsh 2020s). Concerns for facilitating a safe reopening process led to a slow rollout of the reopening plans (Walsh 2020s).

Contradictions in the reopening process were evident in May 2020, with Premier Ford stating that the province was prepared for further reopening alongside plans within stage one of reopening Ontario's economy (Walsh 2020u). Ontario's Chief Medical Officer, however, did not share the sentiment that Ontario was ready for entering stage one of reopening (Walsh 2020u). The challenge in reopening was that the curve had not been reduced as rapidly as needed for safely entering into stage one for reopening (Walsh 2020u). These concerns were passed over by Premier Ford as "bumps in the road" in the process of reopening (Walsh 2020t, 2020u). Moreover, in the process of Ontario's reopening, the Declaration of Emergency was extended to 2 June 2020, despite Ontario's plans for gradual reopening (Walsh 2020u).

Although the federal government had also planned to open the U.S.–Canada border by 20 April 2020, it extended the closure for another month (Walsh 2020c; Walsh 2020i), and repeated this throughout 2021 (Walsh 2020y). The Prime Minister noted that Canada was in no rush to reduce nonessential travel restrictions between the United States and Canada (Walsh 2020u). In the province of Ontario, on 26 April 2020, the provincial government extended schools closures based on expert advice from the Chief Medical Officer of Health and health officials on the COVID-19 Command Table (Government of Ontario 2020b; Walsh 2020c; Walsh 2020p). As of May 2020, cases of COVID-19 also broke out at other healthcare sectors, such as publicly funded hospitals. The University Health Network (UHN) spokesperson Gillian Howard confirmed that four separate outbreaks of COVID-19 affected both patients and staff at Toronto Western Hospital (Fox 2020a). This demonstrated that Canada was also vulnerable to community spread, and the new variant. Despite these facts, one of the most controversial moments in Canada's history during the COVID-19 pandemic came on 23 May 2020, when 10,000 people (mostly young) gathered in Trinity Bellwoods Park, including brief visit by Toronto's Mayor John Tory (Hendsbee 2020; Powell, 2020).

The gathering followed on from similar demonstrations in Queen's Park in April 2020 in which demonstrators argued that COVID-19 was a hoax and fake news (Walsh 2020i). In the process, these demonstrators placed the lives of others at risk (Walsh 2020i). For the 23 May 2020 incident, tickets were issued by the police, but it was for public urination (Walsh 2020i) as opposed to breaking social distancing rules. In response to the gathering, Toronto Board of Health chair Joe Cressy and Toronto's Medical Officer of Health, Dr. Eileen de Villa, along with the City of Toronto, issued warning statements about the adverse impacts of such gatherings (Ritchie 2020). Ontario government and Premier Ford also urged restraint against having such mass gatherings (Rushowy and Ferguson 2020). Toronto's Mayor also apologized after the incident. Thereafter, the City of Toronto implemented and painted "social distancing circles" in the park the following week, modeled after similar tactics used in San Francisco and New York City (Fox 2020b). The Premier expressed his shock at the crowding of people over the weekend and emphasized the importance of testing upon potential or actual exposure to COVID-19, pending the development of a vaccine (Walsh 2020ac). By 25 May 2020, Ontario announced more than 400 new cases of COVID-19 in a single day for the fifth day in a row, attributing the higher rates to the holiday weekends and the gathering of people in groups (Walsh 2020ad).

Several policy changes and events occurred at the end of May and into June, which were spilled over from events from the previous month. For example, on 30 May, the Retirement Homes Act of 2010 was amended to increase the emergency payment that could be made to eligible retirement home residents, applicable not only during COVID-19 but also beyond the pandemic (Walsh 2020ai). On 31 May, $30 million allocated originally to foreign travel to Canada was used to encourage holiday travel by Canadians within Canada (Walsh 2020ai). Additionally, on 1 June 2020, the City of Toronto announced two phases for reopening park washrooms with the first phase reopening about 50 washroom sites by 6 June 2020, and the remaining by mid-June in response to public urination and tickets issued on 23 May, 2020 at Trinity Bellwoods Park (City of Toronto 2020). On 8 June, as the incidence of COVID-19 cases also dipped, the Ontario government allowed Stage 2 reopening in various cities effective 12 June 2020 with the exception of Toronto (Feinstein 2020). This meant that gatherings would increase from 5 to 10 people (except in Toronto, where cases were deemed to be too high to allow loosening of restrictions and Stage-2 reopening was delayed

(Feinstein 2020). On 16 June 2020, the CAF also left LTC homes, including the privately owned Eatonville Care Centre in Etobicoke (a Toronto) LTC facility (DeClerq 2020b). On 22 June 2020, the Province of Ontario announced that it would allow Stage 2 reopening in Toronto effective 24 June 2020 (DeClerq 2020c). Finally, on 30 June 2020, Toronto City Councillors vote on requiring mask requirements at all public settings, including public transit, such as the Toronto Transit Commission (Pagliaro 2020). This policy went into effect on 7 July 2020 (Pagliaro 2020). Three weeks later, on 29 July 2020, Stage 3 reopening was allowed in Toronto and Peel effective 31 July 2020 (Daily Hive 2020).

In early August 2020, the Ontario government requested public health or public health units for guidance about the appropriate delivery and approach for reopening schools for the beginning of the 2020–2021 school year (Government of Ontario 2020c). By 10 August 2020, certain municipalities in Canada announced improvements in cases. For example, Toronto Public Health stipulated that the pandemic stage was upgraded to green (Passafiume 2020).

In the fall of 2020, however, schools in major municipalities had a delayed start. For example, Toronto public schools delayed their start to 15 September 2020 (Fox and Freeman 2020). Normally, schools would have otherwise begun the day after Labor Day. From October to November, many provinces continued to be in lockdowns. For example, Ontario was in a gray lockdown. Wave 1 cases increased again after Stage 3 reopening had occurred (Tubb 2021). In particular, Toronto's "local trend" revealed that the pandemic had a "disproportionate impact on lower-income and racialized communities" (Tubb 2021, para. 4). On 4 November, the Ontario Government's Education Ministry (headed by Ontario Education Minister Stephen Lecce) announced that school boards would decide about the closures, and stated that all boards must offer virtual classes for students who chose to study at home (Miller 2020). The province of Ontario also changed its staging system from a numbered one to a color code system. For example, in late November, it declared a white zone, meaning a complete shutdown and stay-at-home order (Tubb 2021).

15.6 New Year, But Pandemic Looms

As of January 2021, some provinces decided to close schools completely. For example, the Ontario Government decided to close schools in Southern Ontario until 25 January, and schools in the following areas: Toronto, York, Peel Windsor, and Hamilton regions (Alphonso 2021). A mandatory stay-at-home order was also in effect at this time as wave 2 infections continued (Tubb 2021). In March, there was a positive shift from the white zone (shutdown) to the gray zone (lockdown) (Tubb 2021). This allowed for 25% retail capacity (ibid). However, this positive trend reversed on 7 April 2021, as case counts increased again in Ontario (Government of Ontario 2020d; Bianchini 2021). This shutdown was worse than previous ones because retail stores were allowed to stay open for curbside pickup and delivery only and nonessential items were taped off so that consumers could not purchase them (Government of Ontario 2020d; Bianchini 2021). In Toronto and the GTA, the TDSB and Peel region in-person classes/schools were also shut down (Government of Ontario 2020e), and remained shut down until June 2021.

Sadly, some notable COVID-19 cases received notable attention, such as the death of 13-year-old Emily Viegas, whose father was an essential worker (Rider 2021). Emily's death was highlighted as preventable, especially if workers had access to paid sick days (Bianchini 2021). The growing calls for paid sick days (Syed and McLaren 2021; Woodward 2021), which were previously ignored, finally led the Ontario conservative government to accept and implement a paid-sick leave policy. However, the government only offered 3 paid sick days (Tsekouras 2021), which was only a third of the 10 days that interest groups were advocating (Nasser and Powers 2021).

15.7 Summary, Limitations, and Concluding Remarks

This chapter described the major events and policies that occurred during the course of Canada's fight against COVID-19. To date, Canada's government has deployed various measures against COVID-19 to respond to the outbreak through general legislative processes and procedures and numerous investments in both proactive and responsive actions. The governments and courts remained functioning despite the health crisis and challenges experienced within the health system. For example, family courts did not hold in-person hearings during the peak of the pandemic, but law and order was never threatened. Some Canadian provinces had curfews, such as Quebec, despite the fact that stay-at-home orders or shutdown-of-the-city orders can undermine normalcy. However, some of the late responses and late deployment of certain policies, as well as the failure to implement a precautionary principle approach at times, have led to stagnation of improvement. At other times, masking fueled anger among angry businesses and restaurateurs.

This chapter included discussion of topics such as: international travel restrictions, restrictions on freedom of movement within Canada (inter-provincially), restrictions on public gatherings, financial incentives and supports for people and businesses, retail and school closures, and a brief discussion on implications for healthcare, including LTC. One of the limitations of this chapter is that it did not explore action footprints or the application of digital technology, such as pandemic prevention tools. The use of such mechanisms, while interesting, might be a starting point for further work. For example, what are the tools that are employed to control COVID-19 information, such as using cell-phone signals to monitor at-home isolation cases? What are the implications on people's right to information and privacy? When personal information that is gathered and linked or integrated by the government be stored or deleted after the epidemic has ended? While Canada was moderately successful in containing the COVID-19 pandemic, given the current delta variant and its potential to impact restrictions and measures, it remains to be seen what the implications of containment measures on long-term security and stability, including economic stability after the pandemic truly ends.

References

Aiello, R. (2020, March 16). Canada shutting the border to most non-citizens due to COVID-19: PM Trudeau. *CTV News*. Available from: https://www.ctvnews.ca/health/coronavirus/canada-shutting-the-border-to-most-non-citizens-due-to-covid-19-pm-trudeau-1.4854503 (accessed 18 October 2021).

Alini, E., and D'Amore, R. (2020, April 28). CEWS vs. CERB: How the two benefits fit together and who may have to return payments. *Global News*. Available from: https://globalnews.ca/news/6876790/canada-coronavirus-cews-cerb/ (accessed 18 October 2021).

Alphonso, C. (2021, January 19). Ontario's decision to keep students at home questioned by critics. *The Globe and Mail*. Available from: https://www.theglobeandmail.com/canada/article-ontarios-decision-to-keep-students-at-home-questioned-by-critics/ (accessed 18 October 2021).

Armstrong, M. (2020, May 24). Operation LASER: a timeline of the Canadian Forces deployment to seniors homes. *Global News*. Available from: https://globalnews.ca/news/6978533/coronavirus-canadian-forces-seniors-homes-operation-laser/ (accessed 18 October 2021).

Bharti, B. (2020, February 26). Coronavirus updates: Stockpile food and meds in case of infection, Canada's health minister says. *The National Post*. Available from: https://nationalpost.com/news/world/coronavirus-live-updates-who-covid19-covid-19-italy-china-canada-wuhan-deaths (accessed 18 October 2021).

Bianchini, E. (2021, April 26). 'Politics are at the ROOT of Emily Viegas' death': Ontario government slammed for 'cold-hearted' response to Brampton teen's COVID-19 tragedy. *Yahoo!News*. Available from: https://ca.style.yahoo.com/brampton-ontario-teen-covid19-death-emily-viegas-doug-ford-paid-sick-leave-225601123.html (accessed 18 October 2021).

BNN Bloomberg (2020, March 24). *Tories will support aid to Canadians, not Liberal 'power grab': Scheer*. Available from: https://www.bnnbloomberg.ca/tories-will-support-aid-to-canadians-not-liberal-power-grab-scheer-1.1411317 (accessed 18 October 2021).

Bronca, T. (2020, April 8). COVID-19: a Canadian timeline. *Canadian Healthcare Network*. Available from: https://www.canadianhealthcarenetwork.ca/covid-19-a-canadian-timeline (accessed 18 October 2021).

Canadian Military Family Magazine (2020, May 26). *Canadian Armed Forces Long Term Care Facility Report Released*. Available from: https://www.cmfmag.ca/todays_brief/canadian-armed-forces-long-term-care-facility-report-released/ (accessed 18 October 2021).

Cho, C. H., and Kurpierz, J. (2020). Stretching the public purse: budgetary responses to COVID-19 in Canada. *Journal of Public Budgeting, Accounting & Financial Management* 771–783. https://doi.org/10.1108/JPBAFM-05-2020-0070.

City of Toronto (2020, June 1). City of Toronto to reopen parks washrooms. Available from: https://www.toronto.ca/news/city-of-toronto-to-reopen-parks-washrooms/ (accessed 18 October 2021).

Connolly, A. (2020, March 24). Trudeau says sweeping coronavirus bill powers needed given 'exceptional situation'. *Global News*. Available from: https://globalnews.ca/news/6724070/coronavirus-canada-economic-measures-vote/ (accessed 18 October 2021).

Corbella, L. (2020, March 28). Trudeau's attempted power grab an alarming breach of trust. *The Calgary Herald*. Available from: https://calgaryherald.com/news/local-news/corbella-trudeaus-attempted-power-grab-an-alarming-breach-of-trust/ (accessed 18 October 2021).

Coronavirus Resource Center (2021, March 26). John Hopkins University & Medicine. Available from: https://coronavirus.jhu.edu/map.html (accessed 26 March 2021) (accessed 18 October 2021).

Daily Hive (2020, July 29). Toronto will enter Ontario's Stage 3 of reopening this week. Available from: https://dailyhive.com/toronto/toronto-stage-3-reopening-ontario (accessed 18 October 2021).

DeClerq, K. (2020a, March 12). Ontario to close all publicly funded schools for 2 weeks after March break due to COVID-19. *CTV News*. Available from: https://toronto.ctvnews.ca/ontario-to-close-all-publicly-funded-schools-for-2-weeks-after-march-break-due-to-covid-19-1.4850653 (accessed 18 October 2021).

DeClerq, K. (2020b, June 16). Military leaves Ontario long-term care home after facility 'remains COVID-19 free'. *CTV News*. Available from: https://toronto.ctvnews.ca/military-leaves-ontario-long-term-care-home-after-facility-remains-covid-19-free-1.4987125 (accessed 18 October 2021).

DeClerq, K. (2020c, June 22). Ontario to allow Toronto and Peel Region to enter Stage 2 this week. *CTV News*. Available from: https://toronto.ctvnews.ca/ontario-to-allow-toronto-and-peel-region-to-enter-stage-2-this-week-1.4994146 (accessed 18 October 2021).

Feinstein, C. (2020, June 8). Ontario to allow gatherings of up to 10 people as province enters Stage 2 of reopening. *Daily Hive*. Available from: https://dailyhive.com/toronto/ontario-gatherings-10-people-stage-2-toronto (accessed 18 October 2021).

Finance Canada and Parliamentary Budget Office (2020). The PBO'S COVID-19 analysis. Available from: https://www.pbo-dpb.gc.ca/en/covid-19 (accessed 13 May 2022).

Fox, C. (2020a, May 5). Four separate COVID-19 outbreaks declared at Toronto Western Hospital. *CTV News*. Available from: https://toronto.ctvnews.ca/four-separate-covid-19-outbreaks-declared-at-toronto-western-hospital-1.4925194 (accessed 18 October 2021)

Fox, C. (2020b, May 28). 'We are not trying to be killjoys:' Crews begin painting physical distancing circles at Trinity Bellwoods Park. *CP24*. Available from: https://www.cp24.com/news/we-are-not-trying-to-be-killjoys-crews-begin-painting-physical-distancing-circles-at-trinity-bellwoods-park-1.4958220 (accessed 18 October 2021).

Fox, C. and Freeman, (2020, August 20). TDSB approves plan that will help lower class sizes; board looking to delay start of classes by a week. Available from: https://www.cp24.com/news/tdsb-approves-plan-that-will-help-lower-class-sizes-board-looking-to-delay-start-of-classes-by-a-week-1.5071774 (accessed 18 October 2021).

Government of Canada (2020). *Official Global Travel Advisories*. Available from: https://travel.gc.ca/destinations/china (accessed 18 October 2021).

Government of Canada (2021). COVID-19 daily epidemiology update. Available from: https://health-infobase.canada.ca/covid-19/epidemiological-summary-covid-19-cases.html (accessed 19 August 2021).

Government of Ontario (2020a, March 23). News Release. Ontario Orders the Mandatory Closure of All Non-Essential Workplaces to Fight Spread of COVID-19. Available from: https://news.ontario.ca/en/release/56435/ontario-orders-the-mandatory-closure-of-all-non-essential-workplaces-to-fight-spread-of-covid-19 (accessed 18 October 2021).

Government of Ontario (2020b, April 17). News Release. Ontario Offers Emergency Child Care to More Frontline Staff. Available from: https://news.ontario.ca/en/release/56696/ontario-offers-emergency-child-care-to-more-frontline-staff (accessed 18 October 2021).

Government of Ontario (2020c, April 26). News Release. School Closures Extended to Keep Students, Staff and Families Safe Students Will Still Be Able to Complete School Year. Available from: https://news.ontario.ca/en/release/56776/school-closures-extended-to-keep-students-staff-and-families-safe (accessed 18 October 2021).

Government of Ontario (2020d). Approach to reopening schools for the 2020-2021 school year. Available from: https://www.ontario.ca/page/approach-reopening-schools-2020-2021-school-year (accessed 18 October 2021).

Government of Ontario (2020e). COVID-19 public health measures and advice. Available from: https://covid-19.ontario.ca/zones-and-restrictions (accessed 18 October 2021).

Grant, K. (2020). 81% of COVID-19 deaths in Canada were in long-term care – nearly double OECD average. *The Globe and Mail*. Available from: https://www.theglobeandmail.com/canada/article-new-data-show-canada-ranks-among-worlds-worst-for-ltc-deaths/ (accessed 18 October 2021).

Hansen, G., & Cyr, A. (2020). Canada's decentralized "human-driven" approach during the early COVID-19 pandemic. *JMIR Public Health and Surveillance*, 6(4), e20343. https://doi.org/10.2196/20343

Harris, K. (2020). Canada to bar entry to travelers who are not citizens, permanent residents or Americans. *CBC News*. Available from: https://www.cbc.ca/news/politics/cbsa-border-airports-screening-trudeau-covid19-coronavirus-1.5498866 (accessed 18 October 2021).

Hayes, T. and Patton, J. (2020, March 2). Stockpiling in face of COVID-19 unnecessary, Ontario health minister says. *Global News*. Available from: https://globalnews.ca/news/6620830/stockpiling-coronavirus-christine-elliott-costco-ontario/ (accessed 18 October 2021).

Hendsbee, T. (2020, May 25). The mayor says sorry. *Newstalk 1010*. Available from: https://www.iheartradio.ca/newstalk-1010/news/the-mayor-says-sorry-1.12498085 (accessed 18 October 2021) Powell, 2020.

Karaivanov, A., Lu, S.E., Shigeoka, H. et al. (2020). Face masks, public policies and slowing the spread of Covid-19: evidence from Canada. National Bureau of Economic Research. Available from: https://www.nber.org/system/files/working_papers/w27891/w27891.pdf (accessed 18 October 2021).

Katawazi, M. (2020). Toronto declares state of emergency amid COVID-19 pandemic. *CTV News*. Available from: https://toronto.ctvnews.ca/toronto-declares-state-of-emergency-amid-covid-19-pandemic-1.4864679 (accessed 18 October 2021).

Miller, J. (2020, November 4). Ontario school boards will make decisions about COVID-19 closures, adjustments. *The Ottawa Citizen*. Available from: https://ottawacitizen.com/news/local-news/local-trustees-can-decide-when-and-if-covid-19-will-close-schools-says-province (accessed 18 October 2021).

Montpetit, J. (2021, April 8). Curfew in Montreal, Laval rolled back to 8 p.m., lockdown measures extended in Quebec City, Gatineau. *CBC News*. Available from: https://www.cbc.ca/news/canada/montreal/legault-covid-update-emergency-measures-1.5979294 (accessed 18 October 2021).

Nasser, S., and Powers, L. (2021, April 28). Ontario details plan for 3 paid sick days after a year of mounting pressure. *CBC News*. Available from: https://www.cbc.ca/news/canada/toronto/ontario-paid-sick-leave-covid-19-april-28-2021-1.6005192 (accessed 18 October 2021).

Pagliaro, J. (2020, June 30). City council votes to make masks mandatory in public in Toronto. *The Toronto Star*.

Passafiume, B. (2020, August 10). Toronto's pandemic response status upgraded to 'green'. *Toronto Sun*. Available from: https://torontosun.com/news/local-news/torontos-pandemic-response-status-upgraded-to-green (accessed 18 October 2021).

Patton, J. (2020, May 27). Coronavirus: Premier Doug Ford says Ontario to take over 5 more long-term care homes in GTA. *Global News*. Available from: https://globalnews.ca/news/6992824/coronavirus-ontario-government-long-term-care-homes/ (accessed 18 October 2021).

Powell, B. (2020). Mayor apologizes for breaking COVID-19 rules at Trinity Bellwoods Park. *The Toronto Star* (24 May). Available from: https://www.thestar.com/news/gta/2020/05/24/trinity-bellwoods-clears-out-as-police-move-in.html (accessed 18 October 2021).

Pringle, J. (2021, January 9). Quebec curfew: What you need to know about the new rules in Gatineau and western Quebec. *CTV News*. Available from: https://ottawa.ctvnews.ca/quebec-curfew-what-you-need-to-know-about-the-new-rules-in-gatineau-and-western-quebec-1.5259482 (accessed 18 October 2021).

Public Health Agency of Canada (PHAC). (2020a, April 13). Public Health Agency of Canada releases interim guidance for infection prevention and control of COVID-19 for long-term care homes. Available from: https://www.canada.ca/en/public-health/news/2020/04/public-health-agency-of-canada-releases-interim-guidance-for-infection-prevention-and-control-of-covid-19-for-long-term-care-homes.html (accessed 18 October 2021).

Reimer, W. (2020, March 3). COVID-19: no need to stockpile food despite earlier warning, Manitoba health minister says. *Global News*. Available from: https://globalnews.ca/news/6625996/covid-19-stockpiling-food-manitoba/ (accessed 18 October 2021).

Rider, D. (2021, April 26). Emily Viegas, 13, is one of the youngest Canadians to die from COVID-19. *The Toronto Star*. Available from: https://www.thestar.com/news/gta/2021/04/26/brampton-teen-reportedly-dies-of-covid-19-in-her-home.html (accessed 18 October 2021).

Riga, A. (2021). COVID-19 updates, March 16: Montreal curfew will begin at 9:30 p.m. as of tomorrow. *The Montreal Gazette*. Available from: https://montrealgazette.com/news/local-news/covid-19-updates-montreal-quebec-new-cases-variant-vaccine-vaccination-curfew-school-legault-march-16 (accessed 18 October 2021).

Ritchie, K. (2020). City of Toronto officials furious at massive crowds in Trinity Bellwoods Park. *Now Magazine*. Available from: https://nowtoronto.com/news/toronto-furious-massive-crowds-trinity-bellwoods-park/ (accessed 18 October 2021).

Rodrigues, G. (2020). University of Toronto, York University, Ryerson move classes online in response to COVID-19. *Global News*. Available from: https://globalnews.ca/news/6672149/toronto-university-classes-coronavirus-covid-19/ (accessed 18 October 2021).

Rushowy, K., and Ferguson, R. (2020). Ford 'shocked' by Trinity Bellwoods Park crowds, urges restraint. *The Toronto Star*. Available from: https://www.thestar.com/politics/provincial/2020/05/24/premier-shocked-by-trinity-bellwood-crowds-urges-restraint.html (accessed 18 October 2021).

Russell, A., and Connolly, A. (2020). Coronavirus: Trudeau announces economic aid package to help Canadians amid outbreak. *Global News*. Available from: https://globalnews.ca/news/6672830/coronavirus-trudeau-economic-aid-package/ (accessed 18 October 2021).

Silverstein, W.K., Stroud, L., Cleghorn, G.E., Leis, J.A. (2020). First case of COVID19 in Toronto: a 56-year-old man presented to our Emergency Department in Toronto, ON, Canada, with fever and non-productive cough, 1 day after returning from a 3-month visit to Wuhan, China. *The Lancet* 395: 794. Available from: https://www.thelancet.com/action/showPdf?pii=S0140-6736%2820%2930370-6 (accessed 18 October 2021).

Slaughter, G. and Bogart, N. (2020). Sophie Gregoire Trudeau tests positive for COVID-19; PM begins 14-day isolation. *CTV News*. Available from: https://www.ctvnews.ca/health/coronavirus/sophie-gregoire-trudeau-tests-positive-for-covid-19-pm-begins-14-day-isolation-1.4850159 (accessed 18 October 2021).

Syed, I.U. and McLaren, J. (2021). COVID-19 outbreaks in long-term care highlight the urgent need for paid sick leave. *The Conversation Canada*. Available from: https://theconversation.com/covid-19-outbreaks-in-long-term-care-highlight-the-urgent-need-for-paid-sick-leave-153538 (accessed 18 October 2021).

Tsekouras, P. (2021, April 28). Ontario announces paid sick leave program to curb COVID-19 transmission. *CTV News*. Available from: https://toronto.ctvnews.ca/ontario-announces-paid-sick-leave-program-to-curb-covid-19-transmission-1.5405853 (accessed 18 October 2021).

Tubb, E. (2021, March 17). Every day of the COVID-19 pandemic in all 34 Ontario health units, in one image. *The Toronto Star*.

Tunney, C. (2020). Support coming for Canadians quarantined due to coronavirus, finance minister says. *CBC News*. Available from: https://www.cbc.ca/news/politics/quarantined-coronavirus-morneau-supports-1.5488062 (accessed 18 October 2021).

Walsh, P. (2020a, April 14). *COVID-19: Key Developments for April 12-13th*. Email Communication. Ontario Public Health Association (OPHA).

Walsh, P. (2020b, April 15). *COVID-19: Summary of Key Developments – April 15th*. Email Communication. Ontario Public Health Association (OPHA).

Walsh, P. (2020c, April 17). *COVID-19: Key Federal and Provincial Developments – April 17th*. Email Communication. Ontario Public Health Association (OPHA).

Walsh, P. (2020d, April 18 and 19). *COVID-19: Summary of Federal and Provincial Developments – April 18 and 19*. Email Communication. Ontario Public Health Association (OPHA).

Walsh, P. (2020e, April 21). *COVID-19: Summary of Federal and Provincial Developments – April 21st*. Email Communication. Ontario Public Health Association (OPHA).

Walsh, P. (2020f, April 22). *COVID-19: Summary of Federal and Provincial Developments – April 22nd*. Email Communication. Ontario Public Health Association (OPHA).

Walsh, P. (2020g, April 23). *COVID-19: Summary of Federal and Provincial Developments – April 23rd*. Email Communication. Ontario Public Health Association (OPHA).

Walsh, P. (2020h, April 24). *COVID-19: Summary of Federal and Provincial Developments – April 24th*. Email Communication. Ontario Public Health Association (OPHA).

Walsh, P. (2020i, April 26). *COVID-19: Summary of Provincial and Federal Developments for April 25–26*. Email Communication. Ontario Public Health Association (OPHA).

Walsh, P. (2020j, April 27). *COVID:19: Guidelines for Reopening the Province and Other Developments for April 27th*. Email Communication. Ontario Public Health Association (OPHA).

Walsh, P. (2020k, April 28). *COVID19: Key Developments on April 28th – Federal Modelling and Criteria for Restarting the Economy*. Email Communication. Ontario Public Health Association (OPHA).

Walsh, P. (2020l, April 30). *COVID-19: Summary of Key Developments – April 30th*. Email Communication. Ontario Public Health Association (OPHA).

Walsh, P. (2020m, May 1). *COVID-19: Summary of Key Developments for May 1*. Email Communication. Ontario Public Health Association (OPHA).

Walsh, P. (2020n, May 4). *COVID-19: Summary of Federal and Provincial Developments – May 4th*. Email Communication. Ontario Public Health Association (OPHA).

Walsh, P. (2020o, May 5). *COVID:19 – Summary of Key Developments for May 5th/Premier's Remarks about Public Health Testing and Reform*. Email Communication. Ontario Public Health Association (OPHA).

Walsh, P. (2020p, May 6). *COVID-19: Key Development for May 6th – Plans for Race Based Data/Premiers Apology to Public Health*. Email Communication. Ontario Public Health Association (OPHA).

Walsh, P. (2020q, May 7). *COVID-19: Summary of Federal and Provincial Developments – May 7th*. Email Communication. Ontario Public Health Association (OPHA).

Walsh, P. (2020r, May 8). *COVID-19: Summary of Federal and Provincial Developments – May th*. Email Communication. Ontario Public Health Association (OPHA).

Walsh, P. (2020s, May 10). *COVID-19: Summary of Federal and Provincial Developments – May 9–10*. Email Communication. Ontario Public Health Association (OPHA).

Walsh, P. (2020t, May 11). *COVID-19: Summary of Federal and Provincial Developments – May 11*. Email Communication. Ontario Public Health Association (OPHA).

Walsh, P. (2020u, May 12). *COVID-19: Summary of Federal and Provincial Developments – May 12*. Email Communication. Ontario Public Health Association (OPHA).

Walsh, P. (2020v, May 13). *COVID-19: Summary of Federal and Provincial Developments – May 13*. Email Communication. Ontario Public Health Association (OPHA).

Walsh, P. (2020w, May 14). *COVID-19: Summary of Federal and Provincial Developments – May 14*. Email Communication. Ontario Public Health Association (OPHA).

Walsh, P. (2020x, May 15). *COVID-19: Summary of Federal and Provincial Developments – May 15*. Email Communication. Ontario Public Health Association (OPHA).

Walsh, P. (2020y, May 19). *COVID-19: Summary of Federal and Provincial Developments – May 19*. Email Communication. Ontario Public Health Association (OPHA).

Walsh, P. (2020z, May 20). *COVID-19: Summary of Federal and Provincial Developments – May 20*. Email Communication. Ontario Public Health Association (OPHA).

Walsh, P. (2020aa, May 21). *COVID-19: Summary of Federal and Provincial Developments – May 21*. Email Communication. Ontario Public Health Association (OPHA).

Walsh, P. (2020ab, May 22). *COVID-19: Summary of Federal and Provincial Developments – May 22*. Email Communication. Ontario Public Health Association (OPHA).

Walsh, P. (2020ac, May 24). *COVID-19: Summary of Federal and Provincial Developments – May 24*. Email Communication. Ontario Public Health Association (OPHA).

Walsh, P. (2020ad, May 25). *COVID-19: Summary of Federal and Provincial Developments – May 25*. Email Communication. Ontario Public Health Association (OPHA).

Walsh, P. (2020ae, May 26). *COVID-19: Summary of Federal and Provincial Developments – May 26*. Email Communication. Ontario Public Health Association (OPHA).

Walsh, P. (2020af, May 27). *COVID-19: Summary of Federal and Provincial Developments – May 27.* Email Communication. Ontario Public Health Association (OPHA).

Walsh, P. (2020ag, May 28). *COVID-19: Summary of Federal and Provincial Developments – May 28.* Email Communication. Ontario Public Health Association (OPHA).

Walsh, P. (2020ah, May 29). *COVID-19: Summary of Federal and Provincial Developments – May 29.* Email Communication. Ontario Public Health Association (OPHA).

Walsh, P. (2020ai, May 30). *COVID-19: Summary of Federal and Provincial Developments – May 30.* Email Communication. Ontario Public Health Association (OPHA).

Webster P. Canada and COVID-19: learning from SARS. *Lancet* 2020;395:936–7. https://doi.org/10.1016/S0140-6736(20)30670-X

Woodward, J. (2021, April 27). 'It breaks my heart': Essential workers in Ontario plead for paid sick days amid COVID-19 wave. *CTV News.* Available from: https://toronto.ctvnews.ca/it-breaks-my-heart-essential-workers-in-ontario-plead-for-paid-sick-days-amid-covid-19-wave-1.5404771 (accessed 18 October 2021).

World Health Organization (WHO) (2020). *WHO Director-General's opening remarks at the media briefing on COVID-19 – 11 March 2020.* Available from: https://www.who.int/director-general/speeches/detail/who-director-general-s-opening-remarks-at-the-media-briefing-on-covid-19-11-march-2020 (accessed 18 October 2021).

Yu, A., Prasad, S., Akande, A., Murariu, A., Yuan, S., Kathirkamanathan, S., Ma, M., & Ladha, S. (2020). COVID-19 in Canada: a self-assessment and review of preparedness and response. *Journal of Global Health* 10(2), 0203104. https://doi.org/10.7189/jogh.10.0203104; Available from: https://www.ncbi.nlm.nih.gov/pmc/articles/PMC7725009/ (accessed 18 October 2021).

16

Coronavirus and the Social State: Austria in the Pandemic

*Donald Abenheim and Carolyn Halladay**

National Security Affairs Department, Naval Postgraduate School, Monterey, California, USA

Whether touted by the black-green cabinet in the Austrian federal chancellery as "protecting our shared liberty"[1] or lambasted by the radical right-wing and dissident elements in the streets of Vienna's 1st and 6th districts or the conspiracy theorists of scenic Tirol as "a gigantic assault on the freedom of Austrians,"[2] the law that the Austrian parliament approved on 20 January 2022, which ultimately required every resident from Vorarlberg to Burgenland over the age of 18 to be vaccinated against Coronavirus, marked a novelty for Europe and its record of law, governance, and the COVID-19 pandemic. While some European Union (EU) states – notably Greece and Italy – had already enacted vaccine mandates for older residents, and other European countries required COVID-19 vaccines of health-care workers, Austria's more-or-less universal *Impfpflicht* (vaccine directive) for adults represented a new milestone in the EU amid the crises of the twenty-first century.[3] Austria stood as the first among its neighbors to impose a broad vaccine mandate. It was, in many ways, a triumph of "social" Austria.

The present study examines the chronology as well as the cause-and-effect of this evolution of the rule of law, state power, public health, and popular will in Austria. Such timing in the

---

* The views expressed in this chapter are the authors' own and should not be construed as the official position of the U.S. Navy, the U.S. Department of Defense, or the U.S. government.

1 An introduction to government and politics in the Second Austrian Republic is: Herbert Dachs, *Politik in Österreich: Das Handbuch* (Vienna: Manz, 2006); Wolfgang Mantl, *Politik in Österreich: Die Zweite Republik: Bestand Und Wandel* (Vienna, Cologne, Graz: Böhlau, 1992); Reinhard Sieder, *Österreich 1945–1995: Gesellschaft, Politik, Kultur,* 2nd ed. (Vienna: Verlag für Gesellschaftskritik, 1996). Also see: Manfried Rauchensteiner, *Unter Beobachtung: Österreich seit 1918,* 2nd ed. (Vienna and Cologne: Böhlau Verlag, 2021). For a summary of events connected with the novel Coronavirus and Austria in the years 2020–2022, see: Markus Pollack et al., eds., *Chronologie zur Corona-Krise in Österreich – Teil 1: Vorgeschichte, der Weg in den Lockdown, die akute Phase und wirtschaftliche Folgen* (Vienna: University of Vienna, 2022). For an overview of laws and regulations on the pandemic in Austria, see: Bundesministerium für Digitalisierung und Wirtschaftstandort, Ausgewählte COVID-19 Rechtsnormen, at https://www.ris.bka.gv.at/RisInfo/COVID_Gesetze_Bund_Land.pdf. For the onset of the compulsory vaccine mandate in February 2022, see: "Nehammer/Edtstadler: Impfpflicht als Chance für unsere gemeinsame Freiheit," Statement from the federal chancellery, 17 January 2022, https://www.bundeskanzleramt.gv.at/bundeskanzleramt/nachrichten-der-bundesregierung/2022/01/nehammer-edtstadler-impfpflicht-als-chance-fuer-unsere-gemeinsame-freiheit.html.
2 "Debatte im Nationalrat zur Impfpflicht: Statement von Herbert Kickl," OE24.TV, 20 January 2022, https://youtu.be/w8_evaw-m58. The statement is about 45 seconds into the address. See also: Vanessa Gaig et al., "Leises Unbehagen in der FPÖ über radikalen Corona-Kurs," *Der Standard*, 7 January 2022, https://www.derstandard.de/story/2000132356309/coronawird-kickl-der-fpoe-zu-radikal.
3 Paragraph 3 of the law lists three fairly circumscribed populations that might qualify as exceptions: pregnant women, persons with particular medical issues with the vaccine, and people who have certifiably recovered from SARS-CoV-2, although this latter category has only 180 days of relief from the requirement.

Impacts of the Covid-19 Pandemic: International Laws, Policies, and Civil Liberties, First Edition. Edited by Nadav Morag.
© 2023 John Wiley & Sons, Inc. Published 2023 by John Wiley & Sons, Inc.

wielding of state authority in crisis, and indeed, the whole vaccine mandate, was entirely – almost predictably – Austrian as to its constitutional tradition and the somehow ever-present shadow of a generalized threat to the state and citizens that requires, in turn, a strong response to meet public needs and expectations.[4] That is to say, the *Impfpflicht* that took effect on 1 February 2022 fits with Austrian law, history, politics, and social expectations, particularly of the *Sozialstaat*'s appropriate response to a crisis. SARS-CoV-2 arrived at a fateful time in the record of the Second Republic, as the Coronavirus forms just the latest in a string of internal and external crises that have roiled Austrian state and society in the last decade or so. This chapter explores this context.

At the same time, this chapter examines the extent and the impact of the entrenched anti-vaccine sentiment in Austria as a constitutional question of citizenship and an open question of antidemocratic movements – which may or may not be peace- or democracy- or community-minded.[5] Especially since the coalition government announced its intentions in November 2021, amid a fourth Coronavirus lockdown, to embark on a vaccine mandate, large anti-vax demonstrations in many Austrian cities – often with some thousands of participants – have become regular occurrences. While these gatherings have remained largely peaceful, police and journalists reported in the course of 2021 growing instances of intimidation and violence.[6] The extreme right, among other detractors of the Sozialstaat, is conspicuous in the protests.

Indeed, when the new minister of the interior, Gerhard Karner, of the center-right Austrian People's Party (Österreichische Volkspartei or ÖVP) – speaking shortly after his taking office on 6 December 2021 to the ministry magazine, *Public Security (Öffentliche Sicherheit)* – vowed to "proceed forcefully against radicals and extremists," the list of such threats began with the pandemic and its most illiberal protestors, only followed by cyber-crime, illegal migration, right-wing extremism, Islamist extremism, and anti-Semitism.[7] Karner's immediate predecessor in the office, Karl Nehammer, also of the ÖVP – who became Austria's chancellor on 6 December after Sebastian Kurz (ÖVP) had left the Ballhausplatz in scandal – had presided over a total overhaul of Austria's office of constitutional protection as a full-fledged domestic intelligence organization, telling the same in-house publication, "Precisely in times of crisis, when extremism is even visible on the streets, the protection of the constitution is more important than ever."[8] As this chapter demonstrates, Austria's constitutional order, originally wrought amid political and social turmoil a century ago, thus far, has weathered the Coronavirus pandemic and maintained the Austrian *Sozialstaat*, a pillar of the Second Republic's democracy. But can the constitutional order continue to absorb the blows?

---

4 See: Arbeitsgemeinschaft Österreichische Rechtsgeschichte, *Rechts- Und Verfassungsgeschichte*, 4th ed. (Vienna: Facultas, 2016); Theo Öhlinger, *Kultur der Demokratie* (Vienna and Graz: Christian Brünner, 2002) p. 217. Also see the bibliographical essay on democracy, state, and law in Erich Zöllner, *Geschichte Österreichs: von den Anfängen bis zur Gegenwart*, 8th ed. (Vienna: Verlag für Geschichte, 1990), pp. 667–697.

5 Julia Partheymueller et al. *Impfbereitschaft: Wer sind die Zögerlichen,* University of Vienna Corona Panel Project, September 2021, https://viecer.univie.ac.at/corona-blog/corona-blog-beitraege/blog128/; Conrad Seidl, "Corona-Impfung spaltet Österreichs Gesellschaft," *Der Standard*, 27 December 2021, https://www.derstandard.at/story/2000132161692/corona-impfung-spaltet-oesterreichs-gesellschaft.

6 Jakob Winter, "'Grausame Energie': Gewaltpotenzial bei Corona-Demos steigt," *Profil*, 7 December 2021, https://www.profil.at/oesterreich/grausame-energie-gewaltpotenzial-bei-corona-demos-steigt/401832307; "Mindestens 10 Festnahmen auf Corona-Kundgebung in Wien," *Frankfurter Allgemeine Zeitung*, 20 November 2021, https://www.faz.net/aktuell/politik/ausland/protest-gegen-impfpflicht-festnahmen-auf-corona-kundgebung-in-wien-17644126.html.

7 Bundesministerium Inneres, "Interview: 'Konsequent gegen Radikale und Extremisten vorgehen," *Öffentliche Sicherheit*, No. 1/2 2022, p. 12, https://bmi.gv.at/magazin/2022_01_02/Interview_Karner.aspx Karner himself in his earlier role as head of the Lower Austrian state diet was, in turn, accused of anti-Jewish statements, a manifestation of the high sensitivity in Austrian public life to what is a feature of Central European political culture and society. ORF News Innenminister Karner wehrt sich gegen Antisemitismusvorwürfe, 13 Dezember 2021, https://orf.at/stories/3240048/.

8 Bundesministerium Inneres, "Verfassungsschutz: Gefahren erforschen und abwehren," *Öffentliche Sicherheit*, No. 1/2 2022, p. 15, https://bmi.gv.at/magazin/2022_01_02/Verfassungsschutz.aspx.

16.1 The *Impfpflicht*

As expected, on the third Thursday of January 2022, the lower house (the Nationalrat or National Council) of the Austrian parliament voted 137–33 in favor of the vaccine mandate. In fact, the law enacted the mandate in three phases.[9] In the initial phase, authorities could ask for and inspect proof of immunization from Austrians, but no penalties were forthcoming amid a general program of mass persuasion. Health officials were required to issue reminders to the unvaccinated by 15 February – and quarterly thereafter.[10]

Phase 2 was planned to kicked in after 15 March 2022 the expected *Impfstichtag* – immunization deadline – if reminders went out to the unvaccinated on time and if the federal government still felt it was necessary.[11] Random inspections by police and other officials now might lead to fines of up to €600 per quarter.[12] In this regard, the law established failure to vaccinate more as a uniform citation, like a parking ticket, with, at most, a foreshortened and limited legal appeal possible.[13] More controversially, the law also stipulated that anyone who challenged the mandate in a full juridical proceeding and lost could then be fined up to €3,600 each quarter until he or she becomes fully vaccinated.[14] With this provision, Austria sought to avoid deluging the court system with anti-vaccine complaints – rather as the fourth lockdown (November 2021–January 2022), which ended for the unvaccinated only the day before the vaccine mandate entered its first phase, aimed to keep hospitals from being overwhelmed with COVID-19 cases.[15] Still, the penalty was purpose-fully more irritating than punitive; the goal was to nudge the nation's 1.5 million or so eligible but unimmunized denizens toward vaccinations.[16]

---

9 "Gesundheitsausschuss gibt Startschuss für Impfpflicht gegen COVID-19 ab Februar für alle ab 18 Jahren," Parlamentskorrespondenz Nr. 42 vom 17 January 2022, https://www.parlament.gv.at/PAKT/PR/JAHR_2022/PK0042/index.shtml.
10 Bundesgesetz über die Impfpflicht gegen COVID-19 (COVID-19-Impfpflichtgesetz – COVID-19-IG), revised version of 17 January 2022, available from the Bundesministerium Soziales, Gesundheit, Pflege, and Konsumentenschutz, "Impfpflicht: Gesetzesentwurf," 16 January 2022, https://www.sozialministerium.at/Corona-Schutzimpfung/Impfpflicht/Gesetzesentwurf.html.
11 Bundesgesetz über die Impfpflicht gegen COVID-19 (COVID-19-Impfpflichtgesetz – COVID-19-IG), revised version of 17 January 2022, available from the Bundesministerium Soziales, Gesundheit, Pflege, and Konsumentenschutz, "Impfpflicht: Gesetzesentwurf," 16 January 2022, https://www.sozialministerium.at/Corona-Schutzimpfung/Impfpflicht/Gesetzesentwurf.html.
12 Para. 11 of Bundesgesetz über die Impfpflicht gegen COVID-19 (COVID-19-Impfpflichtgesetz – COVID-19-IG), revised version of 17 January 2022, available from the Bundesministerium Soziales, Gesundheit, Pflege, and Konsumentenschutz, "Impfpflicht: Gesetzesentwurf," 16 January 2022, https://www.sozialministerium.at/Corona-Schutzimpfung/Impfpflicht/Gesetzesentwurf.html.
13 Alternately, the enforcement of the Austrian vaccine mandate might function as an administrative infraction. "Festgehalten wird, dass auch eine verpflichtende Impfung nicht durch unmittelbare Befehls- und Zwangsgewalt durchgesetzt werden darf, sondern durch Verwaltungsstrafen sanktioniert wird." See the overview at COVID-19-Impfpflichtgesetz – COVID-19-IG (164/ME), https://www.parlament.gv.at/PAKT/VHG/XXVII/ME/ME_00164/index.shtml.
14 Bundesgesetz über die Impfpflicht gegen COVID-19 (COVID-19-Impfpflichtgesetz – COVID-19-IG), revised version of 17 January 2022, available from the Bundesministerium Soziales, Gesundheit, Pflege, and Konsumentenschutz, "Impfpflicht: Gesetzesentwurf," 16 January 2022, https://www.sozialministerium.at/Corona-Schutzimpfung/Impfpflicht/Gesetzesentwurf.html.
15 "Gesundheitsausschuss gibt Startschuss für Impfpflicht gegen COVID-19 ab Februar für alle ab 18 Jahren," Parlamentskorrespondenz Nr. 42 vom 17 January 2022, https://www.parlament.gv.at/PAKT/PR/JAHR_2022/PK0042/index.shtml.
16 See, for example, the comments of Minister for Constitutional Affairs Karoline Edtstadler, at a press conference with Health Minister Wolfgang Mückstein, Bundeskanzleramt Österreich, "Pressekonferenz zum Thema 'Impfpflicht'," 9 December 2021, https://youtu.be/EMMhqJPHxfs. See also Reuters, "Austria plans to fine vaccine holdouts up to 3,600 euros a quarter," 9 December 2021, https://www.reuters.com/world/europe/austria-announce-details-planned-covid-19-vaccine-mandate-2021-12-09/.

If, however, the country's vaccination rate – variously reported at 75-ish percent when the Nationalrat passed the measure[17] – failed to reach satisfactory levels, then the full mandate would go into effect. The law specified no particular date or threshold for this third phase, nor did it set a level of *Durchimpfung* (full vaccination) that might qualify as sufficient, though this latter omission at least banished unlovely jargon like "herd immunity" from both the law and the public discussion of it. A commission in the federal chancellery – to include at least two legal scholars and a minimum of two medical experts – would monitor the situation and report quarterly.[18] A sunset clause anticipated the mandate ending by January 2024.[19]

The measure enjoyed the broad support of members of the conservative-green governing coalition; the chancellor himself had, in late January 2022, just recovered from a breakthrough COVID-19 infection, and he spoke effusively to the press about vaccination, which he credited with keeping him out of the hospital.[20] It also drew many votes from the opposition Social Democrats (Sozialdemokratische Partei Österreichs or SPÖ) – the party leader at the time, Pamela Rendi-Wagner, was a physician with professional and research experience in infectious disease and epidemiology – as well as the parliamentary caucus of the liberal NEOS. The upper house, the Bundesrat (Federal Council), took up the mandate on 3 February 2022, but this approval – ultimately 47–12 – as well as the final signature by Federal President Alexander Van der Bellen on 4 February 2022 mostly formalized the long-expected outcome: The vaccine mandate was law.[21]

Drafts of the law had circulated for review and comment until mid-January, and for the most part, the final measure reflected these well-publicized and -discussed provisions. For example, the law allows exceptions for pregnant women, people who cannot be immunized for other documented health reasons, and anyone who has certifiably recovered from COVID-19 (though this latter exception extends only for six months after the illness).[22] Popular and political concerns did effect some changes to the law, though. For one thing, the draft approved by the Nationalrat fixed at 18, rather than 14, the minimum age to which the mandate applied.[23] For another, the definition of "fully

---

17 Reuters reported about 72% – see, for example, Francois Murphy, "Austria set to make COVID shots compulsory after bill clears parliament," 20 January 2022, https://www.reuters.com/world/europe/austria-introduces-lottery-covid-vaccine-incentive-2022-01-20/ – up from about 68% the month before. ("Austria plans to fine vaccine holdouts up to 3,600 euros a quarter," 9 December 2021, https://www.reuters.com/world/europe/austria-announce-details-planned-covid-19-vaccine-mandate-2021-12-09/.) The Associated Press put the figure at 75.4% – "Austria to lift lockdown for unvaccinated residents," 26 January 2022, https://abcnews.go.com/Health/wireStory/austria-lift-lockdown-unvaccinated-residents-82480785. Also see the Austrian state broadcasting site: https://orf.at/corona/.
18 "Gesundheitsausschuss gibt Startschuss für Impfpflicht gegen COVID-19 ab Februar für alle ab 18 Jahren," Parlamentskorrespondenz Nr. 42 vom 17 January 2022, https://www.parlament.gv.at/PAKT/PR/JAHR_2022/PK0042/index.shtml.
19 Para. 20 of Bundesgesetz über die Impfpflicht gegen COVID-19 (COVID-19-Impfpflichtgesetz – COVID-19-IG), revised version of 17 January 2022, available from the Bundesministerium Soziales, Gesundheit, Pflege, and Konsumentenschutz, "Impfpflicht: Gesetzesentwurf," 16 January 2022, https://www.sozialministerium.at/Corona-Schutzimpfung/Impfpflicht/Gesetzesentwurf.html. In the event, the Austrians dropped the vaccine mandate on 9 March 2022.
20 Bundeskanzleramt, "Nehammer/Edtstadler: Impfpflicht als Chance für unsere gemeinsame Freiheit," 17 January 2022, https://www.bundeskanzleramt.gv.at/bundeskanzleramt/nachrichten-der-bundesregierung/2022/01/nehammer-edtstadler-impfpflicht-als-chance-fuer-unsere-gemeinsame-freiheit.html.
21 It merits mention here that Van der Bellen, for one, had come out in favor of a vaccine mandate as early as mid-November 2021, when political and public health leaders first proposed it.
22 Para. 3 of Bundesgesetz über die Impfpflicht gegen COVID-19 (COVID-19-Impfpflichtgesetz – COVID-19-IG), revised version of 17 January 2022, available from the Bundesministerium Soziales, Gesundheit, Pflege, and Konsumentenschutz, "Impfpflicht: Gesetzesentwurf," 16 January 2022, https://www.sozialministerium.at/Corona-Schutzimpfung/Impfpflicht/Gesetzesentwurf.html.
23 "Gesundheitsausschuss gibt Startschuss für Impfpflicht gegen COVID-19 ab Februar für alle ab 18 Jahren," Parlamentskorrespondenz Nr. 42 vom 17 January 2022, https://www.parlament.gv.at/PAKT/PR/JAHR_2022/PK0042/index.shtml.

vaccinated," which, in the December 2021 version, had expressly included a booster no more than 270 days old, now was up to the determination of relevant health authorities.[24] Such amendments imparted some flexibility to the enforcement regime, in part to accommodate legal and technological concerns about data collection, accuracy, and privacy. The built-in wiggle room also provided an "emergency brake" for the federal government to interrupt the mandate's staged progression at any point – for legal, public health, or political reasons.

16.2 The Freedom Party's Liberties

Thus, by the time that the vaccine mandate took effect in February 2022, Austria was largely ready for it, save for the vocal minority who saw such a law as a monstrosity of globalized puppet masters, or, perhaps, merely stated in their doubt in the face of legal duty to public health and government a well-known national trait of skepticism of unexpected change and the stubborn will of subjects to court and curia. The vote in the Nationalrat perhaps revealed more enthusiasm for the *Impfpflicht* among parliamentarians than among the general public; still, the most-cited survey data from early December 2021 showed a slight majority of Austrians (53%) in favor of a vaccine mandate; about a third – 32% – against it; and another 13% unsure at the time of the inquiry.[25]

But even this much support did little to quell the controversy and outcry that attended the vaccine mandate as, in fact, every step in the Austrian pandemic response had seen in the years 2020–2022. In parliament as well as in the new and old media, the most prominent objectors to the vaccine mandate hailed from the populist nationalist-right Freedom Party of Austria (Freiheitliche Partei Österreichs or FPÖ),[26] at the time the third-largest party in parliament. The FPÖ consistently and constantly disrupted the otherwise more-or-less united voice and message of the government about the efficacy of any and all Coronavirus measures, reaffirming, if not energizing, the throngs of vaccine resisters, rugged individualists, conspiracy theorists, and neo-Nazis at the demonstrations.

There is some precedent here. In the first decades of the Second Republic, the FPÖ established its own very special heritage of the so-called third camp (*drittes Lager*) between the center-right Christian Social Party and the Socialists.[27] It was a far-right party, but it operated within the bounds of postwar Austrian democracy. Thus, it gave refuge to ex-Nazis who roughly adjusted to democracy (or not) as well as classic national liberals. Since the 1990s, the FPÖ has staked its reputation on resistance to European unity and defiance of a globalized neoliberal capitalist economy, a position that gained supporters especially since the financial crisis of 2008.

---

24 For the earlier wording, see Para. 4 of "Bundesgesetz über die Impfpflicht gegen COVID-19 (COVID-19-Impfpflichtgesetz–COVID-19-IG), 164/ME XXVII." GP – Ministerialentwurf, 9 December 2021, https://www.parlament.gv.at/PAKT/VHG/XXVII/ME/ME_00164/index.shtml. The final version of the relevant language appears in Para. 4 of Bundesgesetz über die Impfpflicht gegen COVID-19 (COVID-19-Impfpflichtgesetz – COVID-19-IG), revised version of 17 January 2022, available from the Bundesministerium Soziales, Gesundheit, Pflege, and Konsumentenschutz, "Impfpflicht: Gesetzesentwurf," 16 January 2022, https://www.sozialministerium.at/Corona-Schutzimpfung/Impfpflicht/Gesetzesentwurf.html.
25 "ATV-Frage der Woche: Mehrheit für Impfpflicht wird starker," 5 December 2021, https://www.ots.at/presseaussendung/OTS_20211205_OTS0002/atv-frage-der-woche-mehrheit-fuer-impfpflicht-wird-staerker.
26 Oliver Gelden, *Diskursstrategien Im Rechtspopulismus: Freiheitliche Partei Österreichs und Schweizerische Volkspartei Zwischen Opposition und Regierungsbeteiligung* (Wiesbaden: Verlag für Sozialwissenschaften, 2006); Thorsten Hoffmann, *Der Organisationale Wandel von Parteien: Eine Diskursive Betrachtung am Beispiel der Freiheitlichen Partei Österreichs im Zeitraum 1986–2002* (Linz: Trauner, 2014); Freiheitliches Bildungsinstitut, *Österreich Zuerst 1956–2016: 60 Jahre FPÖ Die Soziale Heimatpartei* (Vienna: FPÖ-Bildungsinstitut, 2016).
27 Andreas Mölzer, *Freiheit Schreibt auf Eure Fahnen! 1848 - 2008: Das Dritte Lager – Erbe und Auftrag* (Vienna: W3-Verlag Geschichte, 2008).

As it happened, the contemporary party leader and scandal-laden ex-minister of the interior and chief ideologue of his party, Herbert Kickl,[28] finally admitted in early January 2022, after several months of dissembling and diversion in front of his restive crowds in Vienna, that he has, in fact, been immunized. He attempted to package the announcement – the "confession," as he deemed it – in terms of an injection of "optimism, strength, confidence, joy, and the will to liberty."[29] The FPÖ rank and file seems, so far, to have accepted the revelation with equanimity, and Kickl continues to use his role on the right wing of parliamentary opposition to disrupt the ÖVP/Green Austrian government's otherwise general concurrence on pandemic-related measures – as well as to endorse fringe COVID "cures."[30]

For example, in his remarks to the Nationalrat on 20 January 2022, laying out his opposition to the vaccine law, Kickl serially derided the measure as "downgrading" Austrians to serfdom, flirting with totalitarianism, and imposing "health-communism."[31] In line with the twenty-first-century myths and canards of the dark invaders and supranational conspiracies favored by the disaffected in the ailing democracies, he also insisted that this "Chinese virus" should not beget a "Chinese model of society" in Austria.[32] His particular complaint concerned the demise of the citizen as individual: "It no longer matters what the individual wants. The only thing that counts anymore is what is good for the masses," Kickl asserted.[33]

Kickl & Co in the Freedom Party continue to press the point of endless individual liberties in Austria amid (and to) crowds of ever more radical demonstrators and their theories of globalized puppet masters. Indeed, Kickl's lament corresponds with the standard falsehoods about hyper-capitalist wire-pullers and lost constitutional rights among skeptics of all things COVID throughout Europe and the West, if not further; in this view, liberty demands that the much-vaunted individual remain maximally unfettered in her/his pursuit of happiness – presumably unmasked, un-distanced, and unimmunized.

This message well may not resonate across all of Austrian society, however. Solidarity across the demarcation of class and estate do matter in Austria, and Austrians expect their state and government to act accordingly for the collective well-being. And the demand for such action in Vienna, Graz, or Linz is hardly to be found in the pages, say, of Ayn Rand's *Fountain Head* or even Friedrich Hayek's *Road to Serfdom*, but in key features of Austrian law and the record of the past.

16.3 A Bundle of Measures

As the parliamentary overview to the December draft of the mandate notes, the law forms part of a "bundle" of measures to manage Austria's Coronavirus response;[34] officials hoped these efforts

---

28 Helmut Brandstätter, *Kurz & Kickl: Ihr Spiel Mit Macht Und Angst* (Vienna: Kremayr & Scheriau, 2019); see also Republic of Austria, Parliament, Wer ist Wer, "Herbert Kickl," https://www.parlament.gv.at/WWER/PAD_35520/index.shtml.
29 "Herbert Kickl hat sich impfen lassen!" *FPÖ TV*, 11 January 2022, https://www.youtube.com/watch?v=irtBnNwirOI.
30 See, for example, "Ivomectin: Entwurmungsmittel in Österreich ausverkauft – weil FPÖ-Chef es bei Corona empfiehlt," *Der Spiegel*, 16 November 2021, https://www.spiegel.de/wirtschaft/unternehmen/ivomectin-entwurmungsmittel-in-oesterreich-ausverkauft-weil-fpoe-chef-es-bei-corona-empfiehlt-a-42689153-8d8b-4e52-bab1-e86a293fd1b8.
31 Wiener TV, "Herbert Kickl zum Impfpflicht Gesetz im Nationalrat am 20.1.2022," 20 January 2022, https://youtu.be/G_FN_RksLkA; see particularly about 3.5 minutes into the speech.
32 Wiener TV, "Herbert Kickl zum Impfpflicht Gesetz im Nationalrat am 20.1.2022," 20 January 2022, https://youtu.be/G_FN_RksLkA; see particularly about 3:45 into the speech.
33 Wiener TV, "Herbert Kickl zum Impfpflicht Gesetz im Nationalrat am 20.1.2022," 20 January 2022, https://youtu.be/G_FN_RksLkA; the comments appear at about 4:00.
34 COVID-19-Impfpflichtgesetz – COVID-19-IG (164/ME), 9 December 2021, https://www.parlament.gv.at/PAKT/VHG/XXVII/ME/ME_00164/index.shtml.

will keep Austria from careening from lockdown to lockdown anymore.[35] Tellingly, Austria did not resort to formal emergency laws, preferring instead to pass new legislation, specific to the present pandemic, amid the customary parliamentary and public debate. (The drearily regular protest demonstrations in the larger cities might charitably be worked into this latter dynamic, but they owe their vehemence as well as their vernacular to other, rather less democratic agendas.)

Most of Austria's national-level legislation concerned such specific issues as education (grade school through university) during the pandemic or financial support or payments or taxes amid lockdowns and broad uncertainty in and around the markets.[36] Most of the state-level legislation effected the national policies, as Austria's fiercely guarded federalism requires. Perhaps the most significant COVID-era law – other than the vaccine mandate – was the "COVID-19 Measures Law" (COVID-19-Maßnahmengesetz) of 21 March 2020.[37] This law, which mostly survived a challenge in the Austrian constitutional court in July 2020,[38] compiled various rules about public gatherings, masking, distancing, and the appropriate roles of the various organs of state, including the intelligence sector, which received some further or more specific access to spaces (like private homes), though explicitly only to further the measures identified in the law.[39]

This provision – that the security sector may only enforce or even investigate cases that involve specific orders or requirements from health authorities – brings the COVID-19 Measures Law in line with Austria's Epidemic Law of 1950.[40] Actually, much of the language of the COVID-19 Measures Law now corresponds more or less exactly to the text of the Epidemic Law. This earlier law, promulgated so soon after the founding of the Second Republic, demonstrates that the founders of Austria's postwar democracy – well experienced with calamity and crisis – arguably had anticipated such a development as a global pandemic, as well as the appropriate official Austrian responses, all with an eye toward the requirements of democracy and rule of law, as well as public safety. Indeed, credible analysis suggests that the 1950 law would have sufficed as the legal basis from which authorities could have managed the Coronavirus in Austria.[41] As Felix Andreaus notes, not only does the COVID-19 Measures Law "add no value" to the Epidemic Law, but the several and frequent amendments to the law – at least 14 in the two years since it was originally promulgated[42] – testify to its defects as a work of (hasty) legal drafting.[43] One might argue, however,

---

35 "This lockdown-to-lockdown action" was the pithy turn of phrase that Constitutional Affairs Minister Edtstadler used in comments to a German regional broadcaster shortly after the Nationalrat vote on the Austrian vaccine mandate. ("Wir wollten aussteigen aus diesem von Lockdown-zu-Lockdown-Handeln.") Christoph Peerenboom and Babette Bauer, "Österreich: Bundesministerin Edtstadler verteidigt Impfpflicht," *BR24*, 25 January 2022, https://www.br.de/nachrichten/deutschland-welt/oesterreich-bundesministerin-edtstadler-verteidigt-impfpflicht, SvbQdLs.

36 Bundesministerium für Digitalisierung und Wirtschaftsstandort, Ausgewählte COVID-19 Rechtsnormen, at https://www.ris.bka.gv.at/RisInfo/COVID_Gesetze_Bund_Land.pdf.

37 "Bundesrecht konsolidiert: Gesamte Rechtsvorschrift für COVID-19-Maßnahmengesetz, Fassung vom 21.03.2020," at https://www.ris.bka.gv.at/GeltendeFassung.wxe?Abfrage=Bundesnormen&Gesetzesnummer=20011073&FassungVom=2020-03-21.

38 Verfassungsgerichtshof Österreich, "COVID-19-Gesetz ist verfassungskonform, Verordnungen über Betretungsverbote waren teilweise gesetzwidrig," 22 July 2020, https://www.vfgh.gv.at/medien/Covid_Entschaedigungen_Betretungsverbot.de.php.

39 See para. 10, sub. 2, "Bundesrecht konsolidiert: Gesamte Rechtsvorschrift für COVID-19-Maßnahmengesetz, Fassung vom 21 March 2020," at https://www.ris.bka.gv.at/GeltendeFassung.wxe?Abfrage=Bundesnormen&Gesetzesnummer=20011073&FassungVom=2020-03-21.

40 "Bundesrecht konsolidiert: Gesamte Rechtsvorschrift für Epidemiegesetz 1950, Fassung vom 14 February 2022," at https://www.ris.bka.gv.at/GeltendeFassung.wxe?Abfrage=Bundesnormen&Gesetzesnummer=10010265. See also Felix Andreaus, *Handbuch des österreichischen Seuchenrechts* (Vienna: Facultas, 2021), p. 260 and p. 277.

41 Felix Andreaus, *Handbuch des österreichischen Seuchenrechts* (Vienna: Facultas, 2021), p. 271.

42 "Bundesrecht konsolidiert: Gesamte Rechtsvorschrift für COVID-19-Maßnahmengesetz, Fassung vom 3 February 2022," at https://www.ris.bka.gv.at/GeltendeFassung.wxe?Abfrage=Bundesnormen&Gesetzesnummer=20011073.

43 Felix Andreaus, *Handbuch des österreichischen Seuchenrechts* (Vienna: Facultas, 2021), p. 271.

that the COVID-19 Measures Law has more to do with Austrians' expectations of their political leadership in a public-health crisis than with acute legal requirements. Specifically, Austria gives pride of place to the social dimension of government and society – the *Sozialstaat*.

Formally speaking, Austria's self-identification as a "social state" marks a relatively recent development; in 2002, a successful popular referendum against cuts to the social safety net sought to add the core social feature of the polity to the existing language of the Federal Constitutional Law that enshrines people as sovereign.[44] More precisely, the referendum was meant as "the defense and renewal of the *Sozialstaat*" against policies that "curtail services, weaken institutions, and undermine the bases of [social] solidarity."[45] In the event, the ÖVP/FPÖ coalition government that was then in power was perceived by the left – and by a considerable number of citizens – as engaged in a neoliberal campaign to wreck the social compact, starting with the scrapping of the 40-hour work week and the social security benefits that it entails.[46]

But in other ways, the referendum merely reaffirmed a long-standing feature of Austrian civics that can be said to reach back to the eighteenth century and the reign of Habsburg Empress Maria Theresia, namely the requirement that state and society organize and act to protect and advance Austrian social welfare. These basic rights include, for instance, a right to work, the entitlement to a minimum income to sustain life, a right to decent shelter, access to education, and the right to a stable, clean natural environment.[47] In practice, this insistence on the *Sozialstaat* expresses itself in far-reaching measures that include social insurance laws, generous support for the unemployed, and subsidized social housing. And it reflects a deeply Austrian expectation that the government and the community must honor and protect through the constitution the basic rights of social welfare.

A word is in order here about the corpus of Austrian constitutional law, which looks very different from the elaborate and elaborated post-World War II constitutions of even Austria's nearest neighbors. On the one hand, the specific federal "constitutional law" (*Bundes-Verfassungsgesetz* or B-VG) of Austria establishes the nation as a democratic republic (Art. 1) and a federal republic (Art. 2).[48] Then, several pages affirm the independence of the judiciary (in no small part thanks to the first-hand influence of Hans Kelsen on the 1920 constitution of the First Republic, which significantly informs the current Austrian constitutional law) as well as the territorial boundaries of the republic and the greater and finer points of the Austrian federal system. Perhaps most striking about the Austrian B-VG, however, is what it does *not* cover. There is no list of individual liberties or human/civil rights in the law – no Bill of Rights. In fact, other than some oblique references to property owners, there is no mention of individuals, their rights, or their responsibilities anywhere in the narrowly drawn B-VG. Also, there are no provisions for a state of emergency or any other circumstances under which certain parts of the constitution might be suspended, even a little, amid a crisis.

But Austria casts a wide net for its constitutional law (somewhat confusingly called the *Verfassungsgesetz* or the *Bundesverfassung* – without the hyphen that distinguishes the specific

---

44 See Bundesministerium Inneres, "Sozialstaat Österreich," https://www.bmi.gv.at/411/Volksbegehren_der_XX_Gesetzgebungsperiode/Volksbegehren_Sozialstaat_Oesterreich/.

45 See the justifications in Bundesministerium Inneres, "Sozialstaat Österreich," https://www.bmi.gv.at/411/Volksbegehren_der_XX_Gesetzgebungsperiode/Volksbegehren_Sozialstaat_Oesterreich/.

46 Erfolg für Volksbegehren, "Sozialstaat Österreich Mit 35.000 Unterstützungs- erklärungen ist Weg für Volksbegehren offen," *Der Standard*, 11 December 2001, at https://www.derstandard.at/story/805134/erfolg-fuer-volksbegehren-sozialstaat-oesterreich.

47 Lando Kirchmair, "Soziale Rechte als Beitrag zur subjektiven Sicherheit. Die Geschichte der sozialen Grundrechte in Österreich." *SIAK-Journal – Zeitschrift für Polizeiwissenschaft und polizeiliche Praxis*, No. 4 2012, pp. 68–79, https://www.bmi.gv.at/104/Wissenschaft_und_Forschung/SIAK-Journal/SIAK-Journal-Ausgaben/Jahrgang_2010/files/Kirchmair_3_2010.pdf.

48 "Bundesrecht konsolidiert: Gesamte Rechtsvorschrift für Bundes-Verfassungsgesetz, Fassung vom 14 February 2022," at https://www.ris.bka.gv.at/GeltendeFassung.wxe?Abfrage=Bundesnormen&Gesetzesnummer=10000138.

B-VG from/within the broader body of constitutional law), including international agreements, so-called constitutional acts, and provisions in other legislation, among other things.[49] So, for example, Austria is a signatory of the Charter of Fundamental Rights of the European Union (2000)[50] and the United Nations Refugee Convention (1951),[51] and it considers both documents to form part of the – comparatively robust – "constitutional" protections of civil liberties and human rights.[52] And although the wording that the 2002 *Sozialstaat* referendum approved does not (yet) appear in the B-VG, the assertion that Austria is a social state has constitutional-level traction.

16.4   A Decade or More of Crises

The other aspect of the *Sozialstaat* in action – and its manifestation in the "bundle" of COVID-19-related laws, including the vaccine mandate of 2022 – concerns the response of state and government to and amid crises. And the fact is that crisis, internal as well as international, has beset what had become a prosperous, stable, and very European Austria for most of the twenty-first century so far. Each individually and, more importantly, all of them together fuel the sense of siege and threat that informs Austria's Coronavirus laws and the popular responses.

Starting in 2009, Austria faced its own share of the sovereign debt misery or eurozone crisis. Interestingly, as the specter of default spread from Ireland and Greece and Spain, observers and participants including, for example, the European Central Bank (ECB) described the sequence of financial turmoil in epidemiological terms – "contagion" or "fever"[53] – that was seen to spread from the periphery of Europe to its center, overturning what for long had become a serene and content life of the average citizen. Austria did not number among the hardest-hit EU nations, but the government stepped in to nationalize at least two "bad banks" in 2009. In later comments to the Nationalrat, then-Chancellor Werner Faymann, a Social Democrat, invoked the legendary Creditanstalt, the Austrian bank that failed in 1931 and precipitated Europe's Great Depression with catastrophic outcome for Austrian democracy and the *Anschluss* to Hitler's Reich in 1938.[54] The billions of euros in debt that thus fell to Austrian taxpayers now still made for a better deal, according to Faymann, than a potential repeat of the "mistakes of the [thirties]," which had first seen the end of democracy in Austria and then of national independence altogether.[55] The reference underscored the expectation on all sides that the Austrian government today would act decisively to foster stability as the basis for the well-being of all citizens in the *Sozialstaat*.

The 2014 Russian annexation of Crimea and the subsequent low-intensity conflict in eastern Ukraine then threatened to chip away at Austria's dual statecraft of neutrality with a role in the foreign and security policy of the EU, a place where war was said to be impossible, although garden-plot holders in the suburbs of Graz could hear the mortar fire from the wars

---

49 See, for example, Republik Österreich, Parlament, "Das Bundes-Verfassungsgesetz," *Parlament Erklärt*, https://www.parlament.gv.at/PERK/VERF/BVG/.

50 https://www.europarl.europa.eu/charter/default_en.htm.

51 https://www.unhcr.org/en-us/3b66c2aa10.

52 Bundeskanzleramt and Bundesministerium Inneres, "Mein Österreich" (preparatory materials for the Austrian citizenship exam), December 2020, https://www.staatsbuergerschaft.gv.at/fileadmin/user_upload/Broschuere/RZ_BMI_StaBuBro_Gesamt-Buch_2020_screen.pdf.

53 Roberto A. De Santis, "The Euro area sovereign debt crisis: safe haven, credit rating agencies and the spread of the fever from Greece, Ireland and Portugal," ECB Working Paper, No. 1419, European Central Bank (ECB), Frankfurt a. M., 2012, https://www.econstor.eu/bitstream/10419/153852/1/ecbwp1419.pdf.

54 "Faymann: Hypo- Verantwortung bei FPÖ," orf. 8 April 2017, at, https://oe1.orf.at/artikel/367349/Faymann-Hypo-Verantwortung-bei-FPOe.

55 "Faymann: Hypo- Verantwortung bei FPÖ," orf. 8 April 2017, at, https://oe1.orf.at/artikel/367349/Faymann-Hypo-Verantwortung-bei-FPOe.

of independence/dissolution in ex-Yugoslavia in the 1990s. Then, in the summer of 2015, SPÖ chancellor Werner Faymann faced the next, far-greater geopolitical and demographic crisis in and around Austria: the human tide of migrants from the Middle East, South Asia, and Africa. At its most acute, in the first days of September 2015, some tens of thousands of people found themselves stranded in nearby Hungary by the right-wing, anti-immigrant government of Viktor Orbán, which initially refused to let the refugees pass through Hungary on their way to Germany and the wider EU. In an improvisation blind to the climacteric of crisis that now became the nemesis of European statecraft, Faymann and his German counterpart, Chancellor Angela Merkel, agreed to help the migrants move along from the Vienna Westbahnhof and the border crossings at Salzburg and Schärding to Munich and beyond,[56] despite the black-letter provisions of the so-called Dublin Regulation that, at the time, required asylum seekers and refugees to stay in the first EU state they reached for processing.[57]

When the first of the migrants arrived at the Austrian–Hungarian border in Burgenland on the Vienna–Budapest highway, they found Austrian volunteers with food and blankets – and hand-drawn signs reading: *Willkommen* (Welcome).[58] In this spirit, private citizens appeared along the road, offering to transport migrants in their personal vehicles, even while the Austrian state railroad laid on hundreds of special trains to bring the migrants to Vienna.[59] When the trains rolled into the capital, they were met with more cheering crowds.[60] In a word, it was the Austrian *Sozialstaat* in full force amid global upheaval.

While many, if not most, of the migrants in this incident and others traveled on to Germany, Austria took in thousands of asylum seekers – in numbers that amount to more than 1% of the national population.[61] The nation had also done so in the wars of Yugoslav succession two decades earlier. But the political and therefore the legal context was changing.

Faymann stepped down in mid-2016; two more Socialist figures held the office in the same year that saw a sharpening party–political conflict. Then, in December 2017, ÖVP foreign minister Sebastian Kurz took office after a meteoric rise. As the new broom, if not the new kid, Kurz – often called Shorty by friends and foes ("*kurz*" means "short" in German), although he stands more than six feet tall – sought to remake the ÖVP for the new millennium in his hipster-netizen image. To this end, he updated the party's symbolic color to turquoise – think: *haute couture* or at least twenty-first-century club chic – from the traditional black of European Christian democracy.

Shorty had begun in a minor role in the Vienna municipal government; then, he became Minister for Integration, responsible for the large foreign-born population present in Austria since the 1960s, especially with the Yugoslav wars and opening of the borders that came with EU membership.

56 DW, "Thousands of migrants welcomed by Austria, Germany," 5 September 2015, https://www.dw.com/en/thousands-of-migrants-welcomed-by-austria-germany/a-18696175.

57 European Parliament, Council of the European Union, EU Regulation No. 604/2013 (26 June 2013), http://data.europa.eu/eli/reg/2013/604/oj.

58 Don Murray, "UNHCR applauds Austria and Germany as refugees march across Hungary," 5 September 2015, https://www.unhcr.org/en-us/news/latest/2015/9/55eae4116/unhcr-applauds-austria-germany-refugees-march-across-hungary.html.

59 "ÖBB-Bilanz: 300.000 Flüchtlinge befördert, 674 Sonderzüge," *Die Presse*, 22 April 2016, https://www.diepresse.com/4973296/oebb-bilanz-300000-fluechtlinge-befoerdert-674-sonderzuege.

60 DW, "Thousands of migrants welcomed by Austria, Germany," 5 September 2015, https://www.dw.com/en/thousands-of-migrants-welcomed-by-austria-germany/a-18696175. Der Standard, "Tausende Flüchtlinge aus Ungarn bereits in Wien und Salzburg angekommen," 5 September 2015, https://www.derstandard.at/jetzt/livebericht/2000021766384/fluechtlinge-werden-in-bussen-nach-oesterreich-gebracht?responsive=false.

61 "Austria says it will stop any migrants trying to rush its border," *Reuters*, 1 March 2020, https://www.reuters.com/article/us-syria-security-austria/austria-says-it-will-stop-any-migrants-trying-to-rush-its-border-idUSKBN20O2CS. Irene Bricker, "Österreich verstärkt Grenzschutz gegen mehr Flüchtlinge und Migranten," *Der Standard* 24 July 2021, https://www.derstandard.at/story/2000128429188/bundesregierung-schickt-400-zusaetzliche-soldaten-an-die-grenze.

Kurz\nobreak then made the leap to the foreign ministry, where his *coup de main* was a policy with no small indirect aid from Hungary's Orbán to close the "Balkan route" for Syrian and Afghan refugees. This reversal came at the expense of Angela Merkel and the Austrian *Wilkommenskultur*. The *Sozialstaat* seemed rather less social.

Officially, the boy-wonder pace-setter Kurz represented the ÖVP, a center-right, big-tent party, but his agenda had a different tenor as well as color. Aligning himself with an old/new xenophobia that the FPÖ had made a central point of its perma-protest, Kurz can be said to have made this fear more mainstream by packaging it in zippy turquoise rather than the Pan-German cornflower blue of the FPÖ. But the rebranding of Kurz's ÖVP might not have been a coincidence on the color wheel; it ultimately revealed a serious departure from the assumptions and expressions of the rule of law and the *Sozialstaat* that formed the heart of the Austrian constitution.

The ÖVP/FPÖ coalition that emerged from the 2017 parliamentary election culminated with Kurz as chancellor and, as vice-chancellor, the FPÖ's Heinz-Christian Strache, a one-time dental technician with equally laddish and romantic-nationalist affectations who also was then the chairman of the Freedom Party. Strache lived in the shadow of Jörg Haider, the man who in the wake of the 1995 accession of Austria to the EU had thrust the FPÖ rightward. Strache, however, was not as good a politician as the canny Carinthian nationalist, who died in a car crash in 2008.[62]

As party leader, Strache gleefully presided over the FPÖ's alignment with Vladimir Putin's Russia and the latter's use of similar political figures in western democracies as multipliers for Russian great-power revisionism. (After the Russian annexation of Crimea in 2014, Moscow stepped up its outreach to the harder-right-wing parties of Europe, and many of them, including the FPÖ – but also the German Alternative für Deutschland [AfD] and Marine Le Pen's *Rassemblement National* [National Rally, the former National Front] – accepted the offer, which may or may not have included cash transfers.[63]) Then in 2019, video footage came to light in the German press, featuring Strache and his party No. 2, Johann Gudenus, in a 2017 campaign meeting on Ibiza in the sunny Mediterranean with a lissome young woman who presented herself as a Russian oligarch's niece in search of ways to donate money meaningfully, or at least without the normal scrutiny, in Austria – that is, to advance Russian strategic aims of Gazprom's sphere of influence far to the west. Gudenus did the translating, up to and including a Red Bull-and-vodka – fueled pantomime of Glock pistols.[64] Ultimately, the parties seemed to focus on how the "Russian" side might invest in Austria's biggest daily newspaper, the tabloid *Kronen Zeitung*. Strache and Gudenus wanted to influence *die Krone's* huge readership sufficiently to garner votes for policies that the FPÖ and, presumably, also Russia prefer – or perhaps to burst the independence of this most prominent media outlet in favor of reliably tame reporting on matters close to the FPÖ's agenda.[65]

In fact, the scene was a deftly mounted sting operation of the enemies of the FPÖ, including, perhaps, those ÖVP members of greater age and girth who begrudged the young Kurz and his turquoise clique for turning the staid center-right party upside down in 2016–2017 – to say nothing of what one might describe as the Austrian deep state, which found Strache and Kickl too awful for public life; the latter well recalled how the revelations that President Kurt Waldheim (1986–1992) had been

---

62 Wolfgang Haserer, *Der Rechtspopulist Jörg Haider – Eine Analyse seines Politischen Erfolges in Österreich* (Munich: Grin, 2001); Klaus Ottomeyer, *Jörg Haider – Mythenbildung und Erbschaft* (Klagenfurt and Vienna: Drava, 2009); Gerd Kräh, *Die Freiheitlichen unter Jörg Haider: Rechtsextreme Gefahr oder Hoffnungsträger für Österreich?* (Frankfurt Am Main and Vienna: Lang, 1996).

63 See especially the embedded video in DW, "Austria finds former vice chancellor guilty of corruption," 27 August 2021, https://www.dw.com/en/austria-finds-former-vice-chancellor-guilty-of-corruption/a-58999760.

64 "Die Videofalle," *Der Spiegel*, 17 May 2019, https://www.spiegel.de/video/fpoe-chef-heinz-christian-strache-die-videofalle-video-99027174.html.

65 "Die Videofalle," *Der Spiegel*, 17 May 2019, https://www.spiegel.de/video/fpoe-chef-heinz-christian-strache-die-videofalle-video-99027174.html.

a member of the Nazi Sturmabteilung (SA) equestrian branch and later an intelligence officer in the Wehrmacht, specializing in anti-partisan operations, in the Balkans had led to Austria's isolation in foreign standing relative to its "unmastered" Nazi past.[66]

Ironically, in the run-up to the presidential election and the chancellor contest in the years 2016–2017, *die Krone* had disgorged histrionic articles in their dozens, depicting threats on the eastern border and sex-crazed Afghan and Syrian emigrant rapists doing their most dastardly in Vienna and elsewhere. In other words, the tabloid was already largely in step with the new FPÖ. Thus, the crass disregard of the newspaper's freedoms – to say nothing of the public's right to truth and transparency in and from the fourth estate – was particularly shocking. Strache ultimately was found to be as corrupt and venal a public figure as any in the halls of power in Vienna since the seventeenth century.[67] Austrians were deeply shaken by this lawlessness at the highest levels of a government.

Still, Kurz, coasting on his *Wunderkind* cache as an upgrader of European conservatism, survived the 2019 Ibiza video affair and, in fact, returned to power in January 2020. So, Shorty presided, with the overweening mass-persuasion flair that has been his consistent if failing bond, over Austria's initial COVID response – including curfews, lockdowns, and the Byzantine "G rules" that governed individual entry into sundry venues and places of business: 2G, meaning fully vaccinated or recovered within the last six months; 2.5G, meaning fully vaccinated or recovered *or* PCR-tested; 2G-plus, meaning fully vaccinated or recovered *and*, additionally, a negative PCR test result; or 3G, meaning fully vaccinated *or* recovered *or* PCR tested or antigen tested.[68]

Then, amid another corruption scandal in October 2021 – probably more profound than the Ibiza video caper and its blowback in 2019 – Kurz left office again, though he momentarily remained the chairman of the ÖVP and a member of parliament. Thus, he appeared for a while to retain significant influence in the ÖVP – until October 2021, when a shocking stream of SMS messages from the "Projekt Ballhausplatz" clique of 2016 came to light, outlining a broad conspiracy for taxpayer-funded pay-to-play public-opinion "research" with predetermined (and politically persuasive) "results."[69] As criminal charges shaped up for the flagrant misuse of public money for partisan propaganda in the tabloids and parliament acted to strip Kurz of his official immunity in

66 Waldheim, who became a top Austrian diplomat after the war, had served as Secretary-General of the United Nations from 1971 to 1982 before being elected president of the Second Republic in 1986. The stories of his wartime record actually began circulating amid his candidacy which coincided with the scandal about Ronald Regan's visit to the German military cemetery in Bitburg that included the graves of Waffen-SS soldiers. As the controversy accelerated, the Austrian government convened an international group of historians – the so-called Waldheim Commission – to look into how Waldheim spent the war years. While the commission found no evidence of Waldheim's direct complicity in atrocities, it concluded that he knew broadly of what was happening and made no effort to intervene, however little he might have achieved at the time. For details, see Cornelius Lehnguth, *Waldheim und die Folgen: Der Parteipolitische Umgang mit dem Nationalsozialismus in Österreich* (Frankfurt am Main: Campus, 2013); the International Commission of Historians (the Waldheim Commission), *The Waldheim Report* (Copenhagen: Museum Tusculanum, University of Copenhagen, 1993). Georg Tidl, *Waldheim: Wie es Wirklich War: Die Geschichte einer Recherche* (Vienna: Löcker, 2015).
67 Strache's young and photogenic wife, Pia Phillipa Strache, as a member of the Nationalrat, also, was hounded out of public life in a hail of misogynistic tabloid invective about pocketing public cash that is a signal part of the polity. See, for example, "Parteischädigend: Strache aus FPÖ ausgeschlossen," *ORF*, 29 October 2019, https://orf.at/stories/3141862/; "Spesen-Affäre Putzfrau belastet die Straches schwer," *Die Kronen Zeitung*, 27 October 2019, https://www.krone.at/2238919.
68 See, for example, Stadt Wien, "Questions and answers regarding coronavirus and the COVID-19 disease," https://coronavirus.wien.gv.at/faq-english/#3GRule. The titular Gs refer to the first letter of most past participles in German, in this case, "geimpft" (immunized); "genesen" (recovered); and "getestet" (tested).
69 "Eine Chronologie der türkis-grünen Krisen(woche)," *Die Presse*, 8 October 2021, https://www.diepresse.com/6044668/eine-chronologie-der-tuerkis-gruenen-krisenwoche. "Projekt Ballhausplatz" refers to the efforts by Kurz & Co. to secure power through eye-wateringly corrupt and antidemocratic means. Sandra Sperber and Zsolt Wilhelm, "Intrigen, Machtspiele und eine Erpressung," *Der Spiegel*, 30 October 2021, https://www.spiegel.de/

the corruption case, however, Kurz abruptly resigned all his political offices in December 2021, in a kind of virtual exit through the stage trap door in a clap of music-pit thunder and gushing of dry ice.[70]

Then, in a reveal worthy of the stage designers of the Vienna Opera, Shorty burst back into view in, of all places, Silicon Valley, now working for the right-wing German-Californian billionaire venture capitalist Peter Thiel, who, in many ways, bears the standard of the hyper-rich realm of global power and finance that looms so large in the Austrian public mind – even more than the pandemic and its millions of deaths and miseries – as the dominant force that threatens national well-being and has done so for a very long time.[71] To say the very least, Shorty had left the *Sozialstaat*; the only question was exactly when.

16.5 The *Sozialstaat* Strikes Back

Despite the *Sturm*, *Drang*, and sordid scandal of the last decade or so, Austria's *Sozialstaat* is neither down nor out. President since the hard-won and protracted election campaigns in 2017, Van der Bellen has embodied in the Corona-crisis in Austrian constitutional practice as head of state certain salient and ameliorating features of public life. Notably, his Dutch/Baltic and Tirolean heritage underscores the factor of Austria integrated into a Europe of human values; his family fled from what is today Estonia to Tirol in the age of total war, and Van der Bellen deems Austria as his home with neither cynicism nor caveats.[72] And at a critical moment in June 2019, amid the searing domestic political trauma of the Ibiza video and its implications, Van der Bellen summoned a cabinet, led by head of the constitutional court, Brigitte Bierlein.[73] The turmoil of the moment made it very important that she was member of no party; her career as a jurist, legal scholar, and especially a member of the highest court further distinguished her as exactly the Kelsenian character – learned, independent, and constitutionally oriented – to nudge government and society away from the sheer cliffs of crisis of party and geopolitics as had doomed the First Republic and had settled like a cloud over the Second. Bierlein and her cabinet during the pivotal six-month period from June 2019 until January 2020 did much to detoxify national life in the all-too-brief period of quiet before the COVID crisis unfolded. Thus, to a meaningful extent, the Austrian *Sozialstaat* – and especially the community orientation that informs it – prevailed and informed the response to these crises in the years 2008–2022, including, as the next in line, SARS-CoV-2.

To be sure, the *Sozialstaat* is something of a double-edged proposition. On the one hand, Austria and Austrians take the social nature of state and society as a fundamental aspect of Second Republic democracy. There is, on the other hand, the phenomenon – perhaps not exclusively but

---

ausland/sebastian-kurz-wie-er-dank-projekt-ballhausplatz-an-die-macht-kam-podcast-inside-austria-a-72b8ae0b-6d77-4a8b-bacd-3c008306f918. The joint *Spiegel/Standard* podcast is very detailed.

70 Anna Giulia Fink, Jan Michael Marchart, Markus Rohrhofer, Gabriele Scherndl, and Colette M. Schmidt, "Der Rücktritt von Sebastian Kurz: 'Bin weder Heiliger noch Verbrecher'," *Der Standard*, 2 December 2021, https://www.derstandard.at/story/2000131601624/kurz-zieht-sich-aus-der-politik-zurueck.

71 "Peter Thiel – Der neue Chef von Sebastian Kurz," *ORF* Oe 1. 21 January 2022, https://oe1.orf.at/artikel/690803/Peter-Thiel-Der-neue-Chef-von-Sebastian-Kurz.

72 "Bundespräsident Alexander Van der Bellen," https://www.bundespraesident.at/aktuelles/detail/lebenslauf-alexander-van-der-bellen. He is credited on the website as proclaiming that his *Heimat* is Tirol, Vienna, Austria, and Europe. *Heimat*, with its connotations of generational belonging, is a notoriously intractable word to translate into English; "home" fails to do justice, though it must suffice for now. Either way, Van der Bellen's statement is both programmatic – his political priorities (federalism, service, state, and the EU) are made clear – and emblematic of the Austrian Sozialstaat at work.

73 Her official biography as federal chancellor is available through the normal web archives; the original URL is: https://www.bundeskanzleramt.gv.at/lebenslauf-bundeskanzlerin.

certainly characteristically Central European – of a somewhat sharp-elbowed and sharp-tongued "community spirit," or what in another time was called *ein gesundes Volksempfinden*,[74] (a healthy public sense – notice the use of the word "health" in this connection), dedicated to the watchful observance other Austrians' compliance or noncompliance with the black letter of the current rules of the building, town, province, or republic. These interactions easily and often transcend the antics of mere nosey neighbors, accompanied by passive-aggressive notes and rebukes laced with the enormous vocabulary of Vienna-dialect insults, if not outright campaigns of harassment, culminating in spurious calls to the police and days or weeks in court with struggles about dogs without muzzles, hedges left untrimmed, or heavy-footed residents upstairs daring to use their own toilets after 10 p.m. Indeed, a whole legal specialty exists in German-speaking Europe under the heading of "neighbor law" (*Nachbarrecht* or *Nachbarschaftsrecht*), and statutory/code volumes, how-to manuals, and practical guides abound on real and virtual bookshelves.[75]

Perhaps the prime exemplar of this aspect of public health in the pandemic – as viewed through the lens of cabaret and political satire – is a puppet called Berti Blockwardt, who takes form in videos from the left-wing Vienna newspaper, *Der Falter*, grouped under the fateful title of "Berti Blockwardt is Watching" – *Berti Blockwardt passt auf*. The main character's name translates to Bert the Block-Warden or Bert the Block-Watcher. During the Third Reich, the *Blockwart* (or *Blockwalter)* was the lowest-level Nazi social-welfare official responsible for the compliance of the denizens of a "block" comprising 50 or so households, a role that relied heavily on neighbor-beggaring and denunciation.[76] As the proliferation of neighbor-law treatises even today might suggest, the term also captures the tendency of many contemporary Austrians to snoop on their neighbors and to tattle to any and all authorities about the tiniest infraction of the rules in the stairwell in communal housing. Berti's creator, Nikolaus Habjan, is a young theater figure from Styria (in fact, a puppet-master in the actual sense) of sublime talent and regional renown in the mode of Johann Nestroy, Karl Kraus, and Helmut Qualtinger. His creation, Berti Blockwardt, is a cranky, liver-spotted pensioner with nothing better to do than to mind everyone else's affairs amid the pandemic lockdowns, anointing himself as the interpreter and arbiter of the federal health guidance.

In Episode 6, for example, Berti takes aim at "the worst endangerers of human life: our dear children."[77] To this end, he appears with Razzia "Raidy" Rat, a puppet rodent, who has declared that her task is to ensure that people are adhering to the regulations "verrrrrry, very exactly."[78] Razzia Rat further promises to disrupt nefarious disease-spreading events – especially children playing ball games outside their housing developments at this time of abject lockdown – by biting the ball "into bits" or, if necessary, gnawing on the calves of any juvenile soccer scofflaws.[79] Obviously, the puppet freak-out about football-playing children – otherwise confined to their dwellings and trying to do school online in the lockdown, but occasionally allowed to run around, as youngsters do, outside

---

74 This term was used as early as 1913 in periodicals close to Christian Social and Jew baiting mayor of Vienna, Karl Lueger, and was later a term of jurisprudence in the Third Reich as part of the repression of persons and groups targeted by the regime as enemies of Nazi people's community. Herlinde Pauer-Studer, *Justifying Injustice: Legal Theory in Nazi Germany* (Cambridge: Cambridge University Press, 2020).

75 Representative titles from Austria include: Gerhard Putz, *Mein Recht als Nachbar: Nachbarschaftsrecht in Österreich* (Graz and Stuttgart: Leopold Stocker, 2012); Elisabeth Kirschner, *Mediation als Methode außergerichtlicher Streitbeilegung im zivilen Nachbarrecht* (Vienna: danzig & unfried, 2022); Julius Ecker, *Nachbarrechtliche Sonderrechtsverhältnisse: Nachbarrecht bei Miete, Mit- und Wohnungseigentum und Dienstbarkeiten*, RdU - Schriftenreihe Recht der Umwelt (Vienna: MANZ, 2021); Ferdinand Kerschner and Erika M. Wagner, *Nachbarschaftsrecht kompakt: Praxis und Theorie anhand von Fällen*, 3rd ed. (Vienna: Linde, 2014).

76 Ulrich Trebbin, "Blockwarte im Nationalsozialismus," *BR Bayern 2*, 3 November 2011, https://www.br.de/radio/bayern2/sendungen/land-und-leute/blockwarte-im-nationalsozialismus-trebbin100.html.

77 Falter.at, "Berti Blockwardt passt auf," ep. 6, 14 April 2020, https://www.youtube.com/watch?v=pYOaQdHeTs0.

78 Falter.at, "Berti Blockwardt passt auf," ep. 6, 14 April 2020, https://www.youtube.com/watch?v=pYOaQdHeTs0.

79 Falter.at, "Berti Blockwardt passt auf," ep. 6, 14 April 2020, https://www.youtube.com/watch?v=pYOaQdHeTs0.

in the same fresh air that was meant to mitigate COVID-19 transmission – is hilariously misplaced. For one thing, the early anti-Coronavirus measures, in particular, with their emphases on lockdown and isolation, did not really accommodate kids' realities or needs in any state or jurisdiction.

But Berti also forms an integral, if unpleasant, part of the community, the crack from the nasty old geezer next door about the neighbor kids being germ-vectors notwithstanding. In other words, community well-being remains important especially in a Vienna or Graz[80] that treasures the merits of its social housing settlements and a cohesive community. While one might not want to make too much of a particular swiftly enacted government anti-COVID guideline (particularly if, à la Berti, one cannot quite manage to keep one's mask over one's ample nose while poking it into everyone else's business), the point remains that Austrians are in this pandemic together.

16.6   Protest, Rhetoric, and the Law

Or perhaps they are not …

Every Saturday in a rhythm that started in the course of further lockdowns in Austria in the year 2021, hundreds, sometimes thousands, of Austrians have gathered in the major cities to protest the state's COVID-19 response measures. They have demonstrated, variously, against masking requirements, curfews, lockdowns, and especially immunization laws; the advent of the vaccine mandate seemed to (re-)energize the resistors, bringing them back to the "demos" and "freedom marches."[81] The protestors comprise a mixed bag of right-wing populists, old and new Nazis, conspiracy theorists, new-agers, late-blooming hippies, and anti-reason – if not anti-intellectual – agitators of all stripes.[82] Little other than the putative dedication to individual liberties, even or especially at the worst of times, unites these crowds; still, to the extent that the demonstrations feature anxious citizens demanding accountability and flexibility from their elected government, they count as a healthy part of a democratic society. On the other hand, events that do, in fact, resemble all too well the civic violence that wracked Austria in the years 1927–1938 have become a prominent feature of many established western democracies, thus the issue lies in the defense of the rule of law that is based on an enlightened constitution. The antidemocratic, to say nothing of anti-*Sozialstaatlich*, bent of the variously organized extremists who predominate at the weekly gatherings in Vienna and Tirol at least merits the top-of-the-list priority of concern that Interior Minister Karner identified in his December 2021 remarks to *Public Safety*.

And the evidence, particularly later in the pandemic, surely problematizes any blithe assumptions that the people – as in "Wir sind das Volk," a motto cadged from the East German Monday

---

80 In the fall of 2021, that is, well into the pandemic, the city of Graz elected to the mayor's office Elke Kahr, a member of the Communist Party of Austria, with a healthy plurality at the expense of the governing parties, in part because of her role in social housing and an attempt to aid the homeless. See her official biography at City of Graz, City Hall, "Lebenslauf Bürgermeisterin Elke Kahr," at https://www.graz.at/cms/beitrag/10041296/7766633/ Lebenslauf_Buergermeisterin_Elke_Kahr.html.

81 A particularly large demonstration – with more than 40,000 participants who were, at one point, addressed by Herbert Kickl – happened on 11 December 2021, amid the fourth lockdown and with the vaccine mandate well under way. See, for example, "Mass protest in Vienna against Austria's controversial COVID restrictions," *Reuters*, 11 December 2021, https://www.reuters.com/world/europe/mass-protest-vienna-against-austrias-controversial-covid-restrictions-2021-12-11/. Organizers had wildly inflated the turnout – originally claiming nearly a half million demonstrators. See "Faktencheck: Keine 450.000 Teilnehmer bei Demo gegen Corona-Maßnahmen in Wien," *Der Standard*, 29 December 2021, https://www.derstandard.at/story/2000132219854/faktencheck-keine-450-000-teilnehmer-bei-demo-gegen-corona-massnahmen.

82 See, for example, Christian Kreil, "Impfgegner: Braun und Bio im Gleichschritt unterwegs," *Der Standard*, 1 December 2021, https://www.derstandard.at/story/2000131464413/impfgegner-braun-und-bio-im-gleichschritt-unterwegs.

demonstrations before the communist regime there collapsed in 1989 – are all operating within a standard deviation of democratic civil sensibilities. Rather, the symbols and slogans at these gatherings form an alarming study of the chameleon-like energy among those persons and political movements that want to junk democracy in Central Europe. For example, the *Staatsverweigerer* – whose name translates literally to "rejectors of the state" – carry the Austrian state flag but not in any show of patriotic enthusiasm. Instead, the *Staatsverweigerer* version features the Austrian coat of arms inverted, symbolic of the group's refusal to recognize the authority of the Austrian Republic (or any other nation-state), which they dismiss as illegitimate "corporations" serving the interests of unnamed dark invaders and inchoate supranational powers. Akin to the "sovereign" movement in North America, the group, also called the *Staatenbund*, numbering perhaps 2700 members, urges its followers to refuse to pay taxes or license their cars; the organization sells alternate identification to go along with its "advice."[83] The threat to Austrian democracy is real, however; in 2017 a regional court in Graz convicted the founding *Staatenbund* leaders of high treason and subversion following a bid to incite the Austrian Bundesheer to overthrow the government, perhaps with the military aid that they reportedly sought from Vladimir Putin, with wacky "orders" given to the then-Austrian Chief of Defense, General Othmar Commenda.[84]

Similarly, the Corona-Querfront[85] group is a new name for an old accumulation of well-known neo-Nazis, including Holocaust-denier turned Corona-denier and far-right activist Gottfried Küssel, who has faced criminal charges several times in an ignominious career of pro-Hitler agitation or, as it is called in Austria, "Wiederbetätigung."[86] Küssel's crony from the long-ago "new right" days, Harald A. Schmidt – a former attorney not to be confused with the German comedian and late-night talk-show host – also operates his IUVALEX group, which purports to be a Society for Juridical Cooperation and Legal Aid, presumably for other extremists[87] – under the umbrella of the Corona-Querfront.[88] The organization's name attests to its ideological overlap with the German

---

83 This entity also more or less corresponds to the now infamous Reichsbürger in the Federal Republic of Germany, whose role as a fifth column of whatever size in the German police and armed forces have been notable since the impact of the refugee crisis in the years 2015–present. Matthias Meisnner, et al. eds. *Extreme Sicherheit: Rechtsradikale in Polizei, Verfassungsschutz, Bundeswehr und Justiz* (Freiburg i.B.: Herder, 2019); Donald Abenheim and Carolyn Halladay, *Germany: An Army in a Democracy in an Epoch of Extremes,* Oxford Research Encyclopaedia, 23 December 2021; https://oxfordre.com/politics/view/10.1093/acrefore/9780190228637.001.0001/acrefore-9780190228637-e-1892.

84 "Jail terms for Austrian far-right group trying to incite coup," DW, https://www.dw.com/en/jail-terms-for-austrian-far-right-group-trying-to-incite-coup/a-47237523. n.a. "Staatenbund": Ex-Generalstabschef des Bundesheeres als Zeuge Commenda: "Es liegt nicht in meiner Kompetenz, jemanden zu verhaften" *Der Standard*, 15 November 2018, https://www.derstandard.at/story/2000091459055/staatenbund-ex-generalstabschef-des-bundesheeres-als-zeuge.

85 See Markus Sulzbacher, "Alte Kameraden in der 'Corona-Querfront'," *Der Standard*, 6 May 2021, https://www.derstandard.de/story/2000126424532/alte-kameraden-in-der-corona-querfront.

86 The most recent trial – in 2012 for glorifying National Socialism on his Alpen-Donau.info website and blog – despite a certain amount of drama and intrigue about jurors (Maria Sterkl, "Geschworene fehlten, Küssel-Prozess vertagt," *Der Standard*, 14 May 2012, https://www.derstandard.at/story/1336696759434/rechtsextremismus-geschworene-fehlten-kuessel-prozess-vertagt), ended with a nine-year sentence, which was later reduced to seven years and two months. Christa Zöchling, "Gottfried Küssel: Prozess wegen Wiederbetätigung," *Profil*, 21 May 2012, https://www.profil.at/home/alpen-donau-gottfried-kuessel-prozess-wiederbetaetigung-323738; Michael Mösender, "Höchstgericht bestätigt Haft für Küssel und senkt Strafen," *Der Standard*, 15 January 2014, https://www.derstandard.at/story/1388651148819/hoechstgericht-bestaetigt-haft-fuer-kuessel-und-senkt-strafen.

87 "Gesellschaft für juristische Zusammenarbeit und Rechtshilfe" – the programmatic subtitle appears in the group's incorporation listing: https://www.firmeninfo.at/verein/iuvalex-gesellschaft-fuer-juristische-zusammenarbeit-und-rechtshilfe/1189692.

88 Colette M. Schmidt and Fabian Schmid, "Virale Querfront: Von QAnon, Neonazis und Wegbegleitern der Schwarzen Witwe," *Der Standard,* 26 September 2020, https://www.derstandard.at/story/2000120272847/virale-querfront-von-qanon-neonazis-und-wegbegleitern-der-schwarzen-witwe. Schmidt became an ex-lawyer for his

Querdenker ("disruptive thinkers," a group that moved from protesting early pandemic measures to ever more dire fantasies about machinations from malevolent national governments, to include the gene-scrambling COVID-19 vaccines), and, of course, with the American import of QAnon, with its increasingly dangerous anti-government conspiracy theories that in so many significant features recycles shopworn canards of anti-Semitism in Central Europe from about 1873 onward that, in another time, were the rage in right-wing circles in Austria prior to 1938.[89]

Q flags dot many of the Saturday demonstrations, as do a smattering of other well-known extremist emblems. Many of the banners and signs proclaim opposition to "globalist filth" and other aspects of neoliberalism.[90] Others feature right-wing extremist, identitarian, and/or white-supremacist slogans like "Deus vult" – "God wills it" in Latin and a battle cry from the First Crusade[91] – or "great replacement," referring to the conspiracy theory that contemporary liberal democratic orthodoxy, particularly as regards migration and multiculturalism, aims to disadvantage and ultimately eradicate white Europeans.[92]

None too few Austrian Corona protestors seem to have seized on modified Nazi-era iconography that breaks established taboos as well as the law, casting themselves as the victims of state terror in place of Europe's Jews 80 years ago, even despite a well-tracked current of anti-Semitic rhetoric among the protests and the protestors.[93] Specifically, they appear at demonstrations wearing versions of the notorious yellow stars that distinguished Jews in the hierarchy of Nazi society after 1941, now "updated" to include the word "unvaccinated" where the originals had "Jew" emblazoned on them in tendentiously racialized script.

This historical misappropriation is more than political theater or group self-pity. In the first instance, it marks an effort to minimalize the crimes and traumas of World War II and the Austrian role in them, removing Jewish Europeans and other victims from the narrative while

role in forging the wills of the wealthy victims of Austria's "black widow" murderess, Elfriede Blauensteiner. He also got seven years in prison for his efforts. "Elfriede Blauensteiner gestorben," *Der Standard*, 19 November 2003, https://www.derstandard.at/story/1486456/elfriede-blauensteiner-gestorben.

89 In late 2021, the independent Austrian Institute for International Affairs (OIIP) presented a lecture from US scholar Mia Bloom on "Q-Anon: From Conspiracy Theory to National Security Threat," 9 December 2021, at https://www.oiip.ac.at/en/events/qanon/. Also see: Brigitte Hamann, *Hitlers Wien: Lehrjahre Eines Diktators* 3rd ed. (Munich: Piper, 1996).

90 The broadsheet Austrian press has made a careful inventory of the extremist symbols and slogans that appear at the demonstrations. See, for example, Christa Zöchling, "Corona-Demos dokumentiert: Die trügerische Vielfalt des Protests," *Profil*, 12 February 2022, https://www.profil.at/oesterreich/corona-demos-dokumentiert-die-truegerische-vielfalt-des-protests/401903185; Colette M. Schmidt, "Corona-Demos: Unter gefährlichen Flaggen," *Der Standard*, 12 February 2022, https://www.derstandard.at/story/2000133302828/corona-demos-unter-gefaehrlichen-flaggen.

91 Colette M. Schmidt, "Corona-Demos: Unter gefährlichen Flaggen," *Der Standard*, 12 February 2022, https://www.derstandard.at/story/2000133302828/corona-demos-unter-gefaehrlichen-flaggen.

92 Christopher J. Adamczyk, *Gods versus Titans: Ideological Indicators of Identitarian Violence*, Master's thesis, Naval Postgraduate School, September 2020, pp. 5–12.

93 See, for example, Markus Sulzbacher, "Der bizarre Antisemitismus auf den Corona-Demos," *Der Standard*, Standard-Watchblog, 18 April 2021, https://www.derstandard.at/story/2000125773958/der-bizarre-antisemitismus-auf-den-corona-demos. The Jewish-star "unvaccinated" emblems started turning up at German anti-vaccination demonstrations around December 2021; see, for example, "Protest gegen Coronaregeln: Unbekannte hängen Zettel mit 'Judenstern' an Geschäften in Bruchsal auf," 6 December 2021, https://www.spiegel.de/panorama/justiz/bruchsal-zettel-mit-judenstern-an-geschaeften-in-bruchsal-aufgehaengt-a-5ac065df-e52c-4b63-a028-5686362b99e4. Austrian law is especially acute in such instances of the misuse of historical symbols associated with the Third Reich and whatever can hint of denial of the Holocaust. See the text of the June 1945 "Verbotgesetz," drafted within weeks of the end of the Third Reich at: https://www.ris.bka.gv.at/Dokumente/BgblPdf/1945_13_0/1945_13_0.pdf. Also see: Brigitte Bailer, "… Um Alle Nazistische Tätigkeit Und Propaganda in Österreich Zu Verhindern," (Graz: Clio, 2018), p. 13; "Rechtsextreme sind nicht nur kahl geschorene junge Männer," *Der Standard*, 20 April 2010, https://www.derstandard.at/story/1271374739677/buch-ueber-nazi-symbole-rechtsextreme-sind-nicht-nur-kahl-geschorene-junge-maenner.

relativizing the Holocaust. In this effort, it also flirts heavily with *Wiederbetätigung*[94] – literally the "reactivation" or glorification of National Socialism, which is a serious crime in Austria, as Holocaust denier and Nazi relativizer David Irving found out to his discomfiture in 2006.[95] Indeed, Austria passed the first version of the *Verbotgesetz* (Prohibition Law) on 8 May 1945, Victory in Europe Day, so central was this provision to the postwar democratic order. The *Verbotgesetz* counts as a constitutional law in Austria. As such, those who break it or bruise it or attempt to water it down with absurd comparisons or ulterior appropriations well may be citizens and individuals, but they work at direct odds with *das Volk* as a century or more of Austrian legal, political, and social practice conceives of "the people."

16.7   Conclusion: Community, Communicability, and the Constitution

Lockdowns permitting in the years 2020–2022, people in Vienna placed lighted candles at the *Pestsäule* – the "Plague Column" on the Graben, a pedestrian-only cobblestone street in the middle of the city's 1st district. Why not? In 1679, after the outbreak of the worst episode of bubonic plague in the early modern era, Habsburg Emperor Leopold I constructed the monument to God in gratitude for salvation. Perhaps a bit of both – gratitude and divine salvation – would go a long way in Austria today.

The baroque *Pestsäule* also well represents the frictions inherent in Austria's current COVID-19 response. That is, the pillar commemorates the plague but also celebrates the victory of the house of Habsburg against the Ottoman empire and its forays up the Danube toward the so-called Golden Apple; the Protestants in the wars of religion; and the regularly scheduled "most-dangerous enemy within": the Jews who at times were permitted to live a benighted existence in or around town and then were hounded out of the city walls or murdered in their hundreds or thousands at the hands of a berserk mob.

On the one hand, before the Coronavirus pandemic, the "Plague Pillar" was often to be seen in the millions of Instagram pictures snapped by frolicking teenaged girls in the 1st district of Vienna, though it suddenly vanished from social media once the lockdowns took hold and a haunting emptiness swept the streets in the passage of winter to spring 2020. On the other hand, the Pestsäule, as a selfie-worthy chapter in the broader story of constitutions and the rights of the individual in the shadow of disease, still provides a gilded warning that often civil rights have been casualties, as well. In the context of Austria's contemporary constitutional answer to the pandemic of 2020-plus, "the word in stone" of the Pestsäule also makes a way to make sense of the changing role of government and the rule of law amid infection and panic.

---

94 Republic of Austria, "Bundesrecht konsolidiert: Gesamte Rechtsvorschrift für Verbotsgesetz 1947, Fassung vom 20.02.2022," StGBl. Nr. 13/1945, Rechtsinformationssystem des Bundes (RIS), https://www.ris.bka.gv.at/GeltendeFassung.wxe?Abfrage=Bundesnormen&Gesetzesnummer=10000207.

95 On David Irving's charges, trial, and sentence, see, for example: "David Irving rechtskräftig wegen Wiederbetätigung verurteilt," *Der Standard*, 7 September 2006, https://www.derstandard.at/story/2574045/david-irving-rechtskraeftig-wegen-wiederbetaetigung-verurteilt; see also Southern Poverty Law Center, "British Holocaust Denier Sentenced to Three Years," *Intelligence Report*, 11 August 2006, at https://www.splcenter.org/fighting-hate/intelligence-report/2006/british-holocaust-denier-sentenced-three-years. In 2007, Irving mounted an appeal of his three-year sentence, arguing in part that his most outright denial of the systematic and specific Nazi plans to murder Europe's Jews lay years back, and, at his advancing age, probation might be a more appropriate sentence. He won, but was deported to Britain to serve out the rest of his sentence. The presiding judge in Irving's appeal, who conscribed Irving's utterances to a fuzzy past and who explicitly doubted that the 68-year-old would re-offend, was Ernest Maurer, the long-time life-partner of Brigitte Bierlein.

As the drafters of the Austrian *Verbotgetz* knew as they committed the law to paper while the bullets were still flying at the end of World War II, a properly functioning *Sozialstaat* (and democracy and federal state, etc.) places certain duties on its citizens as well as endowing them with enlightened rights, because the survival of the *Sozialstaat* (and democracy and federal state, etc.) represents the most efficacious way to ensure the most liberties remain with the most people. In much the same way, the preservation of Austrians' lives through the various Coronavirus measure – to include the vaccine mandate of February 2022 – forms the clear priority and directive of the Austrian government. In this view, the most extreme attacks on the response (and the Freedom Party's ceaseless support for even the fringiest of weird arguments against the Austrian government's COVID policies gains in extremism because the FPÖ is the third-largest party in parliament) have an antisocial charge that belies the real intent.

As of this writing, however, despite the failings of certain persons in power because of the combination of money and social media glitz as well as the ill-effects of disease on a global scale on the rule of law, an enlightened Austrian *Sozialstaat* has upheld a standard that seeks to inoculate the Second Republic against the danger manifested not only by the effect of the pandemic on constitutions, but the even more destructive political disease of fascism in its twenty-first-century guise.

Afterword

Impacts of the Covid-19 Pandemic: International Laws, Policies, and Civil Liberties

Nadav Morag

Department of Security Studies, Sam Houston State University, Texas, USA

This volume has attempted to provide the reader with a sampling of the response to the Covid-19 pandemic in 16 countries in Europe, Asia, and North America. Some of the countries (the Netherlands, Ireland, Switzerland, Germany, and the United Kingdom) put an emphasis on trying to ensure that any measures would be in keeping with normal (nonemergency) laws and that dealing with the effects of Covid would not significantly impact the civil liberties (including the right to privacy) enjoyed by their respective populations. A second group of countries (Italy, Spain, Romania, and France) took a much more securitized approach, viewing the threat of Covid-19 as a major national security challenge that clearly warranted the use of emergency laws as well as the use of military forces domestically as needed. A third group of countries (Taiwan, Vietnam, and Singapore) employed primarily existing nonemergency laws in dealing with the pandemic, but they had fewer qualms about intensively monitoring their respective populations and restricting freedom of movement in order to reduce transmission. Finally, the fourth group of countries (Sweden, Japan, Canada, and Austria) focused less on the enforcement of laws and more on an attempt to foster popular buy-in for social distancing and other measures and were able to rely, at least to a degree, on widespread trust in government.

Each country's laws and policies, as well as its approach to civil liberties matters such as freedom of movement and privacy, are, of course, a product of its history, institutions, and culture. Both Germany and Japan, for example, were reluctant to impinge upon their respective citizens' civil liberties in dealing with the pandemic because, in part, their laws, institutions, and systems of governance were designed to ensure respect for civil liberties and limitations on governmental power. Taiwan, Vietnam, and Singapore, each have cultures that emphasize social needs, sometimes over individual prerogatives. Moreover, these countries had the experience of coping with the 2002-03 SARS pandemic as they had some of the highest case rates outside of China and thus were primed to respond quickly with a focus on reducing spread. It is not surprising that countries such as Italy, Spain, and France would employ emergency laws and turn, in part, to the military. In their recent history, these countries have experienced significant threats to domestic security and they also have a long tradition of using the military domestically to police the population and in other contexts. As another example, Canada and Switzerland, as befitting their history of strong local and regional (provincial and territorial in the first instance, and cantonal in the second) did enhance the power of their respective federal governments during the pandemic, but this was still balanced by regional power, including, in Canada's case, the power to institute public health measures. The United Kingdom too, with its devolved administrations for Wales, Scotland, and Northern Ireland, respected the authority given these "nations" to regulate internal security and public health.

Ultimately, there were a wide range of laws, institutions, and policies that American and other policymakers can learn from in improving preparedness to cope with new variants of Covid-19 as well as the next pandemic. Each country surveyed here presents a different approach to balancing health security with civil liberties, but they have all attempted to find some balance between the two. The key for any policymaker in looking at these models is to determine:

1. Which laws, policies, institutions, and best practices may be of use in better preparing for pandemics?
2. What are the barriers (legal, sociocultural, institutional, or other) to using another country's model in terms of?
   a. Legislating a particular law
   b. Establishing a particular institution
   c. Adopting a particular best practice
3. How can those barriers be addressed, either through modifying that foreign law, institution, or best practice; or, by modifying, to the degree possible, the laws, institutions, and/or policies in one's country?

Hopefully, this volume and the significant contributions of the chapter authors therein, will be of use to scholars and practitioners dealing with Covid-19 and preparing for future pandemics.

Index

Printed and bound by CPI Group (UK) Ltd, Croydon, CR0 4YY

09/06/2025

14685914-0001